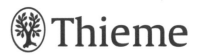

# Basic Otorhino-laryngology

A Step-by-Step Learning Guide

2nd Edition

Rudolf Probst, MD
Professor and formerly Director
Department of Otolaryngology –
Head & Neck Surgery
University Hospital Zurich
Zurich, Switzerland

Gerhard Grevers, MD
Professor
Private Practice
Starnberg, Germany

Heinrich Iro, MD
Professor and Director
Department of Otolaryngology –
Head & Neck Surgery
University Hospital Erlangen
Erlangen, Germany

With contributions by

Frank Waldfahrer
Frank Rosanowski
Ulrich Eysholdt

405 illustrations

Thieme
Stuttgart • New York • Delhi • Rio de Janeiro

**Library of Congress Cataloging-in-Publication Data**
is available from the publisher.

Illustrator: Karin Baum, Paphos, Cyprus

3rd German edition 2008
1st Greek edition 2006
1st Russian edition 2011
1st Turkish edition 2010

© 2006, 2018 by Georg Thieme Verlag KG

Thieme Publishers Stuttgart
Rüdigerstrasse 14, 70469 Stuttgart, Germany
+49 [0]711 8931 421, customerservice@thieme.de

Thieme Publishers New York
333 Seventh Avenue, New York, NY 10001 USA
+1 800 782 3488, customerservice@thieme.com

Thieme Publishers Delhi
A-12, Second Floor, Sector-2, Noida-201301
Uttar Pradesh, India
+91 120 45 566 00, customerservice@thieme.in

Thieme Publishers Rio, Thieme Publicações Ltda.
Edifício Rodolpho de Paoli, 25º andar
Av. Nilo Peçanha, 50 – Sala 2508
Rio de Janeiro 20020-906 Brasil
+55 21 3172 2297 / +55 21 3172 1896

Cover design: Thieme Publishing Group
Typesetting by DiTech Process Solutions, Mumbai, India
Printed in Germany by CPI books GmbH, Leck   5 4 3 2 1

ISBN 978-3-13-132442-9

Also available as an e-book:
eISBN 978-3-13-203472-3

**Important note:** Medicine is an ever-changing science undergoing continual development. Research and clinical experience are continually expanding our knowledge, in particular our knowledge of proper treatment and drug therapy. Insofar as this book mentions any dosage or application, readers may rest assured that the authors, editors, and publishers have made every effort to ensure that such references are in accordance with **the state of knowledge at the time of production of the book.**

Nevertheless, this does not involve, imply, or express any guarantee or responsibility on the part of the publishers in respect to any dosage instructions and forms of applications stated in the book. **Every user is requested to examine carefully** the manufacturers' leaflets accompanying each drug and to check, if necessary in consultation with a physician or specialist, whether the dosage schedules mentioned therein or the contraindications stated by the manufacturers differ from the statements made in the present book. Such examination is particularly important with drugs that are either rarely used or have been newly released on the market. Every dosage schedule or every form of application used is entirely at the user's own risk and responsibility. The authors and publishers request every user to report to the publishers any discrepancies or inaccuracies noticed. If errors in this work are found after publication, errata will be posted at www.thieme.com on the product description page.

Some of the product names, patents, and registered designs referred to in this book are in fact registered trademarks or proprietary names even though specific reference to this fact is not always made in the text. Therefore, the appearance of a name without designation as proprietary is not to be construed as a representation by the publisher that it is in the public domain.

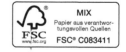

# Contents

# Preface

This preface aims to provide you with some background information on this textbook: Who can benefit most from this book? What is the teaching approach that is used— i.e., how are the contents presented to make them easier to learn? Who are the members of the "textbook team"? What is new in this completely revised second edition?

## Approach

*Who is the book written for?* The classic textbook still has its value, particularly when a new subject area is introduced for learning and basic material is presented. This book is primarily intended for students exposed to otorhinolaryngology, but it is also written for physicians, especially those taking part in further training and looking for basic information.

True learning means understanding, and so teaching means explaining. An essential part of learning is the understanding of basic concepts and potentially complex interrelationships. Moreover, learning should be interesting, and it should convey enjoyment of the material and its fascinating aspects. In this sense, this book aspires to be more than an exam review or a quick reference to specific questions. It was our goal to create an educationally compelling, graphically attractive, yet affordable textbook.

*Structure:* One of the main goals was to present the material in an easy-to-learn, user-friendly format. The result is a textbook in which the material is broken down into brief **study units** (🕮) representing cohesive learning units. Subdividing the contents into manageable portions makes it possible to present thematic highlights that would have been more difficult to incorporate into chapters with a traditional structure.

Each study unit begins with a **starter** in boldface type. This states the topics that are covered in the unit and the way in which they fit into the overall scheme. Special points are noted, and the material is related to other study units. The starter is not a summary.

The topics in each study unit are presented on **facing pages.** For clarity, "open-book" logos are shown at the bottom corner of the right-hand page: the number of logos (from one to six) indicates the number of facing-page sets that are contained in the current study unit. The red-colored logo shows where you are in the unit.

*Subject matter:* This textbook conforms to the latest developments in otorhinolaryngology and head and neck surgery. All main information that is needed for the basic understanding of a topic is contained in the main text, figures, and tables.

---

🔍 1   Knowledge in depth

Boxes marked with this symbol provide information that goes beyond a basic understanding. This may include operating techniques, illustrative case descriptions, historical information, or repetitions from earlier study (e.g., in embryology). If you are in a hurry, you can skip the in-depth boxes and still understand the material in the main text.

---

⚑ Points of emphasis are meant to indicate "caution" or "take note," and serve to direct attention to key points.

*Terminology:* Efforts have been made in various areas of otorhinolaryngology to establish a standard international nomenclature. The most up-to-date terms are used in the current text, while older or less commonly used terms are noted as *synonyms*.

**Fig. 1   Color code for flowcharts**

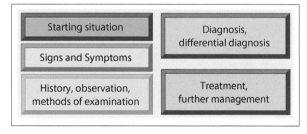

| Starting situation | Diagnosis, differential diagnosis |
| Signs and Symptoms | |
| History, observation, methods of examination | Treatment, further management |

## Acknowledgments

We are excited about our continued collaboration on this book, which first appeared in German in the year 2000. The current second edition of the English version has been completely revised. Both the text and the illustrations have been substantially changed in many chapters, reflecting the many—and sometimes fundamental—advances in otorhinolaryngology since the first English edition was published in 2006. The same team of authors has worked on the current edition, and our continued collaboration has resulted in a text that is greater than the sum of the authors' individual contributions. Anne Lamparter and Martina Habeck, our project managers at Thieme Publishers for the second English edition, have made substantial contributions to this outcome through their enthusiasm and commitment. Stephan Konnry at Thieme Publishers has been the Executive Editor for the English version from the beginning of this project. He continues to contribute his skill and experience to this book, keeping in mind all the cultural aspects associated with a foreign language edition. We are also grateful to the publishers, Thieme, for promoting the project and fostering its development. Finally, our thanks go to Karin Baum for her skillful artwork and her significant additions to the new edition.

Special gratitude is owed to our families. A great deal of time that should really have belonged to them was spent preparing this project. Even so, they supported our lengthy work on the book with the encouragement that only a family can provide.

## What Can We Improve?

Our goal was to tailor this book to meet our readers' needs. Only you, the reader, can judge whether we have accomplished this aim. We would therefore be delighted for you to contact us or the publishers regarding any changes that you would like to see in the next edition. We wish you much enjoyment and every success with this book.

*Rudolf Probst, MD*
*Gerhard Grevers, MD*
*Heinrich Iro, MD*

# Contributors

**Ulrich Eysholdt, MD, PhD**
Professor
Department of Medical Physics and Acoustics
University of Oldenburg
Oldenburg, Germany

**Frank Rosanowski, MD**
Professor
Private Practice
Nuremberg, Germany

**Frank Waldfahrer, MD**
Department of Otolaryngology – Head & Neck Surgery
University Hospital Erlangen
Erlangen, Germany

# I Nose, Paranasal Sinuses, and Face

# 1 Anatomy, Physiology, and Immunology of the Nose, Paranasal Sinuses, and Face

## 1.1 Basic Anatomy of the Nose, Paranasal Sinuses, and Face

The shape and appearance of the external nose affect not only the overall appearance of the face, but also the functional processes that take place inside the nose. The structural anatomy of the nose is important for both aesthetic and functional reasons, since the nose, as the gateway to the respiratory tract, performs a variety of physiologic functions.

### Facial Skin and Soft Tissues

For the effective surgical treatment of soft-tissue defects in the face, whether of a traumatic or neoplastic nature, it is important to consider some distinctive features of the morphology and topographic anatomy of the face, since this is a highly conspicuous region in which the faulty or inadequate treatment of tissue changes will have obvious consequences. One such feature involves the **tension lines** of the skin (**Fig. 1.1a**), known also as the relaxed skin tension lines. Scars can be made less conspicuous by taking these tension lines into account when suturing facial skin injuries. The **aesthetic units** of the face are an important consideration in the treatment of larger soft-tissue defects (**Fig. 1.1b**). Failure to take these units into account will produce a poor cosmetic result.

### The Facial Skeleton

Knowing the various components of the bony facial skeleton (**Fig. 1.2**) and their relationship to one another is important in trauma management and also in the diagnosis and treatment of inflammatory diseases of the facial skeleton and their complications. The upper jaw bone, or *maxilla*, houses the maxillary sinus and articulates laterally with the *zygomatic bone* (zygoma) via the zygomatic process (**Fig. 1.2**). The upper part of the maxilla borders the *nasal bone*, and its frontal process projects upward to the *frontal bone*. The zygoma also has a frontal process that connects superiorly with the frontal bone lateral to the orbit. The zygoma communicates posteriorly with the *zygomatic arch*.

### External Nose

The shape of the external nose is defined by the *nasal bones*, a pair of rectangular bones in the upper nasal dorsum, and by the paired *lateral cartilages* (upper nasal cartilages) and *alar cartilages* (major alar cartilages) in the central and lower portions of the nose (**Fig. 1.3**). The lateral portions of the nasal alae also contain several small accessory cartilages, called the *minor alar cartilages*, which are embedded in the lateral soft tissues of the nose.

The shape and stability of the alar cartilages, each of which consists of a *medial and lateral crus*, chiefly

**Fig. 1.1 Skin tension lines and aesthetic units**

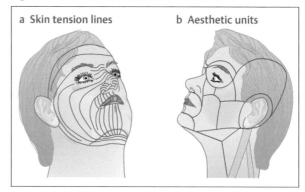

a Skin tension lines     b Aesthetic units

The incisions in facial operations should be placed along skin tension lines (**a**) whenever possible. The aesthetic units (**b**) should be considered in the closure of soft-tissue defects to achieve a satisfactory cosmetic result.

**Fig. 1.2 The cranial bones**

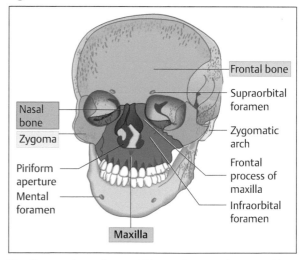

Nasal bone · Zygoma · Piriform aperture · Mental foramen · Maxilla · Frontal bone · Supraorbital foramen · Zygomatic arch · Frontal process of maxilla · Infraorbital foramen

The diagram shows the cranial bones that are relevant to rhinologic disorders.

**Fig. 1.3   Structure of the external nose**

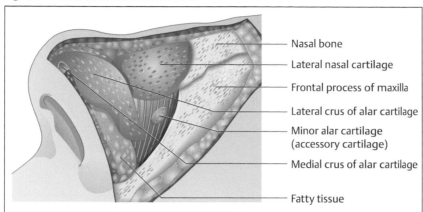

Nasal bone

Lateral nasal cartilage

Frontal process of maxilla

Lateral crus of alar cartilage

Minor alar cartilage
(accessory cartilage)

Medial crus of alar cartilage

Fatty tissue

Various bony and cartilaginous structures define the appearance of the external nose.

**Fig. 1.4   Anatomy of the nasal base**

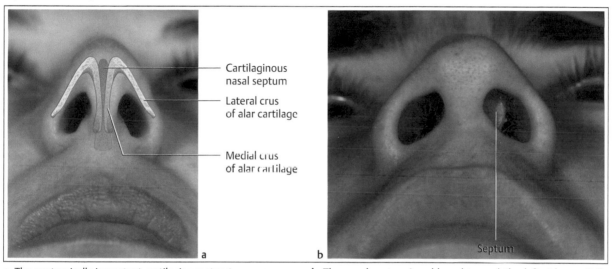

Cartilaginous
nasal septum

Lateral crus
of alar cartilage

Medial crus
of alar cartilage

Septum

**a** The anatomically important cartilaginous structures are projected onto the nasal base.

**b** The nasal septum is subluxed toward the left side, partially obstructing the nasal airway.

determine the appearance of the nasal tip and the shape of the nares. As a result, they are also important in maintaining an effective nasal airway. Besides the medial crura, the inferior septal margin and the connective-tissue septum (*columella*) are also responsible for stabilizing the base of the nose (**Fig. 1.4a**). Subluxation of the inferior septal margin can also hamper nasal breathing by partially obstructing the nasal airway (**Fig. 1.4b**).

## Nasal Cavities

The **nasal cavities** begin anteriorly at the *nasal vestibule*, which is bordered posteriorly by the internal *nasal valve* (limen nasi) located between the posterior border of the alar cartilage and the anterior border of the lateral cartilage. This valve area is the narrowest portion of the upper respiratory tract and, as such, has a major bearing on the aerodynamics of nasal airflow (see also ✥ 1.3). The anterior bony opening of the nasal cavity, called the *piriform aperture*, is bounded

laterally and inferiorly by the maxilla and superiorly by the nasal bone (see **Fig. 1.2**). The interior of the nose behind the nasal valve is divided by the *nasal septum* into two main cavities. The **nasal septum** is composed of an anterior cartilaginous part and two posterior bony parts. Abnormalities in the shape of the nasal septum (see also ✥ 3.2, Septal Deviation), which may consist of a deviated septum, tension septum, spurs, or ridges, are a frequent cause of nasal airway obstruction.

The *choanae* are the paired posterior openings through which the nasal cavities communicate with the nasopharynx.

The nasal cavity is bounded laterally by the lateral nasal walls, which are formed by the *ethmoid bone* and *maxilla*, and posteriorly by the *palatine bone* and the *pterygoid process* of the sphenoid bone. Several functionally important structures are located on the lateral nasal wall: the **nasal turbinates** and their associated passages (meati), sinus ostia, and the orifice of the nasolacrimal duct (**Fig. 1.5**).

**Fig. 1.5 Structure of the lateral nasal wall**

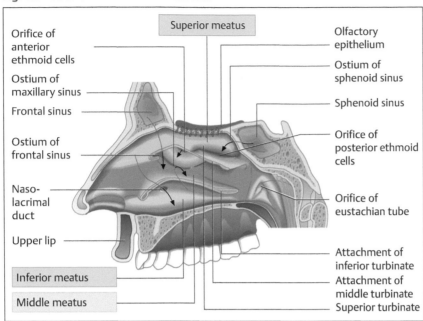

Orifice of anterior ethmoid cells

Ostium of maxillary sinus

Frontal sinus

Ostium of frontal sinus

Naso-lacrimal duct

Upper lip

Inferior meatus

Middle meatus

Superior meatus

Olfactory epithelium

Ostium of sphenoid sinus

Sphenoid sinus

Orifice of posterior ethmoid cells

Orifice of eustachian tube

Attachment of inferior turbinate

Attachment of middle turbinate

Superior turbinate

The relationship of the middle meatus to the sinus ostia is of special importance. See also ◯ **1.3**, Anatomy of the Ostiomeatal Unit.

The *inferior turbinate* consists of a separate bone that is attached to the medial wall of the maxillary sinus. The opening of the nasolacrimal duct is located in the corresponding *inferior meatus* (◯ **1.1**). The middle and superior turbinates are part of the ethmoid bone. In rare cases, a rudimentary "supreme turbinate" is also present above the superior turbinate.

The *middle turbinate* has by far the greatest functional importance, because most of the drainage tracts from the surrounding paranasal sinuses open into the middle meatus (see also ◯ **1.3**, Anatomy of the Ostiomeatal Unit).

The nasal cavity is bounded superiorly by the *cribriform plate* of the ethmoid bone. This thin bony plate has numerous openings for the passage of the *fila olfactoria* and also forms the boundary of the anterior cranial fossa. The floor of the nasal cavity is formed mostly by the *hard palate*, which is formed in turn by the two palatine processes of the maxilla and the horizontal laminae of the palatine bone.

## Paranasal Sinuses

The *paranasal sinuses* are air-filled cavities that communicate with the nasal cavities (**Fig. 1.6**). All but the sphenoid sinus are already present as outpouchings of the mucosa during embryonic life, but except for the ethmoid air cells, they do not develop into bony cavities until after birth. The frontal sinus and

---

◯ **1.1 Nasolacrimal duct**

The *nasolacrimal duct* is part of the lacrimal apparatus, which also includes the lacrimal gland, the lacrimal ducts, and the lacrimal sac. It runs in a bony canal between the medial canthus of the eye and the inferior nasal meatus.

---

**Fig. 1.6 Paranasal sinuses**

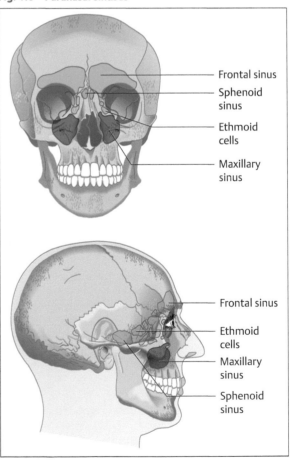

Frontal sinus

Sphenoid sinus

Ethmoid cells

Maxillary sinus

Frontal sinus

Ethmoid cells

Maxillary sinus

Sphenoid sinus

Diagram of the sinuses projected onto the cranial surface.

## 1.2 Ethmoid roof and cribriform plate

The roof of the ethmoid labyrinth is formed mainly by the portion of the frontal bone that covers and closes the ethmoid cells superiorly. The ethmoid roof is continuous medially with the cribriform plate, the lateral lamina of which represents the continuation of the attachment of the middle turbinate and is very easily injured during surgical manipulations in this region (**Fig. 1.7**). The levels of the ethmoid roof and cribriform plate can vary considerably, even in the same patient, depending on the vertical extent of the lateral lamina. Computed tomography scans should be taken preoperatively to define the individual anatomy of the anterior skull base region (**Fig. 1.8**).

**Fig. 1.7  Ethmoid roof and anterior ethmoid at the level of the crista galli**

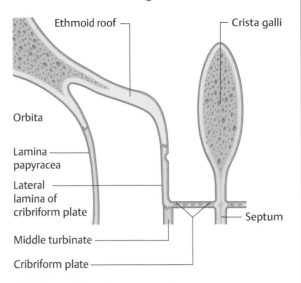

**Fig. 1.8  Computed tomography (consecutive coronal scans) in a patient with recurrent nasal polyps**

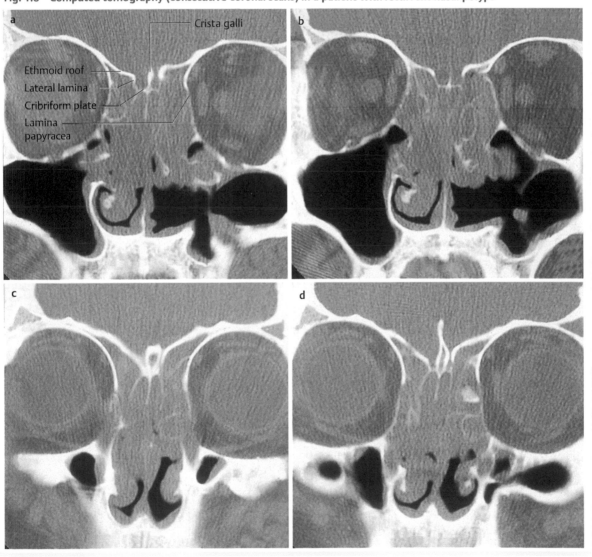

sphenoid sinus reach their definitive size in the first decade of life. The maxillary sinus is present at birth but remains very small until the second dentition, because the presence of tooth germs in the maxilla limits the extent of the sinuses. The maxillary sinus, frontal sinus, and anterior ethmoid cells drain into the nasal cavity through the middle meatus—i.e., below the middle turbinate (**Fig. 1.5**). The posterior ethmoid cells drain into the nasal cavity through the superior meatus. The ostium of the sphenoid sinus is located in the anterior wall directly above the choanae. The anatomic connections between the nasal cavity and paranasal sinuses are functionally important and play a key role in the pathogenesis of many rhinologic diseases that involve the paranasal sinuses (see also 🔎 **1.3**, Anatomy of the Ostiomeatal Unit).

The **maxillary sinus** borders the nasal cavity laterally, and the orbital floor separates the upper part of the sinus from the orbit. Behind the maxillary sinus is the *pterygopalatine fossa*, which is traversed by the maxillary artery along with branches of the trigeminal nerve and autonomic nervous system. The floor of the maxillary sinus is closely related to the roots of the second premolar and first molar teeth. This creates a potential route for the spread of dentogenic infections, and a tooth extraction may create a communication between the oral cavity and maxillary sinus (oroantral fistula).

Superior and medial to the maxillary sinus are the **ethmoid air cells**—a labyrinthine system of small, pneumatized sinus cavities that are separated from one another by thin bony walls and extend posteriorly between the middle turbinate (medial border) and orbit to the sphenoid sinus. The orbital plate of the ethmoid bone, also called the *lamina papyracea*, forms the lateral bony wall that separates the ethmoid air cells from the orbit. Paranasal sinus inflammations can spread through this lamina to involve the orbit (orbital complications). The posterior ethmoid cells are closely related to the *optic nerve*. The ethmoid roof and cribriform plate (🔎 **1.2**) form the bony boundary that separates the ethmoid cells from the *anterior cranial fossa*. The surgeon who operates in this region must have a detailed knowledge of the relations of these structures to the ethmoid labyrinth. The **sphenoid sinus** is located at the approximate center of the skull above the nasopharynx. Its posterior wall is formed by the clivus. It relates laterally to the *cavernous sinus*, the *internal carotid artery*, and *cranial nerves II to VI*, and it is very closely related to the optic canal.

📖 The optic nerve and internal carotid artery may run directly beneath the mucosa of the lateral wall of the sphenoid sinus, without a bony covering.

The sphenoid sinus is bordered superiorly by the sella turcica and pituitary and by the anterior and middle cranial fossae.

The **frontal sinus** is located in the frontal bone, its floor forming the medial portion of the orbital roof. The sinus, which is highly variable in its extent, is bounded behind by the anterior cranial fossa. Inflammations of the frontal sinus can give rise to serious complications because of its close proximity to the orbit and cranial cavity (orbital cellulitis, epidural or subdural abscess, meningitis).

## Vascular Supply

The external nose derives most of its **blood supply** from the *facial artery*, which arises from the external carotid artery, and from the *ophthalmic artery*, which springs from the internal carotid artery. The internal nose receives blood from the territories of the external and internal carotid arteries: the terminal branches of the *sphenopalatine artery*, which arises from the maxillary artery, and the *anterior and posterior ethmoid arteries*, which arise from the ophthalmic artery. A detailed knowledge of the vascular supply is particularly important in the management of intractable epistaxis (nosebleed), which requires vascular ligation or angiographic embolization as a last recourse (see also ✍3.3, Treatment). The **venous drainage** of the facial region is handled by the facial vein, retromandibular vein, and internal jugular vein. The **regional lymphatic drainage** of the face and external nose is handled mainly by the submandibular lymph nodes, while the nasal cavity is additionally drained by the retropharyngeal and deep cervical lymph nodes.

## Nerve Supply

The facial skin receives its **sensory innervation** from terminal branches of the *trigeminal nerve* that enter the facial region through the supraorbital, infraorbital, and mental foramina (see **Fig. 1.2**). Only the skin over the mandibular angle and the lower portions of the auricle are supplied by the great auricular nerve. The facial muscles are classified as mimetic or masticatory, each of these groups receiving different **motor innervation**. While the mimetic muscles of the face develop from the blastema of the second branchial arch (the hyoid arch) and accordingly are supplied by the *facial nerve*, the masticatory muscles trace their embryonic development to the first branchial arch (the mandibular arch) and are therefore supplied by mandibular nerve branches arising from the *trigeminal nerve*.

📖 **1.3 Anatomy of the ostiomeatal unit**

The term *ostiomeatal unit* describes the area on the lateral nasal wall where the ostia of the paranasal sinuses (except for the sphenoid sinus) open into the nasal cavity in a ductlike fashion. Even minor changes (e.g., anatomic variants, mucosal swelling) can hamper ventilation in this region, leading to pathologic sequelae in the paranasal sinuses (see below). The functionally significant anatomic structures of the ostiomeatal unit are the uncinate process, the semilunar hiatus, the frontal recess, the ethmoid bulla, the ethmoid infundibulum, and the maxillary sinus ostium (a coronal section is shown in **Fig. 1.9**). The **frontal sinus** is connected to the ostiomeatal unit via the frontal recess, which has an hourglasslike shape. The **uncinate process** is a thin fibrous or bony process on the lateral nasal wall that arises slightly behind the anterior border of the middle turbinate and may narrow the passage from the nasal cavity to the ostiomeatal complex, depending on its degree of development. Located between the posterior border of the uncinate process and the first ethmoid cell (the **ethmoid bulla**) is another slitlike passage within the ostiomeatal complex, known as the **semilunar hiatus**. The space between the uncinate process, ethmoid bulla, and lamina papyracea of the ethmoid bone is called the **ethmoid infundibulum**. The ostiomeatal unit is bounded medially (toward the nasal cavity) by the middle turbinate and laterally by the lamina papyracea.

The main *clinical significance* of this region relates to the sites of narrowing in the ostiomeatal unit. For example, hyperemia and swelling of the mucosa in the setting of a common cold can obstruct the narrow passages in the ostiomeatal unit, preventing adequate ventilation of the dependent paranasal sinus system and setting the stage for a rhinogenic inflammation of the paranasal sinuses (sinusitis).

**Fig. 1.9   Anatomy of the ostiomeatal unit**

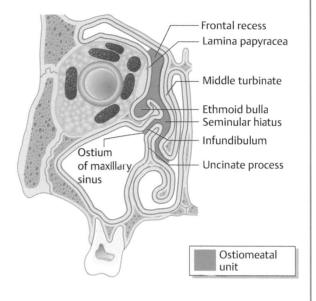

- Frontal recess
- Lamina papyracea
- Middle turbinate
- Ethmoid bulla
- Seminular hiatus
- Infundibulum
- Uncinate process

Ostium of maxillary sinus

☐ Ostiomeatal unit

## Functional Anatomy of the Ostiomeatal Unit

The nose and paranasal sinuses are regarded as a functional unit. Many rhinologic disorders are transmitted from the nasal cavity into the paranasal sinus system. The ostiomeatal unit is the collective term for various anatomic structures located about the middle meatus. It represents the region on the lateral nasal wall that receives drainage from the anterior ethmoid cells, frontal sinus, and maxillary sinus (📖 **1.3**). It is important to know the anatomic details of this region to understand the pathophysiology of acute and especially chronic paranasal sinus inflammations and the surgical procedures that are used in the causal treatment of these conditions.

# 1.2    Morphology of the Nasal Mucosa

Besides the anatomic structure of the external nose and nasal cavity, the nasal mucosa plays an essential role in numerous functions of the nose owing to its "gateway" location in the respiratory tract (see also ✎ 1.3, Basic Physiology and Immunology of the Nose). This ✎ deals with the morphologic structure of the nasal mucosa. Understanding this structure is necessary for an understanding of functional processes.

The anterior part of the nasal cavity (the nasal vestibule), like the external nose, is covered by skin composed of a multilayer, keratinizing **squamous epithelium**. Anterior to the head of the inferior turbinate, this keratinized epithelium gives way to a nonkeratinized squamous epithelium, a nonciliated columnar epithelium, and finally a **ciliated respiratory epithelium**. Along with the submucous tissue, this ciliated epithelium forms the typical mucosal lining of the nasal cavity and paranasal sinuses (**Fig. 1.10**). A small area on the upper nasal septum, superior turbinate, and part of the middle turbinate, located adjacent to the cribriform plate, is covered by **olfactory mucosa** and is called the *olfactory region*.

## Respiratory Mucosa

### Epithelium

The epithelium of the respiratory mucosa is composed of ciliary cells, goblet cells, and basal cells and provides an initial, mechanical barrier against infection. The **ciliary cells** dominate the surface of the respiratory epithelium. Each ciliary cell has about 150 to 200 cilia, which are composed of microtubules and are interlinked by "dynein arms." This cytoskeleton of the ciliary cells and the activity of dynein, a specialized protein, enable the typical, synchronous beating of the cilia in the respiratory epithelium. This ciliary action propels a blanket of mucous secretions (from the **goblet cells**) and serous secretions (from the **nasal glands**) toward the

nasopharynx, mechanically cleansing the inspired air in a mechanism called *mucociliary transport* (see also ✎ 1.3, Basic Physiology and Immunology of the Nose). The **basal cells** represent the morphologic connection between the columnar epithelium and goblet cells on the one hand and the epithelial basement membrane on the other. They are distinguished from the other epithelial cell types by an increased expression of certain adhesion molecules (e.g., intracellular adhesion molecule-1, ICAM-1) and increased cytokine synthesis (e.g., interleukin 1). Besides the four cell types mentioned, the epithelium also contains **immunocompetent cells**, mostly CD8-positive T cells, along with smaller numbers of mast cells, macrophages, and MHC-II-bearing dendritic cells, which function as antigen-presenting cells.

### Lamina Propria

The **lamina propria** of the nasal mucosa is separated from the epithelium by a basement membrane. Some areas of the lamina propria, especially about the inferior turbinate, show a marked preponderance of vascular structures known as **venous erectile tissue** or sinusoids. They consist of thin-walled and thick-walled venous capacitance vessels, which are important not only in warming the inspired air and producing secretions but also in controlling the tumescence of the nasal mucosa. Besides the venous capacitance vessels, there are capillaries and, in deeper areas, arterial vessels. The lamina propria also contains numerous **nasal**

Fig. 1.10    Respiratory nasal mucosa

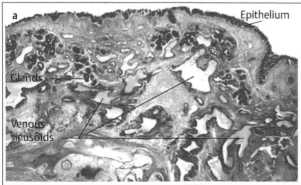

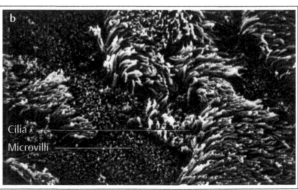

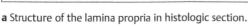

**a** Structure of the lamina propria in histologic section.    **b** Scanning electron micrograph of cilia and microvilli.

**glands**, which mainly produce a serous secretion. The **immunocompetent cells** in the lamina propria consist of CD4-positive T lymphocytes along with CD8-positive cytotoxic cells and suppressor cells such as CD4-/CD8-negative T lymphocytes, mature B lymphocytes, Ig-plasma cells, mast cells, and macrophages. These cellular elements demonstrate the importance of the nasal mucosa, which acts in concert with local host reactions to mediate inflammatory and allergic responses in the nose (see also 🕮 1.3, Basic Physiology and Immunology of the Nose).

## Nerve Supply

Finally, the nasal mucosa is endowed with a rich nerve supply. It receives its sensory innervation from the trigeminal nerve and its autonomic innervation from the pterygopalatine ganglion. The parasympathetic fibers of this ganglion induce vasodilation and stimulate the secretory activity of the nasal glands, while the sympathetic fibers produce vasoconstriction and inhibit glandular secretion. In addition, nitric oxide (NO) influences neurotransmission and neuromodulation of nasal blood vessels and glands of the nasal mucosa.

## Olfactory Mucosa

**Topography:** The olfactory mucosa (see 🔎 **1.4** for details on structure and function) covers the olfactory region, which occupies the anterosuperior part of the nasal septum and adjacent areas of the lateral nasal wall, including the side of the superior turbinate facing the septum and part of the middle turbinate. The olfactory mucosa has the capability to regenerate lifelong. The junction of the olfactory mucosa with the respiratory mucosa is variable in its location.

**Stimulus processing system:** Although it covers an area of only a few square centimeters, the olfactory mucosa contains between 12 and 30 million olfactory receptor neurons (ORN). These ORN are bipolar sensory cells and have dendritic epithelial processes, which protrude into the mucus layer and possess up to 20 cilia with integrated receptor proteins (see also 🕮 1.3, Olfaction). The ORN also have basal axons that

> 🔎 **1.4 Olfactory mucosa**
>
> **Microscopic anatomy**: Besides olfactory receptor cells (ORN), the epithelium of the olfactory mucosa is composed of microvilli, supporting cells, and basal cells (mainly of the globose type, globose basal cells). The lamina propria additionally contains serous glands (olfactory glands) and vessels. The **function** of the microvilli and of the olfactory glands located in the lamina propria of the olfactory mucosa is not yet fully understood.
>
> The *microvilli* most likely represent extra chemoreceptors in the olfactory epithelium, which perform their function along with the classic receptor cells.
>
> As for the *olfactory glands*, it is assumed that the secretions from these glands, released at the surface of the epithelium, also play a role in mediating the olfactory sense. Recent studies have shown that the secretion layer on the epithelium contains a specific protein that has a high affinity for most odorous substances, and thus could facilitate or even mediate their binding to the sensory cells.

pass through the basement membrane between the supporting cells (sustentacular cells) and basal cells and then join into bundles that are encompassed by olfactory ensheathing cells of Schwann's cells' or astrocytes' character. These axon bundles, called the fila olfactoria, pass through foramina in the cribriform plate of the ethmoid bone and enter the cranial cavity. There they unite to form the olfactory nerve and pass to the olfactory bulb in the brain, the *primary olfactory center*. The latter is connected via the olfactory tract to the *secondary olfactory center* in the temporobasal cortex, which is responsible for the perception of smells and their association with other sensory impressions. The secondary olfactory center also has projections to the limbic system that connect with the autonomic centers in the thalamus and hypothalamus; this creates a pathway that mediates the emotional and affective phenomena that are associated with smells. The olfactory cortex has connections with the *tertiary olfactory centers* (including the hippocampus, anterior insular region, and reticular formation), which are believed to have polysensory associative functions.

# 1.3   Basic Physiology and Immunology of the Nose

To understand the pathologic processes that are important in inflammatory and allergic diseases of the nose, it is necessary to first understand the physiologic functions. As the threshold of the respiratory tract in humans, the nose is of major importance in conditioning the air before it reaches the lower airways. To understand this complex process, we must know something about the physics of nasal airflow, which also affects the warming and humidification of the inspired air. Due to its exposed position, the nasal mucosa is in constant primary contact with the environment and thus with a variety of potential pathogens. As a result, the nose is equipped with a variety of defense mechanisms (mechanical defenses, specific and nonspecific immune responses). As part of the supraglottic vocal tract, the nose also contributes to speech production (see 18.1). Finally, the nose contains the olfactory sensory cells, giving it an essential role in olfaction.

## Physical Principles of Nasal Airflow

During inspiration, the air stream enters the nasal vestibule in an oblique vertical direction. Aerodynamically, this air is in a state of *laminar flow*, meaning that there is no mixing of the different air layers. When the inspired air reaches the nasal valve located between the vestibule and nasal cavity, it passes through the narrowest site in the upper respiratory tract (limen nasi); just past the nasal valve, the cross-section of the airway becomes greatly expanded, creating a "diffuser effect" that transforms most of the laminar flow of the inspired air into *turbulent flow*, in which different air layers are swirled together. Besides the velocity of the air, the degree of change in airflow characteristics at this stage is very strongly influenced by the specialized anatomy of the nasal cavity, which is subject to substantial individual differences. Septal deviation and cartilaginous or bony spurs on the septum can be as significant in this regard as turbinate hyperplasia or septal perforation. To a degree, the transition from laminar to turbulent flow within the nose is functionally desirable because it slows the flow velocity of the inspired air. This prolongs its contact with the nasal mucosa, contributing to olfaction and making it easier for the nose to clean, humidify, and warm the inspired air (see below).

## Nasal Cycle

The "nasal cycle" is a physiologic phenomenon marked by an alternation between luminal narrowing and widening of the nasal cavities. This alternate congestion and decongestion of the nasal mucosa is effected mainly through reactions of the venous capacitance vessels of the inferior and middle turbinates, which are regulated by the autonomic nervous system (**Fig. 1.11**).

## Conditioning of the Inspired Air

Inspired air is warmed and humidified in the nose before reaching the lower airways. Turbulent flow and

**Fig. 1.11   The nasal cycle**

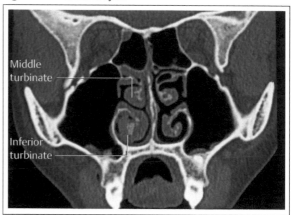

Middle turbinate

Inferior turbinate

This coronal computed tomography scan shows mucosal swelling in the right nasal cavity, predominantly on the inferior and middle turbinates, and mucosal decongestion in the right nasal cavity.

other special physical conditions promote the necessary contact of the inspired air with the nasal mucosa. Moreover, the favorable relationship between the relatively small nasal cavity and the comparatively large mucosal surface area, which is further enlarged by the turbinates, also promotes the functionally important interaction between the inspired air and the mucosa. **Humidification** is accomplished by secretion and transudation from the nasal glands, the epithelial goblet cells, and the vessels of the lamina propria. **Temperature regulation** is controlled by the intranasal vascular system and especially the venous erectile tissue, which is particularly abundant in the inferior turbinates. The temperature in the anterior portions of the nasal cavity is lower than in the posterior regions. This temperature gradient produces a gradual warming of the inspired air, while on expiration moisture and heat are returned to the nose through condensation. The warming capacity of the nasal mucosa is so efficient that even with ambient temperatures below zero, the temperature of the inspired air is raised by

25°C on entering the nasopharynx, with a relative humidity of over 90%.

Disturbances in the conditioning function of the nose can result from age-related drying of the mucosa due to involution of the goblet cells and glands. They can also result from chronic inflammatory changes or extensive resections of the mucosa during intranasal surgery.

## Protective Functions of the Nasal Mucosa

Here the protective functions of the nose are separated into two parts to facilitate learning, although in life the various defense mechanisms are interrelated and should not be thought of as separate entities.

### Nonspecific Defense Mechanisms

**Mechanical defenses**: The most important mechanical defense mechanism of the nasal mucosa is the *mucociliary apparatus*, which physically cleanses the inspired air. The mucociliary transport system consists of the cilia of the respiratory epithelium and a mucous blanket composed of two layers: a deeper, less viscid "sol layer" in which ciliary motion occurs, and a superficial, more viscid "gel layer" (**Fig. 1.12**). The physiology of ciliary movements is described in ⌕ **1.5**. Disturbances of mucociliary transport can have

Table 1.1 Nonspecific protective factors in nasal secretions

| Substance group | Example |
| --- | --- |
| Interferon | |
| Proteases | Cathepsin, elastase, chymase, tryptase |
| Protease inhibitors | $\alpha_1$-Protease inhibitor, C1 inactivator |
| Lysozyme | |
| Antioxidants | Catalases, glutathione, ascorbic acid |

various causes, such as increased viscosity and thickness of the periciliary sol layer, hampering ciliary movements, or changes in the viscoelasticity of the gel layer resulting in ineffectual mucus transport. Finally, various pathogenic mechanisms can produce changes in the cilia themselves, regardless of the viscosity of the mucous blanket. For example, an acute viral infection of the upper respiratory tract can lead to desquamation of the epithelium, with a loss of ciliated cells. Also, certain microorganisms can directly affect ciliary motility by reducing the beat frequency of the cilia. Finally, ciliary dyskinesia syndromes are congenital disorders based on morphologic changes in the cilia such as absence of the dynein arms. This results in uncoordinated, dyskinetic ciliary movements that prevent effective mucus transport (see also ⌕ 3.8).

**Nonspecific protective factors**: The nasal mucosa also has several other, nonspecific defense mechanisms in the form of protective factors in the mucous blanket (**Table 1.1**).

**Cellular defenses**: The mucosa has nonspecific defense mechanisms at the cellular level as well. The predominant phagocytic cells are neutrophilic granulocytes, monocytes, and macrophages. They are accompanied by "natural killer cells," which comprise a small percentage of the peripheral lymphocytes and protect mainly against viral infections of the nasal mucosa.

### Specific Immune Responses

Besides the nonspecific defense mechanisms of the nasal mucosa, the nose possesses a specific immune system that can be viewed as a separate immunologic unit. It is made up of the *nasal mucosa* itself and the lymphoepithelial tissue of *Waldeyer's ring* (see below). Recent discoveries indicate that the structures of Waldeyer's ring, especially the pharyngeal and palatine tonsils, function as inductive components that are active in the absorption, processing, and presentation of antigens, whereas the nasal mucosa itself is purely an effector organ in which, for example, foreign material is phagocytized by immunocompetent cells.

**Fig. 1.12   Mucociliary transport**

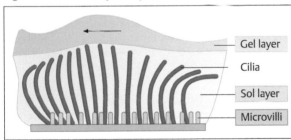

Gel layer

Cilia

Sol layer

Microvilli

Cilia on the respiratory epithelium beat in a coordinated, metachronous pattern in the periciliary fluid (deeper sol layer), which transports the superficial gel layer toward the nasopharynx (arrow).

⌕ 1.5 Physiology of ciliary motion

Ciliary motion consists of three phases and is initiated by adenosine triphosphate (ATP)–splitting proteins, which cause a movement of the filaments within the cilia (sliding filament theory). The superficial gel layer is propelled toward the nasopharynx by a coordinated but metachronous beating of the cilia. The dynamics of ciliary motion has been likened to a "field of grain swaying in the wind." The cilia beat at a high frequency (10–20 times per second), but their motion is influenced by external factors such as temperature and humidity.

The local, specific immune system of the nasal mucosa is based on the actions of antibodies, which are responsible for the humoral immune response, and of immunocompetent cells, which are responsible for the cellular immune response.

**Humoral immune response**: Antibodies are formed in the paraglandular plasma cells. Most notably, IgA is an immunoglobulin that is characteristic of the respiratory mucosa and therefore of the nasal mucosa. The plasma cells also synthesize IgM and the less common IgC. When released, the immunoglobulins (especially IgA) are absorbed by the glandular cells of the lamina propria, provided with a secretory component, and re-released as *secretory antibodies* (sIgA).

**Cellular immune response**: Representatives of the cellular immune response of the nasal mucosa include *mast cells, macrophages*, various *polymorphonuclear leukocytes* (neutrophils, basophils, eosinophilic granulocytes), *lymphocytes*, and the *cells of the reticuloendothelial system*, which occur chiefly as dendritic (Langerhans') cells in the nasal mucosa. T lymphocytes are of special importance in the control and memory functions of the immune response, while B lymphocytes can differentiate into plasma cells and thus have a key role in the humoral immune response of the mucosa in connection with local antibody production. Eosinophilic granulocytes are found mainly in association with chronic sinusitis and nasal polyps. Their granules contain cytotoxic substances that can damage tissues by the lysis of cell membranes. Basophilic granulocytes are involved in immediate allergic reactions, although the mast cells are by far the most dominant cell type in this phase. The mast cells are also chiefly responsible for histamine release in the early phase of an allergic reaction. Basophilic granulocytes (the only representatives of polymorphonuclear leukocytes) and mast cells also have a specific receptor (FcεR) for binding IgE. On contact with the corresponding allergenic substance, this can incite a devastating allergic reaction that may culminate in anaphylactic shock.

The *epithelial cells* of the nasal mucosa also have an immune function. In particular, the adhesion molecule ICAM-1, expressed by the epithelial cells, helps to prevent viral infections by acting as a receptor for more than 90% of rhinoviruses.

Finally, the *endothelial cells* of the blood vessels play an important role in the specific immune responses of the nasal mucosa. The vascular endothelial cells are activated by various inflammatory mediators—for example, interleukin 1, tumor necrosis factor-α (TNF-α)—and they regulate the transendothelial diapedesis of immunocompetent cells into the surrounding tissue through the expression of various adhesion molecules (**Fig. 1.13, Fig. 1.14**).

**Fig. 1.13 Transendothelial migration of immunocompetent cells**

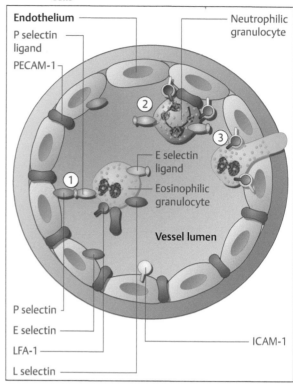

The interaction between immunocompetent cells and endothelial cells in an inflammatory reaction is mediated by various adhesion molecules and proceeds in the following steps:

1. Inflammatory mediators trigger the release of endothelial selectins. The interaction with their ligands initiates the migration of cells along the endothelium.
2. Activated integrins on the cells allow firm binding to the endothelial ligand, usually a member of the immunoglobulin supergene family.
3. The interaction between ICAM-1 and LFA-1 appears to play an important role in the extravasation process. The cells migrate between endothelial junctions, where expressed PECAM-1 is decreased during activation.

ICAM = Intercellular adhesion molecule
LFA = Lymphocyte function–associated antigen
PECAM = Platelet/endothelial cell adhesion molecule

## Speech Production

Various organ systems are involved in the production of voice and speech. The anatomically separate functions of the respiratory tract, glottis, supraglottic vocal tract, and central nervous system must be coordinated to produce a normal voice sound. The term *supraglottic vocal tract* refers to the air-containing regions located above the level of the vocal cords. The rigid portions of this tract, whose condition is subject to only minor variations under physiologic conditions (e.g., due to mucosal swelling), include the nose, paranasal sinuses, and portions of the nasopharynx. Their role in articulation

**Fig. 1.14   Chronic inflammation of the nasal mucosa**

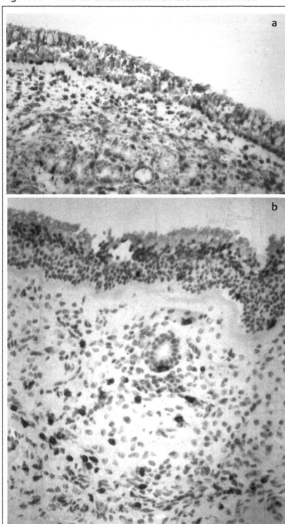

Sections from the lamina propria of the nasal mucosa. Increased numbers of lymphocyte function–associated antigen-1 (LFA-1)–labeled leukocytes (brown stain) resulting from transendothelial diapedesis are found in the setting of a chronic inflammatory reaction (**a**) compared with a control specimen (**b**) (immunohistochemistry, ABC method with hemalum counterstain).

is most apparent under pathologic conditions. "Hyponasal speech" (rhinophonia clausa) occurs when these segments of the vocal tract contribute less to sound production as a result of partial or complete nasal obstruction or mass lesions in the nasopharynx. Conversely, "hypernasal speech" (rhinophonia aperta) develops when the nasopharynx and nasal cavities overcontribute to sound production. This occurs when velopharyngeal closure is absent or incomplete (cleft palate, velar palsy due to various causes).

## Olfaction

The human olfactory system consists of the intranasal olfactory mucosa with its specialized olfactory epithelium and associated central pathways. The sensory cells consist of bipolar ORN whose distal processes (cilia) have receptor proteins in their cell membranes, which are involved in the bond of scents. So far, 200 to 400 receptor protein types have been identified in humans. A scent can connect to different receptors with any of its different molecular components. Vice versa, different scents can bond to the same receptor type. The proximal processes of ORN join to form the fila olfactoria, which are relayed through additional neurons and are distributed to the primary, secondary, and tertiary olfactory centers (see ☞ 1.2, Olfactory Mucosa). From a purely functional standpoint, an olfactory impression can be received only during inspiration, and only water-soluble and lipid-soluble substances are perceived. Even subtle changes in the chemical properties of a molecule can produce a clearly perceptible difference in the quality and quantity of the olfactory impression. The precise sequence of events that are involved in olfaction is still uncertain.

It is important clinically to differentiate between olfactory disturbances and taste disorders, because the senses of smell and taste are closely interrelated. Patients often believe that they have a dysfunction of both senses, even though an olfactory disturbance is the sole cause of the complaints in more than two-thirds of cases (see **Table 2.2**).

# 2    Diagnostic Evaluation of the Nose and Paranasal Sinuses

## 2.1    History and Clinical Examination of the Nose

Aside from special rhinologic tests, which are reviewed in ☞ 2.2, the specific rhinologic history and clinical examination of the nose play a key role in further diagnostic and therapeutic decision-making.

### History

Before the examiner asks about specific rhinologic symptoms, patients should be given an opportunity to describe their complaints "in their own words," as in any history.

The history should begin with questions about general, relatively nonspecific symptoms such as obstructed nasal breathing and nasal discharge. It is important to determine, for example, whether the **nasal obstruction** ("stuffy nose") has been present for some time or is of recent onset, possibly in connection with trauma to the nose. Additional questions should elicit whether the complaints are unilateral, bilateral, or alternate between the sides and whether they are seasonal or present year-round.

In patients with nasal **discharge**, the consistency of the secretions should be assessed: is the discharge watery, mucopurulent, or blood-tinged (which may suggest a tumor)? To exclude allergic rhinitis, the patient should be questioned about sneezing attacks, itchy eyes (conjunctival irritation), cough, and respiratory complaints (evidence for allergic involvement of the lower respiratory tract).

If the history suggests that the disease may have an allergic cause, a **specific allergy history** should be taken. This includes the family and personal history (bronchial asthma, atopic dermatitis, food allergies) as well as details on the household and occupational environments, giving particular attention to pets, indoor plants, and potential allergen exposure at the workplace (e.g., in a bakery or hair salon).

**Headaches** may signify an accompanying paranasal sinus inflammation. Dryness of the nasal mucosa is a common finding in colds but can also result from changes in air quality, previous nasal surgery, or the chronic use of vasoconstricting nose drops or sprays that contain corticosteroids. **Olfactory dysfunction** is another possible symptom of rhinologic diseases, and the patient should always be questioned about this.

### Clinical Examination

#### Inspection

The clinical examination begins with a visual inspection. Findings such as mouth breathing may direct the examiner to suspect nasal airway obstruction. The shape of the external nose may suggest intranasal abnormalities (e.g., a cartilaginous nasal deviation with a tension septum). It is particularly important to evaluate the *nasal base* (see **Fig. 1.4**), for which the patient's head should be tilted back. In this position, the examiner can also test the stability of the nasal alae. If the alar cartilages are too soft, they will be indrawn even during normal, unforced inspiration. Skin changes such as erythema or swelling can occur with orbital complications of paranasal sinus inflammations (erythema and swelling of the upper and lower lids), in erysipelas ("butterfly"-shaped erythema of the midfacial skin), or with nasal furuncles, which present with circumscribed redness and swelling in the nasal vestibule.

#### Palpation

Palpation is most useful for detecting bony discontinuities. In patients with suspected neuralgias, it is also done to check for tenderness over the supraorbital, infraorbital, or mental foramina. In patients with a recent trauma history, palpation of the external nose will disclose any mobility or crepitus suggesting a fracture of the nasal pyramid. The midfacial bones (especially the bony orbital rim) are also palpated to check for step-offs indicating a fracture line. Soft-tissue swelling can limit the accuracy of this examination, however.

#### Anterior Rhinoscopy

The rhinologic examination itself begins with anterior rhinoscopy to evaluate the nasal vestibule and the anterior portions of the nasal cavity (**Fig. 2.1**).

*Technique*: The examiner holds the nasal speculum in the left hand and braces the index finger on the patient's right nostril. The speculum is inserted into the nose with the blades closed. During the examination,

**Fig. 2.1  Anterior rhinoscopy**

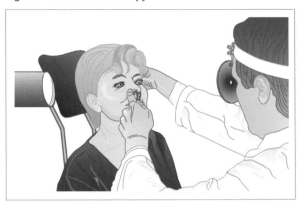

Technique for inspecting the nasal cavity.

**Fig. 2.2  Nasal endoscopy**

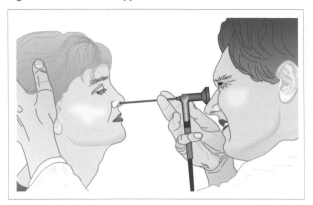

Positions of the patient and examiner.

the physician uses the right hand to position the patient's head and gently opens the speculum to spread open the nostril to allow inspection of the nasal cavity. The speculum should not be opened too far, as this would cause discomfort. The head should be tilted slightly forward for evaluating the nasal floor, inferior turbinate, and the anterior portions of the septum. The head is tilted backward to obtain a limited view of the middle meatus and middle turbinate. Often, this region cannot be adequately assessed by anterior rhinoscopy alone due to anatomic constraints. As a result, endoscopy is commonly used to examine this region as well as the posterior portions of the nasal cavity and the nasopharynx (see below). When anterior rhinoscopy has been completed, the speculum is carefully withdrawn with the blades slightly open to avoid avulsing hairs from the nasal vestibule.

In many cases, the nasal mucosa should be decongested with vasoconstrictors prior to the examination, as this makes it easier to examine the interior of the nose. At the same time, it is also important to assess the "original" condition of the nasal mucosa, and so the nose should be examined before and after decongestion of the mucosa.

*Indication*: Anterior rhinoscopy is used not only for nasal examination but also for minor therapeutic procedures such as intranasal packing for epistaxis, foreign-body removal, and polypectomy.

*Children:* Smaller instruments (pediatric specula) are available for anterior rhinoscopy in children. Moreover, aural specula can be used to examine the nose in infants or small children.

ɤ Decongestants should always be properly diluted when used in children.

## Posterior Rhinoscopy

Posterior rhinoscopy was formerly done to evaluate the nasopharynx and posterior nasal cavity (choanae, posterior ends of the turbinates, posterior margin of the vomer). With the establishment of endoscopic examination techniques in rhinology, this procedure, which requires special patient cooperation, is now considered obsolete.

## Nasal Endoscopy

Nasal endoscopy has become the most important and rewarding clinical examination method in rhinologic diagnosis.

*Prerequisites*: Nasal endoscopy requires practice because, unlike anterior rhinoscopy, it provides only close-up views of small intranasal areas. Besides rigid endoscopes, which are available in 4-mm and 2.8-mm diameters and assorted viewing angles (e.g., 0, 30, 120 degrees), flexible endoscopes are also available for inspecting the nose and nasopharynx and exploring all of the pharynx and larynx in one sitting. Their main disadvantages compared with rigid scopes are their weaker light intensity and poorer image resolution. Also, it takes two hands to operate a flexible endoscope, while a rigid scope leaves one hand free for manipulating instruments.

The patient is seated for the examination (**Fig. 2.2**). As in anterior rhinoscopy, the preparations include decongestion of the nasal mucosa. A topical anesthetic should also be applied. Diagnostic nasal endoscopy is performed with a 4-mm 30-degree telescope. The 2.8-mm scope is used only in a very narrow nasal cavity or in children.

**Fig. 2.3    Nasal endoscopy**

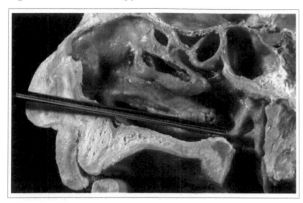

Nasal endoscope shown in an anatomic specimen (sagittal section). The tip of the scope is in the nasopharynx.

**Fig. 2.4    Endoscopy of the nasopharynx**

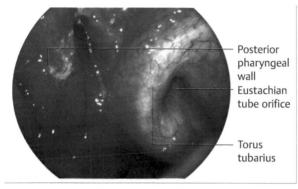

Posterior
pharyngeal
wall

Eustachian
tube orifice

Torus
tubarius

Transnasal endoscopic appearance of the nasopharynx.

**Fig. 2.5    Endoscopy of the middle meatus**

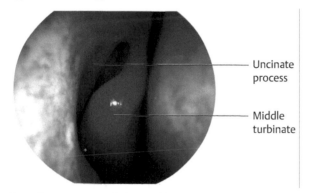

Uncinate
process

Middle
turbinate

Normal appearance of the middle meatus, with the middle turbinate and uncinate process. The asterisk marks the narrow passage through which the endoscope can be advanced into the ostiomeatal unit.

*Technique*: First, the examiner advances the endoscope into the *nasopharynx* (**Fig. 2.3**) and inspects the eustachian tube orifice, torus tubarius, posterior pharyngeal wall, and roof of the nasopharynx (**Fig. 2.4**). While the transnasal nasopharyngeal inspection can provide very detailed views (e.g., for early detection of nasopharyngeal cancer), it should still be supplemented by transoral postrhinoscopic endoscopy (see 5.2, Mirror Examination and Endoscopy).

Nasal endoscopy is particularly useful for evaluating the *ostiomeatal unit* (see 1.3), as this pathophysiological important region generally cannot be adequately evaluated by anterior rhinoscopy alone. To inspect the middle meatus, the endoscope is first advanced toward the head of the middle turbinate. This should provide a good overview of the middle meatus (**Fig. 2.5**).

To advance farther into the ostiomeatal unit, the scope must negotiate the narrow passage between the uncinate process and the middle turbinate (asterisk in **Fig. 2.5**). Normally, this can be done only with a narrow-gauge scope (2.8 mm). The 4-mm endoscope can be used at this site only in patients who have had previous intranasal sinus surgery with resection of the uncinate process.

Direct endoscopic inspection of the *paranasal sinuses* is possible only to a limited degree. In some cases, the sphenoid sinus can be examined with a thin telescope passed through the natural ostium in the anterior sinus wall. If endoscopic exploration of the maxillary sinus is required (e.g., for a suspected tumor), it can be done either through the inferior meatus after perforating the lateral nasal wall or by a transfacial approach with incision of the maxillary sinus mucosa and perforation of its anterior wall.

# 2.2    Special Rhinologic Tests

While the examination methods described thus far are practiced routinely, special rhinologic test procedures are performed only if there is specific evidence that suggests a particular disorder.

## Testing Nasal Patency

Simple methods can be used for the preliminary assessment of nasal patency. One such method is to hold a reflective metal plate under the nose; the degree of fogging will give a crude impression of the patency of the tested nasal cavity. Nasal patency in infants can be tested subjectively by holding a wisp of cotton in front of each nostril.

Today, the most standardized procedure for the assessment of nasal patency is **active anterior rhinomanometry** (**Fig. 2.6**). This procedure measures and graphically records the difference in pressure ($\Delta P$) from the naris (P2) to the nasopharynx (P1) and the respiratory air volume per unit time (V). One nostril is occluded for this test while the nasal air stream is measured on the opposite side. The accuracy of this test is most limited in patients with severe nasal airway obstruction, and the test cannot be performed when one nasal cavity is completely obstructed. **Acoustic rhinometry** is described in 🔎 **2.1**.

The differential diagnosis of nasal airway obstruction is outlined in **Table 2.1**.

## Allergy Testing

While the history and nasal endoscopic findings can provide initial, relatively nonspecific evidence of an allergic etiology for rhinitis, allergy testing is used to verify and differentiate this condition. Various in vivo and in vitro methods are available for allergy testing.

### Skin Tests

When a small amount of allergen is placed in contact with the skin, it can evoke a local or systemic (!) allergic reaction in a previously sensitized individual. The most widely used method is the **prick test**, in which the skin is superficially pricked with standard test substances that contain the suspicious antigens. The local skin reaction is compared with the reaction to a simultaneously applied positive control (histamine solution) and negative control (saline solution).

🖋 A positive skin prick test proves that sensitization has occurred but does not prove an allergic etiology for the rhinitis.

🔎 **2.1 Acoustic rhinometry**

Acoustic rhinometry is a measuring technique that is based on the principle of acoustic reflection and can be used to determine intranasal cross sections. Unlike rhinomanometry, it does not measure dynamic respiratory function but the cross sections of the nasal cavity at various sites, which are averaged together. The main advantages of this method over rhinomanometry are that it is faster and easier to perform and does not depend on patient cooperation. While these features are desirable in the examination of pediatric patients, it should always be considered that acoustic rhinometry measures static parameters and, unlike rhinomanometry, does not assess the patency of nasal airflow.

**Table 2.1  Differential diagnosis of nasal airway obstruction**

- Acute and chronic rhinitis (e.g., allergic, atrophic)
- Sinusitis
- Deviated septum (congenital, acquired)
- Nasal pyramid fracture
- Septal perforation
- Nasal polyps
- Cephalocele
- Adenoids
- Tumors of the nose, paranasal sinuses, and nasopharynx
- Foreign bodies (especially in small children)
- Drugs
  - **Adverse effects:** oral contraceptives, antihypertensive agents (e.g., reserpine, propranolol, hydralazine), antidepressants (e.g., amitriptyline)
  - **Drug abuse:** imidazoline derivatives (e.g., oxymetazoline hydrochloride, xylometazoline hydrochloride)

### Serologic Tests

The total immunoglobulin E (IgE) assay—e.g., paper radioimmunosorbent test (PRIST)—can be used for the quantitative determination of nonspecific total IgE, and various tests are available for specific IgE determination—e.g., radioallergosorbent test (RAST), enzyme allergosorbent test (EAST), etc. Specific IgE testing is recommended because of the low sensitivity and specificity of the total IgE assay.

**Fig. 2.6 Active anterior rhinomanometry**

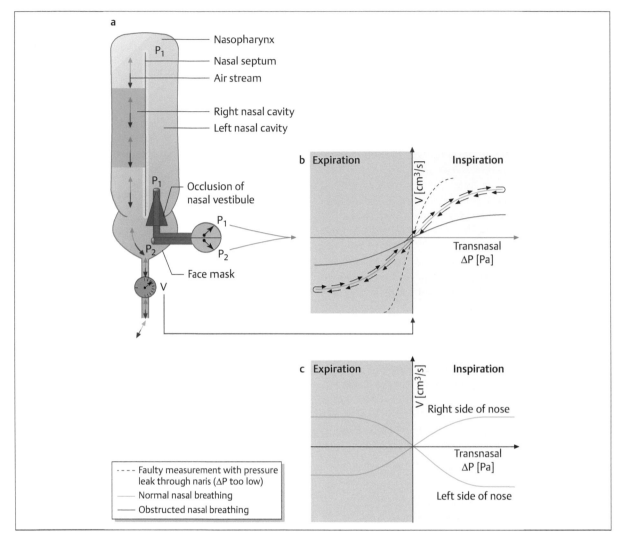

**a** In this example, the left nostril has been occluded. A pressure sensor measures the pressure P1 in the left nasal cavity (= pressure in the nasopharynx), and a second sensor measures P2 in a firmly attached face mask. The difference between the pressures, ΔP, is plotted against the respiratory volume flow V.

**b** The curve (green) starts at the zero baseline. It passes through the right upper quadrant during inspiration, crosses back over the baseline at the end of inspiration, passes through the lower left quadrant during expiration, and returns to the origin at the end of the respiratory cycle. A flatter curve (shown in red) indicates a stenosis in the shaded area of the diagram.

**c** When patency is tested in the left nasal cavity, it is customary to draw the curve in the left upper and right lower quadrants. In practice, the measurements from both nasal cavities are charted in one diagram.

Source: Rasp 1997.

**Nasal provocation test:** This test is of greatest value in allergic rhinitis, as it is the only method in which a specified allergen is placed in direct contact with the nasal mucosa. The technique involves the selective application of an allergen solution to the head of the inferior turbinate. Rhinomanometry (see above), performed before and 20 minutes after application of the allergen, confirms the local allergenic effect of the test substance by showing a significant reduction of nasal patency due to reactive mucosal swelling.

⚕ Since provocative testing involves placing the allergen directly on the turbinate, it may incite a severe allergic response or even anaphylactic shock, and proper emergency equipment should be easily accessible in the examination room.

## Olfactometry

Smelling disorders are common; 5 to 6% of the general population are suffering from an olfactory dysfunction, and complaints become more frequent with aging. They may be caused by a variety of underlying disorders (**Table 2.2**, **Table 2.3**).

🖉 Because it is difficult for laypeople to differentiate between smell and taste, many patients initially complain of a taste disturbance when they actually have an olfactory disturbance.

Pure taste disorders are very rare. The relationship between taste and smell must be considered during the diagnostic work-up, and therefore both sensory modalities should be tested (see also ✍4.2, Taste Testing). After a detailed history has been taken, the patient is examined by anterior rhinoscopy or endoscopy to rule out anatomic and functional obstructions of nasal airflow to the olfactory groove.

### Olfactory Screening Tests

The classic subjective smell tests have increasingly been supplanted by standardized screening tests over the last years. Currently, there are several well-vali-

Table 2.2  Causes of olfactory disturbances

| Classification | Example |
|---|---|
| **Transport of odorants** | |
| Nasal obstruction | Deviated septum, mucosal swelling, polyps, tumor |
| Scar tissue occluding the olfactory groove | After intranasal surgery |
| **Perception:** damage to the olfactory epithelium caused by: | |
| Toxic substances | $SO_2$, NO, ozone, heavy metals, varnishes |
| Drugs | See **Table 2.3** |
| Viral infections | Influenza |
| Radiotherapy (rare) | |
| **Stimulus conduction and processing** | |
| Avulsion of fila olfactoria | Skull base fracture |
| Aplasia of the olfactory bulb (rare) | Kallmann's syndrome |
| Injury to olfactory centers | Contusion or hemorrhage due to head injury |
| Neurodegenerative diseases | Alzheimer's disease, Parkinson's disease, diabetes mellitus (rare) |
| Olfactory hallucinations | After epileptic seizures, in schizophrenia |

Table 2.3  Medications that have been associated with smelling disorders

| Drug class | Examples |
|---|---|
| Antibiotics | Streptomycin |
| Antirheumatic agents | Gold |
| Antihypertensive agents | Diltiazem, nifedipine |
| Antidepressants | Amitriptyline |
| Anticancer agents | Methotrexate |
| Local anesthetics | Cocaine |
| Opioids | Remifentanil, morphine |
| Psychoactive substances | Amphetamine, alcohol |
| Sympathomimetic drugs | Chronic use of local vasoconstrictors |
| Others | Sildenafil |

Source: Hummel et al 2011.

dated tests available which can be performed quickly and easily (e.g., "Cross Cultural Smell Identification Test," **CCSIT**; "Sniffin' Sticks"; "European Test of Olfactory Capabilities," **ETOC**). These screening tests are based on easy handling and perceivability between examiner and patient; another advantage is a better reproducibility compared with the classic subjective smelling tests. Still, these tests require a minimum of cognitive and verbal skills, and the informational value is limited considering the complex process of olfaction.

### Objective Olfactory Testing (Electrophysiological Testing)

Objective olfactory testing is far more costly and is generally performed only at large centers. Pure odorants and trigeminal nerve stimulants are presented separately to the patient, and the responses are measured by the computer-controlled recording and analysis of olfactory evoked potentials. Objective olfactometry is used mainly in disability examinations.

### Functional Magnetic Resonance Imaging

Another way to measure the olfactory capability is by functional magnetic resonance imaging (fMRI), a special imaging technique, which measures the BOLD (blood oxygen level–dependent) effect. Once the person under examination receives an olfactory stimulation, the neuronal activity leads to an increased blood supply, which can be measured by fMRI. Currently fMRI is rather used for research purposes than clinical routine.

# 2.3 Imaging of the Nose and Paranasal Sinuses

Imaging procedures are an important tool in the diagnostic work-up of rhinologic diseases. Besides conventional sinus radiographs, the most important imaging modalities at present are computed tomography (CT) and magnetic resonance imaging (MRI).

## Conventional Radiographs

### Indications

Standard paranasal sinus radiographs in the occipitomental projection (**Fig. 2.7a, b**; Water's projection) and occipitofrontal projection (**Fig. 2.7c, d**; Caldwell's projection) are rarely performed these days due to their limited informational value compared with imaging techniques such as CT.

Conventional radiographs may still be indicated in selected cases, to verify postoperative results after surgery of displaced midfacial fractures (see **Fig. 3.25**).

## Computed Tomography

### Indications

Besides an occasional malformation, the main indications for CT scanning of the nose and paranasal sinuses are chronic sinusitis, trauma (especially frontobasal fractures), and tumors. CT sinus scans are compromised by metal-bearing dentures, which cause beam-hardening artifacts that can significantly degrade the image quality.

### Scan Planes

CT of the paranasal sinuses should be performed in three planes, with coronal (**Fig. 2.8**), axial (**Fig. 2.9**), and sagittal images (**Fig. 2.10**), to provide optimum depiction of all anatomic structures. CT scans in three planes are also frequently used in navigation systems for paranasal sinus surgery (**Fig. 2.11**).

### Scan Acquisition

Scans can be acquired using the sequential, single-slice technique (*conventional CT*) or a continuous spiral technique (*spiral* or *helical CT*). The advantages of spiral CT are complete coverage with no interslice gaps ("volume scan") and a shorter examination time (~20 seconds), making the images less susceptible to respiratory and motion artifacts.

### Documentation

CT images documented on radiographic film should occupy the whole frame, displaying only the structures that are relevant for making an interpretation.

**Fig. 2.7  Standard radiographic projections of the paranasal sinuses**

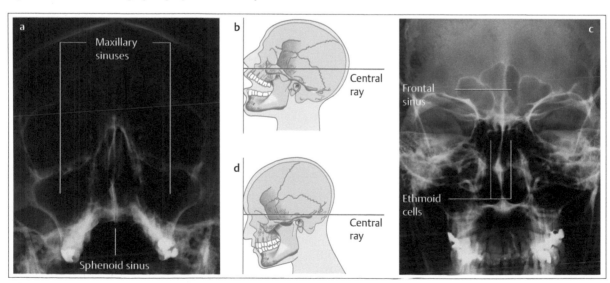

**a,b** The occipitomental projection demonstrates the maxillary sinus and gives a limited view of the sphenoid sinus.

**c,d** The occipitofrontal projection is better for evaluating the ethmoid cells and frontal sinus.

**Fig. 2.8 Computed tomography of the paranasal sinuses**

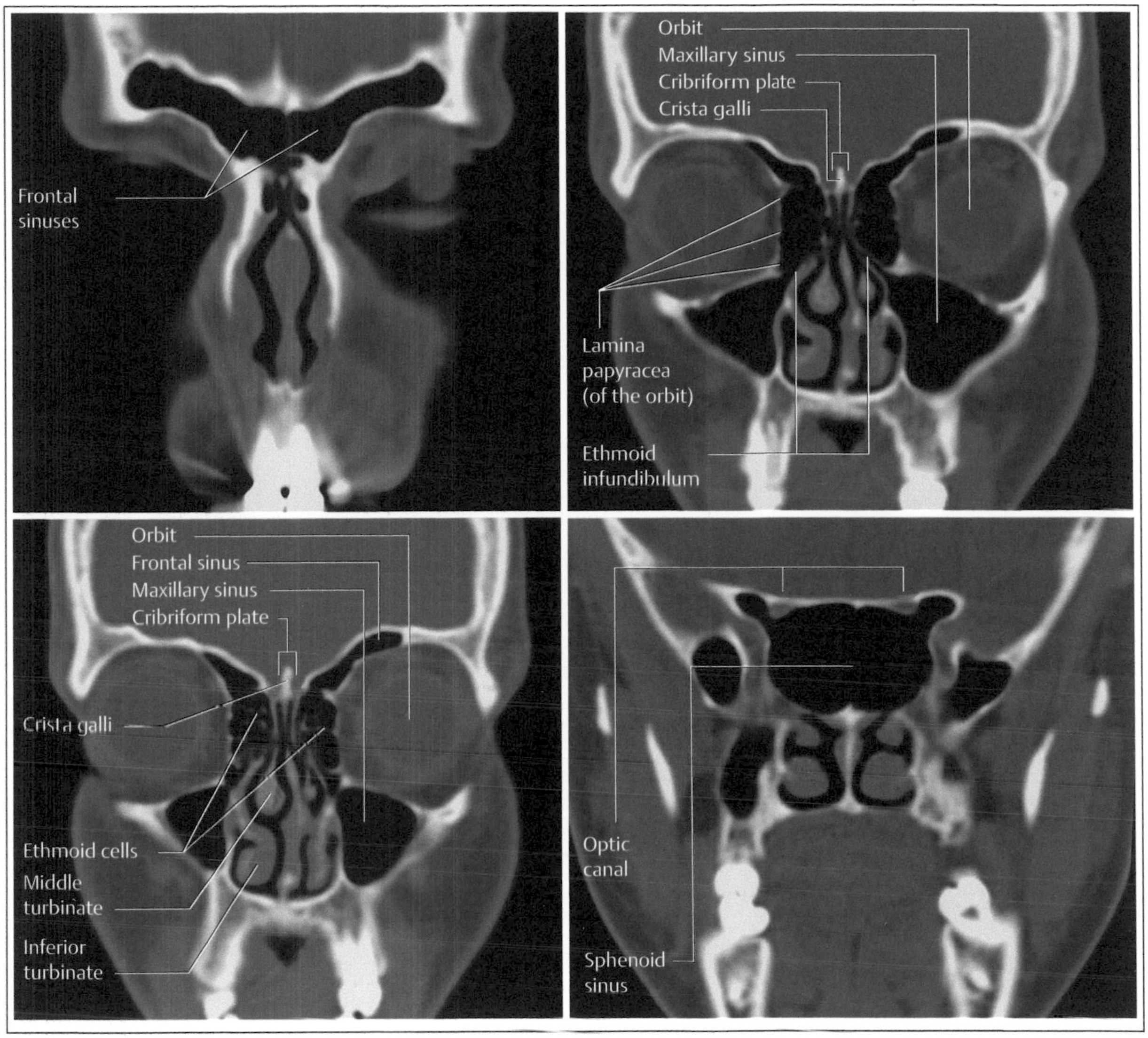

Coronal scans.

## Interpretation

Normally aerated paranasal sinuses exhibit air density on CT scans—i.e., they appear black. The normal mucosal lining of the sinuses is not visualized. The bony sinus walls appear hyperdense (white).

## Cone Beam Tomography

Cone beam tomography (CBT; **Fig. 2.12**) was primarily used in dental medicine. Over the past years, this technique has been increasingly used in patients with inflammatory paranasal sinus disease as an alternative to CT. The major advantage of CBT compared with conventional CT is a reduced radiation dose. Disadvantages include a poor soft-tissue discrimination, which disqualifies the technique for the diagnostic manage-

ment of paranasal sinus tumors and complications of inflammatory sinus disease. Up to now, there is no clinical and only limited research experience with the use of contrast agents in CBT according to the literature.

## Magnetic Resonance Imaging

### Indications

MRI has fewer indications than CT in patients with paranasal sinus disease. This is primarily because MRI is markedly inferior to CT in defining the bony boundaries of the sinuses. The strength of MRI lies in its superior soft-tissue discrimination (**Fig. 2.13**). MRI is indicated in diseases that involve the paranasal sinuses in addition to the cranial cavity or orbit (e.g.,

**Fig. 2.9 Computed tomography of the paranasal sinuses**

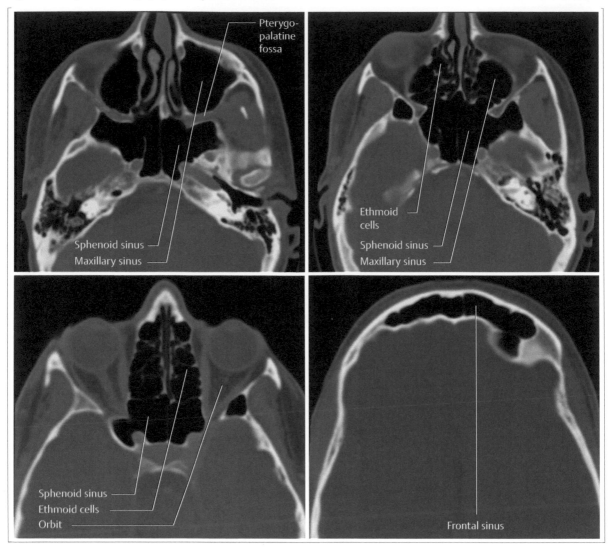

Axial scans.

tumors and congenital malformations such as encephaloceles). It can also supply information that is useful in differentiating soft-tissue lesions within the paranasal sinuses (mucocele, cyst, polyp), and it can distinguish between solid tumor tissue and inflammatory perifocal reaction.

## Contraindications

🖉 Before ordering an examination, the physician should consider the basic physical principle of MRI: the use of magnetic fields and radiofrequency energy.

At present, MRI is contraindicated in most patients with electrically controlled devices such as a cardiac pacemaker, insulin pump, cytostatic pump, or cochlear implant. By contrast, modern internal fixation materi-

als such as titanium are usually nonmagnetic and therefore MRI-compatible.

## Method

The standard imaging protocol employs a *T1-weighted spin-echo sequence* before and after intravenous contrast administration in addition to a *proton- and T2-weighted turbo spin-echo sequence.*

## Slice Thickness

The slice thickness should not exceed 3 to 4 mm, and the slice increment should be no greater than 0.6 mm. Imaging of the frontal skull base, orbit, parapharyngeal space, and pterygopalatine fossa requires the highest possible spatial resolution with a thin slice thickness (3 mm).

**Fig. 2.10 Computed tomography of the paranasal sinuses**

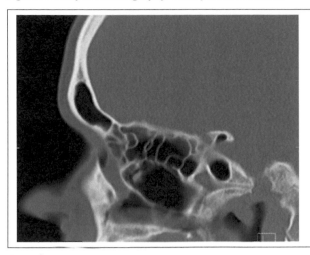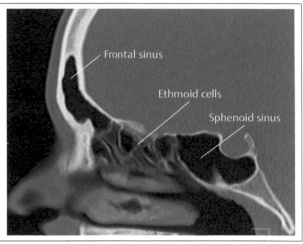

Sagittal scans.

**Fig. 2.11 Computed tomography in navigation surgery**

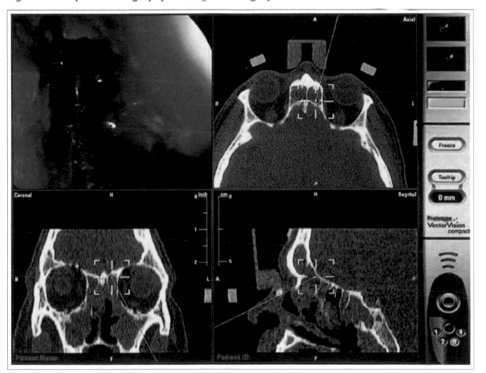

All three CT planes are shown on the same screen with the corresponding endoscopic image. Source: Grevers et al 2002.

**Fig. 2.12 Cone beam tomography of the paranasal sinuses**

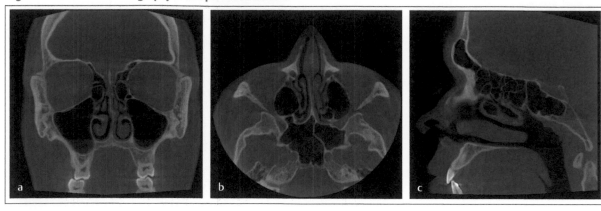

Coronal (**a**), axial (**b**), and sagittal (**c**) planes are shown. Source: Dr. A. Grevers-Kürten, HNO-Zentrum Neuss, Neuss, Germany.

**Fig. 2.13 MRI of the paranasal sinuses**

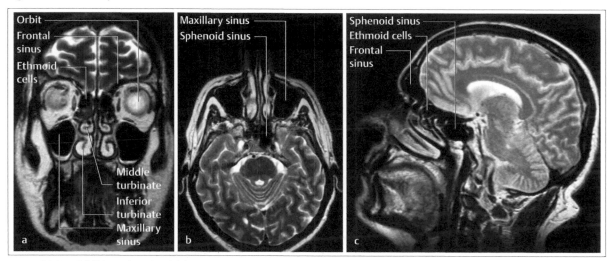

Coronal (**a**), axial (**b**), and sagittal (**c**) magnetic resonance images.

## Imaging Planes

Primary scan acquisition in MRI can be done in three planes: axial, coronal, and sagittal (**Fig. 2.13**). Plain, unenhanced T1-weighted images are excellent for defining normal craniofacial anatomy.

## Ultrasound

The paranasal sinuses can also be visualized with ultrasound (A and B mode).

**Advantages**: Ultrasound is particularly useful in the follow-up of acute inflammatory processes, as it can eliminate the need for extra radiographic views. It is also used in children and pregnant women for the same reason.

**Disadvantages**: Ultrasound yields much less detailed images than CT and MRI, and it cannot provide three-dimensional rendering.

## Indications

The *frontal and maxillary sinuses* are most easily accessible to ultrasound imaging. The *anterior ethmoid cells* can be scanned via the medial canthus of the eye, but it should be added that these cells can be examined from this site only by using a small A-mode transducer or a more costly, specialized B-mode transducer; a large linear array (7.5 MHz) cannot be used. Scanning the *middle and posterior ethmoid cells* by the transocular route is extremely challenging and requires a highly experienced examiner.

The sphenoid sinus is inaccessible to ultrasound imaging because of its location.

# 3   Diseases of the Nose, Paranasal Sinuses, and Face

## 3.1   Malformations of the Nose, Paranasal Sinuses, and Face

**Malformations involving the nose may be caused by developmental abnormalities of the nasal floor, palate, nasal roof, and internasal region. A variety of** disorders can result, depending on the affected anatomic structures.

### Choanal Atresia

*Epidemiology:* Choanal atresia has an incidence of 1 in 5,000 to 1 in 10,000 births and is more often unilateral than bilateral. The atresia is bony in 90% of cases and membranous in only 10%.

---

**3.1  Embryology of choanal atresia**

The choanae are the posterior openings that connect the nasal cavities with the nasopharynx. They develop between the third and seventh embryonic weeks, following rupture of the vertical epithelial fold between the olfactory groove and the roof of the primary oral cavity (pronasal membrane). If this process is disturbed, rupture of the oronasal membrane will be absent or incomplete, resulting in the partial (stenosis) or complete closure (atresia) of one or both choanae.

---

*Symptoms:* Bilateral choanal atresia is an acutely life-threatening emergency because the neonate, except when crying, is an obligate nasal breather until about the sixth week of life. As a result, the infant experiences episodes of asphyxia at rest when its mouth is closed, especially during periods of sleep, and also during feeding. The resulting hypoxia is manifested by cyanosis, bradycardia, and an erratic respiratory rate with the mouth open or closed. Cyanosis that is present at rest and improves with exertion is called **paradoxical cyanosis** because of its opposite pattern relative to cyanosis with a cardiac cause.

Unilateral choanal atresia may be manifested by a purulent nasal discharge on the affected side. Choanal atresia may be associated with various other anomalies, with fully developed cases presenting as the CHARGE syndrome (coloboma; heart disease; atresia of the choanae; retarded growth and development and/or central nervous system anomalies; genital hypoplasia; ear anomalies or deafness).

*Diagnosis:*

- Both choanae in newborns should be routinely catheterized in the immediate postnatal period (e.g., with the suction catheter) to exclude choanal atresia.

The clinical suspicion of choanal atresia can be confirmed by examination with a rigid or flexible endoscope (**Fig. 3.1**).

*Treatment:* The acute care of choanal atresia in asphyxia consists of intubation followed by perforation of the atresia plate. Recurrent stenosis is prevented by inserting a stent and securing it with a suture (to prevent aspiration). The definitive surgical repair of bilateral choanal atresia is performed during the first weeks or months of life. Surgery for unilateral atresia can be postponed until school age, when the anatomy of the region is more similar to that encountered in adults.

### Frontobasal Dysraphias

The incidence of dysraphias involving the anterior skull base is approximately 1 in 20,000 to 1 in 40,000 births. The familial pattern of occurrence suggests a genetic component to the disease. For further details on the embryology, see 3.2.

**Manifestations:** Congenital dysraphias of the anterior skull base can have various manifestations that include dorsal nasal fistulas (3.3), dermoids (3.4), frontonasal extracerebral gliomas, and cephaloceles (3.5).

**Fig. 3.1   Choanal atresia**

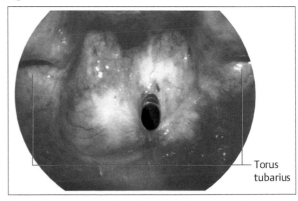

Torus tubarius

Postrhinoendoscopic view shows partial closure (stenosis) of the left choana accompanied by complete closure (atresia) of the right choana (contrast with normal-appearing choanae in **Fig. 2.4**.)

## 3.2 Embryology of frontobasal dysraphias

The skull base may be affected by congenital closure defects, analogous to a dermal sinus or spina bifida involving the lumbar portion of the spine. Dysraphic anomalies of the anterior skull base are caused by exposure to teratogenic agents during the second or third week of embryonic development, when the neural tube is forming from the neural plate, or during the fourth week, when the cerebral ventricles and central canal are forming and the central nervous system is separating from the epidermis and migrating to a deeper level.

## 3.3 Dorsal nasal fistula

*Morphology:* A dorsal nasal fistula consists of a fistulous tract that is lined by keratinized squamous epithelium and forms a tiny opening on the dorsum or tip of the nose. The fistula may terminate blindly or even extend into the cranial cavity, creating an open communication with the subarachnoid space.

*Symptoms:* Fistulas that terminate blindly are usually manifested clinically at an older age due to inflammation around the fistulous opening. If the fistula communicates with the subarachnoid space, it can lead to severe complications such as cerebrospinal fluid leakage, meningitis, or brain abscess.

## 3.4 Nasal dermoid

Nasal dermoids, like dorsal nasal fistulas, are lined by keratinized squamous epithelium. Sites of predilection are the dorsal nasal midline and nasal flank, where the lesions present as cystic protrusions. A nasal dermoid may coexist with a dorsal nasal fistula in rare cases. Abscesses may develop as an inflammatory complication. Diagnosis and treatment are the same as described in 3.3.

*Diagnosis:* The diagnosis is established by computed tomography or magnetic resonance imaging. Diagnostic catheterization or contrast injection is contraindicated due to the risk of intracranial complications.

*Treatment:* Treatment consists of complete removal of the fistulous tract, which may include excising the dural defect and repairing it by duraplasty. Incomplete removal of the fistula will predispose to recurrent infections.

## 3.5 Cephalocele

Cephaloceles are herniations of intracranial contents through a bony defect in the skull. Several types are distinguished according to the structures involved: *meningocele* (congenital protrusion of the leptomeninx; see **Fig. 3.2**), *meningoencephalocele* (leptomeninx and brain tissue), and *meningoencephalocystocele* (meningocele plus portions of the ventricular system).

*Etiology:* Most cephaloceles are congenital, but rare cases are posttraumatic (e.g., after a frontobasal fracture).

*Classification:* Cephaloceles of the anterior skull base are classified into two groups. *Sincipital* cephaloceles are located near the glabella, forehead or orbit, while *basal* cephaloceles are found mainly in the nasal cavity or nasopharynx.

*Presentation:* Most cephaloceles are manifested clinically during childhood. The *sincipital forms* appear as a pulsating mass near the glabella, often associated with a broad nasal dorsum and hypertelorism (**Fig. 3.2a**). The *basal forms* present as an intranasal mass, typically with associated nasal airway obstruction. They closely resemble intranasal polyps and should be considered in the differential diagnosis of children with suspected nasal polyps, which are rare in this age group.

*Diagnosis:* Computed tomography and magnetic resonance imaging can supply information on the location and extent of the mass and the associated bony defect (**Fig. 3.2**).

*Treatment:* Treatment is always surgical and consists of removing the cephalocele and repairing the dural defect. Any associated anomalies of the orbit and facial skeleton should also be corrected.

**Fig. 3.2   Meningocele**

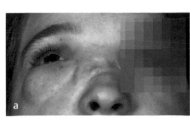
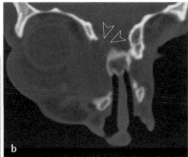
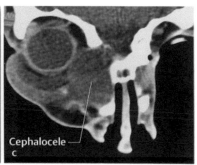

**a** Clinical picture of a girl with an extensive meningocele.
**b** Corresponding coronal CT scan (bone-window setting) displaying the bony defect in the ethmoid roof (arrows).

**c** The coronal CT scan in the soft-tissue window setting more clearly distinguishes the cephalocele from adjacent soft-tissue structures.

# 3.2    Nasal Deformities

A basic distinction is drawn between deformities of the external nose and intranasal deformities. They are frequently combined, however, as deformities of the external nose are generally associated with a variable degree of nasal septal curvature and may even be caused by them (e.g., cartilaginous nasal deviation with a deviated septum, humped nose with a tension septum). For learning purposes, however, septal deviation is classified as an intranasal deformity and is described separately from the various external deformities.

## Septal Deviation

*Definition:* This is defined as a congenital or traumatically acquired bending or bowing of the nasal septum.

*Symptoms:* Almost everyone has some degree of bowing, spurring, or ridging of the cartilaginous or bony nasal septum. Mild forms do not cause symptoms and have no pathologic significance (**Fig. 3.3 a**).
More pronounced degrees of septal curvature can obstruct nasal breathing and may also cause olfactory impairment due to inadequate ventilation of the olfactory groove. Deficient nasal airflow can also lead to paranasal sinus sequelae such as headaches and recurrent sinusitis. A large septal spur that comes into contact with the nasal turbinates can cause epistaxis (**Fig. 3.3 b**).

*Diagnosis:* Septal subluxation is a special form in which the anterior septal margin is displaced from the median plane (**Fig. 1.4 b**). This condition is readily identified by external inspection of the nasal base. Further clinical examination consists of external inspection, anterior rhinoscopy, or endoscopy (**Fig. 3.3 a–d**), which can verify the morphologic changes in the nasal septum. The degree of nasal obstruction can be objectively evaluated by *rhinomanometry* (see **Fig. 2.6**). For medicolegal reasons, *olfactory testing* should always

Fig. 3.3   **Septal pathology**

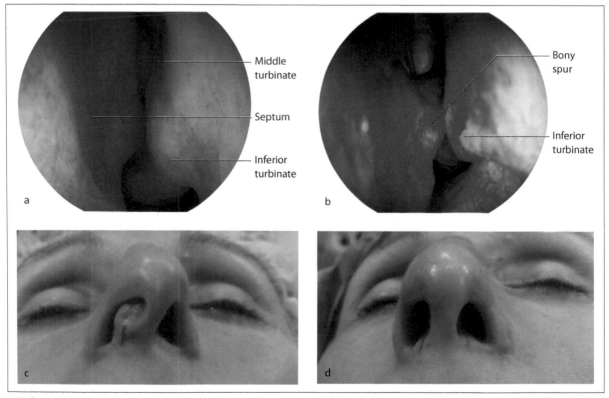

Middle turbinate

Septum

Inferior turbinate

Bony spur

Inferior turbinate

a Endoscopic appearance of a nasal septum deviated toward the left side, partially obstructing the nasal airway.
b Endoscopic appearance of a bony septal spur that touches the inferior turbinate, causing epistaxis (left nasal cavity).

c, d External appearance of posttraumatic septal deviation and subluxation before (c) and after (d) surgery.

be done prior to surgical treatment (see 📖2.2, Olfactometry).

***Treatment:*** The treatment of choice is surgical straightening of the deviated septum (**septoplasty**). This procedure involves removing the deviated cartilaginous and bony portions of the septum along with any spurs and ridges and reimplanting them as needed until the septum occupies a tension-free position in the median plane.

The *indication* for septoplasty is basically any septal deviation that is causing subjective complaints with functional impairment of nasal breathing.

☞ The indication for septoplasty should be weighed very carefully in children and adolescents younger than 15 to 17 years, and a very conservative approach should be taken in patient selection. Indiscriminate use of this procedure in younger patients can damage the growth zones of the septum, causing long-term problems.

## Deformities of the External Nose

***Causes and forms:*** Deformities may be congenital or traumatically acquired. Virtually any bony and cartilaginous structures of the external nose may be affected. An accompanying septal deviation is present in many cases.

The most common deformities are a crooked nose, humped nose, saddle nose, and broad nose, which may occur separately or in combinations (**Fig. 3.4**).

***Diagnosis:*** Besides *inspection* of the external nose, in which the affected cartilaginous and bony structures are identified, the diagnostic work-up should include *anterior rhinoscopy* or *endoscopy* to evaluate the shape and position of the nasal septum.

☞ Photographic documentation should always be obtained preoperatively for medicolegal reasons.

***Treatment:*** Since deformities of the external nose are frequently associated with intranasal changes, most cases have both a functional and an aesthetic indication for corrective surgery.

The treatment of choice is "functional septorhinoplasty," with correction of the nasal septum and external nose. In most cases the bony nasal skeleton has to be osteotomized at multiple sites to achieve the desired nasal shape and position. The humped nose additionally requires dorsal hump removal. Saddle nose is corrected by filling the dorsal concavity with a cartilage graft taken from the septum, auricle, or rib.

**Fig. 3.4  Deformities of the external nose**

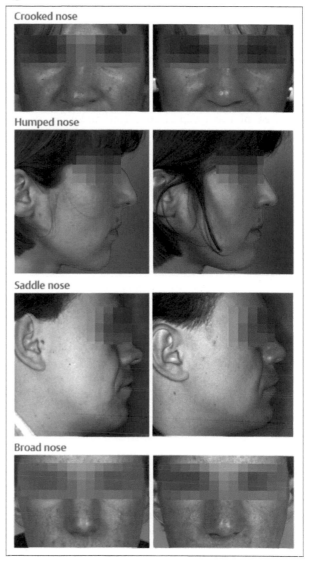

The preoperative appearance of various nasal deformities is shown on the left side, the postoperative appearance on the right side.

# 3.3 Nosebleed (Epistaxis)

**Nosebleed is a relatively common, usually harmless symptom that may reflect several diseases of variable** severity. By knowing the potential causes, the physician can react appropriately in threatening cases.

## Causes

Nosebleed may have a local or systemic cause. Possible **local causes** (**Table 3.1**) include mucosal hyperemia due to an acute inflammation (rhinitis), allergies, and ambient conditions that dry the mucosa, increasing the fragility of the intranasal vessels (e.g., air conditioning). Local manipulations (nose picking) can also cause a nosebleed, usually in Kiesselbach's area (a richly vascularized area of septal mucosa at the junction of the nasal cavity and vestibule; **Fig. 3.5 a–c**). Other possible local causes of epistaxis are congenital or acquired abnormalities of the nasal septum, such as pronounced septal spurs or ridges (see **Fig. 3.3 b**), as well as benign and malignant neoplasms of the nose, paranasal sinuses, and nasopharynx (see 3.10). Finally, nosebleed can result from a septal perforation (**Fig. 3.6**). A perforated septum can have several causes, including a septal fracture with a superinfected septal hematoma (septal abscess), autoimmune disease (e.g., granulomatosis with polyangiitis/Wegener's granulomatosis; see 3.10), or a previous septoplasty (see 3.2, Septal Deviation) leading to mucosal perforation and cartilage necrosis. Epistaxis may also be symptomatic of an underlying systemic disease (**Table 3.2**). Besides vascular and circulatory diseases, typical examples are the various forms of hemorrhagic diathesis (e.g., Osler's disease; see 3.7), infectious diseases, and endocrinopathies.

**Fig. 3.5 Bleeding from Kiesselbach's area**

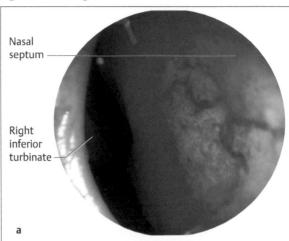

Nasal septum

Right inferior turbinate

a

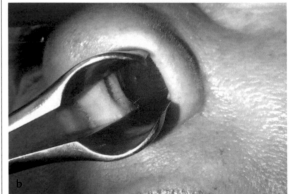

b

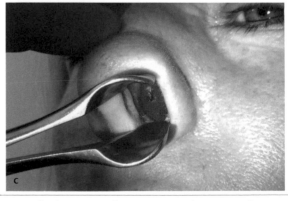

c

**a** Kiesselbach's area on the anterior septal mucosa is the site at which epistaxis typically occurs due to a local cause. The right inferior turbinate is visible in the background.
**b, c** If an isolated vessel can be identified (**b**), electrocauterization (**c**) can be performed as targeted therapy. Under local anesthesia, this is an almost painless procedure.

| Table 3.1 Local causes of epistaxis | |
|---|---|
| *Classification* | *Examples* |
| Change in the nasal septum | Perforation (**Fig. 3.6**): traumatic, iatrogenic, inflammatory; spurs or ridges (**Fig. 3.3 b**) |
| Mucosal or vascular injury | Foreign bodies, rhinoliths, trauma (including nose picking), allergy, acute rhinitis, traumatic aneurysm of the internal carotid artery (very rare) |
| Neoplasia | Benign and malignant neoplasms of the nose, paranasal sinuses, and nasopharynx |
| "Idiopathic" | |

## ⌕ 3.6 Alternatives to anterior nasal packing and complications

A double-lumen **balloon catheter** is introduced and inflated with water to produce local compression in the nasal cavity and nasopharynx.

If the bleeding persists, a **posterior nasal pack (Bellocq's pack)** can be inserted, but it should be used with caution due to the risk of aspirating the pads in the nasopharynx.

**Systemic complications** of anterior and posterior nasal packing:

- Arterial hypoxia: fall of oxygen partial pressure with pulmonary dysfunction due to an impaired nasopulmonary reflux mechanism.
- Toxic shock: focal staphylococcal infection develops within 24 hours after nasal packing, with generalized shock symptoms caused by bacterial toxins.

## Diagnosis

⚐ Nosebleed requires a simultaneous, coordinated protocol of diagnostic and therapeutic actions. One possible algorithm is shown in **Fig. 3.7**.

The diagnostic work-up begins with **blood pressure measurement**. Except in very minor cases, the Hb should also be determined, and a **coagulation disorder** should be excluded by determining the platelet count, bleeding time, thromboplastin time (formerly: Quick), partial thromboplastin time, and thrombin time.

**Bleeding site:** The nasal cavity is inspected by anterior rhinoscopy or endoscopy following decongestion and local anesthesia of the mucosa. In most cases the bleeding site is in Kiesselbach's area (**Fig. 3.5a**). It can be difficult to locate the bleeding source, however, when there is profuse bleeding from the posterior parts of the nasal cavity, which are less accessible to inspection.

## Treatment

*General measures:* The intensity of the bleeding and risk of aspiration can be reduced before the cause and location have been established. The nostrils are compressed against the nasal septum, and the patient is told not to swallow blood running down the pharynx. The patient is kept in an upright posture to reduce blood flow to the head and inhibit the swallowing of blood. An ice bag can be placed on the back of the neck to induce reflex vasoconstriction (see **Fig. 3.8**). An intravenous line should be placed if bleeding is severe.

*Silver nitrate cautery or electrocautery:* Mild epistaxis from Kiesselbach's area can often be controlled by selective local cauterization of the bleeding site with silver nitrate. In some patients, an isolated, pulsating vessel can be identified, which should be electrocauterized (**Fig. 3.5 b, c**).

**Fig. 3.6 Septal perforation**

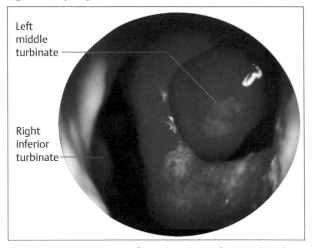

Left middle turbinate

Right inferior turbinate

The bleeding in this case is from the edges of a septal perforation. The endoscope was introduced into the right nasal cavity. The left middle turbinate and right inferior turbinate are visible in the background.

**Table 3.2 Systemic causes of epistaxis**

| Classification | Examples |
|---|---|
| Vascular and circulatory diseases | Atherosclerosis, arterial hypertension |
| Infectious diseases | Influenza, measles, typhus |
| Endocrine changes or diseases | Pheochromocytoma, pregnancy, diabetes mellitus |
| Hemorrhagic diathesis<br>• Coagulopathies | *Congenital:* e.g., hemophilia A and B, von Willebrand's disease<br>*Acquired:* e.g., anticoagulant therapy, hepatocellular insufficiency |
| • Platelet disorders<br>– Thrombocytopenias | Idiopathic thrombocytopenic purpura, platelet proliferation disorders, platelet distribution disorders |
| – Thrombocytopathies | Congenital<br>Acquired: uremia, dysproteinemia, adverse effects of dextran and acetylsalicylic acid (ASA) therapy |
| • Vasopathies | Schönlein–Henoch purpura, Osler's disease (⌕ 3.7) |

Fig. 3.7    Flowchart for the diagnosis and treatment of epistaxis

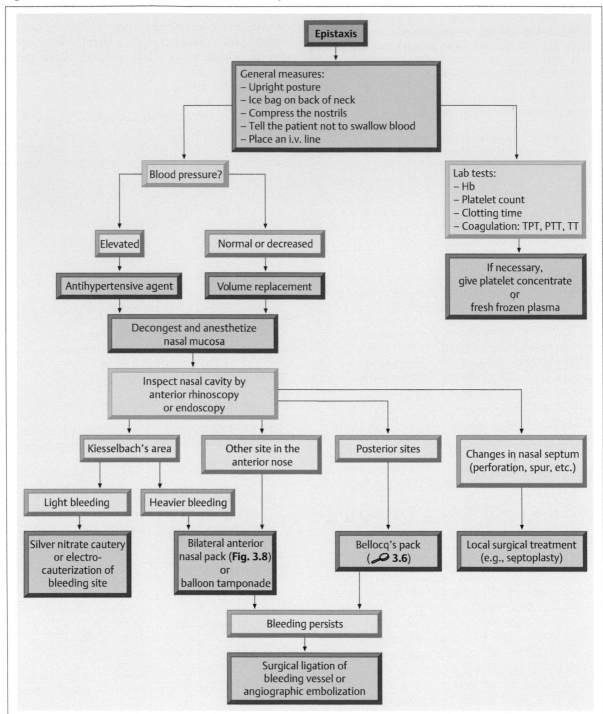

📖 Opposing sites on the nasal septum should not be cauterized due to the risk of septal perforation.

***Nasal packing:*** For severe epistaxis, the anterior nasal cavity can be packed with ointment-impregnated gauze strips (see **Fig. 3.8**) or with ready-made foam packs that expand on contact with fluid.

📖 Both nasal cavities should always be packed to produce adequate counterpressure.

Alternatives to anterior nasal packing are shown in 🔎 **3.6**.

Intranasal packing should not remain in place for more than 2 to 3 days. Balloon catheters should be progressively deflated starting on the second day; otherwise, they may cause irreversible tissue necrosis. Long-term mucosal hygiene should be maintained after the packing is removed.

***Vascular ligation or embolization:*** The most common source of bleeding from the posterolateral part of the

### Fig. 3.8    Anterior nasal packing

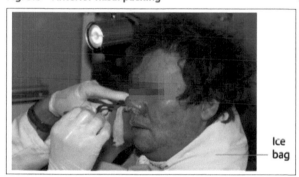

Ice bag

Treatment of a patient with epistaxis. Ointment-impregnated gauze strips are layered into both nasal cavities. An ice bag is placed on the back of the patient's neck.

### Fig. 3.9    Vascular ligation for severe epistaxis

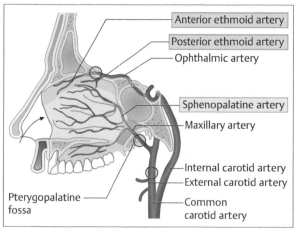

Anterior ethmoid artery
Posterior ethmoid artery
Ophthalmic artery
Sphenopalatine artery
Maxillary artery
Internal carotid artery
External carotid artery
Pterygopalatine fossa
Common carotid artery

Depending on the bleeding source, various vessels can be ligated through a cervical approach, by the transnasal endoscopic route, or by a transmaxillary route in the pterygopalatine fossa.

nasal cavity is the sphenopalatine artery (branch of the maxillary artery), which can be coagulated or clipped under endoscopic control. The ligation or angiographic embolization of a larger arterial trunk may be considered as a last recourse. When this is done, the source of the bleeding must be accurately identified since the nasal lining is supplied by various arteries (**Fig. 3.9**).

Prevention of recurrent bleeding: Besides the conservative treatments noted above, some causes of epistaxis require surgical treatment since nasal packing alone is of only temporary, symptomatic benefit (🔎 **3.7**).

🔎 **3.7   Surgical prevention of recurrent epistaxis**

The main indications for surgery are changes in the nasal septum such as **septal spurs** (**Fig. 3.3 b** and **Fig. 3.10**), ridges, and perforations (**Fig. 3.6**). Treatment consists of straightening the nasal septum (septoplasty, see 📖 3.2, Septal Deviation) or closing the septal perforation (e.g., by implanting an auricular cartilage graft and using local mucosal flap advancement).

In diseases that are associated with **vascular changes**, such as *Osler's disease*, telangiectatic areas on the septal mucosa can be treated with a surgical laser. The figure shows numerous punctate telangiectasias in the left nasal cavity in Osler's disease.

If laser treatment is inadequate, other surgical options are available. In a Saunders dermoplasty, for example, the telangiectatic septal mucosa is resected and replaced with a free skin graft (e.g., from the supraclavicular area).

### Fig. 3.10  Septal spur causing recurrent epistaxis

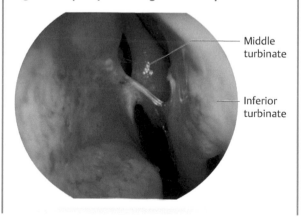

Middle turbinate

Inferior turbinate

# 3.4    Soft-Tissue Injuries and Plastic Surgery

**Facial soft-tissue injuries are still a common occurrence in recreational and traffic accidents. When improperly managed, they can result in disfiguring scars and deformity. Poor cosmetic results are particularly** **objectionable in this very conspicuous region. This 📖 deals with necessary diagnostic measures and also reviews the most important techniques of facial plastic surgery.**

## Diagnosis

*Before* a traumatic facial wound is treated, possible co-existing fractures should be excluded by clinical examination and, if necessary, by imaging studies such as biplane skull films, standard sinus projections (see **Fig. 2.7**), and computed tomography (CT) scans. Especially with bite wounds, a smear should be taken for microbiologic examination.

📙 Every patient with facial injuries should be asked about tetanus immunization.

## Treatment

Prior to surgical treatment, measures are taken to reduce microorganism counts and prevent infection (tetanus, rabies), especially in patients with bite wounds.
In the interest of maximum tissue preservation, only tissues that are definitely necrotic should be debrided from facial wounds.

📙 Wound margins should never be reapproximated under tension, as this would result in aesthetic and functional deficits such as incomplete eyelid closure.

In most soft-tissue injuries to the nose, adequate treatment consists of primary reapproximation and suturing of the wound margins.

## Scar Camouflage

Two fundamental local principles in facial soft-tissue surgery are the relaxed skin-tension lines (RSTLs; see **Fig. 1.1 a**) and the aesthetic units (see **Fig. 1.1 b**). The RSTLs are a particularly important consideration when there are no soft-tissue or skin defects and only a direct closure is required, since scars are easier to camouflage when they are oriented along the RSTLs. The techniques described below are also useful for revising a functionally and/or aesthetically objectionable result, such as lengthening a heavily contracted scar.
Z-plasty (**Fig. 3.11 a, b**): When a wound margin runs perpendicular to the RSTLs, it can be reoriented with a single or multiple Z-plasty and lengthened in the direction of the scar axis.

**Fig. 3.11 Closure of facial soft-tissue wounds**

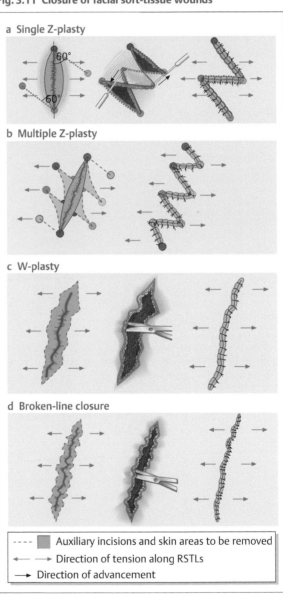

a  Single Z-plasty

b  Multiple Z-plasty

c  W-plasty

d  Broken-line closure

- - - - ▨ Auxiliary incisions and skin areas to be removed
◄──── ──► Direction of tension along RSTLs
──► Direction of advancement

The techniques of scar revision can also be used in primary wound care. The wound area should be broadly undermined to eliminate tension on the reapproximated wound margins. The colored dots mark the original and transposed location of the skin areas. The solid lines represent the wound margins. Broken lines indicate auxiliary incisions.

**Fig. 3.12 Local flap techniques**

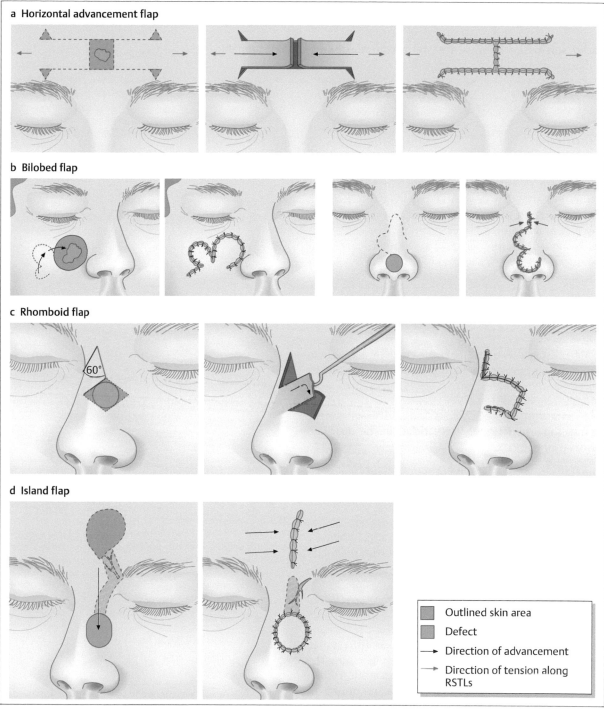

**a Horizontal advancement flap**

**b Bilobed flap**

**c Rhomboid flap**

60°

**d Island flap**

| | |
|---|---|
| ▨ | Outlined skin area |
| ▨ | Defect |
| → | Direction of advancement |
| → | Direction of tension along RSTLs |

**a** Small "Burow triangles" are excised at the ends of the incisions, allowing the two rectangular flaps to be advanced for defect closure.
**b** The bilobed flap is a butterfly-shaped advancement flap used to close a defect.

**c** The rhomboid flap can be used on the nasal flank, as illustrated, or on the cheek.
**d** The skin between the defect and superficial flap is undermined, and the island flap is pulled into the defect on its subcutaneous pedicle.

**Fig. 3.13 Forehead flap**

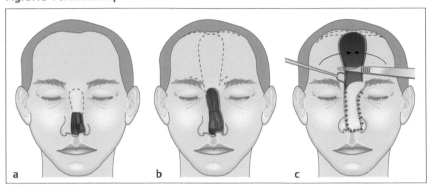

Larger defects of the nose can be reconstructed with a forehead flap based on the supraciliary and supratrochlear arteries. **a** The skin surrounding the defect is circumscribed, mobilized, and turned downward to provide intranasal lining. **b** Next the forehead flap is raised and partially backed with cartilage (composite graft) for coverage of the external defect. **c** The forehead defect can usually be closed directly.

W-plasty (**Fig. 3.11 c**): The principal effect of this technique is to lengthen the scar.

Broken-line closure (**Fig. 3.11 d**): The effect of this technique is to "optically disperse" the scar, making it more irregular and less noticeable.

### Repair of Tissue Defects

Soft-tissue defects (traumatic or post-tumor resection, see 📖 3.9 and **Fig. 3.57**) often cannot be adequately managed by primary wound closure with reapproximation of the skin margins.

*Smaller tissue defects* can be repaired with **local flaps** such as a sliding flap, bilobed flap, rhomboid flap, or island flap (**Fig. 3.12**). A larger defect of the nose can be covered by turning down a forehead flap (**Fig. 3.13**), if necessary after first reconstructing the nasal skeleton with cartilage and bone grafts.

Local flaps are often inadequate for *more extensive defects* of the external nose (e.g., tumor, dog bite), which may require more complex **reconstructive procedures** using an autologous transfer. This may consist of a pedicled flap (e.g., the myocutaneous pectoralis major flap; **Fig. 3.14**) or a microvascular free flap. In a microvascular free transfer, the autologous tissue is removed with its supply vessels, which are anastomosed to corresponding arteries and veins at the recipient site. *Very extensive defects* in the nasal region, like those created by a tumor resection, are repaired in multiple sittings using more complex flap transfers from the scalp (**Fig. 3.15**).

If the graft must also provide a degree of *stability* (e.g., alar cartilage of the external nose), this can be accomplished with a **composite graft** harvested from the auricle (**Fig. 3.16**) or from the costal or septal cartilage.

**Fig. 3.14 Pedicled myocutaneous flap**

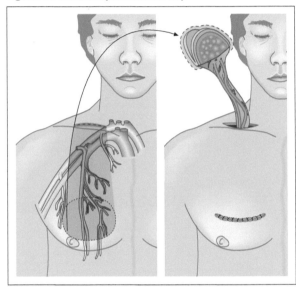

The myocutaneous pectoralis major flap is frequently used in the head and neck and is useful for repairing large defects in the facial region. Based on the thoracoacromial artery, the flap is composed of skin, subcutaneous soft tissue, and portions of the pectoralis major muscle. It is mobilized, swung into the tissue defect, and sutured into place.

**Fig. 3.15  Scalp flap**

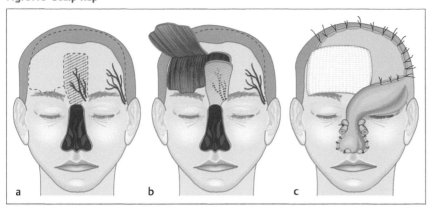

The Converse scalp flap is usually based on the superficial temporal artery. Owing to its size and width, one of its applications is for total nasal reconstruction. Backing material (e.g., costal or auricular cartilage) should be added to the flap when it is mobilized and inset in order to obtain proper nasal height.

**Fig. 3.16  Composite graft**

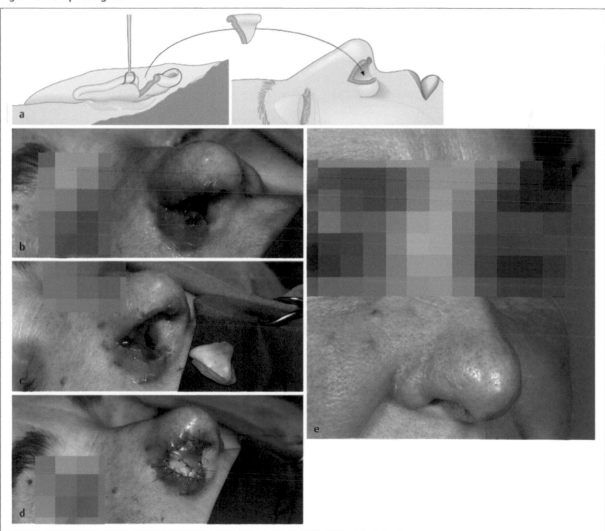

**a** The nasal alar defect is repaired with a composite graft of cartilage and skin from the auricle to restore adequate stability to the nasal vestibule.
**b, c** A woman with a nasal alar defect caused by a dog bite, shown before (**b**) and after (**c**) debridement of the wound margins.

**d** Appearance after inset of the auricular composite graft.
**e** Appearance 6 months later. The healed graft shows an excellent color and texture match with its surroundings.

# 3.5    Fractures of the Nasal Pyramid and Lateral Midface

Bony injuries to the nasal pyramid and midface are still common in sports and traffic accidents. Most of the injuries are closed fractures. The initial findings may be deceptive, due to hematoma-induced soft-tissue swelling.

## Nasal Pyramid Fracture

The nasal pyramid is predisposed to fractures because of its exposed location. The fractures are classified as open or closed on the basis of concomitant soft-tissue injuries.

*Diagnostic procedure:* **Inspection** may show obvious deviation of the external nose (**Fig. 3.17 a**) or a simple depression of the lateral nasal wall. Swelling of the surrounding soft tissues is also present, usually caused by a hematoma. *Intranasal inspection* by anterior rhinoscopy or endoscopy is done to check for concomitant mucosal injuries and especially to evaluate the nasal septum, which also may be fractured. Crepitus noted on **palpation** confirms the suspicion of a fracture. Further diagnostic measures might include **radiographs** of the nose in the lateral projection (**Fig. 3.17 b**) and standard sinus projections or CT scans to exclude bony involvement of the lateral midface (see below and **Fig. 3.22**, **Fig. 3.23**, **Fig. 3.24**, **Fig. 3.25**). Coronal CT scans will also visualize a depressed fracture of the nasal pyramid (**Fig. 3.17 c**).

*Complications:* When a septal fracture is covered by an intact soft-tissue envelope, there is a danger of subperichondrial hemorrhage with hematoma formation (**Fig. 3.18 a**). The hematoma may become infected, giving rise to a septal abscess (**Fig. 3.18 b**), which in turn can lead to cartilage necrosis with loss of the nasal septum and dorsal saddling. Alternatively, the infection may spread to the cranial cavity by the vascular route, causing meningitis.

*Treatment:* Surgical treatment is generally indicated due to the potential for permanent nasal deformity. An open fracture requires immediate surgical care accompanied by tetanus prophylaxis or a tetanus booster. If the fracture is displaced and closed, it can be safely reduced during the initial week after the injury. The displaced or depressed bone fragments can be reduced manually or with the aid of a special instrument (elevator) (**Fig. 3.19**). After the reduction, the nasal cavities should be packed to provide "internal splinting," and a plaster cast is applied externally.

Fig. 3.17 Nasal pyramid fracture

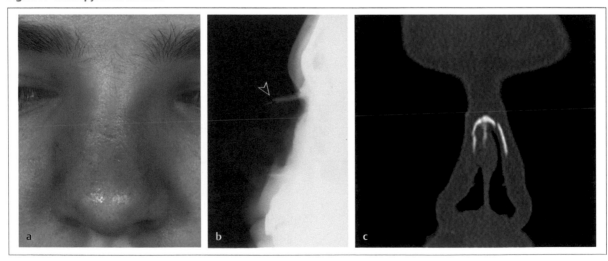

**a** The clinical appearance, showing deviation of the external nose with an intact soft-tissue envelope.
**b** The lateral radiograph of the nose demonstrates a fracture line (arrow).

**c** Depressed fracture of the nasal pyramid with dislocation of the bony fragments toward the left side.

**Fig. 3.18 Complications of septal fracture**

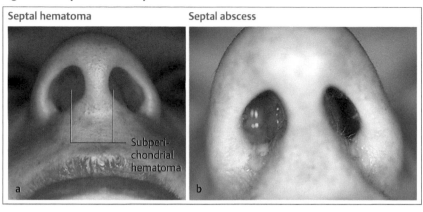

Septal hematoma    Septal abscess

Subperi-
chondrial
hematoma

a      b

**a** Symmetrical sites of boggy swelling over the nasal septum following a septal fracture, with subperichondrial bleeding under the intact mucosa.
**b** Septal abscess with symmetrical bulging and erythema of the mucosa, with a purulent nasal discharge.

**Fig. 3.19 Reduction of a nasal pyramid fracture**

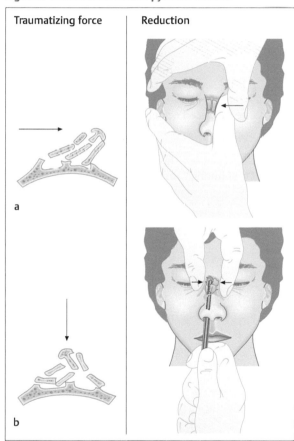

Traumatizing force    Reduction

a

b

**a** Laterally displaced fragments are reduced by external digital pressure.
**b** If the nasal pyramid is depressed, the fragments have to be elevated with an instrument from within the nasal cavity.

## Lateral Midfacial Fractures

Lateral midfacial fractures are usually caused by blunt trauma to the side of the face. Affected structures of the bony facial skeleton are the maxillary sinus, orbit, and the zygoma or zygomatic arch (see **Fig. 1.2** and **Fig. 1.6**).
An isolated fracture of the orbital floor with a partial herniation of the orbital contents into the maxillary sinus is a special type of lateral midfacial fracture called a **blowout fracture** (see **Fig. 3.22 b**).

*Symptoms:* A depressed fracture of the zygoma presents clinically with *facial asymmetry.* Depression of the zygomatic arch frequently causes *limited mouth opening.*
Fractures of the orbital floor can cause *diplopia* on upward gaze due to entrapment of the inferior rectus muscle.
*Sensory disturbances* involving the cheek, ipsilateral upper lip, and lateral nasal wall suggest a direct or indirect fracture-induced lesion of the infraorbital nerve, which enters the buccal soft tissues below the infraorbital margin and is commonly involved by fractures of the orbital floor.

*Diagnosis:*
**Inspection:** Swelling is usually present due to subcutaneous hemorrhage (periorbital or "monocle" hematoma; **Fig. 3.20**). Asymmetry of the affected facial half is most likely to occur with depression of the zygoma or zygomatic arch, depending on the location and extent of the fracture (**Fig. 3.21**).
Enophthalmos signifies involvement of the orbital floor (herniation of orbital contents).

📖 It is prudent to seek ophthalmologic consultation in these cases.

**Fig. 3.20  Unilateral periorbital hematoma**

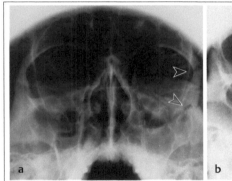

The periorbital hematoma in this patient is the superficial sign of a lateral midfacial fracture.

**Fig. 3.21  Facial asymmetry caused by a depressed fracture of the zygoma**

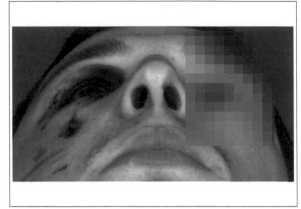

The right cheek is flattened relative to the opposite side due to a depressed fracture of the zygoma.

**Fig. 3.22  Radiographic imaging of lateral midfacial fractures**

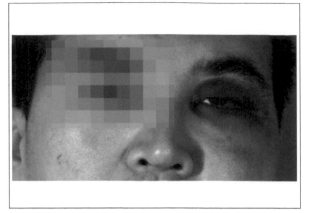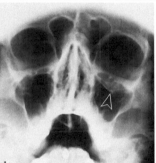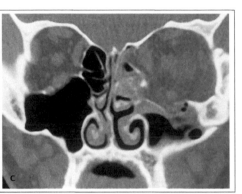

**a** Sinus radiograph demonstrates the displaced bone fragments (arrows).
**b** Sinus radiograph of a blowout fracture shows a typical soft-tissue density (arrow) caused by herniated orbital contents ("hanging drop" sign).

**c** Coronal CT scan of a blowout fracture.

**Palpation:** Concomitant soft-tissue swelling can make it difficult or impossible to palpate sites of bony discontinuity or displacement. The following areas should be examined:

- Frontozygomatic suture (upper part of the lateral orbital rim).
- Infraorbital margin (anterior bony margin of the orbital floor).
- Zygomatic arch (often difficult to evaluate due to soft-tissue swelling).

**Sensory testing:** Wisps of cotton can be used to test sensory function on the healthy and affected sides.

**Radiographs:** Whenever a lateral midfacial fracture is suspected, CT scans should be obtained for an optimum view of the fracture and also to exclude an involvement of the anterior skull base (see 📖 3.6,

**Fig. 3.22 c**, **Fig. 3.23 b**, **Fig. 3.24 b**). Standard sinus radiographs, as shown in **Fig. 3.22 a, b**, **Fig. 3.23 a**, and **Fig. 3.24 a**, provide a comparatively less accurate information and should only be performed nowadays if there is no CT on hand. They are still indicated, however, to verify the postoperative result in displaced midfacial fractures (**Fig. 3.25 a, b**).

*Treatment:* Surgical treatment is unnecessary for undisplaced, asymptomatic fractures, but it is indicated for displaced fractures or fractures that are causing symptoms such as sensory deficits in the distribution of the infraorbital nerve, diplopia on upward gaze, enophthalmos, restricted jaw opening, or facial asymmetry. Treatment consists of reduction and fixation of the bone fragments using miniplates, interosseous wiring, or both (**Fig. 3.25 b** and **Fig. 3.26**). In all cases the patient should be cautioned to avoid nose blowing.

**Fig. 3.23 Depressed fracture of the zygoma**

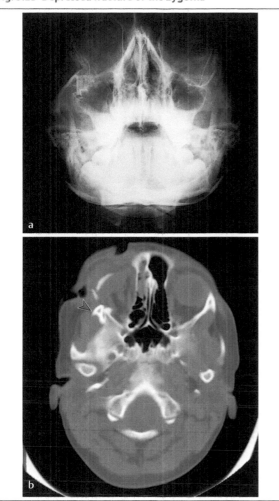

**a** Sinus radiograph of a depressed zygomatic fracture on the right side (the patient had been kicked by a horse).
**b** Axial computed tomogram in the same patient shows the displaced body of the zygoma (arrow), which has penetrated the orbital cone from the lateral side.

**Fig. 3.24 Depressed fracture of the zygomatic arch**

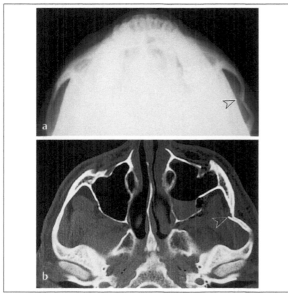

Depressed fracture of the zygomatic arch (arrows), demonstrated by the bucket-handle view (**a**) and axial CT scan (**b**).

**Fig. 3.25 Displaced lateral midfacial fracture on the left side**

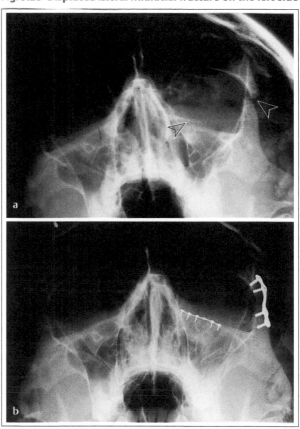

The sinus radiographs show a displaced lateral midfacial fracture on the left side with separation of the frontozygomatic suture and a displaced orbital floor fracture before (**a**) and after (**b**) reduction and stabilization with miniplates.

**Fig. 3.26 Internal fixation of an orbital rim fracture**

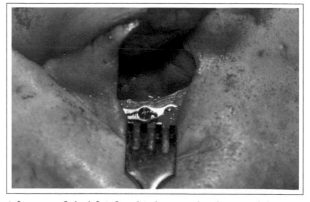

A fracture of the left infraorbital margin has been stabilized by wire and miniplate fixation. The orbital contents are retracted upward with a spatula.

# 3.6    Fractures of the Central Midface and Anterior Skull Base

Although fractures of the central midface and anterior skull base (frontal skull base, rhinobase) are separate entities, they are on a clinical continuum and are therefore discussed in the same 📖.

*Classification:*
**Central midfacial fractures:** The *Le Fort* classification (**Fig. 3.27**) describes various midfacial fracture patterns ranging from isolated detachment of the alveolar process (Le Fort I; **Fig. 3.28**) to separation of the midfacial bones from the anterior skull base (Le Fort III).

**Frontobasal fractures:** These are bony injuries to the anterior skull base and adjacent paranasal sinuses (frontal and sphenoid sinuses, ethmoid labyrinth). The *Escher* classification distinguishes four types of frontobasal fractures based on the location and extent of the fracture lines (**Fig. 3.29**).

*Etiopathogenesis:* Fractures of the central midface and frontal skull base generally occur in multiply injured patients (usually vehicular accidents), but they can also result from "trivial" trauma or even a surgical procedure (e.g., endoscopic sinus surgery), since some bony portions of the anterior skull base are quite thin (e.g., the cribriform plate of the ethmoid bone). Frontobasal fractures occupy a special place among skull fractures because they are usually an "indirectly open" injury that creates a communication between the cranial cavity and the environment.

> 🗓 Ascending infection can occur via the adjacent paranasal sinuses in frontobasal fractures and can lead to life-threatening intracranial complications (e.g., meningitis, brain abscess).

The dura along the fracture line tends to become torn at sites where it is firmly adherent to the bone of the skull base (e.g., cribriform plate, sphenofrontal suture, sellar tubercle, spheno-occipital synchondrosis).

*Symptoms:* Most patients present with a **unilateral** (see **Fig. 3.20**) or **bilateral periorbital hematoma**, depending on the nature and direction of the traumatizing force. A **dish face** is seen in combined fractures (Le Fort II–III, Escher III) where the midface has been separated from the skull base and displaced inward.
**Cerebrospinal fluid (CSF) rhinorrhea** is one of the few reliable signs of an anterior skull base fracture with associated dural injury. It can also occur with petrous bone fractures, in which case CSF leakage occurs via the eustachian tube.

> 🗓 Particularly in fresh head injuries, CSF leak from a dural tear may be obscured by heavy bleeding or may be contained by bone fragments, prolapsed brain tissue, swollen mucosa, or foreign bodies.

Severe craniocerebral trauma can also result in **vision loss** caused by ocular destruction or injury to the optic nerve (nerve contusion, rupture of the nerve in an intact sheath due to sagittal brain motion within the skull). **Diplopia** due to oculomotor palsy from damage to the third, fourth, or sixth cranial nerve is somewhat rare and occurs only if the fracture line runs through the cavernous sinus. Extensive injuries with sites of bone dehiscence can lead to **cerebral prolapse**, with brain tissue herniating externally or into the nasal

**Fig. 3.27 Le Fort classification**

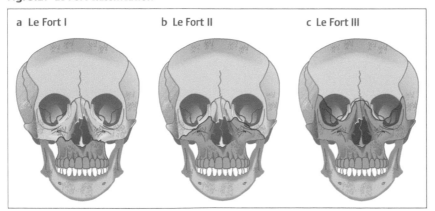

a  Le Fort I        b  Le Fort II        c  Le Fort III

Central midfacial fractures are classified into three groups:
**a** Le Fort I: isolated detachment of the alveolar process (see also **Fig. 3.28**).
**b** Le Fort II: pyramidal fracture with detachment of the maxilla.
**c** Le Fort III: craniofacial dysjunction.

**Fig. 3.28 Le Fort I**

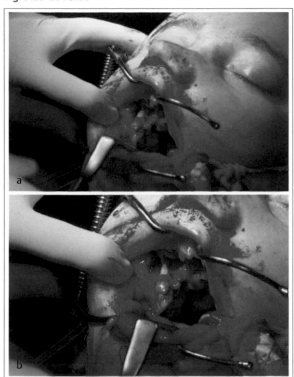

Intraoperative photos of a multiply injured patient with a Le Fort I fracture on the right side.

cavity. **Anosmia** can result from a fracture of the cribriform plate with avulsion of the fila olfactoria, or it may signify damage to more central structures in the setting of a cerebral concussion or contusion.

*Diagnosis:*

🖉 Patients with craniocerebral trauma require inter-disciplinary care.

Before an ENT examination is performed, the patient's vital functions should be stabilized by the anesthesiologist or neurosurgeon.

Facial soft-tissue injuries are often extensive but may provide little information on possible associated bony injuries at the level of the skull base.

A basic impression is gained by **palpation** of the facial bones (**Fig. 3.30**) and **inspection** of the *nasal cavity* by rhinoscopy or endoscopy. Profuse bleeding from soft-tissue injuries, including intranasal lesions, often makes it difficult to adequately evaluate the injury in the acute stage, and it may not be possible at this time to confirm or exclude a CSF leak in multiply injured patients, many of whom are intubated. The next step after nasal inspection is to inspect the *oral cavity* and *oropharynx. Otoscopy* or *otomicroscopy* should also be performed to exclude a concomitant petrous bone fracture.

A clear, watery nasal discharge should raise suspicion of a CSF leak (**Fig. 3.31**), which requires differentiation from ordinary nasal mucus. Various **CSF tests** (e.g., glucose test, $\beta_2$-transferrin assay) are available for this purpose (🔎 **3.8**).

🖉 Intracranial complications (especially bleeding) should also be excluded.

**CT** supplies additional important information on the location and extent of injuries. Neurosurgeons order CT scans with a *soft-tissue window* as an initial study for excluding intracranial bleeding, hematoma, and pneumocephalus. This type of study is not useful for the assessment of bony lesions. While indirect signs such as the presence of intracranial air (**Fig. 3.32 c**) suggest a strong likelihood of dural injury with a frontobasal fracture, only a *bone-window* CT scan can reliably evaluate or exclude a fracture. So whenever a frontobasal fracture is suspected, *high-resolution CT scans* (2-mm slice thickness, bone window) of the paranasal sinuses should be obtained in the *axial* and *coronal projections.* The axial scans are for evaluating

**Fig. 3.29 Escher classification**

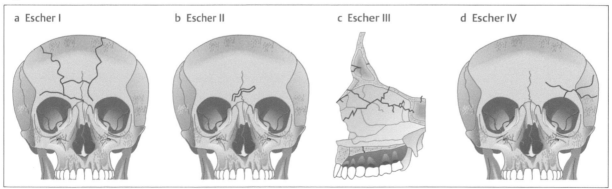

a Escher I    b Escher II    c Escher III    d Escher IV

Frontobasal fractures are classified into four groups:
a Escher I: high fracture.
b Escher II: central fracture.

c Escher III: low fracture.
d Escher IV: latero-orbital fracture.

**Fig. 3.30 Palpation of the bony facial skull**

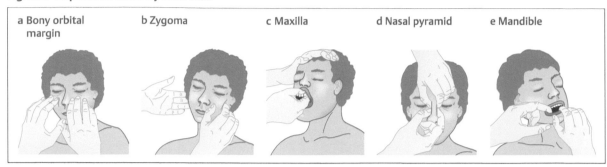

a Bony orbital margin     b Zygoma     c Maxilla     d Nasal pyramid     e Mandible

**Fig. 3.31 Cerebrospinal fluid (CSF) rhinorrhea**

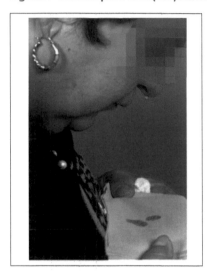

CSF rhinorrhea appears clinically as a watery nasal discharge.

---

**🔍 3.8 Detection of cerebrospinal fluid**

In the **glucose test**, a dipstick is used to test the glucose content of the collected discharge. The presence of blood in the sample can give a false-positive reading, since blood has twice the sugar content of cerebrospinal fluid CSF. This test is therefore very nonspecific.

The immunoelectrophoretic determination of **$\beta_2$-transferrin** is a more accurate method. This protein is normally present only in CSF. Since it is also detectable in the serum in very rare cases, the patient's serum should additionally be tested for comparison. The advantages of this method are that it is noninvasive, supplies a result within 24 hours, and can be repeated as often as needed (for follow-up). The test procedure is relatively costly and complex, however. Over the past years, another specific brain protein, $\beta$-trace-protein ($\beta$ TP), has been described for the detection of CSF leaks. The sensitivity and specificity are similar to those of $\beta_2$-transferrin, but the test is less expensive.

---

the anterior and posterior walls of the frontal sinuses (**Fig. 3.32 a**) and sphenoid sinus (**Fig. 3.32 b**), while the coronal scans more clearly define the ethmoid roof and cribriform plate (**Fig. 3.32 c, d**).

The preliminary **testing of hearing and balance** is possible only if the patient is conscious and responsive to verbal commands.

**Olfactory testing** to exclude anosmia often cannot be performed in the acute stage but should be done at a later time. For medicolegal reasons, it should always precede surgical treatment (see 📖 2.2, Olfactometry).

*Treatment:* Every confirmed fracture of the anterior skull base should be treated surgically in operable patients, regardless of whether or not a CSF leak has been detected. The patient should also be instructed not to blow the nose. With an isolated central midfacial fracture that does not involve the anterior skull base, surgical treatment of the maxilla should be provided by a maxillofacial surgeon to ensure the restoration of normal occlusion. The urgency of surgical intervention for a frontobasal fracture is shown in **Table 3.3**.

Three main **surgical approaches** to the anterior skull base are available (**Fig. 3.33**). The choice depends on the individual situation and is made in consultation with the other involved specialties (e.g., neurosurgeon, maxillofacial surgeon, ophthalmologist).

**Fig. 3.32 Computed tomography examination of frontobasal fractures**

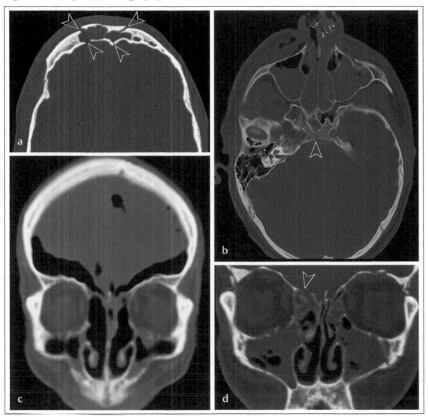

Axial CT scans demonstrate a fracture of the anterior and posterior walls of the frontal sinuses (arrows) (**a**) and a clivus fracture (arrow) that extends anteriorly into the sphenoid sinus (**b**). The coronal scans show air in the cranial cavity (**c**) and a fracture of the ethmoid roof (**d**) (arrow).

**Fig. 3.33 Surgical approaches to the anterior skull base**

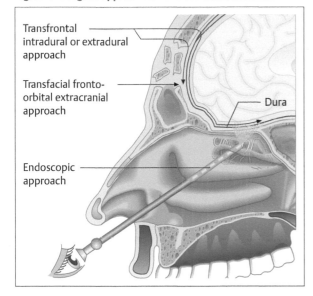

Transfrontal intradural or extradural approach

Transfacial fronto-orbital extracranial approach

Dura

Endoscopic approach

**Table 3.3   Indications for the surgical treatment of frontobasal fractures**

**Vital indications (operate immediately)**
- Life-threatening rise of intracranial pressure due to intracranial hemorrhage
- Bleeding from the nose or sinuses that is refractory to conservative treatment
- Bleeding from an open skull injury that is refractory to conservative treatment

**Absolute indications (operate as soon as possible)**
- Open brain injury
- Dural tear from an indirectly open head injury
- Penetrating foreign bodies and impalement injuries
- Early complications (e.g., meningitis, encephalitis, brain abscess)
- Late complications (e.g., meningitis, brain abscess, osteomyelitis)
- Orbital complications

**Relative indications (operate in 1–2 wk)**
- Displaced bone fragments
- Fractures involving the drainage tracts of the paranasal sinuses ("ostiomeatal unit")
- Acute or chronic sinusitis at the time of the injury
- Post-traumatic sinus inflammation, mucopyocele formation
- Supraorbital nerve injury due to an adjacent fracture
- Fractures involving the drainage tracts of the paranasal sinuses ("ostiomeatal unit")
- Acute or chronic sinusitis at the time of the injury
- Posttraumatic sinus inflammation, mucopyocele formation
- Supraorbital nerve injury due to an adjacent fracture

# 3.7    Inflammations of the External Nose, Nasal Cavity, and Facial Soft Tissues

*Inflammatory diseases of the nasal skin* usually have a bacterial cause and may be manifested on the exposed skin and the dermal appendages. Although these diseases fall primarily within the scope of dermatology, the otolaryngologist is frequently faced with inflammations of this type that can lead to life-threatening complications unless adequately treated. *Inflammation of the nasal cavity* (rhinitis) predominantly involves the nasal mucosa. While it can have a variety of causes, it always exhibits a more or less pronounced combination of characteristic symptoms. Although rhinitis and sinusitis are on a continuum owing to the special anatomical and physiological relationships of the nose and paranasal sinuses (see ▨ 1.1, 1.2, and 1.3), the diseases are covered separately in this unit for learning purposes. The various forms of rhinitis are discussed according to their etiology, noting that the great majority of cases seen in clinical practice are mixed forms that have more than one cause.

## Purulent Inflammations of the Hair Follicles

Pyodermas of the hair follicles are common purulent inflammations that can occur at almost any age. The main causative organisms are staphylococci. If the disease is confined to the hair follicles, it is termed **folliculitis**. If the infection spreads to deeper tissues and forms a central core of purulent liquefaction, it is called a **furuncle**.

*Symptoms:* Nasal furuncles present as painful, tender, erythematous swellings about the nasal tip and nares (**Fig. 3.34**). There may be concomitant edematous swelling of the upper lip. The changes are confined to the outer skin and do not involve the mucosa. Fever is sometimes present.

*Treatment:* The treatment of choice is high-dose parenteral administration of an antibiotic that is active against staphylococci, such as flucloxacillin sodium or dicloxacillin sodium, combined with the local application of an antibiotic-containing ointment (chlortetracycline HCl). Also, the upper lip should be moved as little as possible, and so the patient should be placed on a liquid or semisolid diet and speak as little as possible.

▯ An essential goal of these measures is to prevent the potentially lethal complication of intracranial spread.

*Complications:* Inadequate treatment or manipulations of the nasal furuncle itself can result in hematogenous spread to intracranial structures, since the veins of the nose and upper lip drain via the angular and ophthalmic veins into the cavernous sinus. If tenderness in the medial canthus of the eye raises a suspicion of thrombophlebitis of the angular vein, the vessel should be surgically ligated and divided.

**Fig. 3.34 Nasal furuncle**

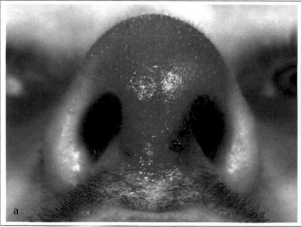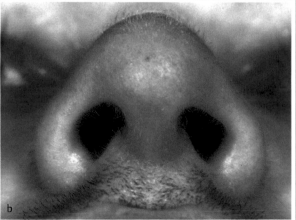

Clinical appearance before (**a**) and after (**b**) antibiotic treatment.

**Fig. 3.35 Facial erysipelas**

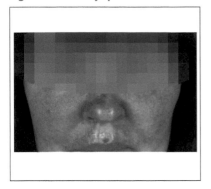

Patients typically present with generalized facial swelling and erythema. The possible portals of entry are visible over the nasal dorsum.

## Erysipelas

*Etiopathogenesis:* The principal causative organisms are β-hemolytic group A streptococci. Less common pathogens are streptococci of other groups, *Staphylococcus aureus*, and gram-negative rods (e.g., *Klebsiella pneumoniae*), which gain entry to the skin through minor injuries (usually on the face and limbs). The inflammation spreads diffusely in the skin and subcutaneous tissue.

*Symptoms:* Facial erysipelas (**Fig. 3.35**) usually begins with a high fever and a feeling of tension in the soft tissues, followed rapidly by broad areas of erythema and swelling, which are sharply demarcated from unaffected skin. The tissue is warm to the touch, and small blisters occasionally form.

- If facial erysipelas spreads lateral to the nose and about the eyelids, there is a risk of intracranial involvement by hematogenous spread of the causative organisms, as with a nasal furuncle.

*Treatment:* The treatment of choice is the parenteral administration of penicillin. Moist compresses soaked in an antiseptic solution can also be applied locally.

---

**⌀ 3.9   Differential diagnosis of facial soft-tissue swelling**

**Lupus erythematosus** (LE) is an inflammatory dermatosis that frequently affects the face, spreading in a butterfly-shaped pattern over the cheeks, forehead, and nose. The differential diagnosis also includes **allergic contact dermatitis**, which may be induced by cosmetics, toilet articles, sun creams, or exposure to airborne plant pollens. In strongly sensitized patients who wear a face mask, even a single contact can incite a severe, acute allergic reaction with erythema and edematous swelling of the facial soft tissues. Finally, the differential diagnosis should include **angioedema**, which is also associated with facial swelling that chiefly affects the eyelids and lips (see also ⟪ 4.4, Angioedema).

---

## Inflammations of the Nasal Cavity

### Acute Rhinitis

*Epidemiology:* Acute rhinitis (common cold) is the most prevalent infectious disease. Given its frequency and the fact that the disease does not confer postinfection immunity, acute rhinitis has assumed major epidemiologic and economic significance.

*Etiopathogenesis:* Rhinoviruses and coronaviruses comprise almost half of the causative organisms of acute viral rhinitis. Other pathogens are influenza viruses and adenoviruses. The infection is transmitted by the airborne route (droplet infection). Cold exposure and other environmental factors can increase the susceptibility of the host to infection. The incubation period is 3 to 7 days.

*Symptoms:* The disease begins with an initial **dry stage** characterized by malaise (lethargy, headache, fever) and local discomfort in the nose and nasopharynx (burning, soreness). This is followed by a **catarrhal stage** marked by a watery, initially serous nasal discharge and nasal obstruction due to mucosal swelling, which mainly involves the turbinates. In addition, patients often complain about a reduction or even loss of smell. The viruses damage the mucociliary transport system, which hampers the normal clearing of secretions. With a profuse nasal discharge, inflammatory changes often develop about the nasal vestibule.

Viral damage to the epithelium promotes bacterial colonization, which alters the consistency of the clear nasal discharge, causing it to become mucopurulent (**Fig. 3.36**). The local and systemic symptoms usually subside in about a week.

**Fig. 3.36  Acute rhinitis**

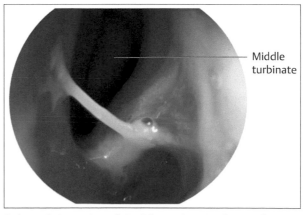

Middle turbinate

Endoscopic inspection of the left nasal cavity shows inflammatory changes in the mucosa with mucopurulent nasal secretions.

**Treatment:** Treatment consists of supportive measures to relieve nasal obstruction and prevent sinusitis and other sequelae by the use of decongestant nose drops.

📋 Nose drops should be used no longer than absolutely necessary (generally no more than 1 week) due to the risk of tachyphylaxis (see also Rhinitis Medicamentosa at the end of this study unit) with severe rebound swelling of the nasal mucosa.

Various other options are available for relieving the discomfort of acute rhinitis, including chamomile steam inhalation, "light baths," and infrared therapy. Antibiotics may also be prescribed in patients with bacterial superinfection or paranasal sinus involvement.

## Nonspecific Chronic Rhinitis

**Etiopathogenesis:** Chronic inflammation of the nasal mucosa can have various underlying causes. Besides recurrent acute inflammations with progressive damage to the mucosa, nonspecific chronic rhinitis can develop due to anatomic changes (e.g., marked septal deviation, septal spur) or other lesions of the nasal cavity (polyps, tumors) and nasopharynx (adenoids, see 📖 5.3). Environmental factors such as sustained extreme temperatures or air pollutants can also bring on this condition.

**Symptoms:** Patients present clinically with obstructed nasal breathing and a mucous nasal discharge. They also complain of frequent throat clearing and occasional hoarseness.

**Treatment:** The most important step is to eliminate the cause by removing chronic irritants from the environment or by surgically correcting any intranasal pathology (e.g., septoplasty, see 📖 3.2, Septal Deviation). Supportive measures such as decongestant nose drops or nasal irrigation with saline solution are of only temporary benefit.

## Specific Chronic Rhinitis

This category includes inflammations of varying causes that may be manifested in the nose (🔍 **3.11**).

## Allergic Rhinitis

Diseases of the nose and paranasal sinuses have undergone a disproportionate rise during the past few decades. Meanwhile, the spectrum of rhinologic diseases has changed from a qualitative standpoint as well. As allergic diseases have become more prevalent, there has also been a notable rise in the incidence of allergic rhinitis. Epidemiological studies indicate that 25 to 30% of the population in industrialized countries have allergic

### 🔍 3.10 Granulomatosis with polyangiitis, GPA (Wegener's granulomatosis, Wegener's disease)

Granulomatosis with polyangiitis (GPA) is a rare autoimmune disease of unknown etiology that starts with the formation of primary granulomas in the connective tissue and later progresses to vascular involvement in the form of a necrotizing vasculitis. In the head and neck region, the nose is predominantly affected. Lesions may also develop in the trachea and middle ear. In some patients, antineutrophil cytoplasmic antibodies (ANCA) can be verified.

The **symptoms** of GPA consist of nasal airway obstruction, a bloody nasal discharge, and severe crusting in the nasal cavity and nasopharynx. As the disease progresses, soft-tissue and cartilage destruction may occur as a result of superinfection or necrotizing granulomas, manifested clinically by mucosal ulcerations, septal perforation, and cartilaginous saddle nose (**Fig. 3.37**).

**Fig. 3.37 Granulomatosis with polyangiitis**

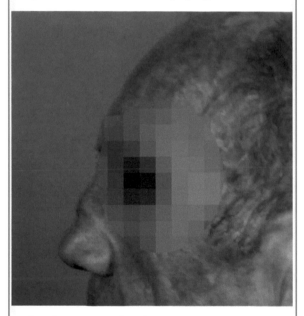

Clinical appearance of cartilaginous saddle nose.

problems; the prevalence of allergic rhinitis is estimated at 10 to 15%. An increase in urbanization as well as improved living standards contributes to more exposure to indoor and outdoor pollutants and allergens, thus increasing the tendency to develop allergies. In children, parental atopy, genetics, and epigenetics apparently influence the development of allergic rhinitis (**Fig. 3.38**).

**Fig. 3.38 Early life determinants in allergic rhinitis**

Source: Schaub 2015.

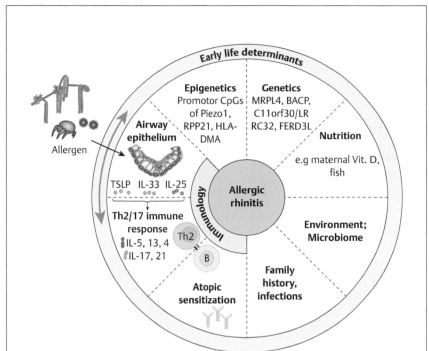

*Etiopathogenesis and classification:* Allergic inflammation of the mucosa is triggered by an immediate, IgE-mediated reaction of the immune system to any of several foreign substances, particularly pollens and animal allergens.

Allergic rhinitis is classified as seasonal (hay fever) or perennial according to the presence of the allergen in the environment.

**Seasonal allergic rhinitis** in Central Europe is caused mainly by pollens from alder, hazel, birch, grasses, rye, mugwort, and plantain. Clinical symptoms appear between February and September, depending on the individual allergen spectrum of the patient, and disappear at the end of the pollen season.

By contrast, **perennial allergic rhinitis** is caused by year-round allergen exposure that incites a permanent inflammation of the nasal mucosa. The predominant causative allergens are house dust, pet dander, and molds. The disease may also be caused by certain foods (e.g., strawberries, nuts, eggs, fish) as well as occupational exposure to allergens (e.g., bakers and hairdressers). A new occupational allergen, especially prevalent in health workers, is latex, which is used to manufacture disposable gloves.

Another classification of allergic rhinitis refers to the duration and severity of the disease and is shown in **Fig. 3.39**.

**Fig. 3.39 Classification of allergic rhinitis according to duration and severity of symptoms**

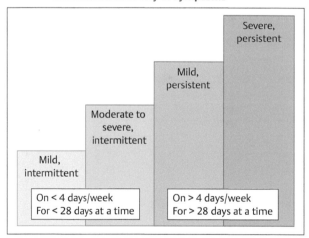

Classification of allergic rhinitis according to duration and severity of symptoms.

*Symptoms:* The clinical manifestations include obstructed nasal breathing and sneezing attacks, a watery nasal discharge, postnasal drip, and itching of the nose and eyes (conjunctivitis). Some patients may also develop oral symptoms to fruit and vegetables (oral allergy syndrome; **Fig. 3.40**). These oral symptoms may include difficulty in swallowing, burning of the tongue, or a sensation of scratching or itching in the throat. The symptoms are usually mild and mainly encountered in patients

**Fig. 3.40 Oral allergy syndrome**

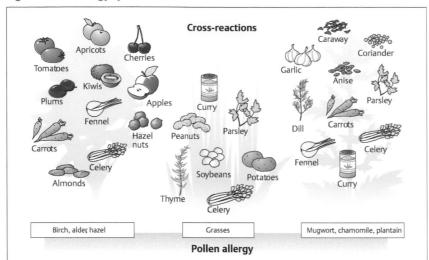

Source: Roecken et al 2003.

### 3.11 Causes of specific chronic rhinitis

#### Tuberculosis

Tuberculosis can involve the nasal mucosa as a primary infection following the inhalation of infectious droplets, forming a *primary complex* approximately 6 weeks after infection.

Another manifestation is **lupus vulgaris**, the most common *postprimary form* of cutaneous tuberculosis. Ulcerative cases are marked by increasing necrosis within the tubercular granulomas, which can cause a mutilating destruction of nasal skin and cartilaginous structures. Lupus vulgaris may also arise from the nasal mucosa itself, causing the contiguous destruction of nasal structures from the inside.

#### Sarcoidosis

Sarcoidosis is a common, granulomatous systemic disease of unknown etiology that predominantly affects women under 40 years of age. Although the lymph nodes, lung, joints, and skin are chiefly affected and involvement of the upper respiratory tract is relatively rare, nasal symptoms may be the initial manifestation of the disease. Involvement of the external nose is called **lupus pernio** because the characteristic skin changes resemble chilblains (pernio). Involvement of the nasal mucosa mainly affects the septum and inferior turbinate, which develop yellowish, submucous nodules that have the gross appearance of intramucosal granulomas.

#### Rhinoscleroma

This chronic inflammatory disease is extremely rare and is manifested in the nose, oral mucosa, and upper respiratory tract. It is transmitted by *Klebsiella pneumoniae* (subspecies *rhinoscleromatis*). Rhinoscleroma presents the features of atrophic rhinitis (see below): fetid nasal discharge, dry mucosa, and crusting. The nasal mucosa shows inflammatory infiltrates that may progress to granulations and also involve the nasal vestibule.

#### Actinomycosis

The gram-positive anaerobe *Actinomyces israelii* can cause this disease, usually in immunocompromised patients. Symptomatic involvement of the nose and paranasal sinuses is somewhat uncommon. Changes in these regions may include firm infiltrates in the nasal mucosa that resemble a nasal furuncle. There have also been sporadic reports of granulations

forming on the nasal mucosa and in the paranasal sinuses. Untreated, the inflammation can spread and cause severe tissue destruction with a fatal outcome.

#### Syphilis

Nasal involvement by syphilis occurs mainly in the tertiary stage of the disease. It is manifested by the appearance of isolated gummata or by diffuse gummatous infiltration of the nasal cavity. Untreated, the disease causes progressive destruction of the surrounding tissue, and eventual bone destruction can occur. Infants with **congenital syphilis** contracted in utero may also manifest nasal changes that include a purulent and sometimes bloody nasal discharge, which may be mistaken for "normal" infant rhinitis.

#### Malleus

Malleus is a rare infectious disease (causative organism: *Pseudomonas mallei*) that is transmitted to humans from horses and occasionally from house pets. When the nasal mucosa is the portal of entry, it exhibits inflammatory swelling, pustule formation, and ulceration with a viscous nasal discharge containing blood and pus.

#### Fungal infections

**Aspergillosis** is the most common fungal infection causing chronic specific rhinitis, with fungal colonization occurring mainly in the paranasal sinuses (see 3.8, Chronic Sinusitis). In rare cases and especially in immunocompromised patients, the infection may take an aggressive, fulminating course with the destruction of surrounding structures, resulting in a very high mortality.

**Mucormycosis** resembles aspergillosis in its symptoms and course. The invasive form of mucormycosis still has a relatively high mortality rate despite the availability of systemic antimycotics, but it mainly affects patients with a weakened immune status.

**Rhinosporidiosis** is another very rare disease caused by the spore-forming fungus *Rhinosporidium seeberi*. Highly vascular, friable granular lesions develop in the anterior portions of the nose and may spread to involve the paranasal sinuses and nasopharynx.

### 🔎 3.12   Nasal hyperreactivity

Because the nasal mucosa is reactive to physical, chemical, and pharmacologic stimuli, which may take the form of allergens, pollutants (cigarette smoke, dust, fumes), or even position changes or exertion, the term *nasal hyperreactivity* (analogous to bronchial hyperreactivity) has lately been coined as a collective term for a heightened reactivity of the nasal mucosa to these agents.

Some of the diseases that lead to nasal hyperreactivity are marked by signs of inflammation and others chiefly by disturbances of autonomic nervous regulation, with an altered response of the associated receptors on vessels, nerves, and glands of the mucosa.

**Fig. 3.41 Allergic rhinitis**

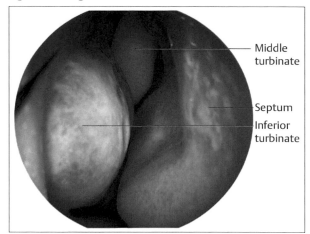

Typical endoscopic appearance of the nasal mucosa in allergic rhinitis.

**Fig. 3.42 Flowchart: pharmacologic treatment of allergic rhinitis according to severity and duration of symptoms**

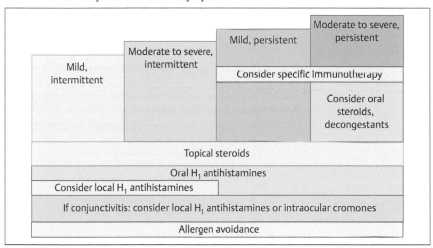

with sensitization to pollen allergens, especially to birch pollen. Nevertheless, there may be life-threatening edema of the base of the tongue or larynx in severe cases.

***Diagnosis:*** The diagnostic work-up should include a detailed allergy history (do the symptoms present year-round or only during contact with certain animals or plants; do they disappear during vacation?). With seasonal allergic rhinitis, inspection of the nasal cavity typically reveals a bluish-purple discoloration of the mucosa (**Fig. 3.41**). With perennial rhinitis, the mucosa is bright red and shows inflammatory changes. Careful allergy testing (see 📖 2.2, Allergy Testing) is necessary to identify the antigens involved.

***Treatment:***

🗲 The best treatment strategy is to **avoid contact with the allergen** or eliminate allergenic irritants from the environment.

Since the avoidance strategy is not always possible for practical reasons, patients with allergic rhinitis receive either specific immunotherapy (🔎 **3.13**), if applicable, or adequate **pharmacologic** treatment according to severity of the symptoms (**Fig. 3.42**). Under certain conditions, surgery might also be helpful as a supplementary therapeutic approach (🔎 **3.13**).

⌀3.13 Long-term treatment options for allergic rhinitis

**Specific immunotherapy or hyposensitization therapy** is a mainstay with allergic rhinitis being one of the most solid indications; the treatment can be applied either subcutaneously (subcutaneous immunotherapy, **SCIT** ) or sublingually (sublingual immunotherapy, **SLIT**). Specific immunotherapy, in the form of hyposensitization, consists of administering increasing amounts of a relevant allergen to eventually silence the disease-induced T cells, thus creating clinical tolerance. The greatest risk for any immunotherapy is an anaphylactic reaction, which can progress to shock. Therefore, this treatment should only be performed in an institution prepared to perform cardiopulmonary resuscitation. Changes in the structure of applied allergens, as well as a specific treatment of the allergen solutions, however, have significantly reduced the risk of severe side effects in recent years. Still, mild local reactions still occur in SCIT. The high cost of specific immunotherapy compared with pharmacologic treatment is a major reason, why many patients still do not benefit from this therapeutic strategy today.

If the response to conservative treatment is unsatisfactory and the principal complaint is nasal obstruction (i.e., hyperplasia of the nasal mucosa, mainly of the inferior turbinates), **surgical treatment** might be a therapeutic option. The main goal in these cases is to reduce the size of the inferior turbinates by radiofrequency therapy, laser treatment, or mucotomy (resecting a tissue strip from the lower edge of the inferior turbinate); turbinate coagulation should not be performed anymore, because of its destructive impact to the nasal mucosa, which results in a prolonged healing process If septal pathology is also present (septal deviation, septal spur or ridge), a concomitant septoplasty should be performed. With associated sinus complaints, endoscopic sinus surgery may also be required (see ⌀3.18).

## Vasomotor Rhinitis

Vasomotor rhinitis resembles allergic rhinitis in its clinical features, but there is no evidence that the patient has been previously sensitized.

The **pathogenesis** of vasomotor rhinitis is believed to involve neurovascular autonomic disturbances in regulating the tonus of the nasal mucosal vessels.

The **symptoms** consist of obstructed nasal breathing, watery nasal discharge, and sneezing. The **history** shows that the symptoms are related to a temperature change, the consumption of hot liquid or alcohol, or less specifically to "emotional stress." On **inspection**, the appearance of the nasal mucosa is similar to that in allergic rhinitis.

Medical **therapy** includes the use of antihistamines or corticosteroid-containing nasal sprays. In the Kneipp system of therapy, ice-cold water is sniffed up the nose as a way of "training" the neuroautonomic regulation of the blood supply to the nasal mucosa.

The last recourse for intractable vasomotor rhinitis is surgical reduction of the turbinates by electrocoagulation, laser ablation, or mucotomy, especially in cases with pronounced inferior turbinate hyperplasia. If significant septal deviation is present, a septoplasty should be performed.

## Atrophic Rhinitis

**Symptoms:** Atrophic rhinitis is characterized by pronounced dryness of the nasal mucosa. Severe cases, especially with secondary bacterial colonization, are marked by a fetid nasal odor that is not perceived by the patient due to degeneration of the olfactory epithelium.

The **etiology** of primary atrophic rhinitis is unknown. Secondary forms can have various causes including an extensive prior tumor resection, the excessive use of nose drops, drug abuse (cocaine), or previous radiotherapy for nasal and sinus tumors. Iatrogenic causes include a botched septoplasty or an excessive turbinate reduction (conchotomy). **Endoscopic examination** reveals a broad nasal cavity lined with dry, crusted mucosa.

**Treatment** should begin with *conservative*, symptomatic measures (saline "nasal douche," soothing mucosal ointments). Under no circumstances should decongestant nose drops be used, as the vasoconstriction would exacerbate the patient's symptoms. If conservative treatments prove inadequate, an attempt can be made to reduce the nasal cavity *surgically* by the submucous implantation of cartilage grafts. This creates a relative increase in surface area in relation to the volume of the nasal cavity.

## Hormonal Rhinitis

Synonym: pregnancy-associated rhinitis.

Hormonal rhinitis occurs mainly during pregnancy and is believed to be caused by estrogen-induced swelling of the mucosa with nasal airway obstruction. The symptoms diminish as term approaches and disappear after the delivery.

## Rhinitis Medicamentosa

This disease occurs mainly as a side effect from the long-term use of decongestant nose drops. It can also result from the use of certain antihypertensive drugs—for example, rauwolfia alkaloids, β-blockers, angiotensin-converting enzyme (ACE) inhibitors—and from oral contraceptive use, in which case the rhinitis is attributed to a vasoactive estrogen effect. Clinical symptoms consist of obstructed nasal breathing, dry mucosa, and occasional olfactory disturbances.

# 3.8    Sinus Inflammations

Sinus inflammations (sinusitis) generally develop in association with rhinitis, and so the term *rhinosinusitis* is often applied to these disorders. Despite the continuum that exists between rhinitis and sinusitis, they are discussed as separate entities in this textbook for teaching purposes. Inflammations that are confined chiefly to the nasal cavity are covered in the previous 📖. This unit deals with acute and chronic sinusitis in addition to nasal polyposis, mucoceles, pyoceles, and rhinosinogenic complications—diseases in which clinical symptoms arising from the paranasal sinuses are the dominant features.

## Acute Sinusitis

See also 🔎 **3.14**.

*Etiopathogenesis:* While acute sinusitis in children predominantly affects the ethmoid cells due to incomplete pneumatization of the other sinuses (see 📖 1.1, Paranasal Sinuses), acute sinusitis in adults affects the following sinuses in descending order of frequency: maxillary sinus, ethmoid cells, frontal sinus, and sphenoid sinus. The inflammation may involve one, several, or all of the paranasal sinuses (pansinusitis). Acute sinusitis generally results from the spread of an intranasal inflammation (rhinitis), since the mucosa of the paranasal sinuses communicates with that of the nasal cavity (**rhinogenic sinusitis**). Accordingly, the causative viruses of acute rhinitis (see 📖 3.7, Etiopathogenesis of Acute Rhinitis) are etiologically important in addition to the common bacterial organisms *Haemophilus influenzae* and *Streptococcus pneumoniae*.

Although rhinitis has a very marked tendency to involve the contiguous sinus mucosae, acute rhinitis does not invariably lead to symptomatic sinusitis. The extent of the inflammation in the sinus system and the associated symptoms depend on various factors:

- Individual functional anatomy (see 📖 1.1).
- Individual immune status.
- Specific virulence of the causative organism.

Besides rhinogenic sinusitis, there are also rare instances of **dentogenic sinusitis** arising from a dental root infection, an apical granuloma, or a maxillary sinus fistula following a tooth extraction (🔎 **3.15**).

*Symptoms:* The clinical picture is marked by the features of acute rhinitis combined with a variable degree of headache, which is exacerbated by bending over. Generally the pain is most intense over the affected sinuses (see also **Fig. 1.6**). Thus, the pain of maxillary sinusitis is greatest over the maxillary sinus and the adjacent midface and temple. Ethmoid sinusitis is most painful over the bridge of the nose and the medial canthus of the eye, and frontal sinusitis over the anterior wall and floor of the frontal sinus, with pain radiating toward the medial canthus.

🔎 **3.14    Clinical definition of acute and chronic rhinosinusitis with and without nasal polyps** (source: Fokkens et al 2012)

**Rhinosinusitis in adults**
Rhinosinusitis in adults is defined as inflammation of the nose and the paranasal sinuses characterized by two or more symptoms, one of which should be either nasal blockage/obstruction/congestion or nasal discharge (anterior/posterior nasal drip):

- with or without facial pain/pressure
- with or without reduction or loss of smell

and either endoscopic signs of:

- nasal polyps, and/or
- mucopurulent discharge primarily from middle meatus, and/or
- edema/mucosal obstruction primarily in middle meatus

and/or CT changes:

- mucosal changes within the ostiomeatal complex and/or sinuses.

**Rhinosinusitis in children**
Rhinosinusitis in children is defined as inflammation of the nose and the paranasal sinuses characterized by two or more symptoms, one of which should be either nasal blockage/obstruction/congestion or nasal discharge (anterior/posterior nasal drip),

- with or without facial pain/pressure
- with or without **cough**

and either endoscopic signs of:

- nasal polyps, and/or
- mucopurulent discharge primarily from middle meatus, and/or
- edema/mucosal obstruction primarily in middle meatus

and/or CT changes:

- mucosal changes within the ostiomeatal complex and/or sinuses.

**Duration of the disease**
- Acute: < 12 weeks, complete resolution of symptoms.
- Chronic: ≥ 12 weeks without complete resolution of symptoms (may also be subject to exacerbations).

🔎 **3.15    Special forms of sinusitis**

Other forms are **nosocomial sinusitis** resulting from prolonged nasal intubation, **barosinusitis** caused by pressure changes during flying or diving, and **swimmer's sinusitis** caused by the entry of infectious microorganisms into the sinus during swimming.

The pain of sphenoid sinusitis is fairly nonspecific, marked by a dull, aching pressure located at the center of the skull and radiating to the occiput.

***Diagnosis:*** Rhinoscopy or nasal endoscopy often reveals pus tracking along the middle meatus of the nasal cavity (**Fig. 3.43**), but a purulent track may not be seen if the mucosa is greatly swollen. With isolated sphenoid sinusitis, pus may be found about the ostium in the anterior wall of the sphenoid sinus or on the posterior wall of the pharynx.

**Sinus radiographs** (see also **Fig. 2.7**) may show partial opacification of the affected sinus due to mucosal swelling (**Fig. 3.44**), but they are not necessary to establish the diagnosis. If imaging is required at all, especially for follow-up and in children and pregnant women, ultrasonography (A-mode or B-mode) can be performed, which avoids radiation exposure.

***Treatment:*** Conservative treatment options should be exhausted before surgery is considered. The latter may be necessary in cases where the complaints of acute sinusitis do not respond to conservative treatment modalities and in cases with persistent sinus empyema.

**Conservative therapy:** Ventilation and drainage of the paranasal sinuses can be improved by the use of decongestant nose drops, nasal spray, or by inserting a cotton pack soaked with nose drops into the middle meatus. In more severe forms associated with fever and significant malaise, *antibiotics* (e.g., amoxicillin) should be administered. *Heat therapy* (electric light bath) and the *inhalation* of chamomile or sage are recommended as adjuncts.

**Surgical therapy:** *Maxillary sinusitis* can be treated by maxillary sinus puncture following decongestion and topical anesthesia of the nasal mucosa. Two approaches are available: first, "sharp puncture" through the inferior meatus, passing the needle below the inferior turbinate; and second, "blunt puncture" via the natural maxillary sinus ostium in the middle meatus. In the sharp puncture technique, there is a significant risk of complications due to air embolism if air is inadvertently injected into the sinus after a medication has been instilled. Another potential danger is perforation of the lateral sinus wall, resulting in a buccal abscess or perforation of the sinus roof causing infection of the orbital contents (**Fig. 3.45**).

A *frontal sinus empyema* can be surgically drained through a "Beck puncture" (⤷ **3.16**). There should be little hesitation in using this procedure, since the frontal sinus directly borders the cranial cavity, posing a risk of meningoencephalitis or frontal brain abscess.

**Fig. 3.44 Acute maxillary sinusitis**

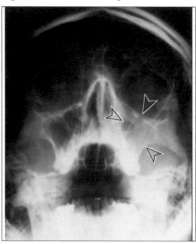

Conventional radiograph of the paranasal sinuses in occipitomental projection showing opacification of the left maxillary sinus (arrows).

**Fig. 3.45 Complication after sharp puncture of the maxillary sinus**

**Fig. 3.43 Acute sinusitis**

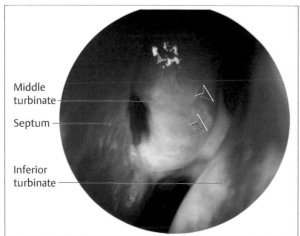

Middle turbinate

Septum

Inferior turbinate

A purulent track (arrows) is visible in the middle meatus of the left nasal cavity.

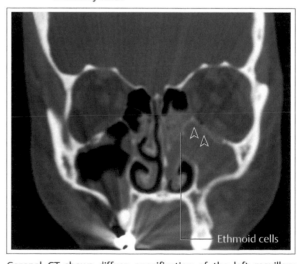

Ethmoid cells

Coronal CT shows diffuse opacification of the left maxillary sinus and left anterior ethmoid bone. The orbit contains two small air bubbles (arrows) signifying perforation of the maxillary sinus roof.

**3.16  Frontal sinus irrigation**

For the Beck puncture, the skin and subcutaneous soft tissues are divided at the medial border of the eyebrow, and the anterior wall of the frontal sinus is opened with a drill. Secretions and pus are aspirated from the frontal sinus, and the sinus is irrigated with decongestant nose drops and an antibiotic solution.

## Chronic Sinusitis

See also 🔖 **3.14**.

*Etiopathogenesis:* Besides intranasal anatomic changes such as septal deviation and septal spurs, a variety of other diseases can lead to chronic sinusitis, in particular chronic inflammatory diseases (see, for example, 🔖**3.17**) and more rarely diseases of an allergic, traumatic, or neoplastic nature. The common pathogenic mechanism is impaired ventilation of the ostiomeatal unit (see 🔖**1.3**) due to stenosis or obstruction of this region. This hampers drainage of the dependent sinus systems, particularly the adjacent maxillary sinus and anterior ethmoid cells. As the mucosa becomes swollen, especially in the narrow anatomic passages of the ostiomeatal unit, a vicious cycle becomes established that initially leads to recurrent bouts of acute inflammation and eventually culminates in a persistent, chronic sinusitis.

Chronic sinusitis frequently affects the maxillary sinus and ethmoid cells, while the frontal and sphenoid sinuses are less commonly involved.

*Symptoms:* The character of the pain is variable and can range from a feeling of pressure to persistent or recurrent headaches. Many patients also complain of nasopharyngeal drainage (postnasal drip), and some complain of obstructed nasal breathing.

*Diagnosis:*
**Rhinoscopy, endoscopy:** The nasal cavity is inspected by rhinoscopy or endoscopy, giving particular attention to changes in the nasal septum, the condition of the turbinates (turbinate hyperplasia, pneumatized middle turbinate, concha bullosa), and the appearance of the ostiomeatal unit (mucosal swelling, polyps, tumors, etc., see also 🔖**1.3**). Other causes of impaired ventilation and drainage in the nasal cavity itself (e.g., tumors) should also be excluded.

**Imaging studies:** Today, CT is considered the only acceptable modality for imaging the paranasal sinuses if chronic sinusitis ist suspected. Conventional sinus radiographs are of very limited value in diagnosing chronic sinusitis due to artifacts from superimposed structures. Also, only CT scans can accurately define

**3.17  Allergic fungal rhinosinusitis**

Allergic fungal rhinosinusitis is a noninvasive chronic fungal inflammation of the paranasal sinuses, with *Aspergillus fumigatus* being the main causative agent involved. Patients often complain about postnasal discharge and other symptoms of chronic sinusitis. On rhinoendoscopic examination, nasal polyps might be visible, as well as mucopurulent secretion (**Fig. 3.46 a**).

Computed tomography scans show the typical, almost pathognomonic "ironlike" signal in the paranasal sinuses or adjacent structures (**Fig. 3.46 b**). Adequate treatment is surgical (functional endoscopic sinus surgery, FESS; 🔖**3.18**). Local or systemic therapy with antimycotic agents showed no improvement in randomized studies.

**Fig. 3.46  Allergic fungal rhinosinusitis (AFRS)**

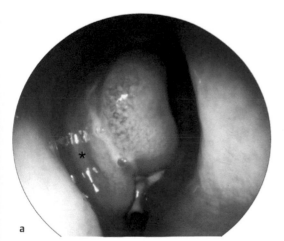 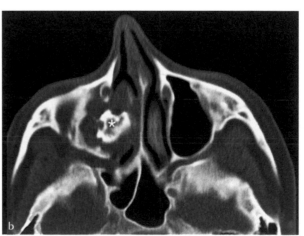

**a** Endoscopy of the right nasal cavity reveals mucopurulent discharge and inflamed, swollen mucosa in the right middle meatus (∗).

**b** Axial CT scan in AFRS. The typical "ironlike" signal (∗) is clearly visible in the pneumatized left maxillary sinus.
Source: Grevers and Leunig 1999.

the key anatomic structures that are important for accurate preoperative planning (**Fig. 3.47**).

**Allergy testing:** If there is evidence of allergic rhinitis, allergy testing should be performed (see 📖 2.2).

*Treatment:* Conservative treatment options include *decongestant nose drops* (for no more than 1 week), *heat therapy* (electric light cabinet, microwaves, infrared), and *broadband antibiotics* (e.g., amoxicillin) for acute exacerbations of sinusitis with fever and malaise. *Mucolytics* can also be administered for supportive therapy.

With an allergic etiology, appropriate antiallergic therapy should also be provided (see 📖 3.7, Treatment of Allergic Rhinitis). All of these conservative therapies are of symptomatic benefit and cannot eliminate the cause of chronic sinusitis. The only definitive treatment is sinus surgery (🔎 **3.18**).

## Nasal Polyposis

*Pathogenesis and morphology:* Nasal polyposis is a very complex condition that develops in response to a variety of noxious stimuli, appearing morphologically as edematous, polypoid hyperplasia of the sinus mucosa (usually in the anterior ethmoid cells and maxillary sinus) and projecting into the nasal cavity in the form of polyps (**Fig. 3.48**).

*Etiology:* Besides genetic causes, nasal polyps are attributed mainly to chronic irritation of the mucosa, like that occurring in chronic rhinitis or sinusitis. They can also form in response to allergic

---

🔎 **3.18  Endoscopic sinus surgery**

The modern surgical treatment of chronic sinusitis is performed intranasally under endoscopic control (functional endoscopic sinus surgery, FESS).

The *principle* of endoscopic sinus surgery is to enlarge the tight passages in the middle meatus and ostiomeatal unit including the natural ostia of the maxillary sinus and, if necessary, the frontal sinus, preserving as much sinus mucosa as possible. A preliminary septoplasty may be necessary in patients with functionally significant septal deviation (**Fig. 3.47 a**).

The *hazards* of intranasal sinus surgery are based mainly on the close proximity of the sinuses to the anterior cranial fossa, optic nerve, and (in the case of the sphenoid sinus) to the internal carotid artery.

The *prerequisites* for any type of intranasal sinus surgery, then, are a detailed knowledge of sinonasal anatomy and technical proficiency in handling the endoscope, which should be gained in diagnostic procedures and by practice on anatomic specimens. The surgeon should also be well versed in the radiographic anatomy of this region.

rhinitis and acetylsalicylic acid (ASA) intolerance (ASA pseudoallergy). The functional anatomy of the ostiomeatal unit, with its slitlike passages, appears to have causal significance in nasal polyposis, as in chronic sinusitis, because it controls the ventilation and drainage of the frontal and maxillary sinuses. The opposing mucosal surfaces in these areas are often separated by a distance of less than 1 mm. If they come into contact, this will impair the mucociliary clearance mechanism and hamper the normal transport of harmful substances toward the nasopharynx. Most polyps form at these narrow passages.

---

Fig. 3.47  **Chronic sinusitis**

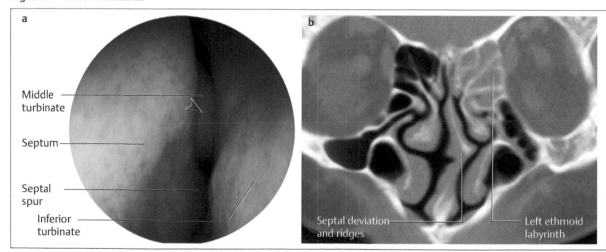

**a** Septal deviation with a prominent septal spur have caused narrowing of the left nasal cavity.
**b** Corresponding coronal computed tomography also demonstrates the marked septal deviation and ridges. The opacifica-

tion of the left ethmoid labyrinth reflects the chronic inflammation resulting from impaired ventilation and drainage of the middle meatus and ostiomeatal unit.

Whether, when, and to what extent these pathologic changes lead to symptomatic polyposis varies in different individuals and may depend partly on the timing of diagnosis and treatment.

Nasal polyps are rarely observed in children. Most occur in a setting of cystic fibrosis.

*Symptoms:* The clinical manifestations of nasal polyps depend on their extent and may consist of obstructed nasal breathing, hyposmia or anosmia (due to obstruction of the olfactory groove), headache (due to impaired ventilation and drainage in the paranasal sinuses), snoring, rhinophonia clausa, and frequent throat clearing due to associated postnasal drainage. Spread to the lower airways can lead to laryngitis with hoarseness and bronchitic symptoms.

*Diagnosis:* As in chronic sinusitis, the diagnosis is established by careful rhinoscopic or endoscopic evaluation of the nasal cavity, giving particular attention to the lateral nasal wall. The imaging modality of choice is CT. Further diagnostic measures consist of allergy tests and olfactory testing.

*Treatment:* Treatment may begin with symptomatic **conservative measures** such as the use of corticoid-containing nasal sprays and systemic antihistamines. Systemic steroids may also be tried. A partial or even complete remission of nasal polyps can sometimes be achieved with these measures alone.

Many cases will require **surgical treatment**, however. Besides intranasal polypectomy, which is performed mainly in older or higher-risk patients, an important current option is intranasal sinus surgery using endo-

### 3.19  Primary ciliary dyskinesia

Primary ciliary dyskinesia is an autosomal-recessive disease characterized by morphologic changes in the cilia (absence of dynein arms, transposition of microtubules), leading to a marked reduction in beat frequency and dyskinetic ciliary movements that are ineffectual for mucus transport. The impaired function of the mucociliary apparatus is manifested by symptoms of primary ciliary dyskinesia, which consist mainly of recurrent sinusitis and nasal polyposis, eustachian tube catarrh, otitis, bronchitis, and bronchiectasis. Life expectancy in affected patients depends mainly on the severity of pulmonary involvement.

scopic or microsurgical technique (see also Treatment of Chronic Sinusitis above).

*Prognosis:* Given the complex and poorly understood etiopathogenesis of nasal polyposis, which is not considered a single entity, the prognosis is guarded even with modern surgical techniques, and even the most meticulous ablative sinus surgery cannot prevent a recurrence. As a result, there is often no alternative to long-term medical *prophylaxis* with topical steroid sprays.

## Mucoceles and Pyoceles

A mucocele is a cystlike, mucus-containing sac that can form within a paranasal sinus. A pyocele is a mucocele that contains purulent material as a result of superinfection.

*Pathogenesis:* A mucocele may be caused by adhesions (postinflammatory, posttraumatic, or postoperative) that obstruct drainage from the paranasal sinus system. Mass lesions (polyps, tumors) can also obstruct and obliterate the drainage tracts, leading to mucocele formation. The outflow obstruction causes the mucocele to exert increasing pressure on the surrounding sinus walls, resulting in progressive thinning of the bone. In this way, the mass can erode into adjacent structures such as the orbit or even the cranial cavity. The most common site of occurrence is the frontal sinus, followed by the ethmoid cells, maxillary sinus, and sphenoid sinus.

*Symptoms:* A frontal sinus mucocele usually presents as an isolated, tense swelling over the anterior wall of the frontal sinus (**Fig. 3.49**). It may also cause inferolateral displacement of the orbital contents, especially if it has eroded through the sinus floor. On the other hand, swelling in the cheek area with upward displacement of the orbital contents is

**Fig. 3.48 Nasal polyposis**

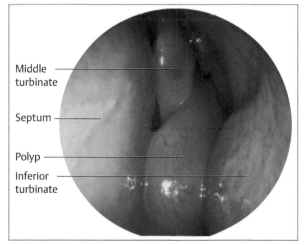

Middle turbinate

Septum

Polyp

Inferior turbinate

A nasal polyp has prolapsed from the middle meatus into the main part of the left nasal cavity.

**Fig. 3.49 Frontal sinus mucocele**

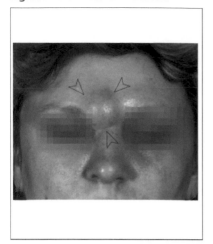

A frontal sinus mucocele appears as a rounded bulge in the anterior wall of the sinus (arrows).

more characteristic of a maxillary sinus mucocele (**Fig. 3.50 a, b**). Proptosis, limited ocular movements, and diplopia may also occur, depending on the location of the mass. In some cases, however, a maxillary mucocele might also erode the medial wall of the maxillary sinus, thus protruding into the nasal cavity and leading to unilateral nasal obstruction (**Fig. 3.50 c–e**). Unlike mucoceles in the frontal sinus, ethmoid cells (**Fig. 3.51**), and maxillary sinus, sphenoid sinus mucoceles (**Fig. 3.52**) often have nonspecific clinical manifestations, with complaints similar to those of sphenoid sinusitis (headache radiating to the vertex and occiput).

*Diagnosis:* A prior surgical history is often helpful in making a diagnosis. The clinical appearance may also be suggestive (**Fig. 3.49** and **Fig. 3.50 a**); sometimes, however, inspection of the nasal cavity by rhinoscopy or endoscopy might also be helpful (**Fig. 3.50 c**). On the other hand, modern sectional imaging modalities (CT, **Fig. 3.50 b**, **Fig. 3.50 d, e**, **Fig. 3.51 a, b**; and magnetic resonance imaging [MRI], **Fig. 3.52**) can make it possible to delineate the mucocele from surrounding tissues and differentiate it from a malignant tumor.

*Treatment:* The treatment of choice is surgical removal of the mucocele.

## Rhinosinogenic Complications

There are various mechanisms by which serious and even life-threatening complications can arise from inflammatory diseases of the paranasal sinuses. Complications with inflammatory involvement of the orbit (orbital complications) are distinguished clinically from bone and soft-tissue complications (osteomyelitis) and from intracranial complications.

## Orbital Complications

Inflammatory complications with orbital involvement most commonly arise from the ethmoid cells or frontal sinus and less commonly from the sphenoid or maxillary sinus. They occur with highest frequency in children younger than 6 years. Four different clinical grades of severity are distinguished, requiring a graded therapeutic approach. Ophthalmologic consultation should be obtained.

**Orbital edema:** The initial stage is marked by a doughy swelling and erythema of the eyelids (**Fig. 3.53**). Ocular mobility is normal, and the globe itself is not displaced. The *differential diagnosis* should include dacryocystitis, the most common disease of the lacrimal sac, which is characterized by tenderness, erythema, and accompanying edema at the medial canthus of the eye. The *treatment* of choice is conservative and relies on nose drops (which may be applied in an intranasal cotton pack; see Treatment of Acute Sinusitis above) and antibiotics. Corticosteroids may also be administered if required.

**Periosteitis:** While lid edema persists, pain develops at the medial canthus of the eye. *Conservative medical treatment* is still adequate at this stage in most cases.

**Subperiosteal abscess:** The inflammatory process has penetrated the bony barrier between the paranasal sinus and orbit, separating the orbital periosteum from the lamina papyracea and raising the pressure within the orbit. This stage is marked by an initial limitation of ocular movement with associated proptosis. Chemosis may already be present in exceptional cases. The *treatment* of choice is surgical drainage of the abscess, which today is done endoscopically. Nose drops and antibiotics are also administered. Ophthalmologic consultation is advised for medicolegal reasons.

**Orbital cellulitis:** The final stage of orbital complications is associated with proptosis and limited eye movements, pain, chemosis, and visual deterioration or even blindness.

⚡ Orbital cellulitis is a life-threatening **emergency** that requires immediate surgical decompression. This should be done with antibiotic coverage, as for a subperiosteal abscess.

An **"orbital apex syndrome"** can develop when the cellulitis spreads to involve the anatomic structures at the orbital apex (cranial nerves II–VI, ophthalmic artery and vein). Progressive thrombophlebitis can also lead to **cavernous sinus thrombosis** and other intracranial complications (see below).

**Fig. 3.50  Maxillary sinus mucocele**

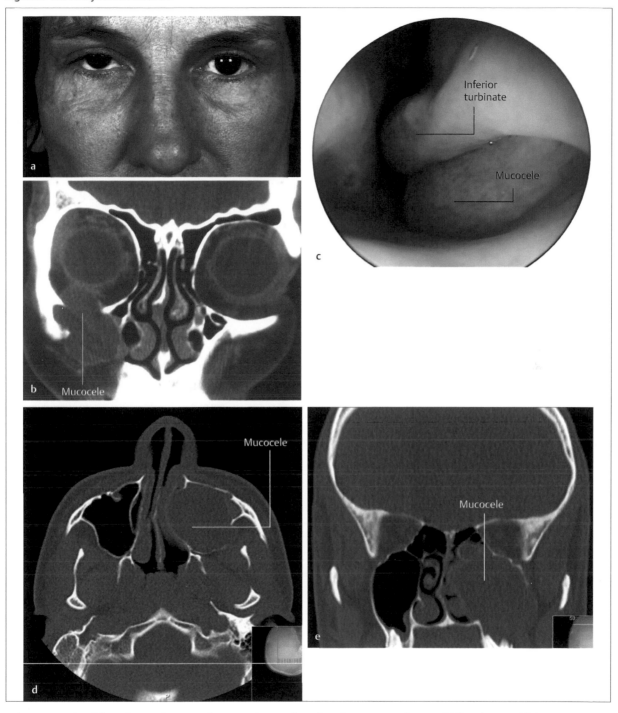

**a, b**  A mucocele of the right maxillary sinus has caused upward displacement of the orbital contents (**a**). The corresponding coronal CT (**b**) demonstrates the sac protruding through the orbital floor.
**c**  Mucocele of the left maxillary sinus protruding into the left nasal cavity.

**d, e** The corresponding axial (**d**) and coronal (**e**) CT scans show almost complete opacification of the left maxillary sinus and the left nasal cavity.
Source **c**: Grevers and Königsberger 2015.

**Fig. 3.51 Ethmoid mucocele**

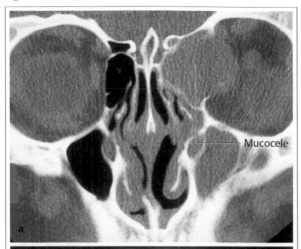

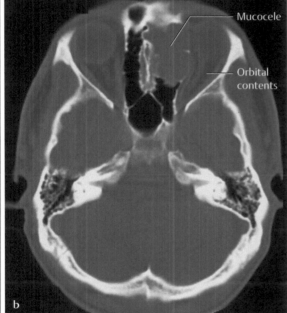

Mucocele

Mucocele

Orbital contents

An ethmoid mucocele on the left side has displaced the orbital contents laterally. Coronal **(a)** and axial **(b)** computed tomography scans.

## Bone and Soft-Tissue Inflammations (Osteitis and Osteomyelitis)

Osteomyelitis occurs mainly as a complication of frontal sinusitis when the bacterial inflammation spreads to the bony anterior wall of the frontal sinus, the frontal bone, and the surrounding soft tissues.

▯ The main danger of frontal osteomyelitis is that the infection may spread to other bony structures of the calvaria.

*Symptoms:* The patient presents clinically with a tender, doughy, erythematous swelling over the forehead (**Fig. 3.54**). The surrounding facial soft tissues are also involved in most cases.

**Fig. 3.52 Sphenoid sinus mucocele**

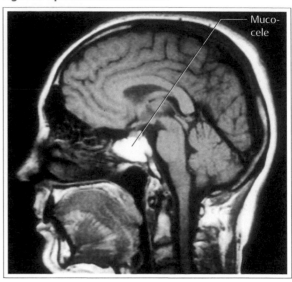

Muco-cele

A sagittal magnetic resonance image demonstrates a sphenoid sinus mucocele.

**Fig. 3.53 Orbital edema**

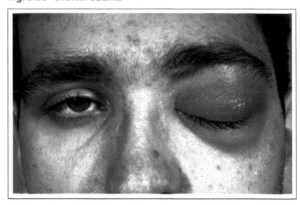

A rhinosinogenic inflammation has spread to the orbit. The initial stage is marked by orbital edema on the left side with an erythematous, doughy swelling of the upper and lower lids.

*Diagnosis:* Cranial CT scans should always be obtained to define the extent of the inflammation.

*Treatment:* The treatment of choice is surgical eradication of the affected bone under antibiotic coverage. Bone affected by inflammatory changes should be generously resected to prevent the further spread of inflammation.

## Intracranial Complications

Intracranial complications also arise from the frontal sinuses in most cases. The ethmoid cells and sphenoid sinus are a more frequent nidus for these complications in children due to their lack of aeration.

**Epidural, subdural and intracerebral abscesses:** The clinical manifestations of these lesions are frequently

Fig. 3.54 Osteomyelitis of the frontal bone

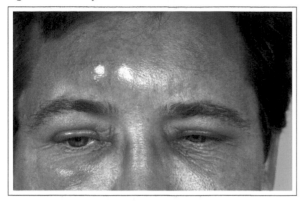

Typical features are a doughy swelling over the forehead with concomitant soft-tissue swelling, especially about the eyelids on both sides.

nonspecific. As the disease progresses, it may produce signs of increased intracranial pressure with nausea, headache, vomiting, and occasional papilledema, somnolence, or seizures. The *diagnosis* relies critically on CT (**Fig. 3.55**) or MRI (**Fig. 3.56**) due to the nonspecific clinical features. The *treatment* of choice for the various types of abscess is surgical drainage with high-dose antibiotic coverage.

**Meningitis:** The main clinical manifestations are stiff neck, headache, fever, nausea, and photophobia. Some cases show increasing somnolence and clouding of consciousness, and seizures are occasionally observed. Cranial CT scans should be obtained whenever meningitis is suspected, particularly to exclude an intracranial abscess. The neurologist confirms the diagnosis by CSF sampling. In rhinogenic meningitis and with other forms, treatment relies mainly on surgical drainage of the affected sinuses under antibiotic coverage. Neurologic therapies may also be indicated (e.g., in patients prone to seizures).

## Sinus Thrombosis and Thrombophlebitis

📙 These complications, while rare, can lead to permanent neurologic deficits if diagnosed too late. They can be fatal in extreme cases.

**Cavernous sinus thrombosis** may present clinically with orbital edema, signs of venous congestion in the optic fundus (ophthalmologist!), chemosis, and occasional diplopia and proptosis with limited ocular movements. MRI should be performed and will often show definite evidence of sinus thrombosis. If MRI is unrewarding in patients with suggestive clinical signs, digital subtraction angiography (DSA) should be performed. As with all other intracranial complications, *treatment* consists of surgical drainage under antibiotic coverage.

Fig. 3.55 Epidural abscess

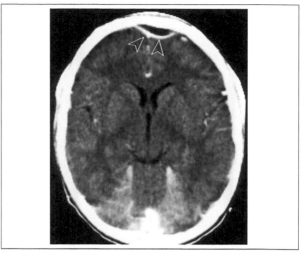

Axial CT scan of an epidural abscess (arrows), which has developed as an intracranial complication of frontal sinusitis.

Fig. 3.56 Rhinosinogenic brain abscess

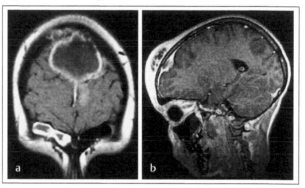

Coronal (**a**) and sagittal (**b**) magnetic resonance images of a pediatric rhinosinogenic brain abscess originating from the right frontal sinus.

# 3.9     Tumors of the External Nose and Face

The majority of facial tumors are malignancies, consisting mainly of basal cell carcinomas and spindle cell carcinomas. Other malignant neoplasms, precancerous lesions, and benign tumors are much less common in this region.

## Benign Tumors

The most important benign facial tumor is **rhinophyma** (**Fig. 3.57a**), a connective-tissue and sebaceous hyperplasia with angiectatic changes occurring over the cartilaginous nose. Most patients have preexisting rosacea, and so concomitant erythema is usually present. Although rosacea is more common in women than men, usually begins after age 20 and has a peak incidence at 40 to 50 years of age, rhinophyma is seen almost exclusively in older men. The *differential diagnosis* should include the cutaneous manifestations of lymphatic leukemia, cutaneous Tcell lymphoma, and sarcoidosis. The *treatment* of choice is surgical ablation of the hyperplastic tissue in layers, allowing the wound area to heal by spontaneous epithelialization (**Fig. 3.57b**).

## Precancerous Lesions

Besides **actinic keratosis** and **Bowen's disease**, a chronic skin inflammation caused by carcinoma in situ, precancerous lesions include **cutaneous horn** and **malignant lentigo**. The latter is attributed to chronic sun exposure, grows slowly, and may progress to malignant melanoma.

Precancerous lesions of the facial skin should be watched closely, as they may progress to a malignant tumor.

Details on these precancerous lesions, which are generally rare, can be found in textbooks of dermatology.

## Malignant Tumors

The most common facial malignancies are of epithelial origin, predominantly basal cell carcinomas and squamous cell carcinomas (spindle cell carcinomas). By contrast, melanomas, sarcomas, lymphomas, and cutaneous infiltration by leukemia are relatively rare in the facial region.

### Basal Cell Carcinoma

Synonym: basalioma.

*Epidemiology:* Basal cell carcinoma has a peak incidence between 60 and 70 years of age but may be seen in patients as young as 40 years.

*Etiology:* The etiology is uncertain. In addition to a genetic predisposition, prolonged sun exposure in people with very sun-sensitive skin appears to have causal significance.

*Clinical manifestations:* The tumor is classified as a malignant neoplasm because of its local invasiveness, but it has no tendency to metastasize. Basal cell carcinomas can vary greatly in their morphologic features. Solid basaliomas are particularly rare in the facial region; they show central crusting and a string-of-beads margin (**Fig. 3.58**).

*Diagnosis and treatment:* After the diagnosis is confirmed by biopsy, treatment consists of surgical *excision* with frozen-section control of all margins. A special form, sclerodermiform basalioma, irregularly infiltrates the surrounding skin and often has ill-defined gross margins. This can lead to problems of surgical excision, as the size of the defect is often underestimated preoperatively. Following tumor removal with a margin of healthy tissue, the surgical defect is *reconstructed* in the same sitting (see 📖 3.4, Repair of Tissue Defects).

### Fig. 3.57 Rhinophyma

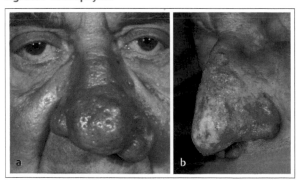

Typical clinical appearance of a rhinophyma before (**a**) and after (**b**) ablation of the hyperplastic tissue areas.

Fig. 3.58 Basal cell carcinoma

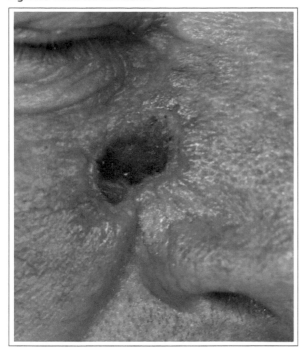

Typical clinical appearance of the lesion.

## Spindle Cell Carcinoma

Synonym: spinalioma.

*Epidemiology:* Spindle cell carcinoma (**Fig. 3.59 a**) is the second most common malignant tumor of the external nose and also tends to occur in older individuals.

*Etiology:* The etiology is uncertain, but it is very likely that exposure to ultraviolet radiation has causal significance.

*Clinical manifestations:* Unlike basal cell carcinoma, spindle cell carcinoma is a "classic" malignant tumor in that it can metastasize to regional lymph nodes.

*Treatment:* Treatment consists of surgical tumor removal. Various plastic reconstructive techniques can be used, depending on the location and size of the defect (**Fig. 3.59 a–d** and **Fig. 3.11**, **Fig. 3.12**, **Fig. 3.13**, **Fig. 3.14**, **Fig. 3.15**, **Fig. 3.16**). Patients with regional lymph-node metastases should undergo a neck dissection in the same sitting, followed by postoperative radiotherapy.

Fig. 3.59 Spindle cell carcinoma of the nose

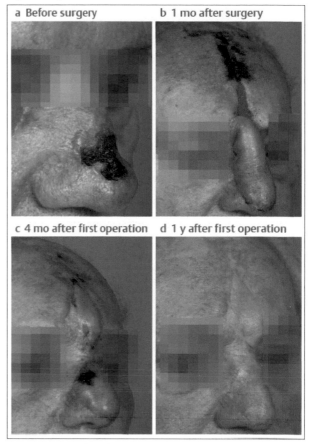

a  Before surgery          b  1 mo after surgery

c  4 mo after first operation    d  1 y after first operation

**a** Preoperative clinical appearance.
**b** Following tumor resection and reconstruction with a midline forehead flap.
**c** Following division of the midline forehead flap and replacement of the flap pedicle.
**d** Final result. The principle of this operation is shown in **Fig. 3.13**.

# 3.10   Tumors of the Nasal Cavity and Paranasal Sinuses

Benign tumors of the nasal cavity and paranasal sinuses are relatively rare. Malignancies of this region occur mainly in older patients and, since they develop in preexisting cavities, may remain asymptomatic for years.

## Benign Tumors

Besides epithelial and connective-tissue neoplasms, benign intranasal and sinus tumors may arise from smooth muscle, peripheral nerves, or blood vessels (**Fig. 3.60**).

### Inverted Papilloma

Sinonasal papillomas, especially inverted papillomas, constitute a special category of epithelial masses. The inverted papilloma has certain characteristics that still prompt discussion on its etiology and appropriate management. It is a locally aggressive tumor, and transformation to squamous cell carcinoma is periodically described. Its growth characteristics resemble those of various virus-induced cutaneous and mucosal lesions (e.g., warts, condylomas, laryngeal papillomas). But while a viral etiology has been discussed, it remains unproved.

*Symptoms and diagnosis:* The clinical manifestations of inverted papilloma are as nonspecific as those of other sinonasal tumors and include nasal airway obstruction, headache, and occasional epistaxis. The lesion often has a polyplike appearance when inspected by nasal endoscopy. In many cases, only histologic examination can establish the diagnosis. Imaging (CT) is helpful in defining the tumor extent.

*Treatment:* The treatment of choice is surgical removal. The special growth characteristics of this tumor require adequate exposure to allow for complete removal.

## Osteomas

Osteomas are benign bone tumors that may occur as isolated masses, especially in the ethmoid cells and frontal sinus, or may form extensive masses that grow along the skull base (**Fig. 3.61**).

*Symptoms and diagnosis:* Many of these tumors are detected incidentally on CT scans performed to diagnose chronic sinusitis. Often, they do not become symptomatic until they obstruct drainage tracts to or from the paranasal sinuses, leading secondarily to headaches and recurrent bouts of sinusitis (**Fig. 3.61 a, b**).

🖉 For medicolegal and other reasons, it is essential to define the relationship of the osteoma to the skull base and other landmarks by multiplanar CT prior to surgical treatment.

*Treatment:* As soon as an osteoma becomes symptomatic, it should be surgically removed. Otherwise there is no need for therapeutic intervention.

## Malignant Tumors

Malignant tumors of the nasal cavity and paranasal sinuses are far more common than benign masses. Histologically, the great majority (>80%) are tumors of the epithelial series (e.g., squamous cell carcinoma, adenocarcinoma, adenoid cystic carcinoma). Neoplasms of mesenchymal origin, such as osteosarcomas and chondrosarcomas, as well as malignant lymphomas are much less common. Metastases from other malignancies are occasionally found, with the primary tumor residing in the kidney, lung, breast, testis, or thyroid gland.

The main sites of predilection are the nasal cavity and maxillary sinus, followed by the ethmoid cells, frontal sinus, and sphenoid sinus.

**Fig. 3.60 Bleeding polyp**

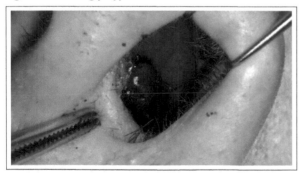

Anterior rhinoscopy of the left nasal cavity reveals a "bleeding polyp" of the nasal septum. This inflammatory hemangioma becomes clinically noticeable by unilateral nasal obstruction and recurrent epistaxis. Bleeding polyps mainly occur in young adults and patients older than 40 years and predominantly originate from the cartilaginous septum. The origin of this benign tumor can be posttraumatic and spontaneous. The treatment of choice is surgical removal of the lesion.

Fig. 3.61   Osteoma

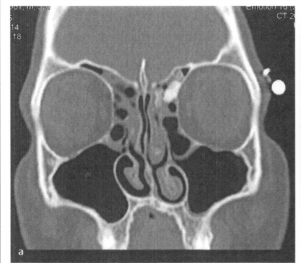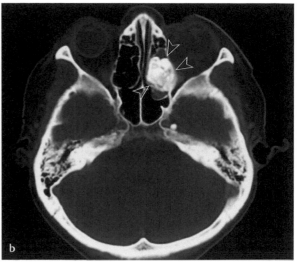

Multiplanar CT scans are crucial to define the exact location of the lesion in relation to the surrounding structures.

**a**   Coronal CT scan displaying an ethmoid sinus osteoma obstructing the left frontal recess (access to the frontal sinus) in a patient with chronic sinusitis.

**b**   Axial CT scan of another patient with ethmoid sinus osteoma (arrowheads).

## Symptoms:

🗹 Because many tumors originate in the paranasal sinuses themselves, they often do not produce clinical manifestations until they have reached an advanced stage.

Symptoms that are suspicious for malignancy include sudden onset of **obstructed nasal breathing** combined with **bloody rhinorrhea** and a **fetid nasal odor**, especially in patients older than 50 years. A malignant tumor should also be considered in the differential diagnosis of unilateral sinusitis that is refractory to treatment. Advanced tumor stages may be marked by swelling of the buccal soft tissues, swelling at the medial canthus of the eye, headache, facial pain, and hypoesthesia or numbness of the cheek due to infraorbital nerve involvement. Orbital infiltration can lead to displacement of the orbital contents, diplopia, or proptosis.

**Diagnosis:** The clinical examination includes external and rhinoendoscopic inspection of the nasal vestibule and cavity (see **Fig. 3.62** and **Fig. 3.64 a**) and a search for regional lymph-node metastases by bimanual palpation of the cervical soft tissues. Since sinus tumors are apt to invade the nasal cavity secondarily, endoscopy alone may provide little information on the extent of the mass. For this reason, CT (**Fig. 3.63 a**,

Fig. 3.62  Squamous cell carcinoma of the anterior ethmoid

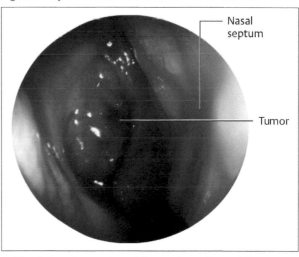

Nasal septum

Tumor

A blood-tinged mass is visible in the right middle meatus between the middle turbinate and lateral nasal wall. The true extent of the tumor cannot be determined from the endoscopic findings alone.

**Fig. 3.64 b**) and/or MRI (**Fig. 3.63 b–d**) should always be performed and should cover the cervical soft tissues to check for nodal metastases. The disease can be staged (**Table 3.4**) based on the results of the examination.

**Fig. 3.63   Imaging of malignant sinonasal tumors**

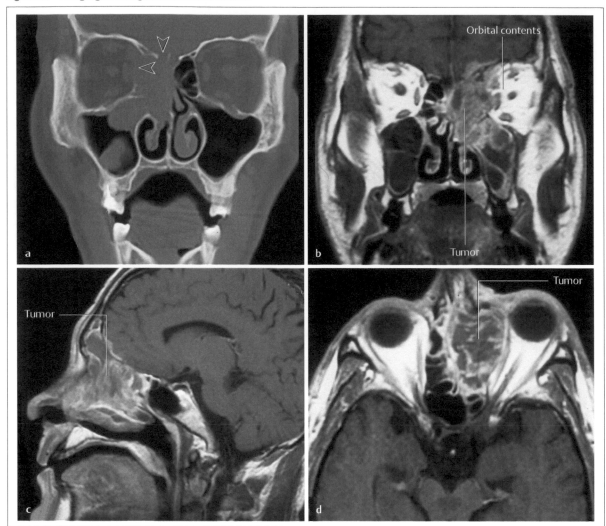

**a** Coronal computed tomography with a bone window demonstrates an extensive sinonasal carcinoma with sites of bone destruction in the anterior skull base and orbit (arrows).
**b** Coronal magnetic resonance (MR) imaging in the same plane more clearly demonstrates the soft-tissue relationship of the tumor to the brain tissue and orbital contents.
**c** Sagittal MR image.
**d** Axial MR image.

*Treatment:* Treatment is individualized according to the histology and extent of the malignant tumor, and the treatment plan should be coordinated with the radiotherapist and medical oncologist. Since the great majority of lesions are squamous cell carcinomas, however, the treatment of choice will usually consist of surgery (**Fig. 3.64 c**) and postoperative radiation. The goal of radical tumor removal may require a very extensive procedure with partial or complete removal of the maxilla or partial resection of the anterior skull base. As a result of close interdisciplinary cooperation with neurosurgeons, maxillofacial surgeons, and ophthalmologists, as well as modern intensive-care options, even very extensive sinonasal malignancies can now be managed by surgical treatment. Since only approximately 20% of sinonasal malignancies metastasize to regional lymph nodes, a neck dissection is necessary only in patients who have clinically positive cervical nodes. Many of these cases will require postoperative radiotherapy (*3.20*).

**Fig. 3.64 Melanoma of the nasal cavity and maxillary sinus**

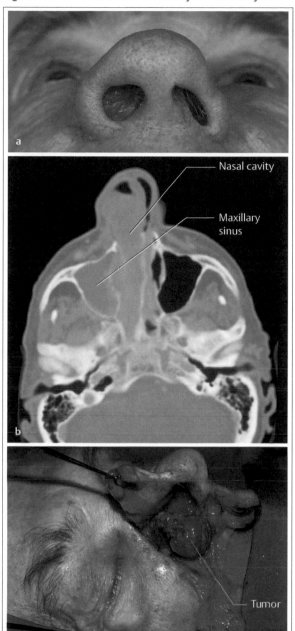

Nasal cavity

Maxillary sinus

Tumor

a

b

c

**🔍 3.20 Esthesioneuroblastoma**

Esthesioneuroblastoma is a rare neurogenic malignancy that arises from the sensory cells of the olfactory region and generally occurs in adults. Its etiology is still uncertain, but it is believed that some cases are embryogenically induced. **Clinically**, esthesioneuroblastoma remains asymptomatic for some time due to its location in the olfactory groove between the upper portions of the nasal septum and the attachment of the middle turbinate. When advanced, the tumor causes obstructed nasal breathing, recurrent epistaxis, and particularly hyposmia or anosmia. Some of these tumors become symptomatic only after invading the cranial cavity or orbit, causing headache or visual deterioration. In a few cases, cervical lymph-node metastases are the primary manifestation of the disease.

The **diagnosis** is based on endoscopy (see **Fig. 3.65**) and especially computed tomography or magnetic resonance imaging; only these modalities can accurately define the tumor extent.

**Treatment** is based on a combination of tumor resection and postoperative radiotherapy.

**Fig. 3.65 Endoscopic examination displays the tumor located between the middle turbinate and the left nasal cavity**

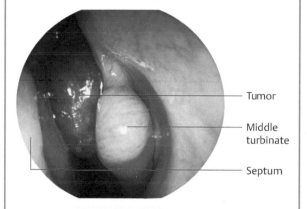

Tumor

Middle turbinate

Septum

**a** The tumor extends into the nasal vestibule, where it is visible to external inspection.
**b** Corresponding axial computed tomography shows tumor tissue occupying the right maxillary sinus and nasal cavity.
**c** During surgery, the tumor is exposed and resected through a lateral rhinotomy.

**Table 3.4** Classification of sinonasal tumors according to the Union for International Cancer Control (UICC) system

| | |
|---|---|
| *Maxillary sinus* | |
| T1 | Mucosa |
| T2 | Bone erosion/destruction, hard palate, middle nasal meatus |
| T3 | Posterior bony wall of maxillary sinus, subcutaneous tissues, floor/medial wall of orbit, pterygoid fossa, ethmoid sinus |
| T4a | Anterior orbit, cheek skin, pterygoid plates, infratemporal fossa, cribriform plate, sphenoid/frontal sinus |
| T4b | Orbital apex, dura, brain, middle cranial fossa, cranial nerves other than V2, nasopharynx, clivus |
| *Nasal cavity and ethmoid sinus* | |
| T1 | One subsite |
| T2 | Two subsites or adjacent nasoethmoidal site |
| T3 | Medial wall/floor of orbit, maxillary sinus, palate, cribriform plate |
| T4a | Anterior orbit, skin of nose/cheek, anterior cranial fossa (minimal), pterygoid plates, sphenoid/frontal sinus |
| T4b | Orbital apex, dura, brain, middle cranial fossa, cranial nerves other than V2, nasopharynx, clivus |
| *All sites* | |
| N1 | Ipsilateral single ≤ 3 cm without ENE |
| N2 | • Ipsilateral single > 3–6 cm without ENE<br>• Ipsilateral multiple ≤ 6 cm without ENE<br>• Bilateral, contralateral ≤ 6 cm without ENE |
| N3 | ENE-positive, or > 6 cm without ENE |

Abbreviation: ENE, extranodal extension.
Source: Brierley et al 2017.

# II Oral Cavity and Pharynx

# 4 Lips and Oral Cavity

## 4.1 Basic Anatomy and Physiology of the Lips and Oral Cavity

The lips and the soft tissues of the cheek function as the outer boundary of the oral vestibule and oral cavity, which form the initial part of the digestive tract. The tongue is situated such that the body of the tongue is within the oral cavity, while the base (root) of the tongue is in the oropharynx, forming its anterior boundary. For learning purposes, however, the tongue as a whole is included in the chapter on the oral cavity. *Functionally*, the lips and oral cavity comprise the initial part of the upper digestive tract and thus play a key role in food ingestion. Speech production additionally developed during the course of phylogenesis. Finally, a large percentage of the taste receptors are located in the oral cavity.

### Anatomy

#### Oral Vestibule

The oral vestibule is bounded externally by the lips and cheeks and internally by the alveolar processes and teeth (**Fig. 4.1**). When the teeth are in occlusion, the oral vestibule communicates with the oral cavity via a space behind the last molar. The oral cavity opens into the pharynx at the faucial isthmus (see ✒5.1, Nasopharynx, Oropharynx, and Hypopharynx).

#### Lips and Cheeks

The lips and cheeks, the morphologic framework of which is formed largely by the mimetic muscles, are lined on their mucosal side by nonkeratinized squamous epithelium.

**Lips:** The longer upper lip and shorter lower lip are connected to each other by the labial commissures at the corners of the mouth. The lips are separated from the cheek by the nasolabial fold, an oblique sulcus that runs laterally and inferiorly from the nasal alae.
The lamina propria of the lips contains numerous seromucous *salivary glands* (see **Fig. 6.2**), the secretions from which drain into the oral vestibule.
The orbicularis oris muscle forms the *muscular foundation* of the lips (**Fig. 4.2**).
The lips receive their *blood supply* from the superior and inferior labial arteries, which arise from the facial artery. The lips are drained primarily by the facial vein, which also communicates with the orbital veins via the angular vein above the upper lip.

▷ With inflammatory lesions of the lip (e.g., furuncles), infectious organisms can spread into the cranial cavity via connections between the orbital veins and cavernous plexus, resulting in complications (see ✒3.8, Rhinosinogenic Complications).

Knowledge about the *lymphatic drainage* of the lips is important for understanding the lymphogenous metastasis of malignant tumors of the lips. The submandibular and submental lymph nodes receive the lymphatic drainage from the lips.
The upper lip receives its *sensory innervation* from the infraorbital nerve and the lower lip from the mental nerve.

**Cheeks:** The cheeks, which form the lateral boundaries of the oral vestibule, also contain small salivary glands in their mucosa. The *buccinator* forms the muscular framework of the cheek. Like the orbicularis oculi, the buccinator is a mimetic muscle (**Fig. 4.2**) and receives its motor innervation from branches of the facial nerve. The *Bichat fat pad* (buccal fat pad) is located between the buccinator muscle and the overlying masseter muscle, the fibers of which run almost perpendicular to the buccinator. This fat pad smoothes the cheek contour by filling in the depression at the anterior border of the masseter muscle. The excretory duct of the *parotid gland* runs through the buccinator muscle and opens into the mucosa of the cheek opposite the upper second molar.

#### Masticatory Muscles

The *masseter muscle*, located in the posterior part of the cheek, covers the vertical ramus of the mandible and the mandibular angle from the outside. It is one of the masticatory muscles, along with the *temporalis muscle* and the *medial and lateral pterygoid muscles* (**Fig. 4.2**). These muscles form both a functional and phylogenetic unit, and accordingly are all supplied by the mandibular nerve (third division of the trigeminal nerve).

**Fig. 4.1 Anatomy of the lips, oral vestibule and oral cavity**

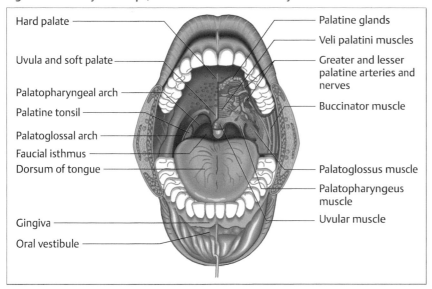

**Fig. 4.2 Anatomy of portions of the mimetic and masticatory muscles**

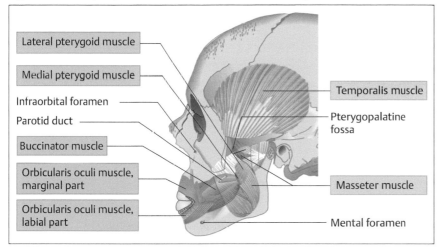

The diagram shows the superficial and deep masticatory muscles, the buccinator muscle, and the orbicularis oculi muscle.

## Teeth

The human dentition consists of two sets of teeth that vary in their individual shapes. The deciduous teeth are replaced by the permanent teeth, eight of which occupy each half of the maxilla and mandible:

- Two incisors.
- One canine.
- Two premolars.
- Three molars.

Each tooth consists of a crown and a root, which terminates at the apex. The area between the crown and root is the neck (cervix), which protrudes from sockets (dental alveoli) in the alveolar processes of the maxilla and mandible. The crown projects freely into the oral cavity and is covered externally by enamel.

Internally, each tooth has a pulp chamber that contains connective tissue, nerve fibers, and blood vessels and is connected to the alveolus via the root canal. The teeth are anchored in the alveoli by the cementum, the bony alveolar wall itself, and the gingiva. These anchoring and supporting structures are known collectively as the periodontium.

§ The alveolar processes in the maxilla also form the floor of the maxillary sinuses—a fact that has major practical relevance.

Normally, the roots of the second premolar and first molar are very closely related to the maxillary sinus (see also **Fig. 1.5** and **Fig. 1.6**). Occasionally, the bony shell between the periodontium and maxillary sinus

**Fig. 4.3    Anatomy of the lingual muscles**

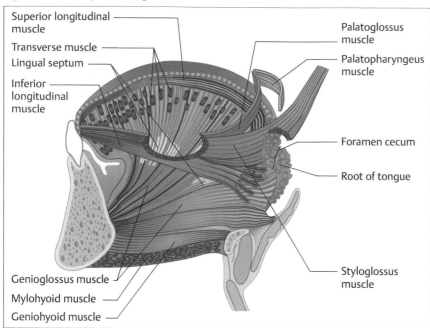

Superior longitudinal muscle

Transverse muscle

Lingual septum

Inferior longitudinal muscle

Genioglossus muscle

Mylohyoid muscle

Geniohyoid muscle

Palatoglossus muscle

Palatopharyngeus muscle

Foramen cecum

Root of tongue

Styloglossus muscle

The diagram shows the intrinsic muscles of the tongue and also the extrinsic muscles, consisting of the genioglossus and geniohyoid. The mylohyoid muscle provides the muscular foundation of the oral floor.

mucosa may even be absent in this region. The *arteries* that supply the maxilla and mandible (inferior alveolar artery, anterior and posterior superior alveolar arteries) arise from the maxillary artery. The upper teeth receive their *innervation* from branches of the maxillary nerve and the lower teeth from branches of the mandibular nerve.

## Oral Cavity

The oral cavity is bounded anteriorly and laterally by the alveolar ridge and teeth, superiorly by the hard and soft palate (**Fig. 4.1**), and posteriorly by the faucial isthmus. This narrow opening between the oral cavity and pharynx is bordered by the soft palate with the uvula and by the dorsum of the tongue at its junction with the tongue base.

**Palate:** The *hard palate* is formed by the palatine processes of the maxilla anteriorly, the incisive bone, and the horizontal plates of the palatine bones posteriorly. The oral cavity is sealed posteriorly by the *soft palate* with its pendulant process, the uvula. The *palatal muscles* that form the framework of the soft palate are the tensor veli palatini and especially the levator veli palatini, which elevates the soft palate during swallowing to keep food from entering the nose. The muscles of the soft palate are completed by the palatoglossus, which runs in the anterior faucial pillar (palatoglossal arch), and by the palatopharyngeus muscle of the posterior faucial pillar (palatopharyngeal arch; **Fig. 4.1**). The uvula also has its own muscle, called the muscle of the uvula. The palatal mucosa, like the

mucosa of the lips and cheeks, contains numerous salivary glands (palatine glands; see also **Fig. 6.2**). The *motor innervation* of the soft palate is described in *4.1*.

The palatal mucosa receives its *sensory* innervation from the greater and lesser palatine nerves (which arise from the second trigeminal nerve division; **Fig. 4.1**). The *blood supply* to the palate is derived from the ascending palatine branch of the facial artery.

**Tongue and oral floor:** The tongue is composed of various muscular systems (**Fig. 4.3**), occupies much of the oral cavity, and is continuous anteriorly and laterally with the floor of the mouth. The muscular foundation of the oral floor is formed by the mylohyoid muscle, which stretches between the anterior portions of the mandible. When the tip of the tongue is raised to expose the undersurface, the sublingual folds and sublingual papillae can be identified on both sides of the frenulum in the anterior part of the oral floor (**Fig. 6.3**).

---

*4.1 Motor innervation of the soft palate*

Developmentally, the individual muscular components of the soft palate are derived from different structures and are therefore supplied by different cranial nerves (mainly by cranial nerves IX and X, see **Fig. 16.4** and **Fig. 16.5**, and to a small degree by cranial nerve V).

Cranial nerve deficits, especially those involving the lower cranial nerves IX and X, tend to restrict the mobility of the soft palate, causing difficulties in swallowing. During phonation ("ah"), the uvula and faucial pillars deviate toward the unaffected side.

**Fig. 4.4   Anatomy of the tongue**

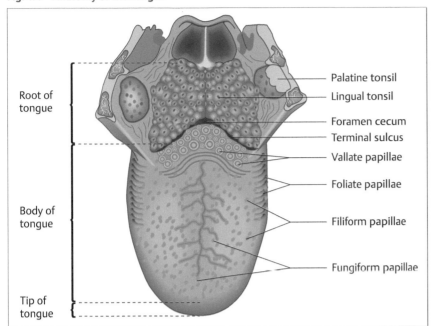

The body and base of the tongue, viewed from the superior aspect.

- Palatine tonsil
- Lingual tonsil
- Foramen cecum
- Terminal sulcus
- Vallate papillae
- Foliate papillae
- Filiform papillae
- Fungiform papillae

Root of tongue

Body of tongue

Tip of tongue

The main anatomic subdivisions of the tongue are the apex, the body, and the base or root. The body of the tongue is separated from the base by a **V**-shaped groove called the terminal sulcus. The tip of this groove is directed toward the tongue base and is formed by the foramen cecum (**Fig. 4.4**).

The *mucosa* of the tongue differs from the rest of the intraoral mucosa chiefly by the presence of numerous *papillae*, which project from the surface of the tongue and give it its characteristic roughness. Four types of papillae are distinguished: filiform, fungiform, vallate, and foliate (**Fig. 4.5**). The latter three types are most important for taste perception. The microscopic *taste buds* are responsible for specific taste reception. They are most numerous on the vallate and foliate papillae and less so on the fungiform papillae. Small numbers of taste buds also occur in other regions of the oral cavity and pharynx (e.g., the soft palate, the anterior pillar, and the posterior wall of the oropharynx). Each taste bud consists of 30 to 80 elongated cells that extend superficially to the gustatory pore. This channel is located between the squamous epithelial cells and communicates with the oral cavity.

The *lingual tonsil* is part of the collection of lympho-epithelial tissue known as Waldeyer's ring (see 5.1, Structure and Function of the Tonsillar Ring).

The tongue and oral floor derive their *blood supply* from the lingual and sublingual arteries, which branch from the external carotid artery. Homonymous accompanying veins provide for drainage via the facial vein to the internal jugular vein.

*Lymphatic drainage* is handled by the ipsilateral and contralateral submandibular and submental lymph nodes, which drain to the lymph nodes at the junction of the facial and internal jugular veins (upper jugular lymph nodes; see **Fig. 16.2**).

▯ The potential for contralateral lymphogenous spread should always be considered in patients with malignant tumors.

Developmentally, the tongue is derived from structures of the first through fourth branchial arches (see 16.5). This accounts for the complex *innervation* of the tongue, which is supplied in varying degrees by cranial nerves V, VII, IX, X, and XII (see also **Fig. 16.3, Fig. 16.4, Fig. 16.5,** and **Fig. 16.6**). The tongue derives its motor innervation from the *hypoglossal nerve*. The terminal sulcus receives its sensory supply from the *lingual nerve*, which branches from the third division of the trigeminal nerve (see **Fig. 6.3**). Sensation to the tongue base region is supplied by the *glossopharyngeal* and *superior laryngeal nerves* (from cranial nerve X). The taste buds (sensory innervation) are supplied by the *chorda tympani* (from cranial nerve VII) in the anterior two-thirds of the tongue and by the *glossopharyngeal nerve* in the posterior third. The central gustatory pathways are described in 4.2.

**Fig. 4.5   Histology of the tongue**

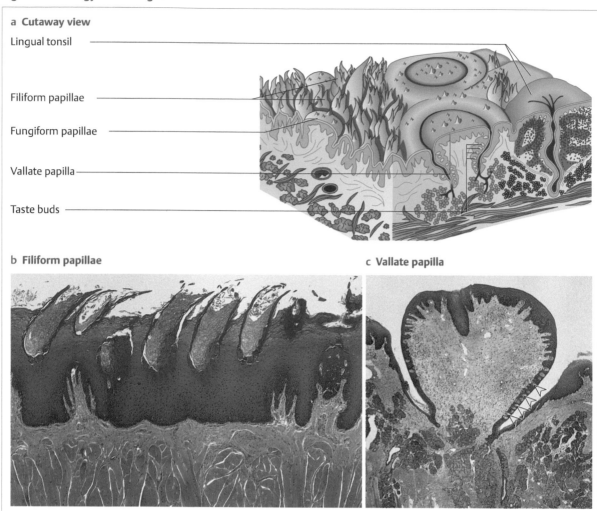

a **Cutaway view**

Lingual tonsil

Filiform papillae

Fungiform papillae

Vallate papilla

Taste buds

b **Filiform papillae**

c **Vallate papilla**

**a** The overall arrangement of the various papillae.
**b** The epithelium of the filiform papillae bears keratinized, threadlike (filiform) structures that are directed toward the pharynx (original magnification ×40).

**c** The vallate papillae are located at the junction of the body and base of the tongue. The epithelium in the pit surrounding the papilla contains numerous microscopic taste buds (arrows; original magnification ×100).
Source (**b, c**): Prof. U. Welsch, Munich, Germany.

## Physiology

### Importance for Food Intake

The **lips** are the gateway to the digestive tract, sealing the oral cavity during chewing and swallowing to prevent the spillage of food. The orbicularis oculi muscle is chiefly responsible for this task. If the function of this muscle is impaired (e.g., due to facial nerve palsy), the resulting deficiency of lip closure can cause eating difficulties as well as drooling from the corners of the mouth at rest.

Within the oral cavity itself, the **tongue** has major functional importance as a "multifunction organ" with both motor and sensory properties. The complex motor functions of the tongue, like its other functions, can be traced to a specialized developmental history,

which accounts for the sophisticated *nerve supply* derived from various cranial nerves (see above and **Fig. 16.4, Fig. 16.5, Fig. 16.6, Fig. 16.7**) and for the specialized muscular structure of the tongue (**Fig. 4.3**). The musculature of the tongue consists of extrinsic and intrinsic muscles. The *extrinsic muscles* are attached to the mandible and to the hyoid bone or styloid process, project into the body of the tongue, and greatly affect the position and movements of the tongue. The *intrinsic muscles* are composed of longitudinal, transverse, and vertical fiber systems and serve mainly to alter the shape of the tongue. The tongue muscles as a whole are distinguished by both their extreme mobility and their considerable strength. These properties play an essential role in swallowing (see 5.1, Physiology of Swallowing); they also influence the normal development of the maxilla and the dentition.

🔍 **4.2 Central gustatory pathways**

All gustatory fibers converge centrally in the area of the ipsilateral solitary tract, which ends at the solitary tract nucleus in the medulla oblongata; there, the signal is relayed to the second neuron (see also **Fig. 4.6**). The further course of the gustatory fibers is not yet fully understood. According to recent discoveries, the axons initially continue on to the medial parabrachial nucleus, where they synapse with the third neuron.

Reportedly, the fibers then travel via the dorsal trigeminothalamic tract, some crossed but most uncrossed, to the thalamus. The cortical taste areas themselves are located in the lateral part of the postcentral gyrus and in the adjacent insular cortex.

**Fig. 4.6 Central gustatory pathways**

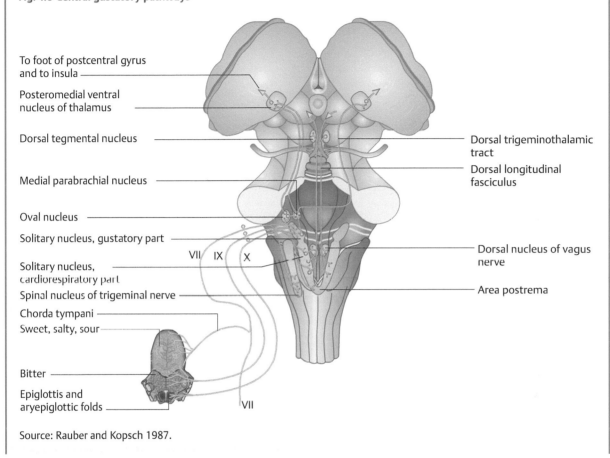

To foot of postcentral gyrus and to insula

Posteromedial ventral nucleus of thalamus

Dorsal tegmental nucleus

Medial parabrachial nucleus

Oval nucleus

Solitary nucleus, gustatory part

Solitary nucleus, cardiorespiratory part

Spinal nucleus of trigeminal nerve

Chorda tympani

Sweet, salty, sour

Bitter

Epiglottis and aryepiglottic folds

VII  IX  X

VII

Dorsal trigeminothalamic tract

Dorsal longitudinal fasciculus

Dorsal nucleus of vagus nerve

Area postrema

Source: Rauber and Kopsch 1987.

The **molars** have the greatest importance in chewing, because they are located closest to the insertion of the masticatory muscles themselves. This allows very high pressure to be developed between their occlusive surfaces.

### Taste

There are only four basic taste sensations: sweet, sour, salty, and bitter. The sensory experience of "taste" is a much more complex phenomenon, however, and results from a combination of olfactory, thermal, mechanical, and sensory impressions.

The precise mechanism that triggers a taste sensation or transmits a gustatory signal at the molecular level remains unknown. Various theories have been advanced

ranging from taste mediation by receptor proteins to taste activation through electrostatic interactions.

### Importance in Phonation and Articulation

The musculature of the lips has an essential role in phonation, while "lingual articulation" controls the production of vowels, certain consonants, and palatal sounds through changes in the shape and position of the tongue. Finally, the oral cavity joins with the pharynx, nose, and paranasal sinuses (see 📖1.3, Speech Production, and 📖18.1, Basic Principles of Speech Production) in forming the "supraglottic vocal tract," which plays a role in the coordination of vocal sounds.

# 4.2    Methods of Examining the Lips and Oral Cavity

Inspection of the lips and oral cavity is an essential part of every otolaryngologic examination. Some problems that cannot be adequately investigated by clinical examination alone (e.g., taste disturbances, tumors) may require additional diagnostic procedures (e.g., taste tests, imaging studies). Disturbances of taste are rare but can be very distressful for the patient. They are reversible in many cases, depending on the cause (see Table 4.1).

## Visual Inspection

After the lips have been inspected, the oral cavity is examined with the aid of a tongue blade. The examiner holds the instrument in the right hand while using the left hand to position and steady the patient's head.

🖉 Dentures should be removed before the examination is started.

The sequence of the examination is shown in **Fig. 4.7**. *Tongue mobility* is assessed by having the patient stick out the tongue. With hypoglossal nerve palsy, the tongue will deviate toward the affected side (**Fig. 4.8**). *Glossopharyngeal nerve palsy*, in which the uvula and palatal arches deviate toward the healthy side ("backdrop sign," **Fig. 4.8b**), is excluded by assessing the mobility of the soft palate. This is done by watching the soft palate while the patient says "ah" several times.

## Palpation

If inspection reveals questionable changes, the affected region or structure should next be palpated to better assess the consistency and depth of the suspicious finding. The cervical lymph nodes should also be palpated.

## Taste Testing

Abnormalities of taste are classified as *hypogeusia* (diminished sense of taste), *hypergeusia* (increased sensitivity of taste), or *ageusia* (absence of the sense of taste).

### Subjective Taste Testing

In the subjective test known as "**whole mouth test**," aqueous solutions of glucose, NaCl, citric acid, and quinine are applied to the tongue and remain in the oral cavity for some seconds to test the taste perception for the four basic qualities of sweet, salty, sour, and bitter. This screening test, while easy to perform, does not provide a high degree of reliability or reproducibility.

Fig. 4.7   Physical examination of the oral cavity

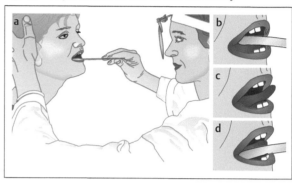

**a** Positions of the patient and examiner.
**b** The lips and cheeks are retracted from the teeth and alveolar ridge with a tongue blade to inspect the mucosa and assess the condition of the parotid duct orifice opposite the second upper molar.
**c** The patient elevates the tongue so that the examiner can evaluate the floor of the mouth and the submandibular duct orifices.
**d** The tongue is retracted with the blade so that the lateral oral floor can be examined.

**Electrogustometry** is another subjective test procedure in which sensations are evoked by applying a constant anodal current to the taste receptors of the tongue.
This test has methodology advantages over chemogustometry, providing better quantitative assessment of side-to-side differences and more accurate localization of responses.

## Objective Taste Testing

Objective taste tests based on gustatory evoked potentials, for example (analogous to objective hearing and olfactory tests), are possible in principle but are very costly. They are practiced only at large centers and are used mainly in examinations for disability assessment.

## Imaging Procedures

Since the anatomic structures of the oral cavity are easily accessible, the diagnosis can often be established by clinical examination alone (inspection, palpation, biopsy, or local excision of a suspected tumor). As a result, imaging procedures tend to have a limited role in

Fig. 4.8 Motor dysfunction of the tongue

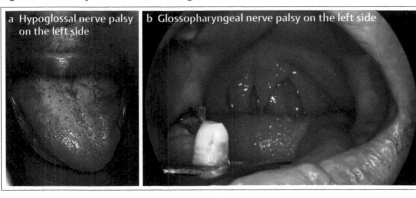

a Hypoglossal nerve palsy on the left side    b Glossopharyngeal nerve palsy on the left side

**a** The tongue deviates toward the affected side when protruded.
**b** The soft palate deviates toward the healthy side during phonation.

diseases of the lips and oral cavity. Nevertheless, there are various clinical situations (e.g., a tumor or extensive inflammatory process) in which a sectional imaging procedure can advance the diagnosis.

## Ultrasound

Basically, only B-mode instruments are useful for ultrasound examinations of the oral floor and tongue (**Fig. 4.9**), and real-time scanning is preferred. Transducers with an operating frequency in the 5 to 10 MHz range are used, depending on the desired penetration depth and resolution. Newer systems have multifrequency transducers that operate at variable frequencies.

## Computed Tomography and Magnetic Resonance Imaging

Normal findings are illustrated in **Fig. 5.9** and **Fig. 5.10**.
Computed tomography and magnetic resonance imaging are not only more cost-intensive than ultrasound but also more invasive in cases where contrast media are used.
**Indications**:
- Pronounced inflammatory changes (e.g., see **Fig. 4.20**).
- Tumors. Information on tumor extent, depth of invasion, and spread across the midline are important parameters in selecting the optimum treatment modality, especially for lesions involving the tongue and floor of the mouth (see ✍5.4, Tumors).

Magnetic resonance imaging offers advantages over computed tomography in its superior soft-tissue discrimination.

▯ If an imaging procedure is performed for confirmation (especially of a suspected tumor), the examination should include the soft tissues of the neck to check for regional lymph-node metastases.

Table 4.1  Causes of taste disorders

| Classification | Examples |
| --- | --- |
| Congenital | Aplasia of the taste buds |
| Endocrine disorders | Diabetes mellitus, hypothyroidism, adrenal insufficiency |
| Drug side effects | For example, D-penicillamine, various lipid-lowering drugs, ACE inhibitors, antifungals |
| Peripheral nerve lesions | Involvement of the chorda tympani by facial nerve palsy, otitis media or previous middle ear surgery; involvement of cranial nerve IX by tumors or fractures of the skull base; very rarely after tonsillectomy |
| Radiotherapy | Radiation damage to the papillae |
| Exogenous chemical agents | Alcohol, nicotine, mouthwashes |
| Central taste disorders | For example, head trauma, carbon monoxide poisoning, Alzheimer's disease, Parkinson's disease |

Abbreviation: ACE, angiotensin-converting enzyme.

Fig. 4.9  Ultrasound (B-mode) image of the tongue and oral floor

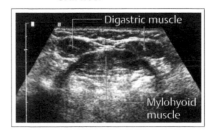

Digastric muscle
Mylohyoid muscle

Normal ultrasound anatomy of the oral floor. The transducer is placed submentally, resulting in an upside-down monitor image.

# 4.3 Malformations of the Lips and Oral Cavity

Malformations of the lips, cheeks, and oral cavity (especially those involving the palate and oral floor) are of epithelial origin. Although they are highly vari-able in their extent and clinical appearance, they are all based on a common teratogenic mechanism.

## Cleft Lip and Palate

*Epidemiology:* Clefts of the lip, palate, and alveolar ridge can occur in various combinations. They are among the most common malformations, with an incidence of 1 in 500.

*Classification:* The following main groups are distinguished:
- Cleft lip and alveolar ridge.
- Cleft lip, alveolar ridge, and palate and isolated cleft palate. The bifid uvula is a very mild variant of the cleft palate (**Fig. 4.10**).

*Symptoms:* Different clefts have a spectrum of clinical manifestations, depending on their morphology and extent:
- Hypernasal speech (rhinophonia aperta) due to incomplete closure of the nasopharynx.
- Recurrent middle ear effusions and inflammations resulting from eustachian tube dysfunction.
- Variable abnormalities of the nasal septum (septal deviation) or in the shape of the external nose.

> 🔎 **4.3 Pathogenesis of cleft lip and palate**
>
> While the pathogenesis of cleft lip and palate is not yet fully understood, basically it involves a developmental anomaly of the embryonic head. In addition to genetic inheritance, clefting can result from several external influences, such as viral infections, placental oxygen deficiency, intrauterine bleeding, and exposure to ionizing radiation.

**Fig. 4.10 Bifid uvula**

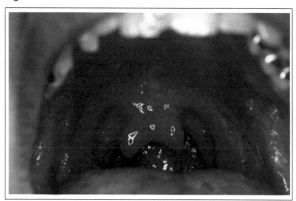

The photograph shows the characteristic appearance of a median cleft in the uvula.

**Fig. 4.12 Basic treatment plan for cleft lip and palate**

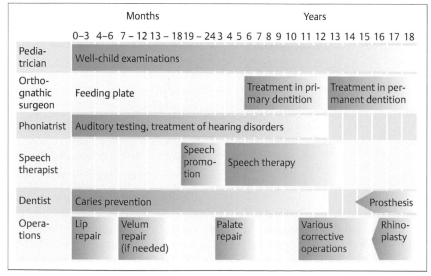

| | Months | | | | | Years | | | | | | | | | | | | | | |
|---|---|---|---|---|---|---|---|---|---|---|---|---|---|---|---|---|---|---|---|---|
| | 0–3 | 4–6 | 7–12 | 13–18 | 19–24 | 3 | 4 | 5 | 6 | 7 | 8 | 9 | 10 | 11 | 12 | 13 | 14 | 15 | 16 17 18 |
| Pedia-trician | Well-child examinations | | | | | | | | | | | | | | | | | | |
| Ortho-gnathic surgeon | Feeding plate | | | | | | | | Treatment in primary dentition | | | | | | Treatment in permanent dentition | | | | |
| Phoniatrist | Auditory testing, treatment of hearing disorders | | | | | | | | | | | | | | | | | | |
| Speech therapist | | | | | Speech promotion | Speech therapy | | | | | | | | | | | | | |
| Dentist | Caries prevention | | | | | | | | | | | | | | | | | | Prosthesis |
| Operations | Lip repair | | Velum repair (if needed) | | | Palate repair | | | | | | | Various corrective operations | | | | Rhino-plasty | | |

📖 4.4 Rare malformations involving the oral cavity

## Malformations of the intermandibular fusion zone

Anomalies of the intermandibular fusion zone are much rarer than cleft lip and palate. They include *dermoids* of the tongue, oral floor (**Fig. 4.11**), and mandible; *superficial median neck clefts*; and *clefts of the lower lip, mandible, and tongue.*

## Transverse facial cleft

Another, very rare anomaly is the transverse facial cleft (*cleft cheek, macrostomia, lateral facial cleft*), caused by either failure of fusion of the maxillary and mandibular processes or failure of the buccal membrane to regress due to fusion of the myoblasts. A transverse facial cleft is marked by bilateral extension of the oral fissure due to lateral displacement of the commissures and is frequently associated with facial dysplasia and auricular dystopia.

### Fig. 4.11 Dermoid cyst of the oral floor

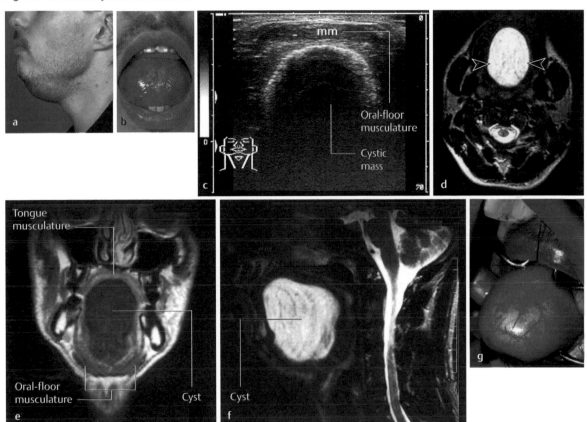

**a, b** The patient presents with submental swelling (**a**) and tense bulging of the entire anterior and lateral oral floor (**b**).
**c** A transverse ultrasound scan reveals displacement of the oral floor musculature by a cystic mass.
**d** An axial T2-weighted magnetic resonance image defines the lateral extent of the mass (arrows).
**e** Coronal magnetic resonance image (T1-weighted, post-contrast) demonstrates the relationship of the mass to the musculature of the oral floor and tongue.

**f** A sagittal T2-weighted image defines the anteroposterior extent of the mass in the direction of the tongue base. The streaky markings within the cystic mass are a motion artifact due to swallowing.
**g** The lesion was surgically removed via the anterior oral cavity, yielding a well-circumscribed, thin-walled mass loosely attached to the surrounding tissue and identified histologically as a dermoid cyst. An important *differential diagnosis* is a dysgenetic salivary-gland cyst (ranula), which also tends to occur in the anterior oral floor (see 📖 **6.2**).

***Diagnosis:*** Particularly with submucous clefts, the examination should include palpation of the hard palate to detect the bony discontinuity in that region.

***Treatment:*** The adequate treatment of cleft lip and palate requires close interdisciplinary teamwork among the pediatrician, otolaryngologist, maxillofacial surgeon, orthognathic surgeon, and phoniatrist (see **Fig. 4.12**).

# 4.4 Inflammations of the Lips and Oral Cavity

Inflammatory diseases of the oral cavity and lips are often on a continuum and can have a variety of causes. An underlying systemic disorder is frequently present. Viral agents, bacteria, fungi, contact aller-gens, and various autoimmune diseases can incite inflammatory changes in this region, which predominantly affect the mucous membranes.

## Viral Infections

### Herpes Simplex Virus

*Epidemiology and pathogenesis:* Herpes simplex virus (HSV) infections of the oral mucosa are most often caused by HSV type 1 (cutaneous and oral-mucosa strain), while infections with HSV type 2 more commonly affect the genital region. The virus may be transmitted by contact or droplet infection or occasionally through superficial skin injuries. About 85 to 90% of the adult population are seropositive for HSV, particularly in urban areas.

*Symptoms:* Primary infection with HSV is usually acquired in early childhood and predominantly affects the oral mucosa as **herpetic gingivostomatitis** (aphthous stomatitis). The appearance of local lesions (bullae) on the oral mucosa is preceded by fever and lethargy consistent with a flulike infection. This is often accompanied by regional lymphadenitis. In rare cases, the nasal mucosa is also involved (herpetic rhinitis). Special clinical forms are reviewed in ⌀ **4.5**. Reactivation of the HSV can occur in response to physical exertion, ultraviolet radiation, a febrile infection, emotional stress, or pregnancy (see also ⌀ **4.6**). Reactivation is most commonly manifested as *herpes labialis*. The site of predilection is the perioral region, especially the mucocutaneous junction of the lips (**Fig. 4.13**), but lesions sometimes occur in the mouth and nasal vestibule or on the cheeks, earlobes, or eyelids.

*Diagnosis:* The diagnosis is generally based on the *history* and *clinical examination.* Ordinarily, there is no need for viral culturing or costly methods of viral identification (electron microscopy, immuno-fluorescence microscopy, polymerase chain reaction). A simple method is to demonstrate classic giant cells by the cytologic examination of a Tzanck smear.

*Complications:* A feared complication is secondary bacterial *superinfection* by *Staphylococcus aureus* or streptococci. This infection frequently heals by scar-ring, in contrast to nonsuperinfected cases (**Fig. 4.14a**). An occasional complication is postherpetic *exudative erythema multiforme*, characterized by skin

**Fig. 4.13 Herpes simplex labialis**

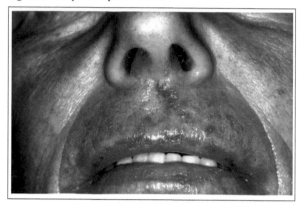

Typical clinical appearance with vesicles about the upper and lower lip.

---

⌀ **4.5 Severe forms of herpes simplex virus (HSV) infection**

A particularly severe form of HSV infection, known as Pospischill–Feyrter aphthoid, can occur in immunocompromised children or as a sequel to measles, rubella, or chicken-pox. A comparable form of this disease occurs much less frequently in immunocompromised adults and especially in HIV-infected patients.

A dreaded *complication of primary HSV infection* in children is **herpetic meningoencephalitis.**

---

⌀ **4.6 Theories on the reactivation of herpes simplex virus (HSV) infection**

The precise etiology of HSV reactivation is uncertain. Besides reinfection due to an exogenous cause, theories have focused mainly on an endogenous reactivation of the virus. The "precipitating factor" may be the integrated viral DNA in the host cells, which often is not detectable during latent periods but is able to induce the production of an "active" virus.

Another theory holds that the herpesviruses persist asymptomatically in the spinal cord, where they may be activated by any of several provocative mechanisms and then travel along sensory nerve fibers to corresponding sites on the skin or mucosa.

**Fig. 4.14 Complications of herpes simplex labialis**

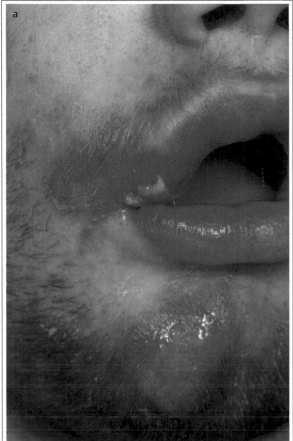

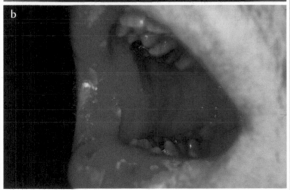

**a** Typical clinical appearance of bacterial superinfection in herpes labialis.
**b** Postherpetic exudative erythema multiforme.

lesions as well as typical ulcerative eruptions on the mucous membranes of the mouth, lips, and genitals (**Fig. 4.14b**).

***Treatment:*** The treatment of herpes simplex labialis should include the use of topical antiseptics to prevent superinfection. Acyclovir, administered as a topical ointment or systemically, is available for severe forms of the disease. Therapy is generally continued for 5 to 7 days, but some cases (especially immunosuppressed patients) may require a more prolonged course of treatment.

## Varicella Zoster Virus

***Pathogenesis:*** Chickenpox (varicella) and zoster are different clinical manifestations of infection with the varicella zoster virus (VZV). **Chickenpox** occurs predominantly in children and results from primary infection with the VZV. After the cutaneous lesions have healed, the virus persists in the ganglion cells of sensory nerves. **Zoster** occurs as a reinfection or results from reactivation of the virus in response to various provocative mechanisms—ultraviolet radiation exposure, infectious diseases, or weakened immune defenses due, for example, to immunosuppressant therapy or human immunodeficiency virus (HIV) infection; hence, it requires previous contact with the virus.

***Symptoms:*** **Chickenpox** presents with a characteristic skin rash consisting of erythematous papules and thin-walled vesicles with watery contents, covering the body but especially pronounced on the head and trunk. Aphthalike vesicles also consistently appear on the oral mucosa and especially on the hard palate, buccal mucosa, and gingiva.
**Zoster** presents clinically as a segmental disease, with cutaneous and mucosal lesions distributed along a sensory nerve segment and often accompanied by systemic signs such as lethargy, fatigue, and occasional neuralgiform pain in the distribution of the affected nerve. With involvement of the second and third divisions of the trigeminal nerve, aphthae or scalloped ulcerations can be found on the buccal mucosa, palate, and body of the tongue (see also ✑10.4, Herpes Zoster Oticus).

***Treatment:*** Zoster, like HSV infection, should be treated with a 5- to 7-day course of acyclovir or famciclovir. Analgesics and anti-inflammatory drugs (especially carbamazepine) can also be beneficial, and antibiotics may be indicated in elderly or immuno- compromised patients to prevent superinfection. The efficacy of adjuvant cortisone therapy for zoster is a controversial issue.

## Herpangina

Synonyms: vesicular pharyngitis, ulcerative pharyngitis.

***Epidemiology and pathogenesis:*** Herpangina is caused mainly by the group A coxsackievirus (CV), less commonly by the group B CV, and occasionally by retroviruses or echoviruses. The disease predominantly

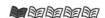

**Fig. 4.15 Herpangina**

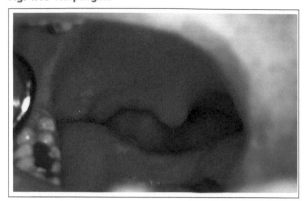

Typical clinical appearance, with aphthous lesions on the anterior faucial pillar.

affects young children but also occurs in adults and is often manifested in the spring and fall.

*Symptoms:* Besides systemic symptoms such as fever, malaise, headache, and muscle pain, bullous eruptions surrounded by a red halo appear on the oral mucosa, particularly affecting the anterior faucial pillars (**Fig. 4.15**), uvula, and palatine tonsils. As a rule, the vesicles rupture in a few days, leaving behind shallow ulcerations.

*Differential diagnosis:* The gingivostomatitis caused by HSV (see above) is considerably more painful and runs a longer course.

*Treatment:* Treatment is purely symptomatic and comprises of anti-inflammatory agents or mouth rinses with chamomile. The disease generally resolves in 14 days without complications.

## Inflammatory Mucosal Lesions in HIV Infection

Inflammatory lesions of the lips and oral cavity, while commonly observed in symptomatic HIV-infected patients, are not caused by the HIV itself but occur secondarily as a result of weakened host defenses.
**Candidiasis:** This disease, caused by *Candida albicans*, is the most common infection seen in HIV-positive patients (**Fig. 4.16**).

> 🔎 **4.7 Hand–foot–mouth disease**
>
> Hand–foot–mouth disease is also caused by coxsackieviruses and predominantly affects small children from 6 months to 5 years of age. *Clinically*, small bullae typically appear simultaneously on the palate, tongue, and gingiva as well as on the palms of the hands, fingers, toes, and soles of the feet. As in herpangina, *treatment* is symptomatic. The disease generally resolves in 1 to 2 weeks without complications.

**Fig. 4.16 Candidiasis in human immunodeficiency virus (HIV) infection**

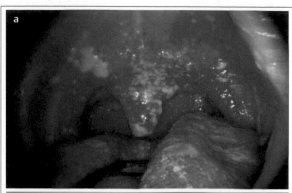

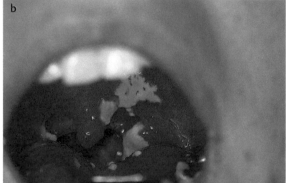

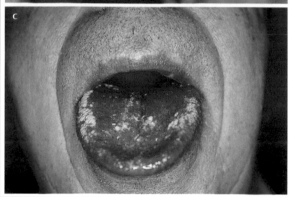

Typical whitish plaques on the oral mucosa.

**Viral infections:**
*Occurrence:* Viral pathogens also play a significant role in the setting of HIV infections. The most common infecting viruses are HSV, VZV, and cytomegalovirus (CMV), all of which can be cultured from mucosal lesions in HIV-infected patients. The occurrence of a CMV infection, like an HSV infection, has been identified as a potential cofactor for the progression of HIV disease and tends to affect patients with an advanced immune deficiency.
*Symptoms:* These diseases warrant special discussion, because their clinical features differ from those of the ordinary forms of these viral infections. This pertains to characteristic morphologic signs (e.g., a herpes simplex infection may have zosterlike manifestations) and to the course of the disease, which is markedly

Fig. 4.17 Cytomegalovirus infection

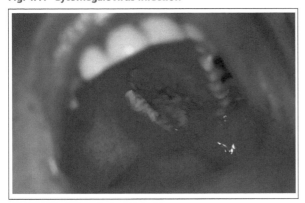

Typical clinical appearance of mucosal ulcerations with grayish-white plaques.

Fig. 4.18 Oral hairy leukoplakia

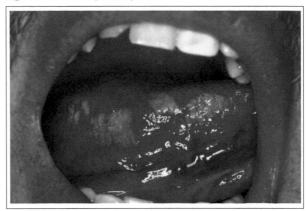

Typical whitish patches on the border of the tongue.

protracted in this subset of patients and is associated with more severe complaints (**Fig. 4.17**).

*Treatment:* Acyclovir is beneficial in HSV and VZV infections, but CMV is much less sensitive to this agent. CMV infections are treated with ganciclovir.

**Special form:** Another disease that has been linked to HIV infection since its initial description and is believed to have a viral cause is **oral hairy leukoplakia (OHL)**. The presence of OHL is basically considered pathognomonic for an HIV infection. Today, it is believed to be caused by the Epstein–Barr virus (EBV). The *clinical presentation* is marked by patchy, whitish, slightly raised lesions occurring predominantly on the border of the tongue (**Fig. 4.18**). Less commonly, the mucosal lesions are found in other regions of the oral cavity (buccal or lip mucosa, oral floor, soft palate). OHL typically runs a painless course, and dysphagia occurs only in cases with *Candida* superinfection. Despite their resemblance to leukoplakia (see **Fig. 4.26**), the lesions have not been known to undergo malignant transformation.

*Treatment* consists of local measures such as the topical application of vitamin A acid and/or podophyllin. Virostatics should not be used due to the high incidence of side effects, and the likelihood that OHL will recur within a few days after the drugs are discontinued.

HIV-infected patients are also predisposed to **bacterial** infections of the oral and pharyngeal mucosa. They have an increased incidence of acute and subacute tonsillitis as well as specific bacterial inflammations such as tuberculosis (see 🔖 5.4, Tuberculosis), atypical mycobacterial infections, and syphilis (50% of HIV-infected patients test seropositive for syphilis; see 🔖 4.10).

## Bacterial and Fungal Infections

### Oral Floor Abscess

Synonym: Ludwig's angina.

*Epidemiology:* Oral floor abscess is a rare disease that can become potentially life-threatening if the inflammatory process spreads to the deep cervical soft tissues and mediastinum.

*Pathogenesis:* In many cases, the inflammation originates from the lower molars. Less commonly, the disease develops from mucosal injuries in the oral floor, leading to abscess formation in the tongue muscles or connective-tissue spaces of the oral floor. The disease can also develop as a sign of impaired host resistance, as in the case of diabetic or immunosuppressed patients (especially children).

*Symptoms and diagnosis:* An oral floor abscess is manifested *clinically* by edematous expansion with a firm, erythematous swelling in the submental to submandibular areas (**Fig. 4.20a**). Patients complain of difficulty swallowing and speaking ("muffled speech"). High fever is also present. The downward spread of infection can lead to dyspnea with acute respiratory distress, and descending infection through the fascial compartments of the neck can incite a life-threatening mediastinitis. *Imaging* is necessary to define the extent of the oral floor abscess (often this cannot be done by physical examination alone due to local pain and induration). The principal options are ultrasonography and computed tomography (**Fig. 4.20b,c**).

*Differential diagnosis:* See 🔖 4.9.

*Treatment:* The treatment of choice is incision and drainage of the abscess via the intraoral and transcervical route. Concomitant antibiotic therapy should be appropriate for a mixed spectrum of aerobic and anaerobic organisms.

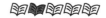

### 🔍 4.8  Recurrent aphthous stomatitis

Synonyms: benign aphthous disorders, canker sores, recurrent aphthous ulceration.

Aphthae are considered the most common inflammatory lesion of the oral mucosa and occur predominantly during the second and third decades of life. Approximately 40% of cases show a familial pattern of occurrence. The **etiology** is still unclear, although viruses of the herpes group (varicella zoster virus, cytomegalovirus) have been identified in some cases.

Various **precipitating factors** have been identified: minor trauma, hormonal changes (e.g., premenstrual), concomitant gastrointestinal disease, and "emotional stress." The disease has also been linked to iron, folic acid, or vitamin $B_{12}$ deficiency.

*Signs and symptoms*: Aphthae are inflammatory, shallow mucosal ulcerations with slightly raised erythematous borders and a tendency to recur. Three clinical variants of recurrent aphthous stomatitis are distinguished:

**Minor aphthae** (~80–90% of cases):

- Superficial, usually small (2–5 mm) ulcerations located in the anterior third of the oral cavity (**Fig. 4.19**).
- Heal without scarring, usually in about 1 week.

**Major aphthae** (~10%):

- Significantly larger (>10 mm) and deeper ulcerations.
- Heal with scarring in about 2 to 4 weeks.
- Greater severity of complaints.
- Often accompanied by tender, enlarged regional lymph nodes.

**Herpetiform aphthae** (~5%):

- Very small aphthae showing a herpeslike arrangement.
- Mild systemic effects.

*Differential diagnosis*: Early differentiation from *Behçet's disease* (see 🔍 **4.15**) is necessary for prognostic reasons and is critical for proper diagnostic and therapeutic management. It is important to watch for accompanying symptoms such as fever, lethargy, joint pain, and ocular signs, since severe oropharyngeal symptoms in themselves can also occur with major aphthae.

The differential diagnosis should also include the various viral diseases of the oral mucosa such as *herpes simplex* (see above), *herpangina* (see above), and *hand–foot–mouth disease* (🔍 **4.7**). The **treatment** of recurrent aphthous stomatitis is symptomatic and may include the frequent topical application of astringents (tincture of myrrh) or mouth rinses with special pain-relieving electrolyte solutions (e.g., Hanks' solution). Deficits can be corrected by means of iron, folic acid, and/or vitamin $B_{12}$ replacement. Chronic recurrent lesions may also benefit from the topical application of corticosteroid gel alternating with antiseptic mouth rinses.

**Fig. 4.19  Typical appearance of a benign aphthous disorder on the tip of the tongue**

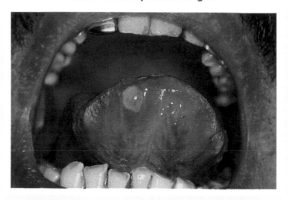

### 🔍 4.9  Differential diagnosis of oral floor abscess

The differential diagnosis of a suspected oral floor abscess should include an abscess of the submandibular or sublingual glands as well as **actinomycosis**, in which subcutaneous infection by the bacterium *Actinomyces israelii* can cause an indurating infiltration of the fatty tissue in the oral floor region. The complaints differ from the symptoms of an oral floor abscess in that actinomycosis is less painful and tends to form an external fistula.

## Lingual Abscess

Overt or covert mucosal injuries to the tongue can become infected, resulting in a lingual abscess (**Fig. 4.21**). The *diagnosis* is established unequivocally by the clinical appearance of the tongue. *Treatment* is surgical and consists of incision and drainage of the abscess with concomitant antibiotic therapy.

## Candidiasis

Candidiasis of the oral mucosa (synonym: thrush) occurs in persons with weakened host resistance due to radiation or cytostatic therapy, diabetes mellitus, long-term antibiotic use, corticosteroid inhalations, leukosis or leukopenia due to a different cause, or HIV infection.

***Symptoms:*** Clinical examination of the oral cavity reveals whitish, firmly adherent plaques that can be scraped from the mucosa, leaving an erythematous, bleeding surface (**Fig. 4.16**).

***Treatment:*** Oral candidiasis is treated with topical antifungal agents such as nystatin solution or amphotericin-B lozenges. Every case should be treated, for otherwise the infection could spread to deeper portions of the alimentary tract (candida esophagitis) causing severe dysphagia, decreased food intake, and rapid weight loss.

**Fig. 4.20  Oral floor abscess (Ludwig's angina)**

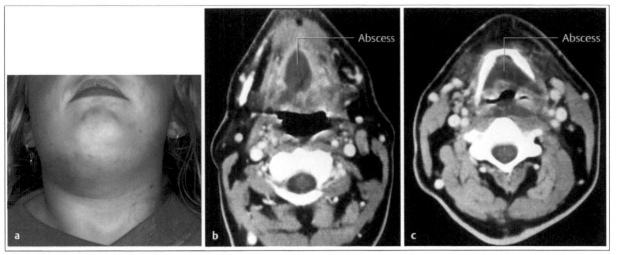

**a** Typical clinical presentation, with erythematous swelling about the oral floor.

**b, c** Sequential axial computed tomography scans show the abscess, which originates from the oral floor (**b**) and extends downward (**c**).

### 4.10  Syphilis

*Clinical features:* Although lesions of the oral and oropharyngeal mucosa can occur in all stages of syphilis, the manifestations in the primary and secondary stages are most important for the differential diagnosis of mucosal lesions in these regions. Three weeks pass until the **primary lesion** appears. The sites of predilection for extragenital primary lesions, after the perianal region, are the oral cavity and oropharynx. Besides the lips and buccal mucosa, the tonsil (unilateral) and tongue are most commonly affected. The primary chancre is painless and appears as an initially papular lesion that gives way to an erosive or ulcerative eruption. Concomitant regional lymphadenopathy (*bubo*) is frequently present and is also painless.

The **secondary stage** begins approximately 6 weeks after the primary lesion appears, as the disease becomes generalized due to hematogenous spread of the microorganisms. The most commonly affected sites are the skin and mucous membranes.

The mucosal syphilids (mucous plaques) are a dangerous source of infection, as they are teeming with infectious organisms.

The syphilitic enanthema in the secondary stage typically consists of patchy, reddish lesions on the hard and soft palate and buccal mucosa. An even more common finding is *specific angina*. In contrast to the unilateral tonsillar changes in the primary stage, both palatine tonsils are inflamed and covered with grayish-white coatings. A sweetly fetid breath odor is also present. A particularly severe form of secondary syphilis is *malignant syphilis*, which occurs predominantly in immunosuppressed and especially HIV-infected patients.

The **tertiary stage** may develop within a period of 3 to 5 years. Lesions of the oral and oropharyngeal mucosae are less common at this stage, but *gummata* (syphilitic granulomas) are occasionally found on the soft palate and uvula and also on the tonsil (unilateral). The tonsillar gumma appears as a sharply circumscribed ulcer with a greasy coating on its base and may initially be mistaken for a primary lesion, but the latter is almost always associated with painless regional lymphadenopathy.

*Interstitial glossitis* is another, rare intraoral manifestation of tertiary syphilis.

*Differential diagnosis:* If specific angina is suspected, the differential diagnosis should include *diphtheria*, in which the mucosal lesions spread to involve the soft palate and uvula. It is important to differentiate interstitial glossitis from the innocuous *fissured tongue* (see **Fig. 4.23**).

*Diagnosis:* **Identification of the causative organism** from the primary lesion can be accomplished with dark-field microscopy (the only reliable test in the early primary stage). **Serologic tests** such as the *Treponema pallidum* hemagglutination (TPHA) test or fluorescent treponemal antibody absorption (FTA-ABS) test are not positive until 3 weeks after the infection is acquired. A good **follow-up test** is the cardiolipin complement binding reaction (CBR), a modification of the Wassermann reaction whose titers correlate with the patient's response to therapy.

*Treatment:* Penicillin G (600,000 IU daily for 14 days) is the drug of choice for all stages of the disease. It is replaced by erythromycin in patients allergic to penicillin.

Syphilis serology should be retested at the conclusion of treatment.

**Fig. 4.21 Lingual abscess**

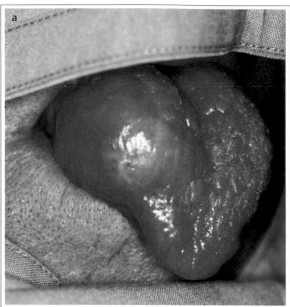

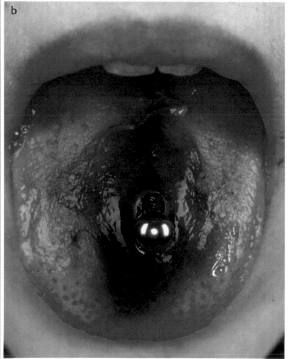

**a** Clinical examination reveals a tense, dorsal swelling on the right side of the tongue.
**b** A dorsal lingual abscess has formed around a foreign body used for tongue piercing.

## Superficial Tongue Lesions

Lesions in the surface of the tongue may reflect systemic diseases and thus provide important clues to the patient's general state of health. Therefore, besides harmless morphologic variants and localized inflammatory lesions, medical disorders should always be considered in the differential diagnosis of these changes.

### Hunter's Glossitis

Synonym: atrophic glossitis.

Hunter's glossitis is an atrophic inflammatory condition of the tongue base. It is an accompanying feature of pernicious anemia. Common **symptoms** are burning of the tongue, dry mouth, and altered sense of taste. Clinically, the tongue presents a typical smooth, shiny appearance with partial atrophy of the filiform papillae.

---

**4.11 Geographic tongue**

Geographic tongue (synonym: benign migratory glossitis) is marked by areas of desquamation of the filiform papillae on the dorsal surface of the tongue. The affected areas are irregularly shaped but are clearly demarcated relative to surrounding areas. The disease is harmless, and histologic examination shows signs of inflammation. Generally, the only symptom is an occasional burning sensation. Treatment is unnecessary.

---

**4.12 Black hairy tongue**

**Features**: Black hairy tongue (synonym: lingua villosa nigra) is due to a hyperkeratosis of the filiform papillae, imparting a furry appearance to the tongue (**Fig. 4.22**).
**Pathogenesis**: The papillary elongation may result from failure of desquamation of the cornified layers or an excessive formation of keratin.
**Etiology**: Various precipitating mechanisms have been discussed. Besides antibiotic and corticosteroid use, they mainly include chronic mucosal irritation from oral hygiene procedures or nicotine abuse as well as metabolic disorders (e.g., diabetes mellitus), vitamin deficiency, and wasting diseases.
**Treatment**: Many cases are adequately managed by eliminating the causal factors or underlying disease.

**Fig. 4.22 Black hairy tongue**

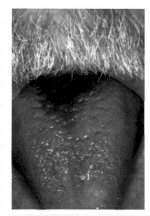

**Fig. 4.23 Fissured tongue**

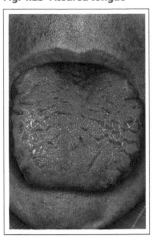

Typical appearance, with conspicuous furrows in the dorsal surface of the tongue

## Fissured Tongue

Fissured tongue, characterized by the presence of numerous furrows on the dorsal surface of the tongue, is a harmless hereditary condition that affects approximately 10 to 15% of the population. Lingual fissures may also be a sign of Melkersson–Rosenthal syndrome (see ✍14.2, Differential Diagnosis of Idiopathic Facial Paralysis).

*Clinically*, the tongue presents a characteristic appearance (**Fig. 4.23**). The *differential diagnosis* should include interstitial glossitis in tertiary syphilis (see ✍ **4.10**).

## Angioedema

*Definition:* Angioedema denotes a transient, frequently pronounced vascular reaction which, in the head and neck region, can lead to swelling of the face, lips, tongue, and larynx (see also ✍17.5, Angioneurotic Laryngeal Edema, Acute Laryngeal Edema).

*Pathogenesis:* This disease occurs as one feature of an anaphylactic or anaphylactoid reaction. Drugs such as acetylsalicylic acid and angiotensin-converting enzyme (ACE) inhibitors are known to precipitate an attack. With ACE inhibitors, bradykinin appears to have a major pathogenic role. By contrast, the forms caused by a C1-esterase inhibitor (C1-INH) deficiency are much less common. Angioedema due to C1-INH deficiency may be hereditary or acquired.

*Clinical manifestations:* The disease is characterized by sometimes massive facial swelling that is most pronounced in the periorbital region but also affects the lips, tongue, tongue base, and laryngeal area. Massive tongue swelling in particular can cause acute obstruction of the upper airways. The hereditary form is additionally characterized by swelling of the extremities and episodes of abdominal pain.

*Treatment:* The cause of the angioedema is a key factor in selecting the appropriate treatment. The treatment of choice for angioedema not induced by a C1-INH deficiency is symptomatic treatment with corticosteroids or epinephrine (especially in the form of the disease induced by ACE inhibitors).

In the form that is induced by a C1-INH deficiency, direct replacement with a C1-inhibitor concentrate should be provided in acutely life-threatening cases with swelling of the tongue and larynx.

> ✂ Antihistamines and cortisone preparations are of little or no benefit in this form of angioedema.

## Immunologic Diseases

Systemic lupus erythematosus, see ✍ **4.13**.
Pemphigus vulgaris, see ✍ **4.14**.
Behçet's disease, see ✍ **4.15**.
Erythema multiforme, see ✍ **4.16**.
Lichen planus, see ✍ **4.17**.

## Fixed Drug Eruption

A fixed drug eruption is a delayed (type IV) allergic reaction that occurs at the same cutaneous or mucosal sites (e.g., the extremities, soles of the feet, palms of the hands, external genitalia, oral mucosa) following repeated drug use. Particularly with mucosal involvement, the disease is characterized by superficial erosions that may resemble an HSV infection due to their scalloped margins. The eruption may be induced by

---

✍ **4.13 Systemic lupus erythematosus**

Systemic lupus erythematosus is a chronic inflammatory systemic disease of the vascular connective tissue with cutaneous involvement and the potential involvement of almost all the organs.

The *etiopathogenesis* of the disease is not yet fully understood. Besides genetic factors (familial incidence in 10% of cases), causal significance has been attributed to hormonal changes (symptoms worsen during estrogen therapy and pregnancy), viral involvement, ultraviolet radiation exposure, and various drugs (e.g., isoniazid, sulfonamide, phenytoin, penicillamine).

*Signs and symptoms:* The oral mucosa is involved in 40% of cases. The lesions appear as edematous erythematous areas, erosions, or ulcerations covered by fibrinous exudate and located on the hard palate, buccal mucosa, and tongue. In rare cases, the oral lesions precede other cutaneous and organ manifestations of the disease (e.g., polyarthritis, serositis, renal involvement, central nervous system involvement, hematologic changes).

*Diagnosis:* Besides further clinical evaluation by a dermatologist, special laboratory tests are necessary to establish the diagnosis (see textbooks of dermatology).

*Treatment* is geared toward the course of the disease and should be directed by the dermatologist.

### 4.14 Pemphigus vulgaris

*Pathophysiology*: Pemphigus vulgaris is an autoimmune disease characterized by the formation of antibodies directed against adhesion proteins in the epidermis. These antibodies can be detected in affected mucocutaneous areas and in the serum.

The *etiology* is uncertain. Besides a genetic disposition, the disease has been attributed to ultraviolet radiation exposure and various medications (e.g., phenylbutazone, indometacin, ibuprofen, tuberculostatic drugs). The disease may also occur spontaneously, however, and it occasionally coexists with other autoimmune diseases (e.g., myasthenia gravis).

*Clinically*, 50% of patients with pemphigus vulgaris show involvement of the oral mucosa with bullous eruptions or saliva-macerated bullae that can make eating extremely difficult.

*Diagnosis* relies mainly on the immunologic detection of pemphigus antibodies; elevated titers correlate with an exacerbation of symptoms. The diagnosis is most quickly established by the histologic or immunohistologic analysis of affected mucosal areas (see textbooks of dermatology).

*Treatment*: Initial treatment consists of systemic corticosteroids, whose use has led to a significant decline in the mortality of the disease. The addition of immunosuppressants is frequently indicated and can reduce the necessary corticosteroid dose. The most widely recommended local measures are oral rinses with anti-inflammatory or anesthetic solutions.

*Prognosis*: Untreated, the disease may lead to death within a period of months or years, generally due to secondary complications such as sepsis or bronchopneumonia.

### 4.15 Behçet's disease

Behçet's disease occurs predominantly in eastern Mediterranean countries (especially Turkey) and in Japan but is becoming more prevalent in Western urban areas as a result of immigration.

*Etiology*: A viral etiology has been suggested in addition to an autoimmune mechanism.

The *major features* of the disease are oral aphthae, aphthous genital ulcers, and hypopyon iritis. The *minor features* are polyarthritis, gastrointestinal symptoms, and vascular lesions.

The *diagnostic criteria* for Behçet's disease are either the presence of the three major features or the presence of two major and two minor features.

*Treatment* depends on disease severity and includes the use of corticosteroids. Cytostatics and immunosuppressants may also be required. Oral mucosal lesions can be treated locally with mouth rinses (chamomile) or pyoktanin (2%).

### 4.16 Erythema multiforme

*Etiology and pathogenesis*: Erythema multiforme (EM) has a multifactorial etiology. Known precipitating causes are *viral infections* such as HSV infections, hepatitis B, mumps, and measles. The main *bacterial agents* are streptococci infecting the upper respiratory tract. The disease may also occur in the setting of diphtheria or syphilis. Other causes are *drug side effects* (sulfonamides, pyrazolone derivatives, barbiturates, penicillins, phenothiazines). *Systemic diseases* such as polyarteritis nodosa, Wegener's granulomatosis, systemic lupus erythematosus, and various malignancies (lymphoma, carcinoma) also have causal significance.

*Signs and symptoms*: A minor form of EM, marked initially by bulla formation on the oral mucosa and lips and later by erosive lesions (see **Fig. 4.14b**), is distinguished clinically from a **major form** (Stevens–Johnson syndrome). Major EM runs a very severe course and may develop following a herpes infection or in response to certain drugs. Besides erythematous

areas on the extremities and buttock, conspicuous mucosal erosions appear predominantly on the lips, oral mucosa, and pharynx. These lesions are very painful and interfere with eating. There may also be ocular involvement in the form of conjunctivitis, keratitis, iritis, or uveitis.

Systemic signs consist of generalized weakness, headache, and high fever. Severe cases may develop renal and cardiopulmonary disorders ranging to renal failure or toxic circulatory collapse.

*Treatment*: Due to the painful involvement of the oral mucosa, adequate food and fluid intake should be stressed (and may necessitate parenteral nutrition). **Milder forms** of the disease may respond satisfactorily to local treatments (rinsing with chamomile solution, local anesthetics if required). Corticosteroids are the agents of choice for the **severe forms**, accompanied by the administration of a broad-spectrum antibiotic to prevent superinfection.

Patients with frequent bouts of severe, postherpetic EM may benefit from **long-term prophylaxis** with acyclovir.

analgesics, anti-inflammatory agents (e.g., pyrazolone, phenylbutazone, phenazone), antibiotics (penicillin, tetracyclines, erythromycin), chemotherapeutic agents, sulfonamides, and certain hypnotics (e.g., barbiturates) and laxatives (phenolphthalein). Treatment consists of avoiding the suspicious substances.

## 4.17 Lichen planus

The **etiology** of lichen planus (LP) is unknown. Besides an immune pathogenesis in the setting of viral diseases (e.g., hepatitis B and C), there appears to be an association with certain medications (e.g., antimalarial drugs, organ arsenic compounds, gold salts). A psychosomatic mechanism is also likely, since lesions often appear following severe emotional trauma or other stressful situations.

**Signs and symptoms:** The disease often affects the skin and mucosae concomitantly, with mucosal involvement occurring in 25 to 70% of patients. Lesions are particularly common on the oral mucosa (**Fig. 4.24**) and the vermilion border of the lips. Diagnosis can be difficult due to the variable clinical manifestations of the disease.

Oral lesions most typically appear as **reticular white markings** on the mucosa of the cheek (**Fig. 4.24**) and tongue (*Wickham's phenomenon—requires* histologic differentiation from leukoplakia!). But **painful ulcerations** may also occur (*erosive LP*), requiring differentiation from the lesions of pemphigus vulgaris, systemic lupus erythematosus, and stage II syphilis.

**Treatment:** A variety of treatments have been recommended for LP ranging from antibiotics and tuberculostatics to antimalarial drugs. Most therapies tried to date have been unconvincing because they were not applied in a controlled-study framework. Corticosteroids are of *symptomatic* benefit, and aromatic retinoid and isotretinoin combined with corticosteroids are recommended for the treatment of mucosal lesions.

Oral rinses with anti-inflammatory and local anesthetic solutions are recommended mainly for very painful, erosive intraoral lesions.

The **prognosis** of LP is guarded in terms of a complete recovery. It is common for oral mucosal lesions to persist for years, especially in the erosive form of the disease. Since it is now believed that LP is a potentially premalignant disease, regular **follow-ups** are also essential.

Fig. 4.24 **Lichen planus of the left cheek**

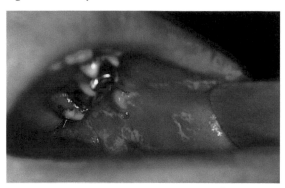

## 4.18 Burning mouth syndrome

Burning mouth syndrome is a symptom complex characterized by a burning sensation and other soreness in the oral cavity, often with an absence of objective mucosal findings. Although the tongue is most commonly affected ("burning tongue"), involvement of the hard palate, alveolar ridge (especially in denture wearers), and other regions of the oral cavity (buccal mucosa, oral floor, mucosal surfaces of the lips) has also been described. Concomitant xerostomia and dysgeusia are occasionally reported.

Burning mouth syndrome is most prevalent in postmenopausal women.

**Causes:**
- Local:
  - Dentures.
  - Candidiasis.
  - Geographic tongue.
  - Allergic mucosal reactions (e.g., to sorbic acid, nicotinic acid, cinnamaldehyde).
  - Toxic mucosal reactions (e.g., to nickel sulfate or mercury).
  - Radiotherapy.
- Systemic:
  - Iron-deficiency anemia.
  - Vitamin $B_{12}$ deficiency.
  - Vitamin $B_1$, $B_2$, and $B_6$ deficiency.
  - Folic acid deficiency.
  - Sjögren's disease.
  - Menopause.
  - Diabetes mellitus.
  - Human immunodeficiency virus infection.
  - Drug side effects (angiotensin-converting enzyme inhibitors).
- Psychogenic:
  - Depression.
  - Cancerophobia.
  - Emotional stress.

# 4.5    Tumors of the Lips and Oral Cavity

Benign tumors of the lips and oral cavity, while rare, can occur as neoplasms of the various epithelial and mesenchymal tissues in this region. Among the precancerous lesions, leukoplakia is particularly important because of its morphologic similarity to carcinoma in situ. Malignant tumors of the lips and particularly the oral cavity have become more prevalent in past decades as a result of alcohol and nicotine abuse and today are counted among the most frequent head and neck malignancies along with pharyngeal and laryngeal cancers (see ✑5.3–5.5 and ✑17.7).

## Benign Tumors

Benign tumors of the lips and oral cavity can arise from all epithelial and mesenchymal tissues in the head and neck region but are relatively rare. Besides papillomas (**Fig. 4.25a**) and pleomorphic adenomas (**Fig. 4.25b**), various mesenchymal tumors can occur such as fibromas, lipomas, rhabdomyomas, leiomyomas, and chondromas. There are also hemangiomas (**Fig. 4.25c**) and lymphangiomas, which are congenital in most cases.

*Treatment:* Treatment is generally surgical and is indicated for patients who describe symptoms and in cases in which it is necessary to exclude a malignant tumor.

*Hemangiomas* and *lymphangiomas* are a special case. Due to the high rate of spontaneous remission during the first years of life, conventional surgical treatment or laser surgery is advised only if the tumor persists beyond that period, provided the patient does not have serious symptoms such as dyspnea or dysphagia that would necessitate earlier surgical intervention. Radiotherapy is no longer advocated for these tumors

**Fig. 4.25  Benign tumors of the oral cavity**

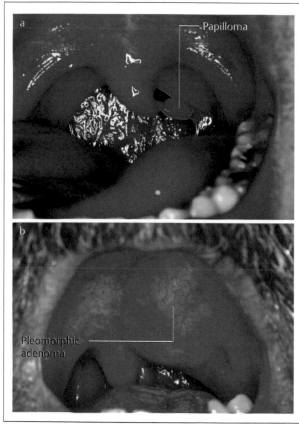

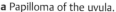

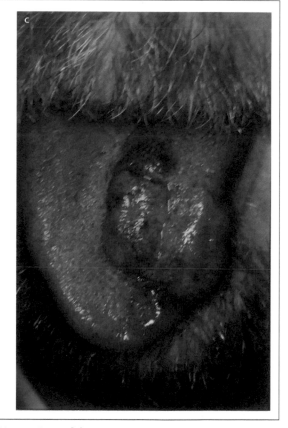

**a** Papilloma of the uvula.
**b** The bulge in the palate is caused by a pleomorphic adenoma arising from the palatal salivary glands.

**c** Hemangioma of the tongue.

**Fig. 4.26 Leukoplakia of the oral mucosa**

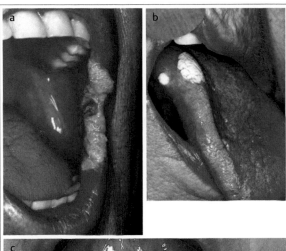
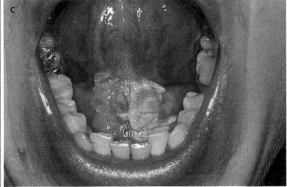

Typical whitish plaques at the oral commissure (**a**), on the tongue (**b**), and on the anterior part of the oral floor (**c**).

due to the potential for adverse sequelae (malignant transformation, growth disturbance).

## Precancerous Lesions

**Leukoplakia** is the most common precancerous lesion of the lips and oral cavity (**Fig. 4.26**). Many of these lesions are asymptomatic and are detected incidentally. Exogenous irritants such as denture pressure or alcohol/nicotine abuse have been most strongly implicated as causal factors. Given their morphologic resemblance to carcinoma in situ and invasive carcinoma and their potential for malignant degeneration, leukoplakic lesions should always be investigated by biopsy. The treatment of choice is complete surgical removal of the neoplasm.

**Bowen's disease** of the oral mucosa, a chronic inflammatory disease caused by an intraepidermal carcinoma, is rare by comparison. Its morphologic features are similar to those of leukoplakia.

**Table 4.2  Classification of malignant tumors of the lip and oral cavity according to the Union for International Cancer Control (UICC) system**

| | Definition | |
|---|---|---|
| T1 | Dimension ≤ 2 cm and depth ≤ 5 mm | |
| T2 | Dimension ≤ 2 cm and depth > 5–10 mm or dimension > 2–4 cm and depth ≤ 10 mm | |
| T3 | Dimension > 4 mm or depth > 10 mm | |
| T4a | *Lip:* | Through cortical bone, inferior alveolar nerve, floor of mouth, skin |
| | *Oral cavity:* | Through cortical bone of the mandible or maxillary sinus, or skin of face |
| T4b | *Lip and oral cavity:* | Masticator space, pterygoid plates, or skull base, or encases internal carotid artery |
| N1 | Ipsilateral single ≤ 3 cm without ENE | |
| N2 | • Ipsilateral single > 3–6 cm without ENE<br>• Ipsilateral multiple ≤ 6 cm without ENE<br>• Bilateral or contralateral ≤ 6 cm without ENE | |
| N3 | ENE-positive or > 6 cm without ENE | |

Abbreviation: ENE, extranodal extension.
Source: Brierley et al 2017.

## Malignant Tumors

### Malignant Tumors of the Lips

Malignant tumors of the lips (for classification see **Table 4.2**) are almost invariably **squamous cell carcinomas** and most commonly affect the lower lip (~90% of cases). They occur predominantly in pipe smokers. Prolonged, intense sun exposure is considered a cofactor.

***Symptoms and diagnosis:*** Early tumors often appear clinically as "intractable" ulcerations in the vermilion border of the lip (**Fig. 4.27a**, **Fig. 4.28a**) but may also consist of large, exophytic lesions (**Fig. 4.27b**). Whenever a tumor is suspected, a biopsy should be taken to confirm the diagnosis.

***Differential diagnosis:*** Differentiation is mainly required from keratoacanthoma and a primary syphilis chancre (see ✑ **4.10**). Basal cell carcinoma (see **Fig. 3.55**) involves the vermilion border of the lip only by secondary spread.

***Treatment:*** The treatment of choice is almost always surgical excision followed by a local primary closure or plastic repair of the defect using various reconstructive techniques (**Fig. 4.27c–g** and **Fig. 4.28b–d**). As a rule,

Fig. 4.27 Malignant tumors of the lower lip

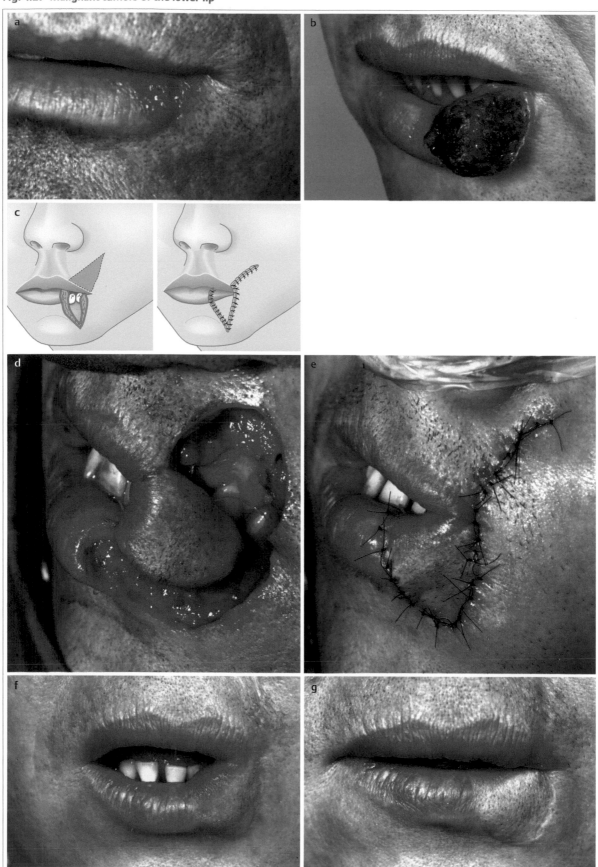

Fig. 4.28 Malignant tumor of the upper lip

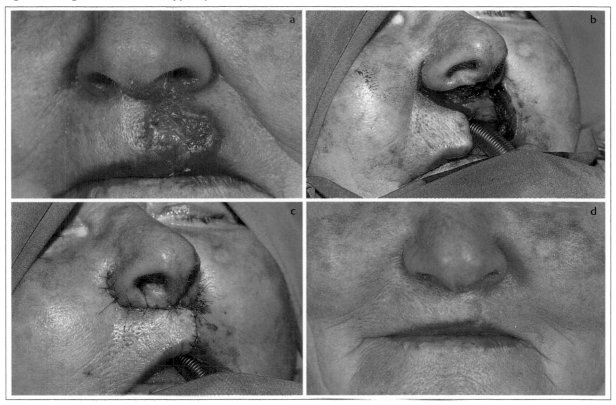

a Ulcerated carcinoma of the upper lip, extending to the nasal base.
b, c The resection defect is closed primarily by mobilizing a flap from the nasolabial fold.

d One year later, the operative site is healed and free of irritation.

even extensive tissue defects can be repaired using regional flap techniques. Carcinomas of the lip have an inherently low rate of metastasis to regional lymph nodes, but a neck dissection should be performed in patients with category 2 or higher tumors (see ✎16.5, Malignant Tumors of the Cervical Lymph Nodeas, and **Fig. 16.23**).

a, b The clinical appearance of T1 (a) and T2 (b)squamous cell carcinomas, which present different morphologic features.
c The diagram illustrates a technique for reconstructing a post-resection defect in the lower lip.
d The flap is mobilized from the upper lip and transposed into the lower lip defect.
e Appearance after flap inset and closure of the donor defect in the upper lip.
f Good flap healing is seen 6 weeks after the operation. A "commissure plasty" can be performed at this stage to extend the obliterated left oral commissure.
g Appearance 3 months after the first operation.

## Malignant Tumors of the Oral Cavity

**Squamous cell carcinomas** also predominate in the **oral mucosa** and are variable in their clinical appearance (**Fig. 4.29**). Approximately 90% of patients have a long history of nicotine and alcohol abuse, and nearly 75% of malignant tumors form in the drainage area of the oral cavity—i.e., the trough between the base of the alveolar ridge and the border of the tongue (**Fig. 4.29a, Fig. 4.30a**).

*Symptoms:* Symptoms vary with the location and extent of the tumor and may consist of painful swallowing, blood-tinged saliva, and a fetid breath odor. Some tumors are completely asymptomatic, however.

*Diagnosis:* **Visual inspection** can raise the suspicion of a malignant neoplasm. This should be followed by **bimanual palpation**, since many tumors infiltrate deeper tissues and the visual impression of superficial findings can be misleading. The clinical examination also includes palpation of the regional cervical lymph nodes to exclude metastases. **Imaging procedures** (ultrasound, computed tomography, magnetic resonance imaging) are generally necessary only for extensive masses, as many tumors can be adequately

**Fig. 4.29  Malignant tumors of the oral cavity**

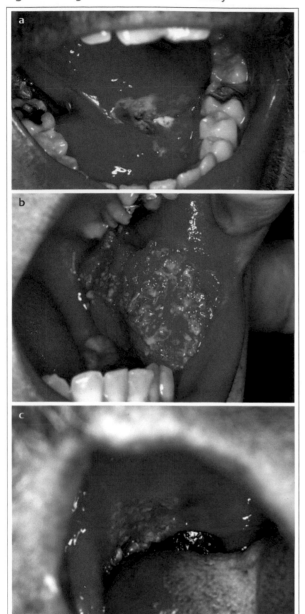

The typical clinical appearance of squamous cell carcinoma of the oral floor (**a**), buccal mucosa (**b**), and soft palate (**c**).

### 4.19  Malignant tumors of the oral cavity in patients infected with human immunodeficiency virus

Human immunodeficiency virus (HIV)-positive patients have a disproportionately high incidence of malignant tumors because of their weakened immune status. Most of these lesions in the oral cavity are **Kaposi's sarcomas**. A smaller percentage are various types of **B cell lymphoma**.

Kaposi's sarcomas were first seen in association with HIV infection in the early 1980s. They are present in approximately 20% of affected homosexual and bisexual men but occur in less than 5% of HIV-infected individuals from other risk groups. The tumor has a variable appearance, depending on its location in the oral cavity. The hard palate is considered a site of predilection in this region (**Fig. 4.31a**). **Fig. 4.31b** illustrates Kaposi's sarcoma of the tongue.

**Fig. 4.31  Kaposi's sarcoma of the hard palate (a) and tongue (b)**

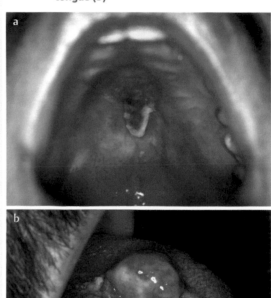

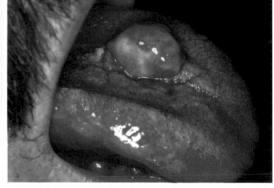

evaluated clinically owing to their exposed location. But with more advanced lesions, imaging is valuable for defining the depth of tumor infiltration and assessing the involvement of adjacent structures (bone). It is also an important tool for excluding regional cervical lymph-node metastases.

***Treatment:*** The treatment of choice in most cases is **surgical removal** of the primary tumor. The resulting defect is either closed primarily or reconstructed using pedicled flaps (see **Fig. 4.30**) or microvascular free transfers (e.g., a radial forearm flap). A unilateral or bilateral neck dissection (see 16.5, Malignant Tumors of the Cervical Lymph Nodeas) may be necessary, depending on the location and T category of the primary tumor (see **Table 4.2**). **Radiation** to the tumor site and lymph areas is frequently indicated following surgery. Primary radiotherapy or combined radiochemotherapy may be considered as alternatives for T3 and T4 tumors.

***Prognosis:*** The prognosis of oral malignancies depends on the location and stage of the disease. The 5-year survival rate varies accordingly, ranging from 0 to 80%.

Fig. 4.30  **Surgical treatment of oral floor carcinoma**

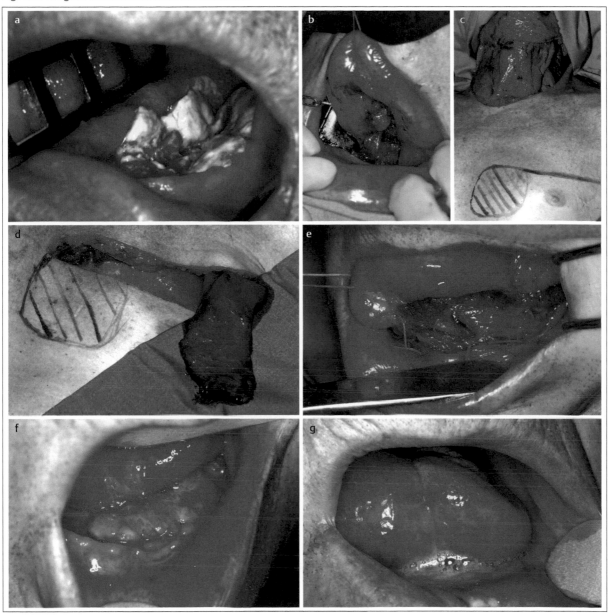

**a** The typical location of an oral floor carcinoma in the drainage area of the oral cavity between the alveolar ridge and border of the tongue. After resection of the tumor, which has infiltrated the tongue (**b**), a pedicled myofascial flap (here a myofascial pectoralis major flap; see also **Fig. 3.14**) is outlined beneath the skin of the chest, mobilized, swung into the tissue defect, and sutured into place (**c–e**). **f** One month later, granulation tissue is still present in the previous tumor defect that was reconstructed with the myofascial flap. **g** The texture of the mucosa appears almost normal 21.2 months after the operation.

# 5 Pharynx and Esophagus

## 5.1 Anatomy, Physiology, and Immunology of the Pharynx and Esophagus

The pharynx is a tubular, fibromuscular space extending from the skull base to the inlet of the esophagus (upper esophageal sphincter). Anatomically and clinically, the pharynx consists of a nasal part (nasopharynx), an oral part (oropharynx), and a laryngeal part (hypopharynx). The entire pharynx is bounded externally by several muscle systems, which perform diverse functions and are continuous distally with the muscles of the esophageal wall.

The primary function of the pharynx and esophagus is to coordinate the act of swallowing, which is regulated by a complex interaction of various cranial nerves and peripheral muscular and connective-tissue structures located in the oral cavity, pharynx, and esophagus. The pharynx also contains the tonsillar ring, a series of lymphoepithelial organs that are important in the immune response to infection. Finally, portions of the pharynx function as a variable resonance chamber for modulating vocal sounds.

### Nasopharynx, Oropharynx, and Hypopharynx

#### Anatomic Extent

**Nasopharynx:** This highest part of the pharynx extends from the bony skull base to an imaginary horizontal line at the level of the velum (**Fig. 5.1**). It communicates with the nasal cavity via the choanae and with the middle ear via the orifice of the eustachian tube. The nasopharynx is bounded *superiorly* by the floor of the sphenoid sinus and pharyngeal roof. Also in this region is the pharyngeal tonsil, which forms part of the tonsillar ring (see below). *Medial* to the eustachian tube orifice, the tubal cartilage forms a projecting lip called the torus tubarius. The concavity behind it is termed the pharyngeal recess (Rosenmüller's fossa) (see **Fig. 5.8b**). The nasopharynx is bounded *posteriorly* by the curve of the first cervical vertebra, with its overlying prevertebral cervical fascia and prevertebral musculature.

**Oropharynx:** The oral cavity communicates via the faucial isthmus (see **Fig. 4.1**) with the oropharynx, which extends inferiorly from the lower boundary of the nasopharynx to the upper margin of the epiglottis (see **Fig. 5.1**). It is bounded anteriorly by the tongue base and lingual tonsil (see **Fig. 4.4**) and posteriorly by the second and third cervical vertebrae with their prevertebral fascia. It is bounded laterally by the faucial pillars (tonsillar pillars; see 4.1), which flank the palatine tonsils.

**Hypopharynx:** The lowest pharyngeal segment is the hypopharynx, which extends from the superior border of the epiglottis to the inferior border of the cricoid cartilage plate of the larynx (**Fig. 5.1**), where it joins with the esophagus. Lying posterior to the hypopharynx are the third through sixth cervical vertebrae. Its anterior wall is formed by the back of the larynx, which protrudes into the hypopharynx and forms two lateral mucosal pouches (piriform sinuses), which rejoin at the level of the esophageal inlet.

#### Mucosal Lining

The mucosa that lines the **nasopharynx** consists of several rows of ciliated epithelium. At the **oropharynx**, this gives way to a stratified, nonkeratinized squamous epithelium, which also lines the **hypopharynx**.

#### Pharyngeal Musculature

The muscular boundaries of the pharynx are formed by the constrictor pharyngis muscle group. The highest of these muscles, the *constrictor pharyngis superior*, begins at the level of the nasopharynx just below

---

🔎 **5.1 Weak points in the wall of the hypopharynx**

Three muscular weak points exist in the lower posterior wall of the hypopharynx. The first is **Killian's triangle**, located between the constrictor pharyngis inferior and the uppermost fibers of the cricopharyngeus muscle. The second area of weakness is the **Killian–Jamieson region** between the oblique and transverse fibers of the constrictor pharyngis. The third is **Laimer's triangle**, which is bounded above by the cricopharyngeus and below by uppermost fibers of the esophageal musculature (see also **Fig. 5.2**). Killian's triangle is a particularly common site for the formation of hypopharyngeal diverticula.

Fig. 5.1 Anatomy of the pharynx

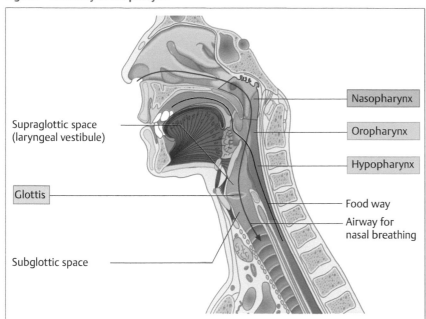

Anatomy of the nasopharynx (blue), oropharynx (yellow), and hypopharynx (green) shown in midsagittal section.

Supraglottic space (laryngeal vestibule)

Nasopharynx

Oropharynx

Hypopharynx

Glottis

Food way

Airway for nasal breathing

Subglottic space

Fig. 5.2 Musculature of the pharynx and esophagus

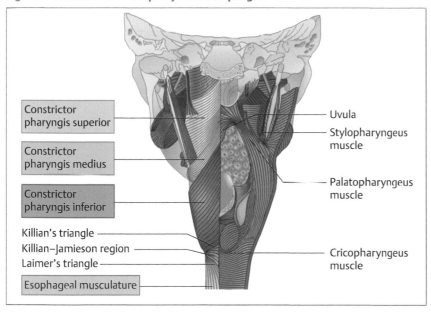

Various muscles contribute to the wall structure of the pharynx and esophagus.

Constrictor pharyngis superior

Constrictor pharyngis medius

Constrictor pharyngis inferior

Killian's triangle

Killian–Jamieson region

Laimer's triangle

Esophageal musculature

Uvula

Stylopharyngeus muscle

Palatopharyngeus muscle

Cricopharyngeus muscle

the tough, fibrous pharyngobasilar fascia, which in turn is suspended from the bony skull base; just below the superior constrictor muscle are the overlapping *constrictor pharyngis medius* and *inferior* muscles, the latter of which joins distally with the esophageal musculature (**Fig. 5.2**).

While most of the constrictor pharyngis muscle fibers run obliquely, the lowest portions of the constrictor pharyngis inferior (cricopharyngeal part) run directly horizontally, creating anatomic weak spots in the pharyngeal wall (*Laimer's* and *Killian's triangles*; 5.1). These weak spots are sites of predilection for the development of pulsion (Zenker) diverticula in the hypopharynx (see **Fig. 5.31**).

Three additional pairs of external muscles are distributed to the pharyngeal wall and assist in controlling vertical movements of the pharynx: the stylopharyngeus, the salpingopharyngeus, and the palatopharyngeus (**Fig. 5.2**).

## Neurovascular Supply

The pharynx receives its *blood supply* from the territory of the external carotid artery (branches of the facial artery, maxillary artery, ascending pharyngeal artery, lingual artery, and superior thyroid artery). The veins of the pharynx drain into the internal jugular vein. The *lymphatic drainage* of the upper portions of the pharynx is through the retropharyngeal lymph nodes, while the lower portions drain to the parapharyngeal or deep cervical nodes.

*Nerve supply:* The muscles and mucosa of the pharynx receive their motor and sensory innervation from the pharyngeal plexus, which in turn receives fibers from the glossopharyngeal and vagus nerves. The plexus itself is located on the outer aspect of the constrictor pharyngis medius muscle.

## Parapharyngeal Space

The parapharyngeal space encompasses an anatomically well-defined region with the shape of an inverted pyramid whose base is formed by the inferior surface of the petrous bone and whose apex is at the lesser horn of the hyoid bone.

The parapharyngeal space is divided anatomically into two parts, the retropharyngeal space and the **lateral pharyngeal space**. The latter in turn is subdivided by the common connective-tissue sheath of the muscles arising from the stylohyoid process (stylopharyngeal aponeurosis) into a prestyloid and a retrostyloid part. The *prestyloid part* communicates with the parotid compartment. It contains the lateral and medial pterygoid muscles, lingual nerve, optic ganglion, and maxillary artery. Its lower part is directly adjacent to the tonsillar compartment. The *retrostyloid part* of the lateral pharyngeal space is traversed by neurovascular bundles made up of the internal carotid artery, internal jugular vein, and lower cranial nerves (IX–XII).

The **retropharyngeal space** contains smaller arterial and venous vessels and, most notably, the retropharyngeal lymph nodes that drain the nasopharynx.

## Esophagus

The esophagus begins at the upper esophageal sphincter, located at the level of the C6 and C7 vertebrae (inferior border of the cricoid cartilage). The esophagus terminates at the gastric cardia in the plane of the T10 vertebra (**Fig. 5.3a**).

The three **physiologic constrictions** of the esophagus are clinically important due to the tendency for ingested foreign bodies to become lodged at those levels (**Fig. 5.3b**):

- *Upper constriction:* in the area of the esophageal inlet between the cricoid cartilage and the cricopharyngeal part of the constrictor pharyngis inferior muscle.

**Fig. 5.3 Anatomy of the esophagus**

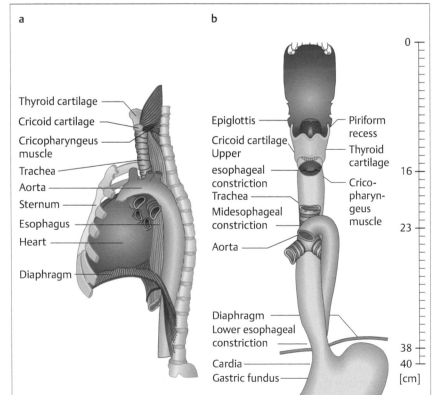

a Thyroid cartilage
Cricoid cartilage
Cricopharyngeus muscle
Trachea
Aorta
Sternum
Esophagus
Heart
Diaphragm

b Epiglottis
Cricoid cartilage
Upper esophageal constriction
Trachea
Midesophageal constriction
Aorta
Diaphragm
Lower esophageal constriction
Cardia
Gastric fundus

Piriform recess
Thyroid cartilage
Cricopharyngeus muscle

0
16
23
38
40
[cm]

**a** The esophagus extends from C6/C7 to the gastric cardia at the level of the T10 vertebra.
**b** The three physiologic constrictions of the esophagus and their relationship to surrounding structures. The numerical scale shows distance in centimeters from the upper incisor teeth.

- *Middle constriction:* where the aortic arch crosses over the tracheal bifurcation.
- *Lower constriction:* where the esophagus pierces the diaphragm.

The **wall structure** of the esophagus adheres to the pattern of the gastrointestinal tract as a whole, consisting of several layers:
- The mucosa, composed of stratified, nonkeratinized squamous epithelium.
- The submucosa.
- The muscularis, consisting of inner circular and outer longitudinal muscle fibers:
  - Upper fourth of the esophagus: striated fibers.
  - Second fourth: mixed striated and smooth fibers.
  - Lower half: smooth fibers.
- The adventitia.

## Neurovascular Supply

*Blood supply:* The cervical part of the esophagus receives most of its blood supply from the inferior thyroid artery (and a lesser amount from branches of the subclavian and vertebral arteries). The thoracic esophagus is supplied by the aorta and intercostal arteries, and the abdominal esophagus by the left gastric artery and left inferior phrenic artery.

Venous blood in the neck is drained by the inferior thyroid vein. Thoracic and abdominal drainage is to the azygos and hemiazygos veins and esophageal veins.

*Lymphatic drainage* is to the lymph nodes of the posterior mediastinum and pulmonary hilum.

*Nerve supply:* The upper, cervical part of the esophagus is supplied with branches from the recurrent nerve and the lower part with unnamed branches from the vagus nerve. Below the tracheal bifurcation is the esophageal plexus, formed by the two vagus nerves.

## Physiology of Swallowing

Normal swallowing requires a coordinated interaction of various anatomic structures in the oral cavity, pharynx, larynx, and esophagus. From a functional standpoint, the voluntarily initiated oral phase of swallowing is distinguished from an "involuntary" pharyngeal phase and esophageal phase, which are controlled through reflex mechanisms (**Fig. 5.4**).

During the **oral phase** of swallowing, food is broken down and moistened to form a bolus that is moved toward the oropharynx. This is accomplished mainly by pressing the food against the hard palate with the tongue (**Fig. 5.4**, ①).

The **pharyngeal phase** begins when the bolus comes into contact with receptors in the throat (especially on the tongue base), eliciting an involuntary swallowing reflex (②). The afferent impulses for this reflex travel through the glossopharyngeal and vagus nerves, while the efferent neurons that supply the pharyngeal muscles arise from cranial nerves V3, VII, IX, X, and XII.

*⧄ The extensive nerve supply highlights the complexity of swallowing as well as the potential vulnerability of this process.*

While the involuntary swallowing reflex is triggered during the pharyngeal phase, the velum is elevated to close off the nasopharynx (③). The larynx is also sealed off by elevation of the epiglottis (④). This is accompanied by a reflex adduction of the vocal cords (⑤), allowing the food to pass through the piriform sinuses toward the esophagus while bypassing the larynx (⑥). The **esophageal phase** of swallowing begins with a primary peristaltic wave, which is reflexly initiated in response to movement of the bolus through the pharynx (cranial nerves IX, X) (⑦). Secondary peristalsis is additionally triggered in the esophagus by the pressure of the bolus against the esophageal wall (⑧).

Through the coordinated action of these mechanisms, the bolus is transported into the stomach within 7 to 10 seconds.

## Structure and Function of the Tonsillar Ring

### Anatomy

The **tonsillar ring** (Waldeyer's ring) is composed of a series of lymphoepithelial "organs" called the tonsils. This tissue is structurally similar to lymph nodes but lacks afferent lymphatic vessels.

The tonsils are named for their location, consisting of a *pharyngeal tonsil*, the paired *palatine tonsils*, and the unpaired *lingual tonsil* at the base of the tongue. Additionally, smaller condensations of lymphoepithelial tissue are found in the pharyngeal recess (see **Fig. 5.8**) and in the "lateral bands" (tubopharyngeal folds) on the posterior wall of the oropharynx and nasopharynx. The **epithelium** of the tonsils also varies by location. While the *pharyngeal tonsil* is covered mainly by multiple rows of ciliated epithelium, the *palatine* and *lingual tonsils* are covered by stratified, nonkeratinized squamous epithelium.

### Structure of the Palatine Tonsil

The palatine tonsil has special immunologic importance among the tissues of the tonsillar ring owing to its distinctive morphology. Its surface is invaginated by crypts–fold-like tissue indentations that are lined by porous epithelium and substantially increase the surface area of the tonsil. This arrangement facilitates

**Fig. 5.4   Physiology of swallowing**

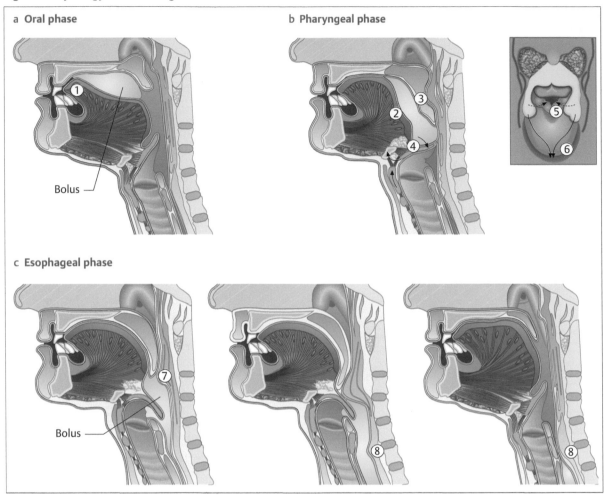

The circled numbers refer to the main text which describes the oral, pharyngeal, and esophageal phases of swallowing. Source: Netter 1975.

contact between inspired or ingested antigens and the subepithelial lymphatic tissue.

Within the lymphatic tissue, *primary follicles* are formed during embryonic development and differentiate into secondary follicles after birth (**Fig. 5.5a**). The secondary follicles mainly contain B lymphocytes at various stages of differentiation, along with scattered T lymphocytes (**Fig. 5.5b–d**).

Besides the lymph follicles, there are also *extrafollicular areas* with B and T lymphocytes that enter the lymphatic tissue through the postcapillary venules.

### Functional Importance of the Tonsils in the Immune System

The palatine tonsil in particular is considered to be an "immune organ" that plays a significant role in the defense against upper respiratory infections. By analogy with comparable lymphoepithelial tissue masses in

the bronchi and intestinal tract, the lymphatic tissue in the tonsillar ring is also termed the *mucosa-associated lymphatic tissue (MALT)* of the upper respiratory tract. Accordingly, this tissue has the ability to mount specific immune reactions in response to various antigens.

The activity of this lymphatic organ is especially pronounced during childhood, when immunologic challenges from the environment induce hyperplasia of the palatine tonsils (**Fig. 5.6**). Following this "active phase" of immune initiation, which lasts until about 8 to 10 years of age, the lymphatic tonsillar tissue becomes less important as an immune organ, and there is a corresponding decline in the density of lymphocytes in all regions of the tonsils. While the tonsils become less important immunologically with aging, the tonsillar tissue continues to perform immune functions even at an advanced age, although this should not alter the decision to remove the tonsils if a valid

Fig. 5.5 **Histology and immunohistochemistry of the tonsils**

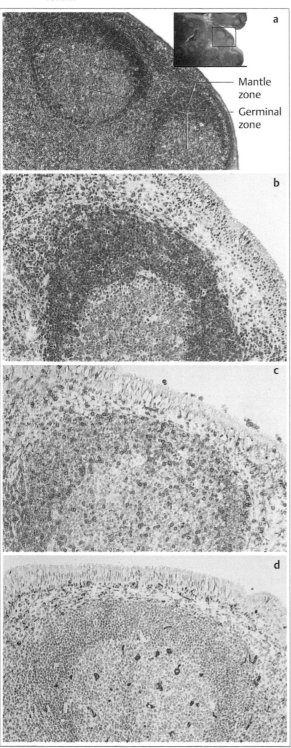

Fig. 5.6 **Tonsillar hyperplasia**

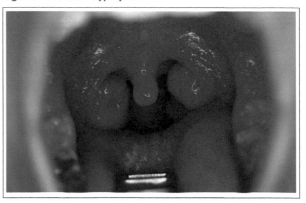

The size and activity of the germinal centers are maximal at ~6–8 years of age, reflecting the immunologic activity of the palatine tonsil. They decline steadily thereafter. Tonsillar hyperplasia develops in many children during this "active immunization phase."

indication for tonsillectomy exists (see 5.4, Chronic Tonsillitis).

While the tonsils are "learning" their immune function during childhood, extreme tonsillar hyperplasia ("kissing tonsils") may develop, leading to functionally significant narrowing of the faucial isthmus, with eating difficulties and obstructed breathing. Especially when recumbent, these children may experience significant respiratory dysfunction, with periods of apnea. They also have an increased long-term risk of developing cor pulmonale. Consequently, there should be little hesitation in recommending tonsillectomy, even in small children.

## Phonation and Articulation

Besides the oral cavity (see 4.1), the pharynx also functions as a variable resonance chamber for phonation and articulation.

**a** The histologic section shows the characteristic epithelium-covered surface invaginations in the palatine tonsil (crypts). The secondary follicles in the lymphatic tissue, which are essential for tonsillar immune function, feature a light-colored germinal zone and a dark mantle zone with mature lymphocytes.
**b–d** Immunohistochemical sections of various antibody-labeled cells in the pharyngeal tonsillar tissue (ABC method with hemalum counterstain).

**b** B lymphocytes (CD22-labeled) outnumber other lymphocytes and are located mainly in the mantle zone.
**c** T lymphocytes (CD3-labeled) are not only distributed throughout the follicle, but are also found in the interfollicular region and epithelium.
**d** Section showing KP1-labeled macrophages.

# 5.2    Methods of Examining the Pharynx

Clinical examination of the pharynx is an essential part of any otolaryngologic examination and relies on various techniques. Besides the classic mirror examination, diagnostic endoscopic procedures have been increasingly utilized in recent years.

Imaging procedures have also assumed major importance in the investigation of various pharyngeal disorders. This trend is due largely to the advent of computed tomography (CT) and magnetic resonance imaging (MRI), while conventional radiographs have become largely obsolete in the investigation of diseases of the pharynx. On the other hand, conventional radiographs are still an essential tool for the investigation of many esophageal disorders.

## Mirror Examination and Endoscopy

### Nasopharynx

The location of the nasopharynx can make it very difficult to access and examine, especially for beginners. Before the advent of endoscopy, the only technique available for examining the nasopharynx was **posterior rhinoscopy** (**Fig. 5.7**). The establishment of endoscopic techniques has dramatically improved the diagnostic evaluation of the nasopharynx.

**Endoscopy:** Nasopharyngeal endoscopy may be performed using a *transoral* or *transnasal technique*. The latter technique is described fully in ✎2.1 and permits the nasopharynx to be examined from the front. It can also provide detailed views of the eustachian tube region, the pharyngeal recess, and other difficult-to-reach sites (see ✎5.1, Nasopharynx, Oropharynx, and Hypopharynx). *Transoral endoscopy* is basically a postrhinoscopic technique that provides the examiner with an excellent overview of the nasopharynx.

*Transoral endoscopic technique:* With the tongue pulled forward (to enlarge the space between the soft palate and posterior pharyngeal wall), the endoscope is introduced into the oral cavity over the left mandibular teeth and advanced past the uvula to the posterior wall of the pharynx (**Fig. 5.8**).

### Oropharynx

Most structures of the oropharynx can also be evaluated during the examination of the oral cavity. The technique is shown in **Fig. 4.7**. The palatine tonsils are evaluated for their symmetry and mobility, and for the presence of any coatings or ulcerations. A laryngeal mirror or telescopic laryngoscope (see ✎17.2) should be used to examine the tongue base and the lateral walls of the oropharynx.

### Hypopharynx

Clinical examination of the hypopharynx (mirror examination, endoscopy) is performed concurrently with the examination of the larynx (see ✎17.2).

### Esophagus

The esophagus can be examined by means of flexible or rigid endoscopy.

**Flexible esophagoscopy** can be performed under local anesthesia, is generally well tolerated, and allows for concomitant examination of the stomach and duodenum. It is the technique generally preferred by internists.

**Rigid esophagoscopy** can also be performed under local anesthesia in principle, but it is more comfortable for the patient and examiner to conduct the procedure under general endotracheal anesthesia. Rigid

**Fig. 5.7    Posterior rhinoscopy**

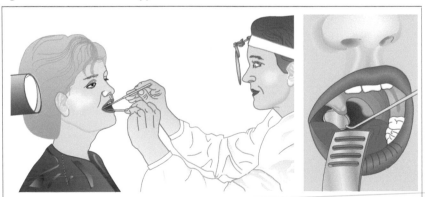

The tongue is carefully depressed with a tongue blade, and then a small, prewarmed mirror is introduced between the soft palate and posterior pharyngeal wall. The mirror should not touch the mucosa to avoid evoking a gag reflex. Structures that can be evaluated with this technique include the posterior ends of the turbinates, the choanae, the posterior margin of the vomer, and the various structures of the nasopharynx (see **Fig. 5.8**).

esophagoscopy provides a better overview, particularly when looking for foreign bodies, because the advancing rigid scope tends to flatten out the mucosal lining, making it easier to detect trapped foreign objects.

## Imaging Procedures

### Conventional Radiographs

In the area of conventional radiography, the **oral contrast examination** is the most valuable technique for diagnosing hypopharyngeal (see **Fig. 5.31**) and esophageal diverticula, tumors, stenoses, and disorders of esophageal motility.

Various contrast media can be used (e.g., barium, Gastrografin, Ultravist, Isovist), depending on the nature of the investigation and any preexisting disorders.

⚕ If there is a risk or suspicion of a perforation, barium should not be used.

Another conventional radiographic technique, used mainly in patients with equivocal swallowing disorders, is **high-speed cineradiography**. This technique can be used to evaluate the different phases of swallowing with high temporal resolution (~50 images per second).

### Computed Tomography and Magnetic Resonance Imaging

The modern sectional imaging modalities of CT and MRI have significantly advanced the diagnosis of pharyngeal tumor masses as well as certain inflammatory processes in this region. MRI (**Fig. 5.9**) has proven particularly effective for the soft-tissue discrimination of tumors in relation to surrounding structures, while CT (**Fig. 5.10**) is the method of choice for confirming or excluding osseous involvement.

**Fig. 5.8 Transoral endoscopy of the nasopharynx**

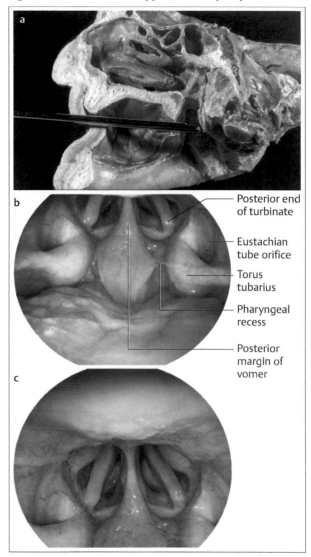

Posterior end of turbinate

Eustachian tube orifice

Torus tubarius

Pharyngeal recess

Posterior margin of vomer

**a** The tip of the endoscope has been positioned between the soft palate and the posterior wall of the pharynx in an anatomic specimen.
**b** Normal view through a 90-degree endoscope, showing the posterior ends of the turbinates, the posterior margin of the vomer, the eustachian tube orifice, and the torus tubarius.
**c** The same area viewed with a 120-degree endoscope.

**Fig. 5.9 Magnetic resonance imaging of the pharynx: normal findings**

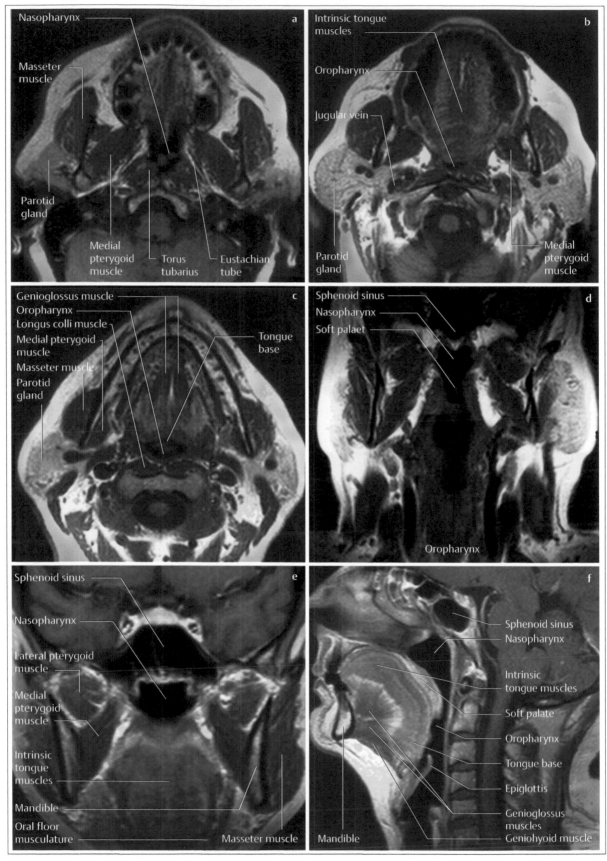

T1-weighted magnetic resonance images. **a** Nasopharynx: axial, without contrast medium. **b** Oropharynx: axial, with contrast medium. **c** Oropharynx: axial, with contrast medium. **d** Oropharynx: coronal, without contrast medium. **e** Oropharynx: coronal, with contrast medium. **f** Oropharynx: sagittal, with contrast medium.

**Fig. 5.10   Computed tomography of the pharynx (axial plane): normal findings**

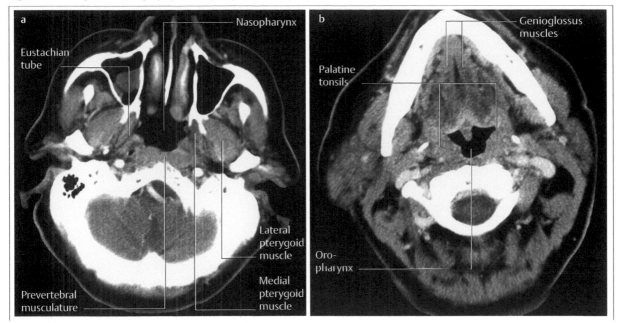

**a** Nasopharynx.
**b** Oropharynx.

# 5.3    Diseases of the Nasopharynx

Diseases of the nasopharynx can have strikingly different causes at different ages. While adenoids are most common in children, tumors predominate in adults. Because lesions of the nasopharynx are difficult to examine and may produce nonspecific symptoms, malignant tumors in particular are apt to go undetected for some time. Modern endoscopic techniques using a high-intensity light source, together with the new sectional imaging modalities, have brought significant improvements, particularly in the early detection of nasopharyngeal lesions.

## Adenoids

Synonyms: polyps, adenoid vegetations.

"Adenoids," the common term for *hyperplasia of the pharyngeal tonsil*, is a very widespread condition in children 3 to 6 years of age. The proliferation of lymphatic tissue in this region is so common in children that it can hardly be considered an abnormal condition, and nearly all children have some degree of adenoid hypertrophy due to the immunologic activity of that tissue. As a result, enlarged adenoids should be considered abnormal and treated accordingly only if they are causing symptoms. Not infrequently, the presence and severity of adenoidal symptoms depend on the relationship between the size of the nasopharynx and that of the adenoids.

*Clinical manifestations:* Common symptoms of adenoids are chronic nasal airway obstruction ("mouth breathing"; **Fig. 5.11a**), nasal discharge ("runny nose"), snoring, anorexia, and a hyponasal voice (rhinophonia clausa). Also, many young patients have frequently recurring infections of the nose and paranasal sinuses with otitis media and chronic impairment of eustachian tube ventilation, caused, for example, by adenoid tissue obstructing the tubal orifices. Prolonged conductive hearing loss (see 9.1), especially during the first 3 to 4 years of life, can lead to delays in speech development. Finally, chronic mouth breathing can lead to maxillary deformity and dental malalignment. Many of these young patients also have enlarged tonsillar lymph nodes at the mandibular angle (**Fig. 5.11a**).

*Diagnosis:* Besides posterior rhinoscopy or endoscopy (see 2.1 and 5.2), the diagnostic work-up includes microscopic examination of the tympanic membrane (otoscopy; see 8.1). Often, this will show retraction of the tympanic membrane or a middle ear effusion resulting from chronic impairment of eustachian tube ventilation, with negative pressure in the middle ear. Additionally, hearing should be tested in adenoid patients (pure-tone audiogram, see 8.3; tympanometry, see 8.4; if necessary, otoacoustic emissions, see 8.4).

*Treatment:* The treatment of abnormally enlarged adenoids basically consists of surgical removal of the adenoids under general endotracheal anesthesia (adenotomy, adenoidectomy). In patients with concomitant middle ear effusion, paracentesis should be performed in the same sitting or a ventilation tube should be inserted for drainage (see 11.3, Otitis Media with Effusion).

## Benign Tumors

### Juvenile Angiofibroma

*Epidemiology:* Benign tumors of the nasopharynx are rare. The most common of these is juvenile angiofibroma, which accounts for less than 0.05% of all ear, nose, and throat (ENT) tumors and occurs exclusively in boys 10 to 18 years of age (**Fig. 5.12**).

*Symptoms:* Typical symptoms are obstructed nasal breathing, recurrent epistaxis, headache, impaired eustachian tube ventilation with middle ear effusion, and conductive hearing loss due to obstruction of the eustachian tube orifice.

*Diagnosis:* The typical endoscopic appearance is that of a well-circumscribed, vascularized mass (**Fig. 5.12a**) with superficial vascular markings, situated in the nasopharynx or posterior part of the nasal cavity.

⚕ If there is clinical suspicion of an angiofibroma, a biopsy should *not* be performed due to the risk of heavy bleeding.

The primary work-up should include MRI or CT, which can accurately define tumor extension into surrounding structures (**Fig. 5.12b**). Digital subtraction angiography (DSA) is useful for identifying tumor-feeding vessels (**Fig. 5.12c**).

Fig. 5.11   Adenoids

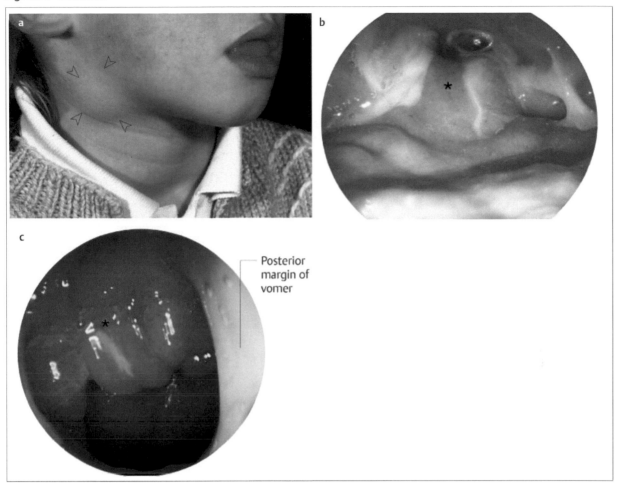

Posterior margin of vomer

**a** Children with enlarged adenoids are "mouth breathers" due to nasal airway obstruction and exhibit a typical facial expression called *adenoid fades*. The arrows point to the enlarged lymph nodes at the mandibular angle.

**b** Postrhinoscopic endoscopy shows the typical appearance of the hyperplastic pharyngeal tonsil (*), which is covered with viscous secretions and almost completely fills the nasopharynx (contrast with normal finding in **Fig. 5.8b**).

**c** The transnasal view shows hyperplastic adenoid tissue (*) partially obstructing the choanae.

***Treatment:*** The treatment of choice is surgical removal of the tumor. Preoperative embolization of the feeding vessels (usually the maxillary artery) should be performed to reduce the intensity of intraoperative bleeding (**Fig. 5.12d**).

## Malignant Tumors

***Epidemiology:*** Carcinomas of squamous cell origin account for the great majority of malignant nasopharyngeal tumors. A basic distinction is drawn between **squamous cell carcinomas** and **lymphoepithelial carcinomas** (Schmincke's tumor).

Much less common tumors of this region are adenocarcinoma, adenoid cystic carcinoma, malignant melanoma (**Fig. 5.13**), sarcoma, lymphoma, and plasmacytoma.

***Etiology:*** The Epstein–Barr virus (EBV) appears to have a key role in the etiology of undifferentiated lymphoepithelial carcinoma.

***Symptoms:*** Early symptoms of nasopharyngeal malignancies are unilateral conductive hearing loss with middle ear effusion.

▸ Any persistent middle ear effusion of long duration in an adult patient with no prior history of middle ear disease is suspicious for a tumor and should be investigated accordingly.

**Fig. 5.12   Juvenile angiofibroma**

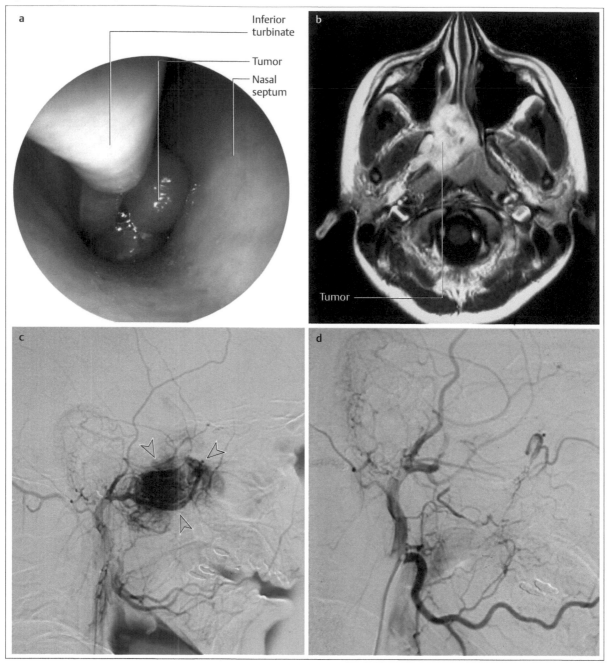

a Endoscopy reveals a spherical, well-circumscribed tumor in the posterior portions of the right nasal cavity.
b Axial T1-weighted MRI after contrast administration demonstrates an enhancing mass in the nasopharynx.

c Digital subtraction angiography shows a well-vascularized tumor (arrows).
d After embolization of the feeding vessels, the tumor is no longer visible.

**Fig. 5.13   Malignant melanoma**

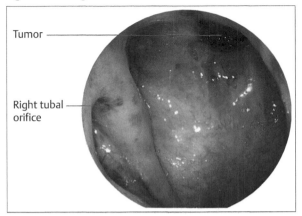

Endoscopic view of a malignant melanoma in the nasopharynx.

**Fig. 5.14   Nasopharyngeal carcinoma**

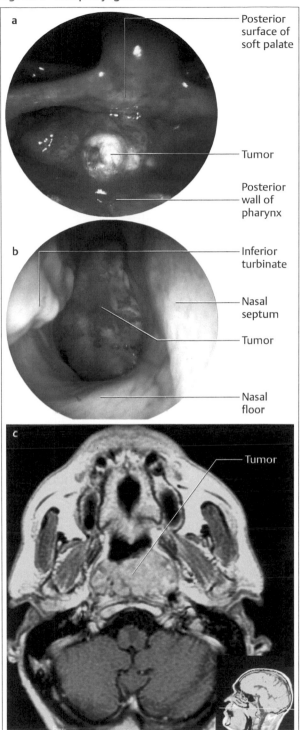

a Postrhinoscopic endoscopy demonstrates a mass that has obstructed the nasopharynx.
b In the transnasal endoscopic view, the tumor completely fills the choanae (only the right side is shown here).
c The corresponding axial T1-weighted magnetic resonance image after contrast administration shows the tumor and its extension into surrounding structures.

Cervical lymph-node metastasis, usually involving the nodes at the mandibular angle, is another common initial finding. Features of advanced disease include nasal airway obstruction, recurrent epistaxis, headaches, and cranial nerve palsies.

*Diagnosis:* The primary study is **endoscopy** of the nasopharynx (**Fig. 5.14a,b**). Nasopharyngeal malignancies can have a variety of appearances ranging from a smooth, well-circumscribed tumor surface to mucosal ulcerations.

⚑ Some of these tumors are initially submucosal and are easily missed at endoscopy.

**Otomicroscopy** reveals unilateral tympanic membrane retraction and a middle ear effusion as a result of impaired eustachian tube ventilation. Given the EBV association of many nasopharyngeal cancers, the **EBV antibody titer** should be determined (this shows an elevated IgA, contrasting with the elevated IgM/IgG that is found in infectious mononucleosis). **MRI** or CT is useful for defining tumor extent (**Fig. 5.14c**).

*Treatment:* The treatment of choice for most nasopharyngeal carcinomas is primary high-voltage radiotherapy, because most of these tumors are very radiosensitive and the unfavorable tumor location and rapid invasion of the skull base preclude curative surgery in many cases.

# 5.4 Diseases of the Oropharynx

The most common diseases of the oropharynx are inflammatory processes. Tumors, especially malignancies, are far less common in this region but should still be considered in the differential diagnosis, especially when certain risk factors are present (heavy smoking, alcohol abuse). Lesions of the oropharynx can also contribute to the development of sleep-related breathing disorders, particularly obstructive sleep apnea.

## Injuries and Foreign Bodies

### Scalds and Corrosive Injuries

*Etiology:* The accidental drinking of hot liquids by children can cause severe scalding of the lips, oral cavity, and oropharynx. Corrosive injuries are more common in adults due to the ingestion of caustic liquids with suicidal intent.

*Symptoms:* The dominant clinical symptoms are severe pain, especially on swallowing, and increased salivation.

*Diagnosis:* Initially, the mucosa appears erythematous on mirror examination. Subsequent blistering may occur, followed by the formation of a whitish fibrin coating. Further tests are aimed at excluding injuries at lower levels of the alimentary tract and in the mediastinum. A chest radiograph should always be obtained (to check for mediastinal widening due to esophageal perforation). An early, careful endoscopic examination can be performed so that the extent of the esophageal injury can be accurately assessed.

*Treatment:* The initial treatment for scalds and corrosive injuries is to rinse the oral cavity with cold water. If the *lips are affected*, they should be treated with a corticosteroid-containing ointment.
Patients with *more severe injuries* can additionally be treated with systemic corticosteroids, antibiotics, and analgesics.
A nasogastric feeding tube should be placed in patients with *severe dysphagia* who are unable to swallow.

🖉 Correct placement of the tube should be checked radiographically before the initial feeding, because the tube may perforate an esophagus that is affected by severe mucosal changes.

### Foreign Bodies

Foreign bodies in the oropharynx are most commonly located in the tonsils and at the tongue base. Typical foreign objects are fish bones (**Fig. 5.15**) and bone fragments, usually with an obvious prior history of oral ingestion. Most patients describe well-localized pain on swallowing.
*Treatment:* The foreign material should be removed as soon as possible due to the risk of superinfection.

Fig. 5.15 Foreign bodies in the oropharynx

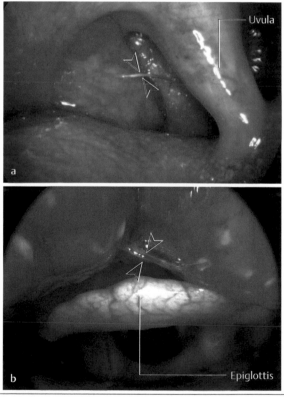

**a** Clinical appearance of a fish bone lodged in the right tonsil (arrows).
**b** A fish bone lodged in the tongue base just above the vallecula (arrows).

# Acute Inflammations

## Acute Tonsillitis

Synonym: streptococcal angina.

***Definition, etiology:*** Acute tonsillitis is an acute bacterial inflammation of the palatine tonsils that is generally caused by group A β-hemolytic streptococci. Rare cases may be caused by staphylococci, *Haemophilus influenzae*, orpneumococci.

***Symptoms:*** This disease is particularly common in children and adolescents and presents initially with high fever and severe pain on swallowing, which often radiates to the ear. Other symptoms are swollen tonsillar lymph nodes and muffling of speech due to oropharyngeal swelling.

***Diagnosis:***
**Mirror examination:** Both tonsils are swollen, bright red, and coated (**Fig. 5.16**).
**Inflammatory parameters:** The *blood count* shows leukocytosis, and the *erythrocyte sedimentation rate (ESR)* and *C-reactive protein (CRP)* are elevated.
**Bacteriologic testing:** A *bacterial culture* is rarely taken from throat smears because it usually takes 2 to 3 days to obtain a definitive result, by which time treatment should already be initiated. It is better to perform a *rapid immunoassay*, which can identify the causative organism as a group A streptococcus in just 10 minutes.

### 5.2    Rapid streptococcal test

This rapid immunoassay makes use of colloid-labeled specific antibodies, which are placed onto reaction strips along with the pharyngeal smear. A color change in the "result window" indicates the presence of streptococcal group A antigen.
The specificity and sensitivity of the various rapid tests available on the market range from 80 to 90%, making them useful tools in deciding whether to administer antibiotics. Note that a correlation exists between the test result and clinical findings—i.e., asymptomatic patients with a positive rapid test should not be placed on antibiotics. Conversely, a culture should be taken in cases where there is clinical suspicion of streptococcal tonsillitis but the rapid test is negative (see also **Fig. 5.17**).

Fig. 5.17    **Bacteriologic testing for group A streptococcus**

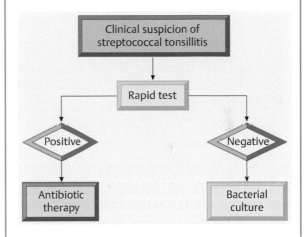

Fig. 5.16    **Acute tonsillitis**

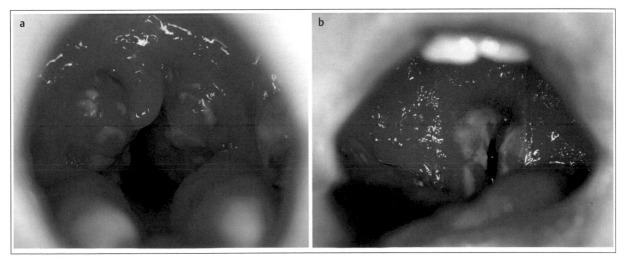

**a** Typical appearance of the palatine tonsils, which are bright red, swollen, and coated.

**b** The tonsils in this patient were so swollen that they caused respiratory distress, necessitating an immediate tonsillectomy.

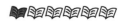

🔎 **5.3 Complications and sequelae of streptococcal tonsillitis**

**Lingual tonsillitis**

In rare cases, the lingual tonsils may become inflamed and greatly swollen, and there may be concomitant edema involving the tongue base and laryngeal introitus. Endoscopic findings (**Fig. 5.18**) include marked hyperplasia of the lingual tonsils, which appear cylindrical with a stippled surface.

Fig. 5.18  **Inflamed and swollen lingual tonsils in lingual tonsillitis**

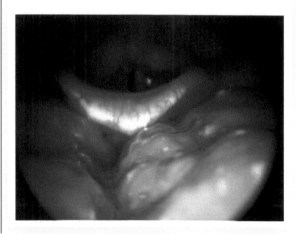

These patients may experience brief periods of progressive respiratory distress, requiring intubation. Patients with lingual tonsillitis should be hospitalized for observation and should receive high doses of antibiotics.

**Streptococcal gingivostomatitis**

In rare cases, tonsillitis may be followed or accompanied by streptococcal gingivostomatitis, characterized by diffuse inflammation and redness of the gingival mucosa and the formation of gingival abscesses. These lesions may also be seen at other sites on the oral mucosa and on the lips.

**Sequelae of streptococcal tonsillitis**

Rarely, a delayed-type antigen-antibody reaction can give rise to poststreptococcal diseases involving the kidneys (**acute glomerulonephritis**), major joints (**acute rheumatic fever**), or heart (**rheumatic endocarditis**). Besides appropriate medical therapy, the treatment of choice is tonsillectomy under antibiotic coverage.

*Treatment:* The standard treatment for streptococcal tonsillitis is a 10- to 14-day course of penicillin V. This regimen should be continued for at least 7 days to avoid late complications (see below). Macrolides or oral cephalosporins can be used in patients allergic to penicillin. Analgesics as well as a single shot of IV corticosteroids might also be administered for pain relief.

*Complications:* See 🔎 **5.3** and Tonsillogenic Complications below.

## Scarlet Fever

The tonsillitis in scarlet fever is also caused by infection with group A β-hemolytic streptococci. These are highly virulent bacterial strains that produce the scarlet fever exotoxin.

*Clinically,* patients present with a rash that begins on the trunk. The area around the mouth is spared ("perioral pallor"). A pathognomonic feature is a bright red tongue with a glistening surface and hyperplastic papillae ("raspberry tongue"; **Fig. 5.19**). The tonsils are greatly swollen with a deep red color. Occasionally, there is an enanthema of the soft palate with hemorrhagic areas. The diagnosis is established by the overall clinical picture combined with a positive rapid streptococcal test (see 🔎 **5.2**).

Medical *therapy* relies on penicillin, as in acute tonsillitis. Additionally, the oral cavity should be rinsed with mild antiseptic solutions, and analgesics should be given for pain.

🔎 **5.4 Complications of scarlet fever**

A feared complication is necrotizing **scarlet fever tonsillitis**, which will cause extensive necrotic areas in the pharynx and oral cavity unless adequately treated. **Septic complications** can also arise, manifested by extensive soft-tissue infections and a toxic shock–like syndrome. As in all infections with β-hemolytic streptococci, late sequelae can develop after an initial period of apparent recovery (rheumatic fever, diffuse hemorrhagic glomerulonephritis, and rheumatoid arthritis) (see 🔎 **5.3**).

Fig. 5.19  **Raspberry tongue**

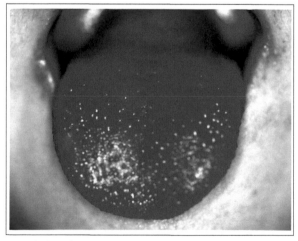

Typical clinical appearance of the tongue in scarlet fever. The bright red coloration and prominent papillae create a raspberrylike appearance.

## Plaut–Vincent Angina

This inflammatory disease is caused by fusiform rods and spirochetes and presents clinically with unilateral dysphagia and a fetid breath odor with very little malaise. Mirror examination reveals a unilateral, fibrin-coated ulcer on the palatine tonsil.

🖉 Differential diagnosis: tonsillar carcinoma.

The causative organisms can be detected by the direct microscopic examination of a Gram-stained smear.

*Treatment:* Local measures (cautery with 10% $AgNO_3$ or 5% chromic acid) are usually satisfactory, but should be supplemented by antibiotics (penicillin) in patients with more severe complaints.

## Diphtheria

*Epidemiology:* Diphtheria was controlled for a time by active immunization, but lately its incidence has been rising due to low vaccination numbers, especially in immigrants from Eastern Europe, and secular fluctuations in the virulence of the toxin.

🖉 All instances of the disease must be reported to health officials.

*Causative organism:* The causative organism is *Corynebacterium diphtheriae*, which is transmitted by droplet inhalation or skin-to-skin contact. The incubation period is 1 to 5 days.

*Pathogenesis:* The bacterium produces a special endotoxin that causes epithelial cell necrosis and ulcerations.

*Clinical manifestations:* Two main forms are distinguished based on their clinical presentation:
• Local, benign pharyngeal diphtheria.
• Primary toxic, malignant diphtheria.

The disease begins with moderate fever and mild swallowing difficulties. The clinical picture becomes fully developed in approximately 24 hours, characterized by severe malaise, headache, and nausea.

*Diagnosis:* Mirror examination of the pharynx reveals typical grayish-yellow pseudomembranes that are firmly adherent to the tonsils and may spread to the palate and pharynx. The underlying tissue bleeds when the coatings are removed. A slightly sweet breath smell is also characteristic. The diagnosis is confirmed by the overall clinical impression, combined with smear findings.

*Treatment:* First, the patient should be isolated. Whenever diphtheria is suspected, even before it is confirmed by smear results, **diphtheria antitoxin** (200–1,000 IU/kg body weight) should be administered by intravenous or intramuscular injection.

🖉 Allergy to the antitoxin should be excluded (with a skin test) before it is administered.

Penicillin G should also be administered.
**Discharge** from the hospital is contingent upon test results: three smears taken at 1-week intervals must all be negative. Two percent of patients continue to carry the bacterium and should undergo tonsillectomy.

*Complications:* Dangerous complications, which occur mainly in association with the primary toxic malignant form, are toxic myocarditis (which may terminate fatally in 10–14 days) and interstitial nephritis. The more severe the diphtheria, the earlier these complications may arise. Electrocardiography and urinalysis follow-ups should be continued for at least 6 weeks after the onset of the disease.

## Tuberculosis

*Epidemiology:* Oral or oropharyngeal manifestations of tuberculosis most commonly occur in the setting of advanced **organ tuberculosis**. Although these lesions are very rare (0.2% of patients with organ tuberculosis), they should be considered in the differential diagnosis as the incidence of tuberculosis has been on the rise. It is even less common to see oropharyngeal involvement by a **primary complex** or in the setting of **miliary tuberculosis**.

*Clinical manifestations:*
**Primary complex:** A primary tuberculous complex in the tonsillar and cervical lymph-node region is most common in children who have become infected by drinking cow's milk contaminated with tubercle bacilli. The primary complex in these cases consists of a typical ulcerative lesion of the oral mucosa and tonsil, associated with regional cervical lymphadenopathy. The swelling in the neck leads most patients to seek medical attention.
**Organ tuberculosis with ulcerative mucocutaneous lesions** occurs mainly in regions that may come into contact with secretions containing infectious organisms, resulting in the formation of ulcerative mucosal lesions that are sometimes necrotic. (Other forms of organ tuberculosis can affect the lung, bowel, etc.)
*Morphologically,* the lesions may appear as mucosal ulcerations on the lips and dorsum of the tongue or as

**Fig. 5.20** "Cold abscess" of the cervical spine in tuberculosis

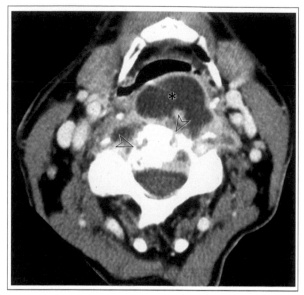

Axial CT scan after contrast administration shows a marked protrusion (*) of the posterior wall of the oropharynx. It also reveals sites of bone destruction in the cervical vertebral body behind the oropharynx (arrows).

slightly raised, nodular eruptions on the palate. Skeletal involvement is also occasionally seen due to hematogenous spread. In this case, "cold abscesses" may form about the cervical spine (**Fig. 5.20**), causing the posterior wall of the pharynx to bulge forward and mimicking the features of a retropharyngeal or parapharyngeal abscess (see below).

**Miliary tuberculosis:** Involvement of the oral mucosa can result from hematogenous spread, appearing as multiple pinhead-sized papules, some of which are hemorrhagic, that form on the oral mucosa.

*Diagnosis:* The diagnosis is established by the **detection of acid-fast rods** in smears, sputum, bronchial secretions, gastric juice, or biopsy material. The diagnostic work-up should include **biplane chest radiographs** to check for pulmonary involvement. The **tuberculin skin test** is also performed to assess the reactivity of the organism to tubercle bacilli. Calcifications detected by **ultrasound** in enlarged cervical lymph nodes are pathognomonic for tuberculosis. If the result is equivocal, a **cervical lymph-node biopsy** should be taken for a histologic and bacteriologic tissue analysis.

*Treatment:* Inpatient antituberculous polychemotherapy is required, consisting either of a triple regimen (isoniazid, ethambutol, rifampicin) or a quadruple regimen with pyrazinamide added.

## Acute Viral Pharyngitis

*Etiology, symptoms:* Acute viral pharyngitis, which is often caused by influenza or parainfluenza viruses, typically presents clinically with sudden onset of fever, sore throat, and headache. There may also be coughing and catarrhal symptoms (e.g., rhinitis, sinusitis). Concomitant cervical adenopathy may also be present.

*Diagnosis:* The pharyngeal mucosa appears red and coated on mirror examination. If a bacterial etiology is suspected, a rapid streptococcal test can be performed (see ⌕ **5.2**).

*Treatment:* Treatment is supportive and consists mainly of analgesic agents. Cold compresses to the neck can also help to relieve pain. The patient should drink copious amounts of warm liquid to ease complaints.

## Infectious Mononucleosis

Synonyms: Pfeiffer's glandular fever, kissing disease.

*Causative organism:* Infectious mononucleosis is caused by infection with EBV. It predominantly affects adolescents and young adults. The incubation period is 7 to 9 days.

*Clinical manifestations:* Although infectious mononucleosis is a systemic illness, it is common to encounter tonsillitis as the initial or cardinal symptom. Besides systemic symptoms such as fatigue, anorexia, and moderate temperature elevation (38–39°C), patients complain of severe pain on swallowing, headache, and limb pains.

*Diagnosis:*
**Clinical examination:** The tonsillar and nuchal lymph nodes, axillary nodes, and inguinal nodes are palpably enlarged. Often, there is concomitant enlargement of the spleen and liver.
On mirror examination, the tonsils are found to be bright red, swollen, and covered with a grayish fibrin coating (**Fig. 5.22**).
**Laboratory tests:** The *blood count* initially shows leukopenia, followed later by leukocytosis (20,000/mL) with 80 to 90% atypical lymphocytes (lymphomonocytoid cells, Pfeiffer's cells). *EBV serology* (especially IgM and IgG) is another important test. The enzyme-linked immunosorbent assay (ELISA) can confirm infectious mononucleosis by quantitatively detecting antibodies against the various EBV antigens (virus capsid antigen, early antigen, Epstein–Barr nuclear antigen). Rapid mononucleosis tests are also available but are less sensitive and specific than ELISA. The serum *hepatic*

**Fig. 5.21  Peritonsillar abscess**

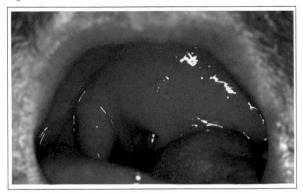

Inspection reveals typical unilateral erythema, swelling, and protrusion of the left tonsil and of the soft palate on the left side.

**Fig. 5.22  Infectious mononucleosis**

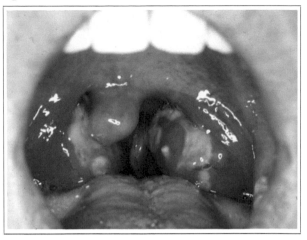

At clinical examination, the tonsils are bright red and swollen, with fibrin coatings.

*enzymes* should be determined to exclude concomitant involvement of the liver or spleen.
**Upper abdominal ultrasound** and an **electrocardiogram** are also recommended.

*Treatment:* Treatment centers on the symptomatic relief of pain and fever. The agents of choice for **pain relief** are acetaminophen or ibuprofen. Aspirin products should not be used, as they could cause bleeding problems if tonsillectomy is required. **Antibiotics** (penicillin V) should be given only if signs of bacterial superinfection are present.

☒ Ampicillin and amoxicillin should be avoided because they frequently induce a pseudoallergic rash (**Fig. 5.23**).

In cases of infectious mononucleosis that run a severe course with persistent fever, respiratory distress, or stridor, a **tonsillectomy** can expedite recovery by eliminating the focus of greatest viral proliferation.

*Complications:* Complications are rare and consist mainly of myocarditis, hemorrhage, nephritis, hepatitis, meningitis, or encephalitis.

**Tonsillogenic Complications**

**Peritonsillar abscess:** Peritonsillar abscess is a unilateral inflammatory process that involves not only the tonsillar parenchyma but also the peritonsillar tissue —i.e., the abscess spreads past the tonsil to involve the connective tissue between the parenchyma and pharyngeal musculature. The *clinical features* are pronounced unilateral redness and swelling of the soft palate (**Fig. 5.21**), muffled speech, and possible trismus. This is frequently accompanied by uvular edema, but the swelling may also spread to the tongue base

and lateral pharyngeal wall, causing respiratory complications.
The *treatment of choice* is removal or incision of the affected tonsil under antibiotic coverage, bearing in mind that most patients harbor a mixed spectrum of aerobic and anaerobic organisms.
Other complications: see ⌕ **5.5**.

## Chronic Inflammations

### Chronic Pharyngitis

*Etiology:* Chronic pharyngitis is often a result of long-term exposure to various noxious agents (nicotine, alcohol, chemicals, gaseous irritants). It can also occur as a result of chronic mouth breathing due to nasal airway obstruction (e.g., deviated septum) or as an accompanying feature of chronic sinusitis.

*Symptoms:* The main clinical manifestations are a dry-throat sensation with frequent throat clearing and the drainage of a viscous mucus. Some patients have a dry cough and a foreign-body sensation in the pharynx.

*Diagnosis:* The **history** will often direct attention to possible noxious agents. On **mirror examination**, the pharyngeal mucosa appears red and "grainy" due to the hyperplasia of lymphatic tissue on the posterior pharyngeal wall (*hypertrophic form*; **Fig. 5.25**). The pharyngeal mucosa may also have a smooth, shiny appearance in some cases (*atrophic form*).
A thorough **nasal examination** should be performed to exclude nasal airway obstruction as the cause of chronic pharyngitis, giving particular attention to possible septal deviation or turbinate hyperplasia. The middle meatus should also be examined endoscopically (see ⌕ **1.3**).

**Fig. 5.23   Pseudoallergic rash in infectious mononucleosis**

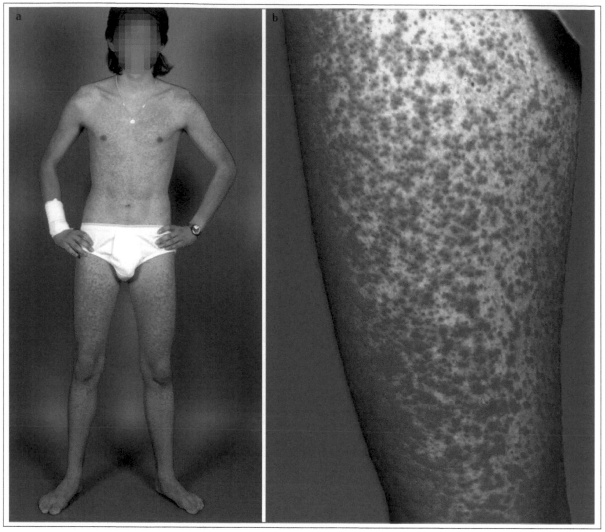

A pseudoallergic rash developed in this patient following treatment with ampicillin.

***Treatment:*** Any agents causing the pharyngitis should be avoided. Also, a herbal product such as sage or chamomile can be used in a steam inhalation to moisten the airways. In patients with nasal airway obstruction due to septal deviation or turbinate hyperplasia, a surgical procedure can be performed to improve complaints.

## Chronic Tonsillitis

***Pathogenesis:*** Like infections confined to the tonsillar crypts, recurrent inflammations of the tonsils and peritonsillar tissue can lead to permanent structural changes with scarring. Bacteria that grow on cellular debris in poorly drained crypts can perpetuate a smoldering inflammation, chronic tonsillitis. In this condition, the palatine tonsils provide a "focus" that can sustain a variety of diseases in other parts of the body (rheumatic fever, glomerulonephritis, iritis,

psoriasis, inflammatory heart disease, pustulosis palmaris and plantaris, erythema nodosum).

***Symptoms:*** Chronic tonsillitis may cause recurrent episodes of pain or may run an asymptomatic course. The most frequent complaints are lethargy, poor appetite, a bad taste in the mouth, and a fetid breath odor.

***Diagnosis:*** **Mirror examination** often reveals small, firm, immobile tonsils with associated peritonsillar redness. Occasionally, a purulent liquid can be expressed from the crypts. **Tonsillar smears** are found to contain group A β-hemolytic streptococci. The McIsaac scoring system can be used to establish the probability of streptococcal tonsillitis (**Table 5.1**).
**Palpation:** The tonsillar lymph nodes at the mandibular angle may be enlarged.

🥄 5.5  Rare tonsillogenic complications

## Tonsillogenic sepsis

Tonsillogenic sepsis has become rare in the antibiotic era. It most commonly affects patients with weakened host resistance. In these cases, bacteria enter the bloodstream by the hematogenous or lymphogenous route, and the bacteremia can lead to full-blown sepsis.

## Retropharyngeal and parapharyngeal abscess

An inflammation or abscess may arise from the prevertebral or parapharyngeal lymph nodes or by hematogenous spread as the result of a minor foreign-body injury or upper respiratory inflammation. This abscess is called a retropharyngeal or parapharyngeal abscess, depending on whether it is located between the spinal column and posterior pharyngeal wall or lateral to the pharyngeal wall.

The **clinical** hallmarks are severe pain on swallowing with progressive dysphagia, muffled speech, and possible trismus and dyspnea.

**Diagnosis**: The *mirror examination* shows pronounced swelling in the oropharynx or hypopharynx, usually at a prevertebral or parapharyngeal location.

The swelling may also spread to the larynx. The *blood count* indicates leukocytosis with a left shift and elevated erythrocyte sedimentation rate (ESR) and C-reactive protein (CRP) values. An *imaging study* should be performed (**Fig. 5.24**) to define the extent of the abscess and exclude the spread of infection through the fascial compartments of the neck to the mediastinum (see 📖 16.4, Deep Neck Infections).

**Treatment** consists of surgical incision and drainage of the abscess under general endotracheal anesthesia. Retropharyngeal abscess is generally approached by the transoral route. Sometimes, it is better to drain a parapharyngeal abscess through an external approach. The surgery is performed under antibiotic coverage, taking into account the mixed spectrum of aerobic and anaerobic causative organisms. Cortisone should also be administered in patients with significant dyspnea. Some patients require prolonged intubation.

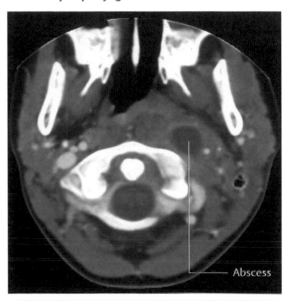

**Fig. 5.24  Postcontrast axial CT scan of a right parapharyngeal abscess**

Abscess

**Laboratory tests:** An elevated *ESR* and CRP and a left shift in the *differential blood count* are present as signs of the inflammatory process.

**Treatment: Tonsillectomy** may be considered if the patient has had six or more inflammatory episodes in the preceding year. Surgery is performed under general endotracheal anesthesia with the head hyperextended.

🖉 Heavy postoperative bleeding may occur on the day of the tonsillectomy, during the first week after the operation, or even later in rare instances.

## Obstructive Sleep Apnea Syndrome

Obstructive sleep apnea syndrome (OSAS), like snoring, is a type of sleep-related breathing disorder that can have serious health effects and social consequences. The history can provide important clues to the presence of OSAS (**Table 5.2**).

**Etiology and pathogenesis (Fig. 5.26):** There is a tendency for the pharynx to collapse during sleep, narrowing the pathway for airflow and causing periods of apnea or hypopnea that can last up to 2 minutes. This leads to frequent arousals from sleep and gasping for air, preventing a normal sleep pattern. Besides disturbing the sleep–wake rhythm, OSAS can have longer-term effects due to a reduction in blood oxygen levels and an increase in the activity of the

**Fig. 5.25  Chronic pharyngitis**

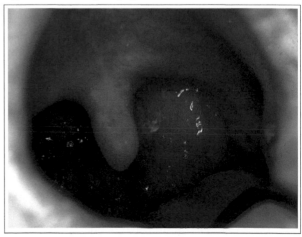

The typical appearance of a granulating inflammation involving the posterior wall of the pharynx (hypertrophic form).

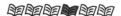

| Table 5.1 McIsaac scoring system to predict infection with group A streptococci | |
|---|---|
| *Scoring system* | |
| *Symptom* | *Points* |
| Body temperature > 38°C[a] | 1 |
| No cough | 1 |
| Swelling of cervical lymph nodes | |
| Tonsillar swelling or exudate | 1 |
| Age 3–14 y | 1 |
|     15–44 y | 0 |
|     ≥ 45 y | –1 |
| *Probability of positive throat culture* | |
| *Total score* | *Probability* |
| –1 or 0 points | 1% |
| 1 point | 10% |
| 2 points | ~17% |
| 3 points | ~35% |
| 4 or 5 points | ~50% |

[a]At the time of examination.

**Table 5.2 Signs in the patient's history that are suggestive of (obstructive) sleep apnea**

- Loud, irregular snoring
- Periods of apnea during sleep (witnessed)
- Unusual daytime sleepiness or fatigue
- Restless sleep
- Intellectual deterioration (poor concentration and impaired memory)
- Personality changes
- Loss of libido, impotence

Source: Günther 1997.

**Symptoms:** Typical symptoms of OSAS are morning lethargy and daytime fatigue, with a tendency to fall asleep during the day. Witnesses additionally report irregular snoring with periods of apnea followed by "gasping" and loud snoring. Obesity is usually present as an accompanying condition.

**Diagnosis:** Mirror examination may demonstrate an elongated uvula, a narrow velopharyngeal passage, and a bulky or low soft palate with a small oropharyngeal lumen. It is also common to find a hyperplastic tongue base and hyperplasia of the palatine tonsils. The nasal airway should also be examined for possible septal deviation, turbinate hyperplasia, or other abnormalities.

sympathetic nervous system, with a potential for significant damage to the cardiopulmonary system. Factors that narrow the pharyngeal airway or lead to decreased muscle tone (**Table 5.3**) can promote or intensify the disease process.

**Fig. 5.26**   Pathophysiology, effects, and clinical manifestations of obstructive sleep apnea

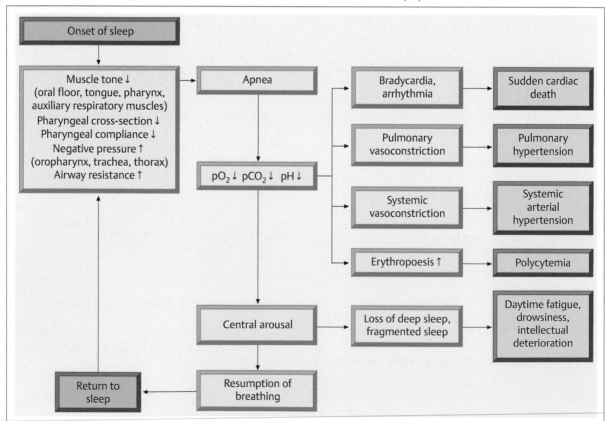

| Table 5.3 | Factors and conditions that promote snoring and apnea |
|---|---|
| *Classification* | *Common factors* |
| Pharyngeal obstruction | • Obesity<br>• Adenoids<br>• Tonsillar hyperplasia, elongated uvula, hyperplasia of base of tongue, low soft palate<br>• Dysgnathia/retrognathia<br>• Tumors in the oral cavity, pharynx, larynx, neck<br>• Acromegaly |
| Nasal obstruction | • Turbinate hyperplasia<br>• Septal deviation<br>• Nasal polyps<br>• Tumors of the nose |
| Decreased muscle tone | • Alcohol<br>• Nicotine<br>• Drugs (sedatives, hypnotics, muscle relaxants)<br>• Shiftwork<br>• Hypothyroidism |
| Other | • Sex (males predominate)<br>• Genetic predisposition: familial occurrence<br>• Sleeping in a supine position |

| Table 5.4 | Differential diagnosis of sleep apnea |
|---|---|
| | • Occasional or habitual nonobstructive snoring<br>• Upper airway resistance syndrome<br>• Narcolepsy<br>• Underlying heart disease with Cheyne–Stokes respiration (e.g., heart failure)<br>• Nocturnal bronchial asthma<br>• Periodic hypersomnia, hypersomniac form of endogenous depression<br>• Insomnia |

Source: Günther 1997.

*Screening:* Reports given by the patient and witnesses can be objectified by recording $O_2$ saturation, respiratory sounds, and heart rate on an outpatient basis during sleep. However, these screening devices alone cannot provide an accurate sleep evaluation, since they do not at present include an electroencephalography (EEG) channel.

*Confirming the diagnosis:* The current gold standard for confirming OSAS and differentiating it from other sleep-related breathing disorders is *polysomnography.* Conducted as an inpatient procedure in a sleep laboratory, it measures thoracic and abdominal respiratory excursions and transcutaneous $PO_2$, and records an EEG, EOG, and EMG of the mentalis muscle to record the different sleeping phases in addition to the usual screening parameters.

*Treatment:* **General treatment measures** consist of weight reduction, abstinence from alcohol and nicotine, and avoiding big meals, especially at night. It is also important to establish a regular sleep–wake cycle and avoid the use of sedatives.

Today, CPAP (continuous positive airway pressure) is the gold standard in the treatment of OSAS.

With this measure, the unstable portions of the airway can be "pneumatically splinted" by means of transnasal continuous positive pressure ventilation; this keeps the tissues from collapsing during sleep and obstructing airflow. A nasal or oronasal **CPAP mask** for this purpose is custom-fitted at the sleep laboratory.

One nonsurgical treatment option is the **Esmarch splint**, an occlusive splint that advances the lower jaw. By moving the tongue base and adjacent pharynx forward, this device widens the airway in the unstable portion of the oropharynx.

**Surgical treatment options** are tailored to the specific pathology causing the apnea.

> Surgical treatment requires very careful patient selection, because many patients will derive little or no benefit from the operation.

An *established procedure* is the uvulopalatopharyngoplasty (UPPP) with tonsillectomy, in which redundant mucosa is resected from the posterior pillars and the remaining mucosa is tightened by suturing it to the anterior pillars. At least part of the uvula is also resected in most cases. The operation may employ conventional instruments, a laser technique (laser-assisted uvulopalatoplasty, LAUP), or radiofrequency therapy. Some patients will also require adjuvant intranasal surgery (septoplasty, septorhinoplasty, turbinate reduction).

*Differential diagnosis:* The differential diagnosis should include various disorders that are associated with snoring or with the hypersomnia that is typical of obstructive sleep apnea (**Table 5.4**).

## Tumors

### Benign Tumors and Precancerous Lesions

The occurrence, incidence, clinical features, and treatment of these lesions are covered in 4.5, Benign Tumors and Precancerous Lesions.

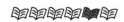

## Malignant Tumors

The overwhelming majority of malignant tumors of the oropharynx are squamous cell carcinomas. Approximately 80% are located in the palatine tonsils or tongue base. Less common sites are the soft palate and posterior wall of the pharynx.

*Etiology:* In most patients, chronic nicotine and alcohol abuse have a major etiologic role in the development of oropharyngeal cancers. Another risk factor for the development of oropharyngeal cancer, especially tonsillar carcinoma, is human papillomavirus (HPV) infection.

*Symptoms:*

 Cancers at some sites in the oropharynx may remain clinically silent for some time.

Otherwise, the symptoms depend on the location and extent of the tumor. Besides dysphagia and odynophagia, the symptoms may include blood-tinged saliva and a fetid breath odor. Advanced stages (**Fig. 5.27a**) often produce trismus, signifying that the tumor has invaded the surrounding musculature (pterygoid muscles).

*Diagnosis:* **Inspection:** Tonsillar carcinomas may appear as exophytic lesions (**Fig. 5.27a**) or may show an ulcerating, infiltrating type of growth. Occasionally, they are not grossly visible (microcarcinomas of the tonsils), and the first presenting symptom of the disease is cervical lymph-node metastasis.

**CT** and **MRI** (**Fig. 5.27b–d**) are useful for defining the extent of tumor growth and detecting the invasion of surrounding structures.

*Treatment:* The **treatment of choice** for most cases is surgical tumor removal. The resulting tissue defect may be closed primarily with local pedicled flaps or by using microvascular free tissue transfers, depending on the size and location of the defect (see **Fig. 4.30**). A neck dissection (see ✎16.5, Malignant Tumors of the Cervical Lymph Nodes) may be necessary on one or both sides, depending on the location and stage of the primary tumor (see **Table 4.2**).

**Postoperatively**, radiation should usually be delivered to the tumor site and lymphatic pathways.

**Alternatives** for the treatment of **advanced tumors** (T3, T4) are primary radiotherapy or combined radiation and chemotherapy.

**Fig. 5.27  Tonsillar carcinoma**

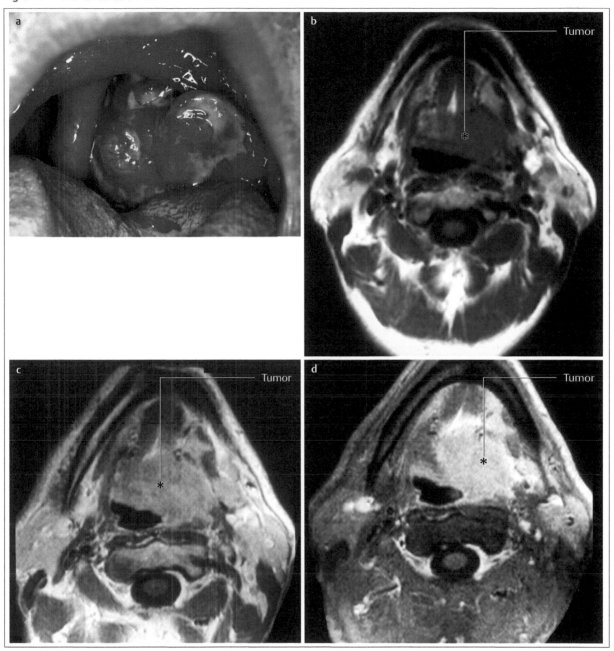

**a** Visual inspection reveals an exophytic mass arising from the left tonsil.

**b, c** T1-weighted axial MR images before (**b**) and after contrast administration (**c**) show that the tumor (*) has deeply infiltrated the lingual muscles.

**d** The corresponding fat-suppression sequence more clearly delineates the tumor from its surroundings.

# 5.5    Diseases of the Hypopharynx and Esophagus

The diseases of the hypopharynx that have the greatest clinical importance are foreign bodies, hypopharyngeal diverticula, and especially malignant tumors, which frequently do not produce symptoms until they have reached an advanced stage. The ENT physician is not often confronted with diseases of the esophagus.

The majority are caused by injuries and foreign bodies. Congenital malformations such as brachyesophagus and tracheoesophageal fistulas are managed by a thoracic or pediatric surgeon, while esophageal tumors are treated by a general surgeon or abdominal surgeon.

## Injuries and Foreign Bodies

### Caustic Ingestion

*Etiopathogenesis:* Caustic ingestion in children is almost always accidental, caused by drinking an alkaline or acidic liquid that has not been properly stored. Most such injuries in adults result from attempted suicide.

While acids cause a coagulation necrosis with the denaturation of proteins, alkalis cause a colliquative necrosis with liquefaction of the necrotic tissue.

Strictures caused by scarring are common sequelae of this type of injury.

⚕ There is a long-term risk of cancer developing in esophageal strictures caused by caustic ingestion.

*Symptoms:* **Acute** cases present with severe pain in the mouth and pharynx and possibly in the retrosternal and epigastric areas. Drooling is also present.

Patients with an *esophageal perforation* may also present with subcutaneous emphysema in the neck or a pneumomediastinum (see **Fig. 5.30**), and mediastinitis may supervene. Symptoms such as high fever and retrosternal or interscapular pain in these cases are accompanied by typical shock symptoms with an elevated pulse rate, a fall in blood pressure, cold sweats, and pallor. Generalized symptoms of *intoxication* such as renal and liver failure, electrolyte imbalance, and hemolysis generally do not appear until 1 to 2 days after the caustic injury.

In the **long term**, patients may develop an esophageal stricture with progressive dysphagia.

*Diagnosis:* **Acute evaluation** begins with a *minor examination* of the oral cavity, oropharynx, hypopharynx, and larynx. The mucosa initially appears erythematous and edematous and later may show epithelial defects and a whitish fibrin coating. It is also important to obtain *radiographs* of the chest and abdomen to exclude a perforation of the esophagus or stomach. If the diagnosis cannot be confirmed by imaging studies, *esophagoscopy* should be performed using careful technique.

⚕ The extent of the injuries to the oral and pharyngeal mucosa does not necessarily reflect the severity of corrosive damage to the esophagus, which may be very severe despite a normal appearance of the oral and pharyngeal mucosae.

**Follow-up:** Caustic injuries to the esophagus require long-term follow-up with imaging studies and periodic esophagoscopy.

*Treatment:* **Acute:** The first priority is to treat the patient for shock. It is important to stabilize the airway, replace fluids, correct electrolyte imbalances, relieve pain, and provide sedation. Treatment should also include high doses of corticosteroids as well as antibiotics to prevent superinfection.

The therapeutic value of "neutralizing" agents (e.g., magnesium oxide for acid ingestion, citric or acetic acid for alkali ingestion) is questionable because the tissue damage occurs on immediate contact with the corrosive substance, and some time passes before the neutralizing agent can be administered.

**Long-term:** Some esophageal strictures can be treated by dilation. In cases with severe caustic injury, early dilation should be started just 1 week after the injury. The dilator should never be introduced blindly but should always be passed over a guidewire (**Fig. 5.28**). If a stricture cannot be expanded by dilation, the stenotic segment should be resected. It may then be necessary to perform a gastric pull-up or interpose a free segment of jejunum with microvascular anastomosis, depending on the length of the esophageal segment that has been removed.

### Foreign Bodies

*Etiology and pathogenesis:* Foreign bodies typically become lodged in the hypopharynx or in the upper constriction of the esophagus (see **Fig. 5.3**). Most patients are *small children* who have swallowed coins, nuts, or toy parts, but in many cases they are *older patients* who have decreased sensation in the hard palate (e.g., due to a maxillary denture). Objects typically swallowed by adults are fish bones or larger bone fragments (**Fig. 5.29a**), pieces of meat (**Fig. 5.29b**), and denture parts.

**Fig. 5.28 Conservative treatment of esophageal strictures**

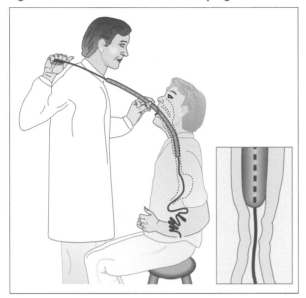

An esophageal stricture is treated with a dilator passed over a guidewire.

***Symptoms:*** Typical symptoms are a feeling of pressure, a "pricking" sensation, or pain in the hypopharynx or retrosternal area. Dysphagia may also be present, depending on the size and location of the foreign body.

***Diagnosis:*** **Inspection** and **palpation** will disclose any cutaneous emphysema caused by perforation of the hypopharynx or esophagus (sharp object!). This is followed by indirect **mirror examination** of the hypopharynx. If this fails to locate the foreign body, diagnostic imaging should also be performed. The imaging procedure of choice depends on the nature of the foreign body suggested by the patient's history. If a radiopaque foreign body is believed to be lodged in the hypopharynx or upper esophageal constriction, the soft tissues of the neck should be imaged with a lateral radiograph (**Fig. 5.29a**). Otherwise, an oral contrast examination (with a water-soluble medium) should be performed (**Fig. 5.29b**). An abdominal plain film can also show evidence of a foreign body in some cases (**Fig. 5.29c**).

 Since there is always a danger of perforation, barium should never be used in oral contrast examinations (risk of foreign-body reaction or pneumonia).

***Treatment:***

 The sun should never rise and set on a foreign body.

Whenever an ingested foreign body is suspected, rigid esophagoscopy should be performed without delay to retrieve the foreign object. With a foreign body that has skewered and cannot be removed endoscopically, it may be necessary to expose the object through an external approach. This may require a transcervical incision or thoracotomy, depending on the location of the foreign body.

## Rupture of the Esophagus

Synonym: Boerhaave's syndrome.

Boerhaave's syndrome refers to a spontaneous rupture in the left posterolateral portion of the terminal esophagus just above the esophageal hiatus caused by forceful vomiting or retching. The condition is most common in patients with habitual vomiting and in alcoholics.

***Symptoms:*** The classic symptoms occur immediately after the rupture and consist of very severe retrosternal or epigastric pain that may be accompanied by the features of an acute abdomen. Patients may also exhibit hematemesis, dyspnea, and progressive shock symptoms.

***Diagnosis:*** First, an anteroposterior chest radiograph should be obtained in the standing or left lateral decubitus position. This will disclose a pneumomediastinum or possible air crescent below the diaphragm caused by air leakage from the ruptured esophagus. Neither of these signs is always evident in the chest radiograph, however, and so CT should be performed if there is lingering suspicion of a rupture (**Fig. 5.30**). Another option is oral contrast radiography of the esophagus, making certain to use only a water-soluble contrast medium (Gastrografin). If imaging procedures do not furnish a definitive diagnosis, the patient should undergo endoscopy.

The ***treatment*** of choice is immediate surgical intervention by thoracotomy with primary closure of the defect and pleural repair, leaving a drain in the pleura or mediastinum. The surgery must be performed under antibiotic coverage.

Fig. 5.29   Various foreign bodies in the hypopharynx and esophagus

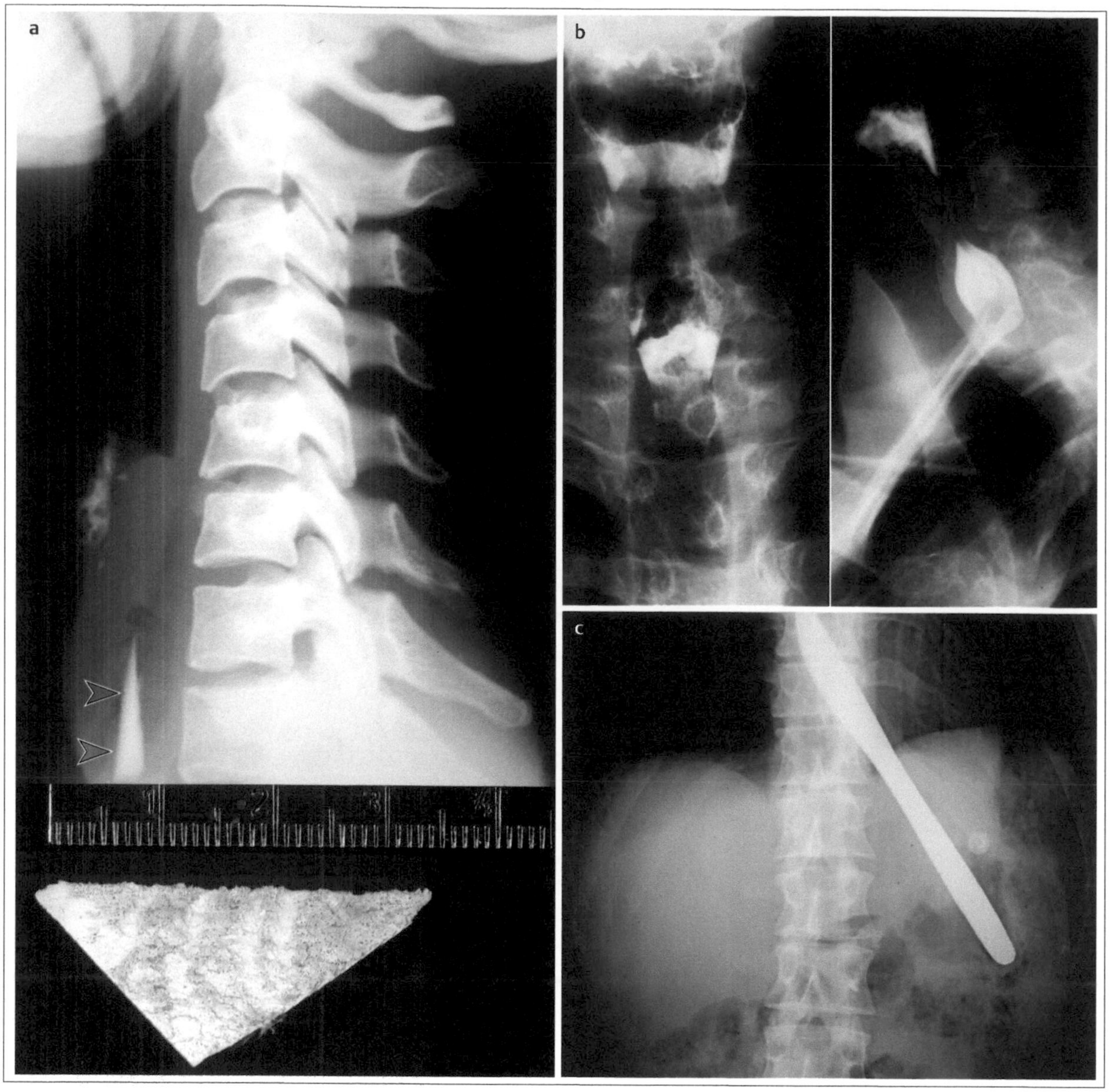

**a** Lateral radiograph of the cervical soft tissues shows a radiopaque foreign body (arrows) in the hypopharynx, corresponding to a sharp-edged *bone fragment*.
**b** Oral contrast examination with a water-soluble medium (Gastrografin) in the anteroposterior and lateral projections shows a nonradiopaque foreign body (lodged *piece of meat*) surrounded by an irregular pool of contrast material.

**c** The radiopaque foreign body in the abdominal plain film is a *knife*, which has become lodged between the lower third of the esophagus and the stomach.

## Diverticula

Two types are distinguished: *pulsion diverticula*, in which the mucosa herniates through a weak point in the muscular coat due to a rise of intraluminal pressure; and *traction diverticula*, which usually form at parabronchial sites due to scar traction following hilar lymphadenitis and involve all layers of the esophageal wall.

The treatment of esophageal diverticula is described in standard textbooks of surgery.

### Hypopharyngeal Diverticulum

Synonym: Zenker's diverticulum.

*Epidemiology:* The hypopharyngeal (Zenker's) diverticulum is the most common diverticulum of the

**Fig. 5.30  Boerhaave's syndrome**

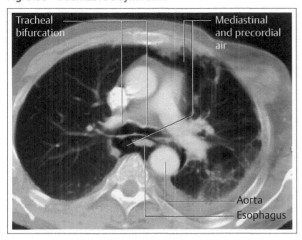

Axial CT scan of a pneumomediastinum resulting from a spontaneous rupture of the terminal esophagus.

**Fig. 5.31  Hypopharyngeal diverticulum: radiographic appearance**

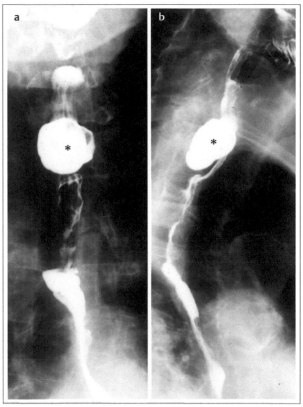

Oral contrast study of the esophagus shows pooling of contrast medium in the diverticular pouch (*) in the anteroposterior (**a**) and lateral (**b**) projections.

esophageal inlet. Most patients are middle-aged or older, with a 3:1 preponderance of males over females.

***Pathogenesis:*** The herniation of esophageal mucosa (pulsion diverticulum) classically occurs at "weak points" in the posteroinferior hypopharyngeal wall located above the cricopharyngeal part of the constrictor pharyngis inferior muscle (see ✎ **5.1** and **Fig. 5.2**). Many patients present with a long history of reflux esophagitis.

✍ In rare cases, a carcinoma may be the cause of a hypopharyngeal diverticulum.

***Symptoms:*** Classic symptoms are dysphagia and the regurgitation of undigested food, especially in the morning and while lying down. Patients also complain of pronounced halitosis caused by food residues trapped in the diverticulum. Smaller diverticula are sometimes manifested only by a foreign-body sensation or may be completely asymptomatic.

***Diagnosis:*** Mirror examination or indirect laryngoscopy (see ✎ 17.2) will occasionally show the pooling of saliva in the piriform sinus, but only an imaging procedure can establish the diagnosis. An oral contrast examination of the esophagus is best for defining the diverticulum (**Fig. 5.31**). If reflux esophagitis is suspected (belching, heartburn, possible epigastric pain, and dysphagia), the imaging study should be supplemented by ambulatory 24-hour pH-metry and esophageal manometry (✎ **5.6**).

***Treatment:*** The treatment of choice is surgery, using either an endoscopic or external approach.

---

✎ **5.6   pH and esophageal manometry**

With the development of special pH electrodes and modern data-storage capabilities, it is now possible to perform pH recordings and long-term manometry in the esophagus on an ambulatory basis over a 24-hour period.

***Indications:*** This study is used to differentiate primary from secondary reflux in patients with reflux esophagitis, investigate motility disorders (achalasia, esophageal spasms), and investigate causes in clinical syndromes such as globus sensation and noncardiac chest pain. The procedure is also used to evaluate response to medical therapy, sphincter dilation, antireflux surgery, and myotomy.

---

**Endoscopic approach:** The endoscope is advanced through the mouth toward the esophageal introitus. The muscular septum formed by the cricopharyngeus is transected using either conventional technique or a $CO_2$ laser (**Fig. 5.32**), thereby reintegrating the diverticular pouch into the hypopharynx or esophagus. The endoscopic technique is particularly suitable for older patients with a high surgical risk, as the procedure is well tolerated and of relatively short duration.

**External approach:** An alternative is to resect the diverticulum through an external transcervical approach (**Fig. 5.33**). In this technique, the cricopharyngeus is exposed and divided through a cervical incision, and the diverticular pouch is removed. A postoperative radiograph should always be taken to assess the integrity of the esophagus (**Fig. 5.34**).

**Fig. 5.32  Hypopharyngeal diverticulum: endoscopic treatment**

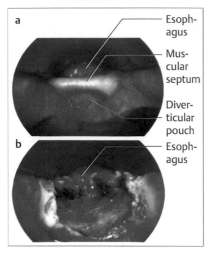

a

— Esophagus

— Muscular septum

— Diverticular pouch

b

— Esophagus

At surgery, the muscular septum is identified endoscopially and (in this case) divided with a $CO_2$ laser.

**Fig. 5.34  Diverticulum after endoscopic removal**

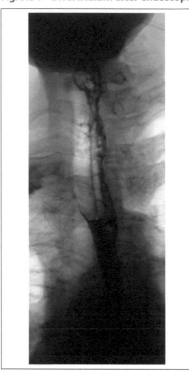

Postoperative radiograph after endoscopic cricopharyngeal myotomy (see **Fig. 5.32**) shows no evidence of a diverticular sac.

**Fig. 5.33  Removal of a diverticulum through an open cervical approach**

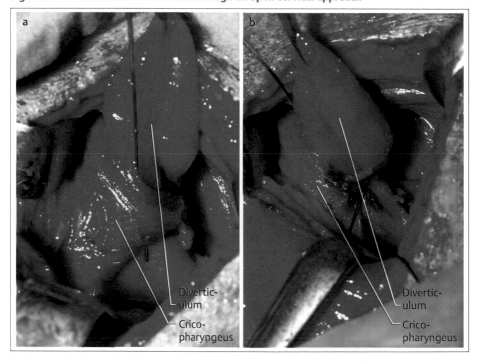

a

b

Diverticulum

Cricopharyngeus

Diverticulum

Cricopharyngeus

The cervical soft tissues are divided, exposing the diverticulum and the cricopharyngeal part of the constrictor pharyngis inferior muscle, before (**a**) and after (**b**) division of the muscular septum. The diverticular pouch is then removed, and the hypopharynx is closed with external sutures.

## Tumors of the Hypopharynx

### Benign Tumors

Benign tumors of the hypopharynx are considered a rarity. They may present clinically with dysphagia, regurgitation, or retrosternal pain. The diagnosis is established with an incisional biopsy taken endoscopically under general endotracheal anesthesia. Treatment consists of surgical removal, depending on the tumor size.

### Malignant Tumors

Histologically, almost all of these tumors are squamous cell carcinomas. As with oral and oropharyngeal carcinomas, there is an etiologic link to chronic alcohol and nicotine abuse.

*Symptoms:* Most malignant tumors of the hypopharynx are diagnosed at an advanced stage because earlier lesions do not produce symptoms.
Initial complaints tend to be nonspecific, depending on tumor size and location (**Table 5.5**), and consist of dysphagia and a fetid breath odor. Later, there may be pain radiating to the ear. Hoarseness and possible dyspnea signify tumor extension to the larynx. In many cases, cervical lymph-node metastasis is noted as the earliest sign of disease.

*Diagnosis:* Besides the mirror examination or indirect laryngoscopy (see 17.2, Indirect Laryngoscopy), the diagnostic work-up should include endoscopic examination under general endotracheal anesthesia, as this is the best way to evaluate tumor extent. A biopsy can also be taken in the same sitting for histologic confirmation. Additionally, sectional imaging modalities can help define the tumor size and check for involvement of adjacent structures while also evaluating the cervical lymph-node status (**Fig. 5.35a**).

*Treatment:* Treatment depends on tumor size but usually consists of local surgical excision with a concomitant neck dissection (see 16.5, Malignant

**Table 5.5** Classification of hypopharyngeal carcinoma according to the Union for International Cancer Control (UICC) system

|  | Definition |
|---|---|
| T1 | ≤ 2 cm and limited to one subsite |
| T2 | > 2–4 cm or more than one subsite |
| T3 | > 4 cm or with hemilarynx fixation/extension to esophagus |
| T4a | Thyroid/cricoid cartilage, hyoid bone, thyroid gland, esophagus, central compartment soft tissue |
| T4b | Prevertebral fascia, carotid artery, mediastinal structures |
| N1 | Ipsilateral single ≤ 3 cm without ENE |
| N2 | • Ipsilateral single > 3–6 cm without ENE<br>• Ipsilateral multiple ≤ 6 cm without ENE<br>• Bilateral, contralateral ≤ 6 cm without ENE |
| N3 | ENE-positive, or > 6 cm without ENE |

Abbreviation: ENE, extranodal extension
Source: Brierley et al 2017.

Tumors of the Cervical Lymph Nodes). Many malignant tumors of the hypopharynx have already spread to the larynx, making it necessary to perform a laryngectomy in the same sitting (see 17.7). The tissue defect is closed primarily whenever possible. This cannot be done with extensive hypopharyngeal resections due to the high risk of stricture formation, and larger defects should be reconstructed by means of a free jejunum transfer with microvascular anastomosis. Surgery should be followed by radiation to the tumor site and lymphatics.
*Alternative treatments* for advanced hypopharyngeal cancers are primary radiotherapy and combined radiation and chemotherapy.

**Fig. 5.35   Hypopharyngeal carcinoma**

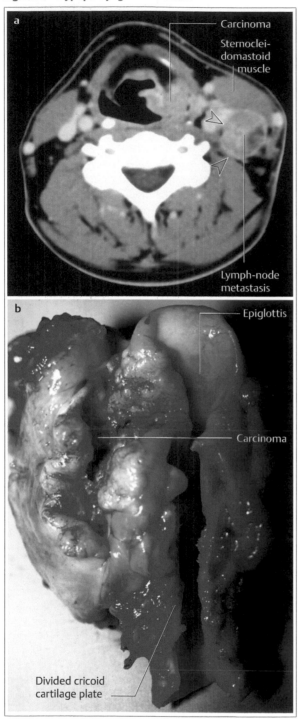

a Carcinoma
Sternoclei-
domastoid
muscle

Lymph-node
metastasis

b Epiglottis

Carcinoma

Divided cricoid
cartilage plate

**a** The axial CT scan demonstrates a mass that is completely filling the right hypopharynx. The arrows point to an ipsilateral
lymph-node metastasis below the sternocleidomastoid muscle.
**b** The surgical specimen includes a posteriorly incised larynx,
which has been resected along with the left piriform sinus. The
left piriform sinus has been completely obliterated by an extensive squamous cell carcinoma infiltrating the larynx.

# 6  The Salivary Glands

## 6.1  Clinical Anatomy of the Salivary Glands

As an introduction, we will review the clinically relevant anatomy of the major and minor salivary glands. A knowledge of salivary gland anatomy is essential for understanding and diagnosing diseases of the salivary glands and providing appropriate treatment.

### Classification

There are three pairs of major salivary glands (**Fig. 6.1**) and several hundred solitary, minor salivary glands distributed throughout the upper aerodigestive tract:
- **Parotid gland:** The largest salivary gland; it mainly produces a serous secretion.
- **Submandibular gland:** Produces a seromucous secretion.
- **Sublingual gland:** Produces a mucoserous secretion.
- **Minor salivary glands (Fig. 6.2):** These consist of labial glands in the mucosa of the lips, palatine glands in the mucosa of the palate, lingual glands in the tongue, and pharyngeal glands in the pharyngeal mucosa. They secrete a saliva that is predominantly mucous.

### Parotid Gland

**Location:** The parotid gland descends into the retromandibular fossa between the vertical ramus of the mandible and the mastoid. Embedded in a subcutaneous pseudocapsule, it lies in contact with the sternocleidomastoid muscle and the posterior belly of the digastric muscle.

**Fibrous capsule:** The subcutaneous pseudocapsule, composed of dense fibrous tissue, is not a discrete tissue layer but blends with the skin and with the parotid gland itself. The capsule is poorly distensible and can cause severe pain when there is acute swelling of the gland. It is less dense inferiorly and medially, facilitating the spread of inflammations and tumors toward the pterygopalatine fossa and parapharyngeal space ("iceberg tumor," see **Fig. 6.5**).

**Parotid duct (Stensen's duct):** This excretory duct, approximately 6 cm long, leaves the parotid gland in its anterior superior third and passes forward over the masseter muscle (see **Fig. 6.1**). It winds around the anterior border of the muscle and pierces the buccinator muscle and buccal mucosa. It opens opposite the second upper molar, forming an orifice with slightly raised edges.

After entering the parotid gland, the **facial nerve** branches into a plexus at the pes anserinus, subdividing the gland into a lateral and medial portion. This anatomic subdivision provides an important landmark

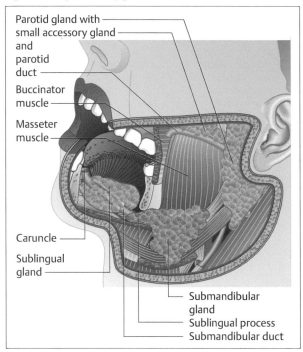

Fig. 6.1  Major salivary glands

Parotid gland with small accessory gland and parotid duct
Buccinator muscle
Masseter muscle
Caruncle
Sublingual gland
Submandibular gland
Sublingual process
Submandibular duct

during surgery of the parotid gland. The facial nerve is identified at its trunk and isolated. Surgical removal of the portion of the gland lateral to the pes anserinus is called a lateral parotidectomy. *Medial* to the pes are branches of the external carotid artery (superficial temporal artery, transverse facial artery) and venous vessels that drain into the internal jugular vein. **Lymphatic drainage** of the parotid gland is through several intraglandular and periglandular lymph nodes to the submandibular and deep jugular nodal chains.

### Submandibular Gland

**Location:** The submandibular gland lies in the submandibular trigone between the two deep parts of the digastric muscle and the mandible. The gland makes a **U**-shaped bend around the posterior border of the mylohyoid muscle. The outer part of the gland extends past the trigone to a variable degree under cover of the outer cervical fascia. Because of this arrangement, the glandular compartment connects the sublingual and posterior portions of the oral floor,

## 6.1 Embryology, malformations, and anomalies

### Embryology
The major salivary glands arise from ectodermal tissues in the foregut between the fourth and eighth weeks of embryonic development. The surrounding mesenchyma segregates the glandular tissue and may include lymph-node primordia. The excretory ducts become patent by the 22nd week of development.

### Malformations
**Aplasia, hypoplasia, duct atresia**: Aplasia of all the salivary glands is extremely rare. Malformations affecting individual salivary glands are also rare. Duct atresia most commonly affects the submandibular glands, and cysts may form.

**Dystopias, accessory and aberrant salivary glands**: Dystopia refers to the abnormal location of an otherwise normally developed salivary gland, such as a parotid gland located anterior to the masseter muscle. Accessory salivary glands are appendages of the major salivary glands that communicate with the duct system and are fully functional. They are most commonly found appended to the parotid gland (see **Fig. 6.1**). Aberrant salivary glands are heterotopic salivary gland primordia that do not have a duct system and are nonfunctional. They occur most frequently in the lateral neck or gingiva and rarely in the middle ear. Salivary gland tumors may develop from these aberrant glands.

**Dysgenetic cysts and ectasias**: These congenital malformations of the excretory ducts require differentiation from similar, acquired abnormalities. They can predispose to recurrent inflammations (see 6.2).

creating a potential route for the spread of infection (abscess or cellulitis of the oral floor).

**Submandibular duct (Wharton's duct):** The excretory duct, approximately 5 cm long, of the submandibular gland passes with the sublingual process of the gland to the sublingual plane of the oral floor and runs forward beneath the mucosa. It crosses over the *lingual nerve* (**Fig. 6.3**) and opens at the sublingual caruncle.

**Nerves and vessels:** The lingual nerve not only closely apposed to the excretory duct but it also forms a genu that runs just above the gland body, where it distributes branches to the submandibular ganglion. The hypoglossal nerve runs inferomedial to the gland. The facial artery and vein loop around the posterior part of the gland.

The **lymphatic drainage** of the submandibular gland is to lymph nodes in the lateral and posteroinferior portion of the gland, which also receive drainage from the face and oral cavity. Because of this, it is usually necessary to remove the submandibular gland when a neck dissection is performed (see "Neck dissection" under Lymph-Node Metastases in 16.5).

**Fig. 6.2  Minor salivary glands**

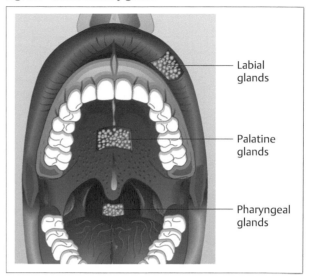

**Fig. 6.3  Submandibular duct**

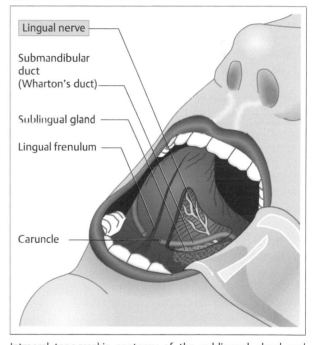

Intraoral topographic anatomy of the sublingual gland and submandibular duct.

## Sublingual Gland

The sublingual gland lies in the anterior, submucous part of the oral floor on the mylohyoid muscle, lateral to the submandibular duct and distributed along the medial surface of the mandible (**Fig. 6.3**). Excretory ducts may drain into the submandibular duct (Bartholin's duct) or may open directly into the oral mucosa as small (Rivini's) ducts.

# 6.2    Functional Morphology and Physiology of the Salivary Glands

To understand disorders of salivary gland function, it is also important to know the common histologic structure of the glands, the physiologic functions of the saliva, and the clinical terms for secretory dysfunction.

## Histologic Structure

All salivary glands are based on a common structural principle: glandular acini connected to a system of salivary ducts (**Fig. 6.4**). The acini and the duct system are embedded in a glandular mesenchyma that contains connective tissue, blood and lymphatic vessels, lymphatic tissue, and nerve fibers.

### Glandular Acini

The acini produce the primary saliva, which contains enzymes (including amylase) and sialomucins. Several histologic types are distinguished based on the relative amounts of enzymes and mucins that are formed:
- Serous glands, which mainly produce enzymes (e.g., the parotid gland).
- Mucous glands, which mainly produce mucin (e.g., the palatine glands).
- Mixed glands (e.g., the submandibular and sublingual glands).

The acini include myoepithelial cells, which form a weblike structure that surrounds the acinus and can extrude its contents through a contractile action.

### Salivary Duct System

The salivary duct system is not a passive transport system but actively modifies the contents and consistency of the primary saliva. The short intercalated ducts secrete mucins and regulate the electrolyte concentration. Next come the striated ducts, which can quickly and actively secrete fluid, followed by the interlobular duct system, which mainly transports the saliva while only slightly altering its properties.

## Composition of the Saliva

The salivary glands constantly produce a certain amount of saliva. In the absence of external stimuli, this production, called the *resting secretion*, probably relates to the basic activity of the salivatory nucleus. External and internal factors, particularly eating and the associated chewing movements, smells, etc., can significantly increase the rate of salivary secretion. In the parotid gland, this *stimulated secretion* is around four to five times greater than the resting secretion (**Table 6.1**).

**Fig. 6.4   Basic structure of the salivary glands**

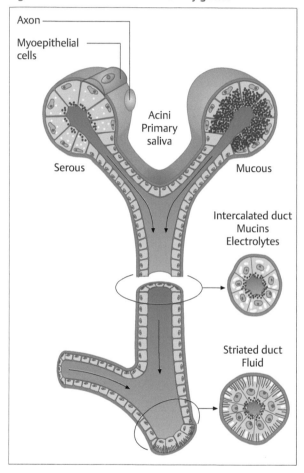

Axon

Myoepithelial cells

Acini Primary saliva

Serous

Mucous

Intercalated duct
Mucins
Electrolytes

Striated duct
Fluid

**Table 6.1   Resting secretion versus stimulated secretion**

|  | Resting secretion | Stimulated secretion |
|---|---|---|
| Origin | Mainly from the submandibular and sublingual glands and minor salivary glands | Mainly from the parotid gland |
| Consistency | Relatively mucous | More serous |
| Contents | Mucins, few enzymes | Enzymes, fewer mucins |

The total daily volume of saliva secreted by all the salivary glands is from 500 to 1,000 mL, subject to influence by numerous factors such as climate, fluid intake, nutrition, age, and gender (**Table 6.2**). The production of saliva is controlled mainly by parasympathetic-cholinergic stimuli. But sympathetic stimuli also exercise a control function via α- and β$_1$-adrenergic receptors, especially in the regulation of α-amylase.

## Physiologic Functions of Saliva

### Nutrition and Digestion

The saliva emulsifies and dissolves food constituents, aiding in the perception of taste. The glycoproteins in the saliva lubricate the bolus to facilitate swallowing. The actual digestive enzyme is α-amylase, a starch-splitting enzyme that is produced mainly by the parotid gland.

### Protective Functions

The quantity and composition of saliva have a major influence on the microbiological and inorganic milieu of the oral cavity. Mechanical cleansing (irrigation) plays a role, as does the secretion of enzymes (lysozyme, muramidases, peroxidases) and immunoglobulins (mainly IgA).
The production of saliva is also important in the prevention of gum disease and dental caries.

### Excretion

Both endogenous and exogenous substances can be excreted in the saliva. Of clinical importance is the excretion of certain *ions* (iodine, fluorine) and of *viruses* that can be transmitted via the saliva—poliomyelitis, hepatitis B, Epstein–Barr virus, cytomegalovirus, coxsackievirus, rabies, human immunodeficiency virus (HIV). The excretion of genetically determined *glycoproteins*, whose antigenic properties are similar to the ABO system but independent of it, can be of forensic importance.

### Secretory Disorders

Disorders of salivary gland secretion, transport, and consumption can lead to changes in the quality and quantity of the saliva. The general term for these disorders is *dyschylia*. Several terms are applied to increased salivary flow and are not always clearly differentiated from one another (**Table 6.3**). In *sialorrhea*, the quantity of the saliva is not necessarily increased (retention sialorrhea due to impaired swallowing). Sialorrhea is particularly common in children with

cerebral palsy and may become a significant nursing problem.
The condition resulting from pronounced hyposalivation may be termed *xerostomia* (dry mouth) or *sicca syndrome* (additionally involving the conjunctiva and other mucous membranes). It is frequently associated with very troublesome complaints.

**Table 6.2 Factors that influence saliva production**

| Hypersalivation | Hyposalivation |
| --- | --- |
| Stimulation | Depression |
| Foods, acids, poisons (mercury, arsenic, lead), nausea, pregnancy | Inflammation of the glands, dehydration, marasmus, radiation exposure |
| Parasympathomimetic agents (e.g., pilocarpine, muscarine, nicotine), sympathomimetic agents (e.g., isoproterenol), iodine, bromide, fluoride, curare, theophylline, caffeine | Anticholinergic agents (e.g., atropine, scopolamine), α-blockers (e.g., phentolamine), β-blockers (e.g., propranolol), antihistamines, antihypertensive agents (e.g., clonidine, reserpine), psychoactive drugs (e.g., antidepressants), topical anesthetics |

**Table 6.3 Terms for disorders of salivary secretion**

| Disorder | Symptoms |
| --- | --- |
| **Dyschylia** | General disturbances of salivary secretion or production |
| **Hypersalivation** Synonym: ptyalism | Increased flow of saliva Causes: see **Table 6.2** |
| Sialorrhea | Excessive flow of saliva from the mouth (drooling, slobbering) Caused by swallowing difficulties due to: <br> • Neurologic diseases (Parkinson's disease, bulbar paralysis, myasthenia gravis, cerebral palsy) <br> • Mechanical obstruction (pharyngeal tumor, esophageal obstruction) |
| **Hyposalivation** Synonym: sialopenia | Decreased flow of saliva Causes: see **Table 6.2** |
| Asialia | Absence of salivary secretion |
| Xerostomia | Dryness of the oral mucosa |
| Sicca syndrome | Dryness of the oral mucosa and other mucous membranes (conjunctiva, genital mucosae) |

# 6.3    Clinical Examination, Imaging Studies, and Biopsy of the Salivary Glands

In many cases, a salivary gland disease can be classified as inflammatory or neoplastic based on a detailed clinical examination. The first-line modality for further investigation is ultrasonography; computed tomography (CT) and—preferably—magnetic resonance imaging (MRI) are available as second-line studies. The histologic diagnosis is particularly important as it provides the basis for treatment.

## Clinical Examination

### History

Particular attention should be given to:
- Systemic diseases, especially metabolic disorders (e.g., diabetes mellitus) and autoimmune diseases (e.g., rheumatoid arthritis, systemic lupus erythematosus, IgG$_4$-related diseases), which can have a systemic effect on the salivary glands.
- Medications (antihypertensive drugs, psychotherapeutic drugs; see **Table 6.2**).
- Prior illnesses, surgical procedures, or therapies (radiotherapy) involving the glands and oral cavity.
- Hypersalivation and hyposalivation, sialorrhea, or sicca syndrome (see **Table 6.3**).

### Inspection

The glands are inspected externally (periauricular and submandibular region) along with the oral cavity and tonsillar region. Facial nerve motor function should also be tested.

**External:** Normally, visual inspection reveals only the flat contour of the submandibular gland in the submandibular trigone if the overlying skin is thin. A normal parotid gland is not visible. *Masseter hyperplasia* can mimic enlargement of the parotid gland but is easily differentiated by having the patient squeeze the jaws together. This activates the masseter muscle, making it easily accessible to inspection and palpation.

**Oral cavity:** The orifices of the excretory ducts (Wharton's and Stensen's ducts) are evaluated for redness and swelling. The flow of saliva, either spontaneous or in response to glandular massage, is an important parameter for differentiating between obstruction, inflammation, and normal findings (saliva clear or absent, flocculent, purulent, blood-tinged).

**Tonsillar region** (**Fig. 6.5**): The parapharyngeal or tonsillar region may appear prominent due to swelling of the deep portions of the parotid gland.

**Fig. 6.5    Deep tumor of the parotid gland**

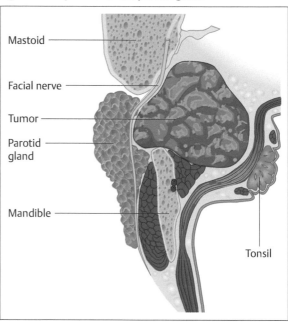

Mastoid

Facial nerve

Tumor

Parotid gland

Mandible

Tonsil

A tumor involving the deep portions of the parotid gland may produce a bulge in the tonsillar region ("iceberg tumor").

**Fig. 6.6    Palpation of the oral floor**

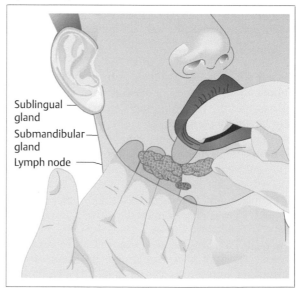

Sublingual gland

Submandibular gland

Lymph node

Bimanual palpation of the submandibular gland.

**Fig. 6.7 Ultrasound examination of the salivary glands**

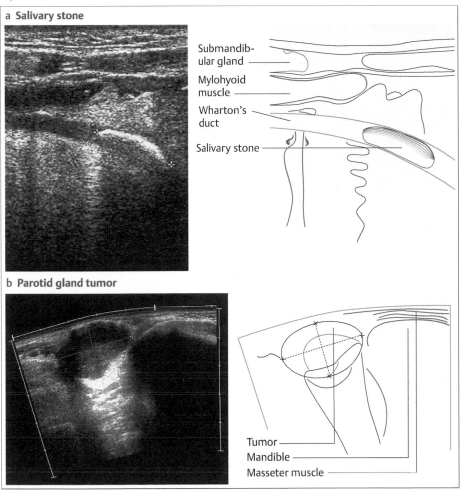

a Salivary stone

Submandibular gland
Mylohyoid muscle
Wharton's duct
Salivary stone

b Parotid gland tumor

Tumor
Mandible
Masseter muscle

**a** Large salivary stone in Wharton's duct. The stone, which casts a distal acoustic shadow, has obstructed and dilated Wharton's duct.
**b** Well-demarcated tumor in the parotid gland.

---

⚕ With changes in the parotid gland, especially neoplastic changes, **facial nerve function** should always be tested and documented in a side-to-side comparison.

## Palpation

A normal parotid gland is barely palpable. The submandibular glands, a swelling of the sublingual glands, and the excretory ducts are palpated bimanually (**Fig. 6.6**), noting the size of any abnormalities in centimeters and assessing their consistency, surface contours, tenderness, and mobility relative to the skin and underlying tissues. A normal sublingual gland cannot be palpated.

The intraglandular, periglandular, and cervical lymph nodes should also be examined.

## Imaging Studies

**Ultrasound examination:** Ultrasound has proved to be a well-tolerated and rewarding study for investigating the salivary glands. It can differentiate among normal glandular parenchyma, inflammatory processes (with or without liquefaction), tumors, lymph nodes, and calculi (**Fig. 6.7**). Generally, the ultrasound examination is the first imaging procedure used. It can be combined with fine-needle aspiration or core needle biopsy.

**Radiographs:** Plain radiographs of the oral floor, submandibular gland, and parotid gland are seldom rewarding because of superimposed structures. To be visible on radiographs, calculi must have a sufficient calcium content and measure at least 2 to 3 mm in size. For this reason, plain radiographs are of low diagnostic value.

**Sialography:** Radiographic contrast examination of the excretory ducts after catheterization gives the most detailed view of the duct systems of the parotid and submandibular glands. Sialography is rarely performed today, however, due to potential complications (infection, abscess formation, extravasation) and the availability of ultrasound, sialendoscopy, and MRI. Its possible indications include the detection of small stones in the excretory ducts, anomalies of the excretory ducts, sialadenosis, and chronic inflammation.

**Fig. 6.8  Abscess of the parotid gland**

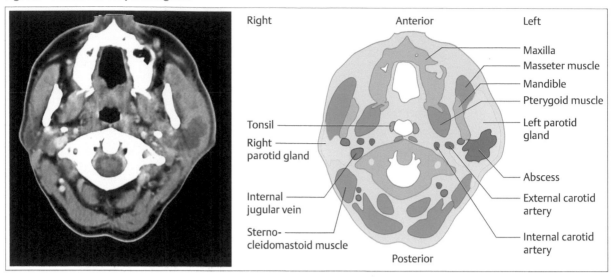

CT scan of an abscess in the left parotid gland, with a correlative drawing. Axial scan at the level of the hard palate (soft-tissue window after contrast administration).

⚠ Sialography is contraindicated in the presence of acute inflammation.

**CT and MRI:** Most lesions of the salivary glands that cannot be adequately diagnosed from the history, palpation, and ultrasound findings must be investigated by CT or MRI. This particularly applies to tumors and masses that transcend the gland boundaries or involve the deep portions of the parotid gland (**Fig. 6.8**). MRI is superior to CT in the diagnosis of salivary gland tumors (**Fig. 6.9a–c**).

### Sialendoscopy

The major excretory ducts (Stensen's and Wharton's ducts) can also be inspected with special endoscopes, which are introduced under local anesthesia after dilation of the papillae. The duct is irrigated during endoscopy, which can demonstrate mucous plugs, calculi, and stenoses. Interventional procedures can also be performed such as dilation or the removal of a stone with a loop or by laser lithotripsy.

### Biopsy

**Fine-needle aspiration biopsy** (FNAB) has established itself as a low-risk, well-tolerated procedure in the preoperative investigation of salivary gland swelling. It can also furnish material for bacteriologic analysis.

More deeply situated lesions can be aspirated under ultrasound guidance.

The main complication of FNAB is secondary infection of the puncture site, which is why the procedure requires meticulous aseptic technique.

**As an alternative, core biopsy** may be performed especially for typing of salivary gland tumors.

**Incisional biopsy and intraoperative frozen section:** In rare cases, an incisional biopsy of the salivary glands may be warranted for the investigation of a chronic inflammatory process. An incisional biopsy is relatively safe for ulcerative lesions and in patients with facial nerve palsy. Otherwise, an incisional biopsy should be avoided, especially in the parotid gland, due to the ever-present risk of facial nerve injury.

⚠ Incisional biopsy is contraindicated for benign salivary gland tumors.

If the tumor is most likely benign (see ✍6.4), the tumor should be completely removed along with its capsule. This involves surgical removal of the gland combined with an *intraoperative frozen section*.

With generalized salivary gland disease (e.g., Sjögren's myoepithelial sialadenitis), the *biopsy of a minor salivary gland* in the lower lip is commonly performed under local anesthesia, but its sensitivity is low. Therefore, open biopsy of the parotid gland seems to be the better alternative.

**Fig. 6.9  Tumor of the parotid gland**

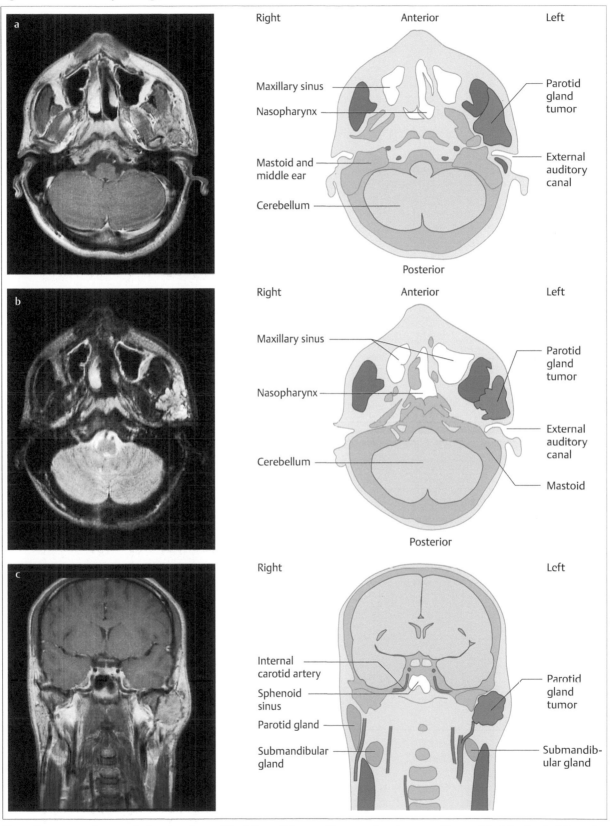

Magnetic resonance images of a lymphangioma of the left parotid gland, with correlative drawings. Axial T1-weighted (**a**) and T2-weighted (**b**) postcontrast images at the level of the external auditory canal, and a coronal image (**c**) at the level of the sphenoid sinus.

# 6.4   Overview: Diagnosis and Management of Salivary Gland Swelling

**Diseases of the salivary glands are often manifested by unilateral or bilateral swelling of the glands. This swelling leads to differential diagnostic considerations in which the history, clinical examination, imaging** studies, and biopsy have an important role (see ✍6.3). This ✍ shows how the various diagnostic options can be effectively coordinated in practice (see also ✍6.7).

The swelling of one or more salivary glands may be a result of duct obstruction, inflammation, or neoplasia. A detailed history and physical examination will usually furnish a differential diagnosis as a basis for further testing. The clinical suspicion of a malignant tumor is particularly important in this regard. The clinical steps involved in making a differential diagnosis are outlined in **Fig. 6.10**. Standard laboratory tests are also helpful in distinguishing between inflammation and a tumor. An elevated white blood cell count, erythrocyte sedimentation rate (ESR), or C-reactive protein (CRP) is suggestive of inflammation. Tumors of the salivary glands generally produce no changes in routine blood tests. A somewhat rare exception to this rule is the situation where an obstructive tumor has caused salivary stasis, leading to an infection.

Generally, an ultrasound examination is the next diagnostic procedure to follow the clinical examination. It can demonstrate changes in the duct system and more accurately characterize the swelling, differentiating between a cyst and solid lesion, for example. This information will usually yield a diagnosis or indicate the need for additional, more specific studies as shown in **Fig. 6.11**.

The definitive diagnosis of a swollen salivary gland is occasionally made at the time of operation, particularly in the case of a tumor. Tumors are manifested clinically by a more or less painless, unilateral swelling with a palpable nodule. It is important to look for signs that are helpful in distinguishing benign and malignant tumors.

Signs suggesting a **benign tumor**:
- Slow growth (months to years).
- Painless, soft or tense nodule that is freely movable.
- No signs of tumor infiltrating the surrounding tissue.
- No additional symptoms.

Signs suggesting a **malignant tumor**:
- Rapid growth (weeks to months).
- Painful, fixed nodule.
- Evidence of tumor infiltrating muscle, skin, or nerves (facial nerve palsy; **Fig. 6.12**).
- Lymph-node enlargement.

**Fig. 6.10   Acute and chronic swelling**

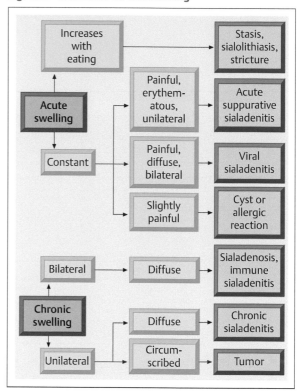

⚡ Facial nerve palsy associated with a tumor in the parotid gland almost always signifies a malignant tumor (and indicates a worse prognosis).

The *location* of a salivary gland tumor can also furnish clues to the differential diagnosis of the tumor.

⚡ Eighty percent of salivary gland tumors occur in the parotid gland, about 10% in the submandibular gland, and 10% in other salivary glands.

A localized swelling of the parotid gland very often signifies a tumor. This is less often the case with the submandibular gland. Only approximately 20% of tumors in the parotid gland are malignant, compared with approximately half of tumors in the submandibular glands and about 80% of tumors in the small salivary glands.

**Fig. 6.11   Flowchart for the investigation of salivary gland diseases**

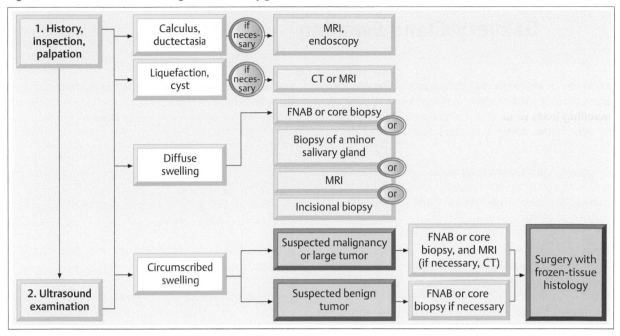

**Fig. 6.12   Facial nerve palsy due to a salivary gland tumor**

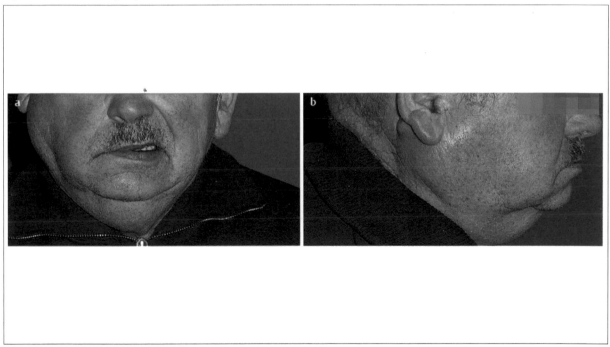

Mucoepidermoid carcinoma of the right parotid gland with facial nerve palsy, signifying invasion of the nerve by the tumor.

⚑ Rule of thumb for salivary gland tumors: the smaller the salivary gland, the greater the likelihood that the tumor is malignant.

FNAB will yield an accurate cytologic diagnosis in approximately only 50 to 60% of tumors. The positive detection of malignant cells has a high correlation with the actual presence of a malignant tumor, and appropriate tests should be initiated at once. It does not justify a radical procedure such as facial nerve resection, however. At the same time, the absence of malignant cells on FNAB does not confidently exclude a malignancy.

# 6.5    Noninflammatory Diseases and Injuries to the Salivary Glands

This 📖 deals with salivary gland diseases other than primary inflammations and tumors. The most important are sialolithiasis, sialadenosis, and injuries.

## Sialolithiasis

Synonym: salivary stone disease.

**Definition:** Stone formation in the excretory duct system of a salivary gland.

**Epidemiology:** Adults in the third and fourth decades are most commonly affected, with males predominating by a ratio of 2:1.

**Location:** Around 60 to 70% of salivary stones are located in the main duct. Generalized lithiasis (urinary stones, gallstones, and salivary stone) is present in approximately 6 to 10% of all cases.

📖 Approximately 70 to 80% of salivary stones occur in the submandibular gland, and about 20% in the parotid gland. A smaller percentage occur in the minor salivary glands or sublingual gland.

**Etiopathogenesis:** Salivary stones result from the secondary calcification of "plugs" that form from enriched organic salivary contents (mucins). A microcalcification can lead to increased salivary stasis and to the precipitation of inorganic compounds.

**Symptoms:** Eating and other gustatory stimuli incite a swelling of the affected gland, often accompanied by severe pain ("salivary stone colic"). There may also be a stasis-induced "salivary tumor." The stasis can lead to infection of the excretory duct and gland, which may present as a primary or secondary symptom (see 📖6.6, Acute Sialadenitis).

**Diagnosis:** Stones are often palpable in the duct system of the submandibular gland. Ultrasound reveals dilation of the duct system with typical acoustic shadowing. Approximately 70% of the stones are radiopaque, particularly those occurring in the submandibular gland. Plain radiographs or sialography are no longer necessary today, as diagnostic sialendoscopy offers an elegant opportunity to confirm the diagnosis.

**Differential diagnosis:** External obstruction of the excretory duct, as by a denture or tumor, is the most frequent differential diagnosis. Also, stricture of the duct without stone is a possible cause of obstructive sialadenitis. Phleboliths are rare, and calcified lymph-node tuberculomas are very rare.

**Complications:** Infection and abscess, particularly of the oral floor.

**Treatment:** Treatment is generally surgical (with inclusion of minimally invasive sialendoscopic procedures).
- With distal submandibular stones, it is sufficient to incise the excretory duct, extract the stone, and suture the duct epithelium to the mucosa (marsupialization; **Fig. 6.13**).
- Intraglandular stones of the submandibular gland and a chronically damaged gland should be excised. In some cases, stones can be extracted by an extended marsupialization.
- Salivary stones located in the duct or near the gland can be removed by endoscopic fragmentation (using a laser beam or ultrasound shock waves) or extracorporeal lithotripsy (ultrasound shock waves).

Stones in the parotid gland can today be treated by sialendoscopy-guided procedures such as loop

Fig. 6.13    **Marsupialization**

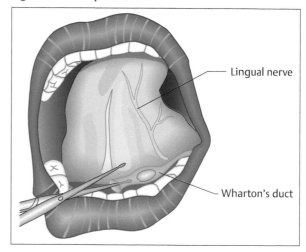

Lingual nerve

Wharton's duct

## 🔍 6.2  Salivary gland cysts

Cysts of the salivary glands require differentiation from tumors and chronic inflammations. Various forms may be encountered:

**Dysgenetic cysts**: These are primary cysts resulting from a developmental abnormality and must be distinguished from secondary, acquired cysts. Dysgenetic cysts occur most commonly in the sublingual gland and its excretory ducts. A cyst at this location is called a ranula ("little frog," after its resemblance to the expanded vocal air sac of a frog; **Fig. 6.14**). Ranulae seem only to appear in cases with presence of a major sublingual duct of Bartholin. A ranula of sufficient size can restrict tongue mobility and cause difficulties with speech and swallowing. It may also become infected. Treatment consists of surgical removal. Dysgenetic cysts of the parotid gland may become inflamed, particularly in children.

**Salivary duct cysts** occur predominantly in the parotid gland. They may be complicated by infection.

**Mucoceles and retention cysts of the minor salivary glands**: Injuries to minor salivary glands may allow saliva to escape into the tissue, forming a pseudocyst. Duct obstructions give rise to true cysts (= retention cysts) with an epithelial lining. Both forms occur predominantly in the mucosa of the lower lip. The differential diagnosis should also include a possible tumor of the minor salivary glands, especially when the mass is located on the palate.

**Lymphoepithelial cysts** probably originate from lymph follicles and therefore occur mainly in the parotid gland. Histologic examination reveals lymphatic tissue in the cyst wall. This type of cyst is particularly common in HIV infections; they tend to be bilateral and occur predominantly in younger patients.

**Fig. 6.14   Ranula (right)**

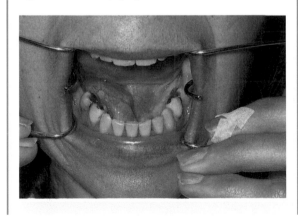

extraction and intraductal lithotripsy. If the stone cannot be removed by these measures, also a combination of sialendoscopy and a small incision of the gland can be performed. A parotidectomy is rarely indicated.

## Sialadenosis

**Definition:** Sialadenosis refers to a noninflammatory, symmetrical swelling of the major salivary glands caused by a systemic, frequently unknown cause. The parotid gland is most commonly affected.

**Pathogenesis:** Sialadenosis can occur in association with:
- Chronic alcoholism.
- Vitamin deficiencies.
- Diabetes mellitus.
- Protein deficiency.
- Anorexia nervosa and other eating disorders.

Sialadenosis is a secretory disorder characterized by enlarged acinar cells. The most likely cause is disordered autonomic innervation of the affected salivary glands. It seems likely that a defect of aquaporins is causative for sialadenosis.

**Symptoms:** The disease causes a painless, usually symmetrical swelling that is unrelated to eating.

**Diagnosis:** A bilateral, symmetrical, painless swelling of the salivary glands is typically noted on clinical examination. MRI or FNAB may be indicated in cases with equivocal clinical findings. The diagnosis can be histologically confirmed by glandular biopsy, but this is rarely necessary.

**Differential diagnosis:** All forms of chronic sialadenitis must be excluded. Less frequent possibilities are masseter hyperplasia and obesity with fatty hypertrophy of the gland.

**Treatment:** Treatment is directed toward the underlying cause. No specific therapy for sialadenosis is required.

## Injuries

### Penetrating or Blunt Trauma

Direct sharp or blunt injuries most commonly affect the parotid gland, which occupies a less protected location than the submandibular gland. It is important to distinguish injuries to the glandular parenchyma alone from injuries involving the excretory duct system or facial nerve.

⚡ Every open salivary gland injury should be surgically explored.

**Bleeding:** Bleeding in the parotid gland is not life-threatening and can usually be managed by primary compression. Coagulation, clipping, or ligation should be avoided in an obscured field (risk of facial nerve injury).

**Duct injuries:** A duct injury can result from trauma to the anterior third of the gland. Whenever possible, a microsurgical end-to-end anastomosis should be performed over a fine plastic catheter. Another option is to suture the duct stump to the mucosa, creating a neo-ostium.

**Facial nerve injuries:** see 🔖 14.2, Traumatic Facial Paralysis. Immediate or early treatment is advised.

## Pneumoparotid

The retrograde entry of air into Stensen's duct is considered a special case of parotid trauma. It results from a high positive pressure in the oral cavity, which may occur during forcible mask ventilation or when blowing a musical instrument, blowing glass, or inflating a balloon. It is marked by transient pain in the region of the parotid gland. Cutaneous emphysema is rarely detectable by palpation. Specific treatment is unnecessary, and the air should be quickly eliminated by reabsorption or leakage from the duct orifice.

# 6.6 Inflammatory Diseases of the Salivary Glands (Sialadenitis)

The inflammation of a salivary gland usually leads to diffuse swelling of the entire gland. Table 6.4 reviews the various forms of sialadenitis, which may be acute or chronic. They may be caused by viral infections, bacterial infections, autoimmune diseases, or ionizing radiation exposure.

## Acute Sialadenitis

### Acute Viral Sialadenitis, Mumps

Various organisms have been identified as the cause of acute viral inflammations of the salivary glands. Rarer causes are cytomegalovirus (*➧ 6.3*), coxsackievirus, influenza virus, and HIV. The most common viral pathogen is the mumps virus. It is the causative organism of **mumps** (see below), which occurs predominantly but not exclusively in children. Synonyms: epidemic parotitis, infectious parotitis.

The causative organism is the mumps virus, from the family of paramyxoviruses. The virus is shed in the saliva, and the infection is spread by droplet transmission. The major salivary glands are infected by the hematogenous route. The incubation period is 18 (±10) days. Fifty percent of cases run a silent course, and the infection confers lifelong immunity.

*Symptoms:* Cases typically present with diffuse, painful, acute swelling of the parotid glands with a doughy edema ("hamster cheeks"). Often, one parotid gland is affected initially, followed several days later by swelling of the cervical lymph nodes, the opposite parotid gland, and the submandibular glands. The duct orifices are reddened and slightly swollen, and the secretions are nonpurulent. Usually, only a mild fever is present, and approximately 30% of patients are afebrile. The infection should resolve in 1 to 2 weeks.

*Diagnosis:* The diagnosis is based on the clinical presentation. Serologic testing is necessary only in doubtful cases. A fourfold rise of antibody titers 2 to 3 weeks after the onset of the disease establishes the diagnosis.

*Differential diagnosis:* Differentiation is mainly required from cervical lymphadenitis and acute suppurative parotitis. Less frequent conditions to be considered are chronic recurrent parotitis, a dentogenic infection or abscess, sialolithiasis, or a tumor.

*Complications:* An abnormal cerebrospinal fluid examination accompanied by serous meningitis is relatively common. Serious but less frequent complications are

---

**Table 6.4 Types of sialadenitis**

**Acute sialadenitis**
Viral:
- Mumps
- Cytomegalovirus (*➧ 6.3*)
- Coxsackievirus, echovirus, parainfluenza viruses, influenza

Bacterial:
- Acute suppurative parotitis
- Obstructive (electrolyte) sialadenitis

**Chronic sialadenitis**
Chronic recurrent parotitis
Chronic recurrent sialadenitis of the submandibular gland, sclerosing sialadenitis (Küttner's tumor)
Radiation sialadenitis
Immune sialadenitis:
- Myoepithelial (Sjögren's syndrome)
- Epithelioid cell (Heerfordt's syndrome; *➧ 6.4*)

Infectious granulomatous sialadenitis (*➧ 6.4*):
- Tuberculosis
- Actinomycosis
- Syphilis

---

*➧ 6.3 Cytomegalovirus sialadenitis*

The second most common viral sialadenitis is caused by cytomegalovirus (salivary gland inclusion disease). The sialotropic virus usually affects the salivary gland with no inflammatory signs and is shed in the saliva. Often acquired perinatally, the infection may run a silent course or may produce various symptoms separate from the salivary glands themselves, such as sensorineural hearing loss. In later stages of life, the infection most commonly occurs in immunocompromised patients and causes systemic symptoms that resemble mononucleosis.

---

meningoencephalitis with permanent cranial nerve deficits, orchitis, and labyrinthitis. Deafness may also occur and is unilateral in most cases. The pancreas and ovaries may also be involved.

*Treatment:* Treatment is supportive, consisting of analgesics, increased fluid intake, and salivary stimulation with lemon drops, etc.

**Prophylaxis:** The best preventive measure is a mumps vaccination program (96% protection rate with proper use).

## Acute Bacterial Sialadenitis

Synonym: acute suppurative sialadenitis.

**Etiology and pathogenesis:** This suppurative infection most commonly affects the parotid gland in debilitated, dehydrated patients. When the submandibular gland is affected, the cause is usually obstructive (sialolithiasis, poorly fitting denture) or dentogenic in nature.
The main causative organism is *Staphylococcus aureus*. Streptococci, *Haemophilus*, and other organisms may also be found. The typical pattern is an ascending bacterial infection in a patient with decreased salivary flow. Usually, there is a general predisposing condition for bacterial sialadenitis such as diabetes mellitus, weakened host defenses, or poor oral and dental hygiene.

**Symptoms:** The patient presents with a painful, diffuse swelling of the affected gland. The skin over the gland may be reddened, and the gland may become fluctuant due to tissue liquefaction (**Fig. 6.15**). The excretory duct orifices are red and swollen. A turbid fluid or pus can be expressed from the gland orifice or may drain spontaneously. Trismus may be present.

**Diagnosis:** The diagnosis is made from the typical palpable findings and suppurative discharge in patients with a corresponding prior illness. The discharge should be tested bacteriologically to determine antibiotic sensitivity.

**Differential diagnosis:** A dentogenic infection can produce similar findings. A less frequent cause is furuncular otitis with a periauricular abscess or lymphadenitis (especially with sialadenitis of the submandibular gland).

**Fig. 6.15  Parotid abscess**

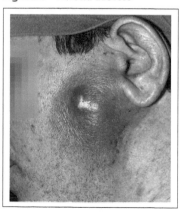

Acute suppurative parotitis with abscess formation.

**Treatment:** Generally, the disease responds well to medical management with antibiotics, analgesics (nonsteroidal anti-inflammatory agents), hydration, salivary stimulation, and good oral hygiene. If an abscess develops, the parotid gland should be incised parallel to the branches of the facial nerve.

## Chronic Sialadenitis

(See also 🔍 **6.4**)

### Chronic Recurrent Parotitis

The *pathogenesis* of recurrent bacterial infections of the parotid gland, which are common in childhood but also occur in adults, is still uncertain, but sialendoscopy showed that strictures and inflammation of the duct system are present in most cases.

**Symptoms:** Usually, there is a unilateral or alternating (rarely bilateral) swelling of the parotid gland, which may be very painful. The saliva is milky, granular, or purulent. Trismus is frequently present. The attacks recur at varying intervals. Between attacks, the patient has no subjective symptoms but the parotid gland may be indurated.

---

🔍 **6.4  Other forms of chronic sialadenitis**

Epithelioid cell sialadenitis and Heerfordt's syndrome: *Sarcoidosis of the salivary glands* is usually characterized by unilateral or bilateral involvement of the parotid gland, which shows a moderately firm, constant swelling. Intraglandular lymph nodes may be affected in addition to the glandular parenchyma. Involvement of the minor salivary glands may occur. Pain is relatively mild, and little or no sialopenia is present. The diagnosis is established by biopsy. Differentiation from tuberculosis is required. The disease is treated with corticosteroids.
Simultaneous involvement of the eyes (mainly the uvea) and salivary glands is known as *Heerfordt's syndrome* (subchronic uveoparotid fever). It is often associated with cranial nerve deficits, especially facial nerve palsy.
**Tuberculosis:** Tuberculosis of the salivary glands is rare. The intraglandular lymph nodes are predominantly affected, and less commonly the glandular parenchyma. The diagnosis is established by bacteriologic testing and/or histologic examination. Treatment relies on tuberculostatic drugs.
**Other chronic forms: Actinomycosis** with a hard, painless swelling and a typical violaceous skin discoloration should be included in the differential diagnosis. It may develop in proximity to the parotid or submandibular gland and may involve the gland secondarily. It is generally rare.
**Syphilis** of the salivary gland is very rare but should be excluded when a granulomatous inflammation is present.
**HIV infection:** Symmetrical enlargement of the salivary glands is relatively common in patients infected with human immunodeficiency virus (HIV salivary gland disease). It is particularly common to find bilateral lymphoepithelial cysts of the parotid glands, and patients with acquired immune deficiency syndrome (AIDS) may exhibit a Sjögrenlike syndrome with marked xerostomia.

In *children*, the symptoms usually resolve during puberty. Cases in *adults* may take a very protracted course in which obliterative scarring of the parenchyma causes saliva production to dwindle and finally cease, with an associated resolution of symptoms.

**Diagnosis:** The diagnosis is made from the history and clinical course. Generally, a normal sonogram is obtained between attacks. Sialendoscopy typically shows inflammation of the duct (sialodochitis) and/or strictures.

**Differential diagnosis:** Differentiation from the less common immune sialadenitis can be difficult in adults and may necessitate an incisional biopsy. Immune sialadenitis occurs predominantly in women.

**Complications:** Abscess formation.

**Treatment:** Exacerbations are treated the same as acute bacterial parotitis. A conservative approach is definitely indicated in children. Sialendoscopy does not only play an important role in the diagnosis but also in the treatment of this disease: the duct is rinsed with saline or corticosteroids, and strictures are dilated. Adult patients may require a parotidectomy, which is difficult in these cases and carries a significant risk of facial nerve injury.

## Chronic Sclerosing Sialadenitis

Synonyms: chronic recurrent sialadenitis of the submandibular gland, Küttner's tumor.

**Definition:** This is the most common form of chronic inflammatory sialadenitis, usually occurring in association with obstruction and sialolithiasis. It may culminate in a permanent, tumorlike swelling of the affected gland.

**Pathogenesis:** Chronic sclerosing sialadenitis was recently recognized as a member of the family of IgGn4-related systemic diseases (**Table 6.5**).

**Symptoms:** Patients present with a firm swelling of the submandibular gland, which undergoes an acutely painful enlargement that is related to eating. The end stage, called a Küttner tumor, is a firm, constant, essentially nontender enlargement of the gland that is difficult to distinguish from a neoplasm by palpation.

**Diagnosis:** The diagnosis is made by demonstrating the duct obstruction with ultrasound. MRI is necessary only in complicated cases. FNAB reveals inflammatory changes and the presence of $IgG_4$-producing plasma cells beneath an obliterative

| Table 6.5 Spectrum of $IgG_4$-related diseases |
|---|
| *Manifestations of $IgG_4$-related disease* |
| • Mikulicz's syndrome (dacryoadenitis and sialadenitis) |
| • Küttner's tumor |
| • Riedel's thyroiditis |
| • Chronic sclerosing aortitis |
| • Abdominal aortitis |
| • Retroperitoneal fibrosis (Ormond's disease) |
| • Autoimmune pancreatitis |
| • Sclerosing cholangitis |
| • Orbital pseudotumor |
| • Eosinophil angiocentric fibrosis of the paranasal sinuses |
| • Multifocal fibrosclerosis |
| • Pachymeningitis |
| • Hypophysitis |

phlebitis. Serum $IgG_4$ may or may be not elevated. The gland can be extirpated as an "excisional biopsy." Patients with local $IgG_4$ disease should be screened for other organ manifestations.

**Differential diagnosis:** Differentiation is required from other causes of excretory duct obstruction such as extrinsic pressure due to tumors, cysts, or other intraoral lesions and from intraductal obstruction by a stone or viscous plug. The differential diagnosis should also include lymph-node metastasis, especially from squamous cell carcinoma of the oral cavity. Differentiation from a dentogenic abscess can be difficult. Actinomycosis and tuberculosis are rare differential diagnoses.

**Treatment:** Chronic sclerosing sialadenitis is treated with corticosteroids for up to 6 months. Excision of the gland is sometimes necessary (**Fig. 6.16**).

## Myoepithelial Sialadenitis and Sjögren's Syndrome

Synonym: benign lymphoepithelial lesion.

**Definition:** This is an autoimmune form of chronic sialadenitis marked by a gradual decline in saliva production. A sicca syndrome may develop (**Fig. 6.17**). *Sjögren's syndrome* consists of myoepithelial sialadenitis accompanied by keratoconjunctivitis sicca (decreased lacrimation), frequently accompanied by a rheumatoid-type disorder (rheumatoid arthritis, lupus erythematosus, polymyositis, scleroderma).

**Pathogenesis:** Myoepithelial sialadenitis is a B cell–driven autoimmune disease characterized by inflammation and the formation of antibodies directed against antigens of the salivary duct epithelium.

**Fig. 6.16   Extirpation of the submandibular gland**

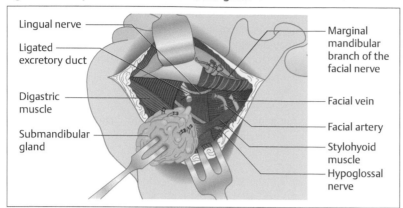

Lingual nerve

Ligated excretory duct

Digastric muscle

Submandibular gland

Marginal mandibular branch of the facial nerve

Facial vein

Facial artery

Stylohyoid muscle

Hypoglossal nerve

Surgical removal of the left submandibular gland. The lingual nerve, the marginal mandibular branch of the facial nerve, and the hypoglossal nerve are vulnerable during the operation. Source: Becker et al 1989.

Histologically, the gland exhibits parenchymal atrophy, interstitial lymphocytic infiltration, and islands of myoepithelial cells.

**Symptoms:** The disease predominantly affects women 50 to 60 years of age. Both parotid glands are diffusely swollen and doughy, with very little pain or tenderness. The end stage presents with atrophy of the gland. Many patients have Sjögren's syndrome with xerostomia, keratoconjunctivitis sicca, and an accompanying rheumatic disease. Sicca syndrome is manifested by troublesome oral dryness, infections of the oral mucosa, and dental caries.

**Diagnosis:** Tests show nonspecific signs of inflammation such as an elevated ESR. Cytoplasmic antibodies against excretory-duct epithelium (parotid antibodies: anti-SS-A/Ro, anti-SS-B/La, anti-α-fodrin, anti-centromere [CENP], anti-M$_3$-acetylcholin-receptor) can generally be detected. Sialography would demonstrate the bare duct system ("leafless tree" pattern) but is rarely necessary. It is often helpful to take an incisional biopsy from the parotid gland, which are involved in approximately 60 to 70% of cases and exhibit typical histologic changes. Lip biopsy should no longer be undertaken, as sensible deficits may occur. Sonography shows a specific "cloudy" pattern (**Fig. 6.17c**). In hepatitis C, a Sjögrenlike disease (called hepatitis C virus–associated sicca syndrome) can occur.

**Complications:** Frequent complications are chronic recurrent parotitis and the sequelae of sialopenia (mucositis, dental caries) and decreased lacrimation (ulceration, infection). There is a highly increased incidence of non-Hodgkin lymphomas (MALT lymphoma) both within and outside the gland.

**Treatment:** Immunosuppressant therapy is indicated only in the setting of a rheumatic disease. Otherwise, treatment is supportive and includes the use of oral

**Fig. 6.17   Sjögren's syndrome**

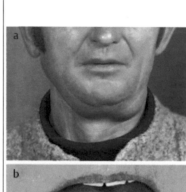

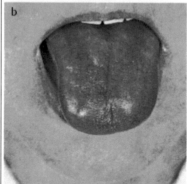

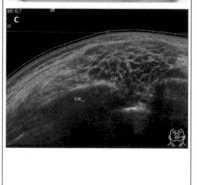

**a** Swelling of the right parotid gland and bilateral swelling of the submandibular glands in a patient with Sjögren's syndrome.
**b** Glossitis in sicca syndrome.
**c** Typical sonographic appearance of the parotid gland in Sjögren's syndrome: cloudy loosening of the parenchyma with echogenic septae and nonechogenic islands.

saliva substitutes and eye drops to replace the lacrimal fluid. A regimen of 3 × 5 mg/day pilocarpine can be tried to stimulate salivation.

## Radiation Sialadenitis

*Pathogenesis:* External irradiation or radioiodine therapy (iodine is excreted in the salivary glands, "radioiodine mumps") incites an inflammation of the salivary glands with atrophy and transient or permanent oral dryness. At doses less than 25 Gy, the injury is reversible. Higher radiation doses cause irreversible injury with a variable degree of partial recovery. The most severe damage is to the serous glandular acini, causing a quantitative decrease and qualitative change in the saliva. Sicca syndrome results in dental caries and mucosal inflammation.

*Symptoms:* The main symptoms are xerostomia and burning of the tongue, frequently combined with hypogeusia or ageusia. A full-blown sicca syndrome may develop. Some degree of recovery may occur over a period of years, but many patients are left with distressful complaints.

*Treatment:* Symptomatic measures should be tried such as stimulating the production of saliva (e.g., 3 × 5 mg/day pilocarpine), administering a saliva substitute, or frequent hydration (e.g., with sage tea).

*Prophylaxis:* If possible, at least one parotid gland should be excluded from the radiation field by using 3D conformal radiotherapy techniques.

# 6.7 Tumors of the Salivary Glands

Approximately 70% of salivary gland tumors are benign. The benign/malignant differentiation of a tumor can generally be accomplished by the history, inspection, and palpation. This was covered in ◈6.4. The present unit describes the most common tumors; less common types are reviewed in Table 6.6.

## Benign Tumors

### General Aspects of Diagnosis and Treatment

*Diagnosis:* The presence of a painless, soft or tense, mobile nodule in the salivary gland, unaccompanied by other symptoms, signifies a benign salivary gland tumor. Clinically benign salivary gland tumors should not be investigated by incisional biopsy due to the risk of tumor cell dissemination and facial nerve injury.

*Treatment:* Biopsy and treatment are generally accomplished in one step. The treatment of benign salivary gland tumors consists of complete removal with a margin of healthy tissue; otherwise, the risk of local recurrence is markedly increased. The specimen provides material for intraoperative frozen-tissue histology and for a definitive pathologic diagnosis.
Since most tumors are located in the parotid gland, extracapsular dissection and *lateral parotidectomy* are the most common procedures done for benign salivary gland tumors. In extracapsular dissection, the tumor is removed with surrounding tissue but without identifying the facial nerve. In lateral parotidectomy, first the facial nerve trunk is identified, and the glandular tissues lateral to the pes anserinus of the nerve are excised. Most benign tumors can be removed in these ways while safely preserving the facial nerve.

🗡 The possibility of temporary or permanent facial nerve injury exists in any type of parotid gland surgery, and the patient must be informed of this prior to the operation.

### Pleomorphic Adenoma (◢6.5)

Archaic name: benign mixed tumor.
Despite its histologic pleomorphism, the epithelial nature of pleomorphic adenoma has been well established (**Fig. 6.18**). It is the most common adenoma of the salivary glands, occurring predominantly in the parotid gland. Women are affected more frequently than men. Generally, the tumor is surrounded by a pseudocapsule. Multifocal tumors are rare, but it is important to appreciate multifocality from a treatment standpoint.

Fig. 6.18 Pleomorphic adenoma

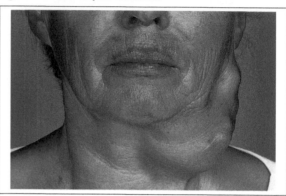

*Symptoms:* The clinical presentation is that of a painless, firm or nodular salivary gland tumor that is freely movable, usually confined to one side, and shows no evidence of malignancy.

*Diagnosis:* The history, inspection, palpation, and ultrasound examination are sufficient for the diagnosis of small and superficial tumors. FNAB (see ◈6.3, Biopsy) can identify the tumor as a pleomorphic adenoma in a fairly large percentage of cases. With larger tumors, CT or preferably MRI will furnish precise information on tumor extent and location. Definitive diagnosis relies on examination of the surgical specimen.

*Treatment:* See above.

*Prognosis:* The prognosis is good following a technically sound tumor resection. Prompt surgery is recommended even for smaller tumors, as this will make it easier to remove the tumor and also preserve the facial nerve. Both can be difficult to accomplish with larger tumors. Carcinoma is known to occur in pleomorphic adenoma but is rare. In very rare cases, patients with removed pleomorphic adenoma develop distant metastases without showing signs of malignancy.

### Cystadenolymphoma

Synonyms: Warthin's tumor, papillary cystadenoma lymphomatosum.

## 6.5 Benign parotid tumor: a case report

*History:* A 52-year-old woman presents with a painless nodule below the right ear. The patient states that the nodule has always been "about the same size" but that it may have gradually enlarged over time. Otherwise the patient feels well.

*Findings:* At examination, a tense nodule approximately 2.5 cm in diameter, freely movable relative to the skin and underlying tissues, is palpable below the right earlobe. The nodule is most clearly visible from behind and is located over the posterior part of the vertical ramus of the mandible. No other palpable abnormalities are noted, and there is no evidence of lymphadenopathy. Otoscopic findings are normal. On intraoral examination, massage of the parotid gland elicits normal salivary flow from Stensen's duct. Facial nerve function is symmetrical.

*Further tests:* Ultrasound demonstrates a solid mass in the parotid gland with no evidence of other abnormalities or enlarged lymph nodes. The next study is fine-needle aspiration biopsy, which is done easily and painlessly since the nodule is directly subcutaneous and easily palpable. The pathologist describes cells from a benign adenoma, most likely a pleomorphic adenoma.

*Recommendation and informed consent:* The patient is advised to have the lesion surgically removed along with the lateral portions of the parotid gland.

The patient is informed about the risk of facial nerve injury, the increase of risk with further tumor growth, an the rare possibility of carcinoma development. The division of cutaneous nerves (great auricular nerve) may cause some degree of numbness in the cheek and auricle. Also, sweating may occur over the parotid gland during eating several months after the operation as a result of nerve damage (gustatory sweating, Frey's syndrome, or auriculotemporal syndrome).

*Treatment:* The patient consents to the proposed surgery. She is hospitalized, and the operation is performed under general anesthesia. Facial nerve function is continuously monitored during the operation by electromyography. This makes it easier to identify the nerve trunk, over which the tumor is located. Following the trunk, the surgeon identifies the facial nerve branches that run medial to the tumor. A lateral parotidectomy is performed, and the intraglandular tumor is completely removed along with its capsule and the surrounding tissue. Frozen-section histology confirms the presumptive diagnosis of **pleomorphic adenoma**. A suction drain is placed at the resection site, and the wound is closed. The patient shows no abnormalities of facial nerve function after the operation. The drain is removed on the second postoperative day. The wound is healing well, and the patient is discharged on the fourth postoperative day.

---

*Definition:* Typically located at the inferior pole of the parotid gland, cystadenolymphoma is the most common monomorphic adenoma and the second most common tumor of the parotid gland. These tumors are occasionally bilateral, and 90% occur in males. Typically, the patients are heavy smokers.

*Pathogenesis:* It is believed that the tumor forms from inclusions of glandular parenchyma in lymph nodes. Recent studies showed that the epithelial component and the lymphatic component of the tumor are of polyclonal origin. Therefore, cystadenolymphoma is identified as a tumorlike lesion. Presently, uncharacterized viruses may also play a role.

*Symptoms:* The typical patient is a man older than 60 years who presents with a relatively soft, indolent swelling of the inferior pole of the parotid gland, which may be nodular in some cases. The swelling is not painful, and there are no functional deficits. Bilateral tumors are present in approximately 10% of cases.

*Diagnosis:* FNAB generally does not contribute to the diagnosis of cystadenolymphoma. Ultrasound may demonstrate one or more typical cystic formations. The definitive histologic diagnosis is made from the surgical specimen.

*Differential diagnosis:* Cystadenolymphoma can be difficult to differentiate from lymphomas in the

parotid gland and from lymphoepithelial cysts (in HIV). Salivary duct cysts and branchiogenic cysts may also be confused with cystadenolymphoma.

*Treatment:* Treatment consists of extracapsular dissection of the tumor in the inferior parotid pole. In cases of multilocular tumors, a lateral or complete parotidectomy is appropriate. An expectant approach may be taken in cases with a typical clinical presentation.

*Prognosis:* The prognosis is good. Malignant transformation does rarely occur, and complaints are rare. The disease may be complicated by an infected cyst.

## Malignant Tumors

### General Aspects of Diagnosis and Treatment

The clinical signs of a malignant salivary gland tumor were discussed in 6.4. The TNM classification is used to describe the clinical spread of malignant salivary gland tumors.

*Diagnosis:* The suspicion of a malignant tumor can often be confirmed by FNAB or core biopsy. If there is clinical suspicion of a malignant salivary gland tumor, *MRI* should be performed to define the extent of the tumor and check for invasion of adjacent structures. Obtaining a specimen for a *definitive histologic diagnosis* is closely related to treatment planning and can

**Tabel 6.6  Overview of benign and malignant tumors of the salivary glands**

|  | Name of tumor | Percentage of all salivary gland tumors | Course and prognosis | Other features |
|---|---|---|---|---|
| **Benign tumors of epithelial origin** | Pleomorphic adenoma | 40–50% | Good prognosis | Most common in the parotid gland |
|  | Cystadenolymphoma | 15% | No malignant transformation | Monomorphic adenoma, most common in the parotid gland, can be bilateral, 90% in men |
|  | Other monomorphic adenomas (e.g., salivary duct adenoma, oncocytoma) | 5% | Good prognosis |  |
| **Malignant tumors of epithelial origin** | Mucoepidermoid carcinoma | 5% | Depends on tumor differentiation; 5-year survival rate for low-grade tumors is 90% | Most common in the parotid gland or minor salivary glands of the palate |
|  | Acinar cell carcinoma | 2–3% | 5-year survival rate 75% | More common in women, usually in the parotid gland |
|  | Adenoid cystic carcinoma | 3% | 5-year survival rate 75% 10-year survival rate 30% | Arises from minor salivary glands in 70% of cases; perivascular and perineural infiltration |
|  | Mammary analogue secretory carcinoma (MASC) | 1% | Intermediate prognosis |  |
|  | Salivary duct carcinoma | 1% | Very poor prognosis | Lymph-node metastasis very common |
|  | Adenocarcinoma NOS | 3% | Poor prognosis |  |
|  | Carcinoma ex pleomorphic adenoma | 5% | Poor prognosis | Develops in 3–5% of untreated pleomorphic adenomas |
|  | Squamous cell carcinoma | 2% | Poor prognosis | Requires differentiation from intraglandular lymph-node metastases |
|  | Undifferentiated carcinoma | 3% | Poor prognosis |  |
| **Benign tumors of nonepithelial origin** | Lipoma | 1–2% | Good prognosis | Usually in the parotid gland, easy to remove |
|  | Hemangioma, lymphangioma | 2% | See "Features" column | Lymphangiomas tend to recur |
|  | Others | <1% | – |  |
| **Malignant tumors of nonepithelial origin** | Sarcoma | <1% | Poor prognosis |  |
|  | Lymphoma | 1–2% | Like other lymphomas | Mostly non-Hodgkin lymphomas: MALT lymphoma (as sequelae of Sjögren's syndrome) |
|  | Others | <1% | – |  |

critically influence management. The pathologist can evaluate frozen sections during the operation. Because frozen-tissue histology is sometimes equivocal, a two-stage surgical procedure may be necessary, especially if the facial nerve must be resected. In this case, the definitive plan of treatment is decided only after the surgical tumor biopsy has yielded a definitive histologic diagnosis.

*Treatment:* The treatment concept for malignant salivary gland tumors is based on removing the tumor as completely as possible and then irradiating the tumor region. Complete tumor removal is not always possible or desirable, however, for a variety of reasons. In the case of the parotid gland, possible resection of the facial nerve must always be considered. The case may require a total parotidectomy with or without facial nerve preservation or the (subtotal) removal of the temporal bone, mandible, skin, vessels, and/or cervical lymph nodes, depending on the extent of the tumor. Reconstructive measures may be considered for the facial nerve (nerve grafting) and skin (advancement flaps; see ✍3.4).

## Mucoepidermoid Carcinoma

*Definition:* Mucoepidermoid carcinoma occurs predominantly in the parotid gland and minor salivary glands of the palate. It is the most common malignant tumor of the salivary glands and can occur even in young patients.

*Pathogenesis:* A distinction is made between well-differentiated *low-grade tumors* (~75% of cases) and more poorly differentiated *high-grade tumors* (~25% of cases). The grade of tumor differentiation determines the prognosis, with higher-grade tumors having a considerably poorer prognosis than lower-grade lesions. Metastasis usually occurs by the lymphogenous route; hematogenous (pulmonary) metastasis is less common.

*Symptoms:* The tumor begins as a nonpainful swelling (see **Fig. 6.12**). Sooner or later it causes pain, facial nerve palsy, and lymph-node metastases, depending on the tumor grade.

*Diagnosis:* See General Aspects of Diagnosis and Treatment above.

*Differential diagnosis:* See **Table 6.6**.

*Treatment:* Treatment consists of complete parotidectomy. The surgery may include the resection and reconstruction of the facial nerve and portions of the temporal bone. If lymph-node metastases are present, a neck dissection (see "Neck dissection" under Lymph-

Node Metastases in ✍16.5) is added. Most patients undergo postoperative radiotherapy.

*Prognosis:* The prognosis depends strongly on the tumor grade. The 5-year survival rate for patients with well-differentiated, low-grade tumors is 90%.

## Acinar Cell Carcinoma

*Definition:* Acinar cell carcinoma is a locally invasive tumor that grows predominantly in the parotid gland and has little tendency to metastasize. The peak incidence is between 40 and 60 years of age, and women are affected more than men.

*Pathogenesis:* As in the case of mucoepidermoid carcinoma, various tumor grades are distinguished. Most acinar cell carcinomas are relatively well differentiated, however. The tumor tissue includes acinar and ductal components. Granules positive on periodic acid–Schiff (PAS) staining and amylase can be detected.

*Symptoms:* The symptoms depend on local tumor growth and infiltration.

*Diagnosis:* See General Aspects of Diagnosis and Treatment above.

*Differential diagnosis:* These tumors mainly require histologic differentiation from other adenocarcinomas and adenoid cystic carcinoma.

*Treatment:* See mucoepidermoid tumor.

*Prognosis:* The prognosis is good following a complete resection (5-year survival rate: 70%).

## Adenoid Cystic Carcinoma

Archaic name: cylindroma.

*Definition:* The clinical picture of adenoid cystic carcinoma is marked by a highly variable course and by perivascular and perineural infiltration. The tumor may take a relatively benign, slow course. Other cases take a fulminating course with rapid recurrence and widespread hematogenous metastases.

*Histology:* Despite its clinical malignancy, this tumor has a relatively benign and well-differentiated histologic appearance. Solid, cribriform, and tubular types are distinguished, and these histologic categories may bear some relationship to the prognosis.

*Symptoms:* The symptoms are dependent on tumor location. Local infiltration leads to pain or nerve deficits caused by typical, early perineural infiltration by the tumor.

*Diagnosis:* See General Aspects of Diagnosis and Treatment above. The lungs and skeleton should be screened for additional sites of hematogenous metastasis.

*Treatment:* Treatment is surgical due to the poor radiosensitivity of the tumor. The value of an ultraradical procedure that sacrifices major structures (facial nerve, temporal bone, carotid artery) is disputed due to the slow growth rate and frequent metastasis, and should be decided on a case-by-case basis. Surgery may be appropriate even when pulmonary metastases are present, depending on the frequently slow growth of the metastases.

*Prognosis:* Aside from a few fulminating cases, adenoid cystic carcinoma generally grows slowly, but cures are infrequent. The 5-year survival rate is 75%, but the 10-year survival rate is only 30%.

## Other Carcinomas and Malignant Tumors

Other malignant tumors are generally rare and, like most tumors, occur predominantly in the parotid gland. The prognosis tends to be unfavorable. These tumors are summarized in **Table 6.6**.

# III   Ear

# 7   Anatomy and Physiology of the Ear

## 7.1   Basic Anatomy and Physiology of the Ear

The goal of this ✍ is to describe the basic anatomic and physiologic principles of the auditory and vestibular apparatus and thus provide a basis for understanding the complex disorders that can affect this sensory organ. Given the complicated structure of the cochlea, its anatomy and function are described in a separate unit (✍ 7.2). Further details, especially pertaining to the vestibular apparatus, are presented in Chapters 10 to 14.

Hearing in humans plays a central role in social communication, while also serving as a warning and orientation system that functions in all spatial directions. The vestibular system is important for maintaining balance and stability and for spatial orientation.
The following systems are responsible for carrying out these functions:

*   The *peripheral auditory and vestibular system* (the "ear"). The function of the peripheral auditory system is to perceive periodic air-pressure variations and process them into neural signals. The vestibular function of the ear is described in ✍ 13.1.
*   The *central auditory system*, which further processes the acoustic information and is particularly instrumental in *directional hearing* and *sound pattern recognition.*

🗒 Speech is the most important sound pattern for human hearing.

*   The *central vestibular system*, which establishes the connections between the vestibular apparatus and the effectors for *spatial orientation* and *balance* (see ✍ 13.1).

The morphologic and anatomic boundary between the peripheral and central systems is located at the site where the vestibulocochlear nerve enters the brainstem. The functional boundary is formed by the central synapse of the peripheral neuron.

### Peripheral Auditory System

The peripheral auditory system is divided into three parts (**Fig. 7.1**):

*   The *external ear*, consisting of the auricle and external auditory canal.
*   The *middle ear*, consisting of the tympanic membrane, tympanic cavity, auditory ossicles, intra-aural muscles, and the air cells of the temporal bone.
*   The *inner ear*, which is embedded in the petrous bone. It is subdivided into the vestibule and the semicircular canal system of the vestibular end organ (see ✍ 13.1) and the cochlea, which is the auditory end organ (see ✍ 7.2).

🗒 The acoustic systems of these three regions are coordinated in such a way that the principal frequencies of speech are transmitted with particular efficiency.

**Fig. 7.1   Peripheral auditory system**

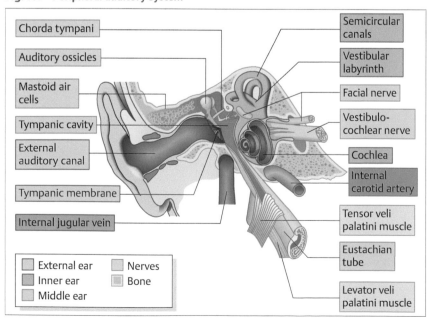

Chorda tympani
Auditory ossicles
Mastoid air cells
Tympanic cavity
External auditory canal
Tympanic membrane
Internal jugular vein

Semicircular canals
Vestibular labyrinth
Facial nerve
Vestibulo-cochlear nerve
Cochlea
Internal carotid artery
Tensor veli palatini muscle
Eustachian tube
Levator veli palatini muscle

☐ External ear   ☐ Nerves
☐ Inner ear   ☐ Bone
☐ Middle ear

The peripheral auditory system can be divided into three parts: the external ear (blue), middle ear (green), and inner ear (red). The vestibulocochlear nerve is shown in yellow.

The *vestibulocochlear nerve* (cranial nerve VIII) is part of the peripheral auditory system. It runs in the internal auditory canal and connects the peripheral end organs to the central nervous system (CNS).

## External Ear

**Anatomy:** The external ear consists of the *auricle* (pinna) and the *external auditory canal* (external acoustic meatus, ear canal). The formative elements of the external ear are composed of flexible cartilage and of bone, which are attached to the skin by their perichondrium and periosteum (see  10.1).

**Physiology:** The function of the external ear is that of an acoustic antenna which transmits sound waves to the sensitive middle ear structures in a discriminating way. The auricle and ear canal together form an acoustic funnel that amplifies selected frequency bands, chiefly in the range from 2 to 4 kHz. This explains why noise in this particular frequency range damage hearing predominantly. The *amplification* does not involve an increase in the amplitude of sound waves but is based on *resonance*, meaning that certain wavelengths vibrate better, similar to the columns of air in a pipe organ. The resonant frequency may be altered by cerumen, insert earphones, or by the earmolds of hearing aids. Owing to the differential refraction of sound waves by the shape of the auricle, two different acoustic pathways exist: a direct route through the conchal cavity and an indirect route via the helix and antihelix. This slightly longer pathway creates a brief sound delay of approximately 0.2 milliseconds, which has a significant role in acoustic analysis, especially for *localizing a sound source* in the vertical plane. The auricle also functions as a *windbreak* by creating air turbulence, thereby diminishing the constant acoustic effects of moving air.

On the whole, however, these effects are of relatively minor importance, and the loss of an auricle does not cause serious functional impairment.

## Middle Ear

**Anatomy:** The middle ear is comprised of air-filled cavities that are subdivided into the *tympanic cavity* and *mastoid air cells*. These cavities communicate with the nasopharynx via the *eustachian tube* (see **Fig. 7.1**). The middle ear, then, may be viewed as a highly specialized paranasal sinus. Like the sinuses, it is lined by a respiratory ciliated epithelium that contains goblet cells.

Topographically, the middle ear borders on or encloses functionally important structures such as the facial nerve, the internal carotid artery, venous sinuses from inside the skull, the dura, and the inner ear. The principal middle ear space is the *tympanic cavity*. It is separated from the external auditory canal by the *tympanic membrane*, which in turn is mechanically linked to the inner ear by a chain of three *auditory ossicles*. The ossicles form the sound conduction apparatus of the middle ear and, together with the *chorda tympani*, make up the actual contents of the tympanic cavity. The auditory ossicles are also connected to the two intra-aural muscles, the stapedius and tensor tympani.

**Physiology:** The main function of the middle ear is *impedance matching*. Due to the different acoustic impedances of air and fluid—i.e., the different resistance that each medium offers to the propagation of sound—the direct transmission of air vibrations to the fluid-filled inner ear would cause more than 99% of the incident sound to be reflected from the fluid surface (**Fig. 7.2**). The task of the middle ear is to keep this transmission loss as small as possible and, at certain frequencies, transmit virtually all of the energy of the vibrating air to the inner-ear fluid. This is made possible by the approximately 20:1 size disparity between the transmitting surfaces of the tympanic membrane and the stapes footplate.

Like the external ear, the middle ear has a resonant frequency at which sound energy is transmitted most efficiently. That frequency is approximately 1 kHz.

But for the middle ear to maintain effective impedance matching at all times, even in the face of *atmospheric pressure changes*, it has a second important function to perform: it must equalize the static air pressure, which is in a constant state of flux due to weather and altitude changes.

The greatest atmospheric pressure variations occur in response to significant altitude changes, as in flying or riding in a cable car. They are many times greater than the dynamic air pressure changes that occur in the acoustic range. An altitude change of 2 m is roughly equivalent to the sound pressure amplitude at 120 dB, bearing in mind that the static pressure, unlike the alternating acoustic pressure, acts in one direction only. Ambient pressure changes are counterregulated by the eustachian tube, which periodically equalizes the pressures between the environment and the tympanic cavity but cannot entirely prevent pressure changes within the middle ear. The articular connections between the auditory ossicles also help to equalize the static pressures. These connections protect the inner ear by preventing extreme displacement of the stapes footplate.

## Inner Ear

Located in the petrous part of the temporal bone, the inner ear consists of multiple interconnected ducts that are collectively called the *labyrinth*.

**Fig. 7.2 Function of the middle ear**

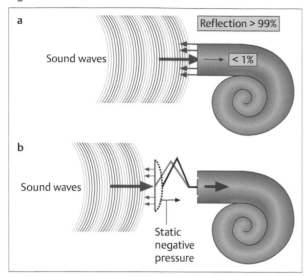

The middle ear is an impedance transformer that also compensates for static pressure differences (air pressure).
**a** Without the interposed ossicular chain of the middle ear, more than 99% of the sound energy would be reflected at the fluid surface of the inner ear.
**b** The impedance is modified by the difference in area between the tympanic membrane and the stapes footplate. The ossicular chain and its joints are shown schematically in green. With static pressure changes that produce a negative pressure in the middle ear (black line), the joints of the auditory ossicles maintain the function of the sound conduction apparatus and protect the inner ear.

**Membranous labyrinth (Fig. 7.3):** The membranous labyrinth is filled with a potassium-rich fluid, the endolymph, and contains cilia-bearing sensory cells that are also known as hair cells. It is divided into the *vestibular labyrinth* and the *cochlea*, which are interconnected by the narrow ductus reuniens. The vestibular labyrinth is composed of three *semicircular canals*, the *utricle*, and the *saccule*. The nature and function of the sensory cells in the vestibular labyrinth are described in ⟁13.1. The utricle and saccule are connected by another duct of the membranous labyrinth, the *utriculosaccular duct*. Another membranous labyrinthine structure arises from the utriculosaccular duct: the *endolymphatic duct* (vestibular aqueduct), which extends to the endolymphatic sac on the posterior surface of the petrous bone (see ⟁7.1 and **Fig. 7.4**). The function of the endolymphatic sac is not fully understood. It appears to have a secretory function and is believed to play a role in endolymph regulation and in the immune processes of the inner ear.
The membranous labyrinth of the cochlea is the *cochlear duct* (scala media), which makes two and one-half spiral turns. The anatomy and physiology of the cochlea are described in the next ⟁ (Structure of the Cochlea), and those of the vestibular labyrinth are covered fully in ⟁13.1.

**Bony labyrinth (Fig. 7.4):** The membranous labyrinth is embedded in the bony labyrinth within the petrous bone. The bony labyrinth is filled with perilymph, in which the membranous labyrinth is suspended. The composition of the perilymph, unlike the endolymph, is very similar to that of the extracellular fluid compartment. The bony labyrinth can be subdivided into three parts: the *semicircular canal system*, the *cochlea*, and the *vestibule*. The bony labyrinth encloses the membranous semicircular canals and reproduces their shape. The cochlear duct is attached between the inner and outer walls of the bony cochlea. This arrangement creates two separate ducts called the *scala vestibuli* and *scala tympani*, which are connected at the cochlear apex by the *helicotrema*.
Between the semicircular canals and cochlea, the vestibule forms a large cavity that contains the saccule, the utricle, the base of the cochlear duct, and the connecting ducts of the membranous labyrinth. The *oval window* is part of the vestibule. It links the inner ear to the middle ear and it is covered by the stapes footplate representing the "acoustic entrance" to the labyrinth. It is the site where impedance-matched acoustic vibrations are transmitted from the middle ear to the perilymph.
Because the entire bony labyrinth is filled with incompressible perilymph, a "pressure valve" is needed so that the vibrations can be effectively transmitted. This function is served by the *round window*. Located inferior to the oval window at the end of the scala tympani and sealed by a mobile membrane, the round window provides a second opening between the bony labyrinth and the tympanic cavity.
The perilymphatic space of the bony labyrinth communicates with the subarachnoid cerebrospinal fluid (CSF) space via the *perilymphatic duct*, known also as

**Fig. 7.3 Membranous labyrinth of the inner ear**

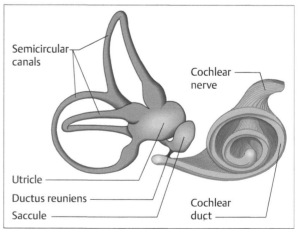

The vestibular labyrinth (gray) and cochlea (green) are interconnected by the narrow ductus reuniens (dark gray). The neural connection to the cochlear nerve is shown in yellow. For clarity, the vestibular nerve and the endolymphatic duct are not shown.

**Fig. 7.4 Bony labyrinth**

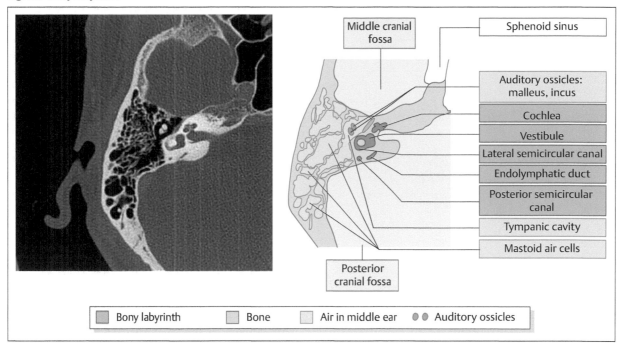

Middle cranial fossa

Sphenoid sinus

Auditory ossicles: malleus, incus

Cochlea

Vestibule

Lateral semicircular canal

Endolymphatic duct

Posterior semicircular canal

Tympanic cavity

Mastoid air cells

Posterior cranial fossa

Bony labyrinth    Bone    Air in middle ear    Auditory ossicles

Computed tomography demonstrates the structures of the bony labyrinth. The turns of the cochlea, the vestibule, the sectioned semicircular canals, and the endolymphatic duct are clearly displayed in this axial scan through the left temporal bone.

the cochlear aqueduct. This duct begins at the scala tympani below the round window and ends at the posterior surface of the pyramid below the internal porus acusticus. Most likely, it is consistently open only in children and is often sealed by fibrous tissue in adults.

**Blood supply:** The inner ear derives its blood supply from the labyrinthine artery, which usually arises from the anterior inferior cerebellar artery or the basilar artery. It runs with the vestibulocochlear nerve through the internal auditory canal, where it divides into the vestibular artery and cochlear artery. These vessels may anastomose with the middle ear vessels. Several veins drain blood from the inner ear to the superior bulb of the jugular vein and to the inferior petrosal sinus.

## Vestibulocochlear Nerve

The vestibulocochlear nerve (cranial nerve VIII) leaves the brainstem as a nerve trunk that has a grossly homogeneous appearance. Functionally, however, it consists of an anterosuperior part, the *vestibular nerve*, which is distinct from the posteroinferior *cochlear nerve*. This subdivision becomes anatomically apparent in the internal auditory canal, where the vestibular and cochlear nerves appear as separate structures. In the fundus of the internal canal, the vestibular nerve forms the *vestibular ganglion* from which various nerve fibers are distributed to the structures of the vestibular end organ (utriculoampullar nerve,

saccular nerve, posterior ampullary nerve). The *cochlear ganglion* (spiral cochlear ganglion) is not located in the internal auditory canal but in the bony modiolus of the cochlea (see ☞7.2 and **Fig. 7.7**).

The vestibulocochlear nerve mainly contains afferent fibers, which lead to the vestibular and cochlear nuclei in the brainstem. Efferent fibers are also present; they are generally less well myelinated than the afferent fibers. The function of the afferent vestibulocochlear nerve can be described as passive information transfer. The information is already transformed into complex neurobiologic signals (action potentials) at the level of the synapses in a process that can be likened to digital data transmission. The precise timing of the transmission is crucial.

The *facial nerve* (see also ☞14.1) is anatomically separate from the vestibulocochlear nerve throughout its course but approaches it very closely in the internal auditory canal.

## Embryology and Development of the Peripheral Auditory System

The auricle, middle ear, inner ear, and internal auditory canal undergo a more or less separate embryonic development. As a result, a malformation affecting one part of the ear is not necessarily combined with malformations of other parts. On the other hand, malformations of the external auditory canal are frequently associated with anomalies of the middle ear.

The germ layers that give rise to the various auditory structures and the timetable of inner ear development are shown in ◢ **7.1.**

## Central Auditory System

The central auditory system begins in the brainstem at the cochlear nucleus, where the cochlear nerve terminates (**Fig. 7.5**). The cochlear nucleus, unlike many other nuclei, receives its afferents entirely from one side. Past the cochlear nucleus, the auditory pathways run mainly but not exclusively via the two inferior olivary complexes, the inferior colliculus of the midbrain, and the thalamus to the contralateral areas of the auditory cortex, which are located mainly in the temporal lobe.

The following systems, while not strictly separate anatomically, are distinguishable in a functional sense:

- *Tonotopic system:* The frequency processing that occurs in the cochlea already assigns certain frequencies to specific fibers in the acoustic nerve. This "tonotopic principle" is maintained in some of the central auditory pathways as far as the cerebral cortex.
- *Nontonotopic system:* Parallel to the tonotopic system are other modes of central processing that are largely independent of frequency analysis and rely on other parameters such as temporal information.
- *Polymodal or polysensory system:* This system establishes connections with other sensory and nonsensory centers at various levels in the CNS. An example is the stapedial reflex, which induces contraction of the stapedius muscle by the stapedius nerve (a branch of the facial nerve) in response to a sufficiently loud acoustic stimulus.

Besides these anatomically and physiologically distinct systems of the ascending auditory pathway, numerous collateral connections are present at all levels. The neurons generally become more numerous at the higher centers; this property of the ascending auditory pathway is called *diversification.*

While the cochlear nerve contains only a few efferent fibers, the efferent fibers outnumber the afferents in many of the connections from higher to lower centers in the CNS. They assist in controlling the flow of information.

### Function of the Central Auditory System

In the peripheral system, auditory information is collected and relayed to the CNS with maximum fidelity as a complex mix of signals. The task of the CNS is to separate and recognize the auditory signals. Two basic functions are distinguished in this process: *sound localization* (where?) and *sound pattern recognition* (what? who?). These two functions are complementary and cannot always be clearly separated from each other. They are very highly evolved in humans, because a human being receives visual information only in the frontal plane and must rely on hearing for orientation in all other spatial planes.

**Sound localization** is based largely on the binaural auditory information pathways in the brainstem: sound reaches the ear closer to the sound source earlier and with greater intensity than the ear farther from the source. Without having to identify the sound source in terms of recognition, this system permits one or more acoustic sources to be localized at the same time.

**Sound pattern recognition**, which involves the naming and identification of a sound source, is a cognitive cerebral function that is based on experience and learning. It relies on the preliminary neural processing of the sound information in the cochlea and brainstem. Directional hearing and its associated functions, then, form an essential foundation for sound pattern recognition. Sound identification or pattern recognition includes the separation of "desired" auditory information or sound sources from "extraneous" sources, or noise. While one picture after another is recognized in the visual system, auditory "picture recognition" is essentially dynamic and transitory. The recognition of speech sounds and their combination into syllables, words, phrases, and sentences in human communication is the most important example of

**Fig. 7.5   Central auditory pathway**

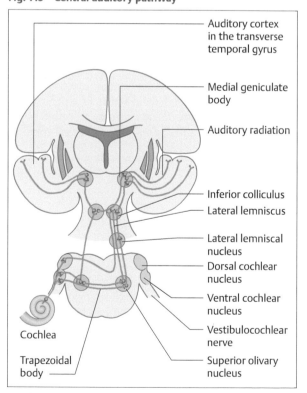

Auditory cortex in the transverse temporal gyrus

Medial geniculate body

Auditory radiation

Inferior colliculus

Lateral lemniscus

Lateral lemniscal nucleus

Dorsal cochlear nucleus

Ventral cochlear nucleus

Vestibulocochlear nerve

Superior olivary nucleus

Cochlea

Trapezoidal body

Simplified diagram of the central afferent auditory pathway on one side. Numerous cross-connections exist at all levels except at the cochlear nuclei, each of which is connected only to the ipsilateral cochlear nerve. The complex efferent system is not shown.

## 7.1 Embryology of the Ear

### Germ layers

The **external ear** develops from the ectoderm and mesoderm. The auricle is formed from six mesenchymal tubercles and migrates cephalad with further development, explaining why malformed auricles tend to occupy a low-set position.

The **auditory canal** starts as a depression in the epidermis, and the tympanic membrane combines all three germ layers with its ectodermal epidermal layer, mesenchymal fibrous layer, and endodermal mucosa. The **auditory ossicles** are of mesenchymal origin, while the **tympanic cavity** and **eustachian tube** develop from the first pharyngeal pouch. The **membranous inner ear** is of ectodermal origin; the **otic capsule** is mesodermal.

### Timetable of inner ear development

The otocyst forms from an epithelial thickening between the cutaneous ectoderm and neural groove in the *third and fourth weeks* of embryonic development. This thickening invaginates and closes off to form a separate vesicle (**Fig. 7.6a**).

In the *fifth week,* the otocyst becomes infolded, forming the upper utriculovestibular part and the lower sacculocochlear part (**Fig. 7.6b**).

In the *sixth week,* the three semicircular canals form from the utriculovestibular part (**Fig. 7.6c**).

In the *seventh to ninth weeks,* the cochlear duct forms as a tubular extension of the sacculocochlear part and becomes coiled (**Fig. 7.6d**).

Development of the labyrinth is paralleled by the essentially independent embryology of the internal auditory canal via development of the vestibulocochlear nerve, which is controlled by the otocyst.

**Fig. 7.6   Embryology of the inner ear**

a Fourth week of development

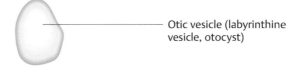

Otic vesicle (labyrinthine vesicle, otocyst)

b Fifth week of development

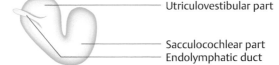

Utriculovestibular part

Sacculocochlear part
Endolymphatic duct

c Sixth week of development

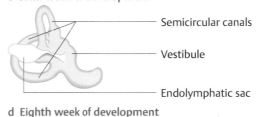

Semicircular canals

Vestibule

Endolymphatic sac

d Eighth week of development

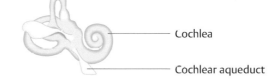

Cochlea

Cochlear aqueduct

recognizing rapidly changing sound patterns. Music may be considered a specialized form of sound pattern recognition. *Auditory hallucinations* or illusions are sound pattern recognition without a physical correlate in the outside world. *Tinnitus* also lacks an external physical correlate but does not involve pattern recognition; only "noise" is perceived.

# 7.2 Anatomy and Function of the Cochlea

As the actual sensory organ for hearing, the cochlea is of key physiologic and clinical importance. The main function of the cochlea is to translate auditory events into a pattern of neural impulses that precisely reflects the nature and timing of the sound stimulus. To perform this neural coding, the cochlea divides the broad frequency spectrum of the sound into narrow frequency bands that are matched to the neural processing capacity of the organ. This 🔖 shows how the cochlea performs this task with the help of the cochlear amplifier and the tonotopic principle. Clinical implications are also discussed.

## Structure of the Cochlea

The bony cochlear canal spirals around the axis of the cochlea (modiolus) for 2.5 turns and a length of 3 to 3.5 cm to the cochlear apex. It contains three separate cavities: the scala media, scala vestibuli, and scala tympani.

The **basilar membrane** (**Fig. 7.7**, **Fig. 7.8**, and **Fig. 7.9**), which is narrow (0.1 mm) and relatively thick at the base of the cochlea and considerably wider (0.5 mm) and thinner at the cochlear apex, stretches radially between the *spiral lamina*, a bony shelf projecting from the modiolus, and the *spiral ligament* of the outer cochlear wall. The mechanical properties of the basilar membrane change along the course of the cochlea. The membrane is markedly stiffer and less compliant at the base of the cochlea than at the apex. Its resonance is tuned to higher frequencies in the basal area of the cochlea and to lower frequencies in the apical area.

> ✒ The formation of the passive traveling wave is based on these mechanical properties of the basilar membrane, with a frequency-dependent maximum amplitude occurring at different sites along the cochlea.

Together with the organ of Corti, the basilar membrane forms the floor of the **scala media** (cochlear duct), which is filled with endolymph. The ionic composition of the endolymph is similar to that of the intracellular space (**Fig. 7.8**).

The **scala vestibuli** lies above the cochlear duct, contains perilymph, and is separated from the endolymphatic space of the scala media by the thin *Reissner's membrane*. Because the composition of the perilymph is similar to that in the extracellular space, a potential difference is created at the membrane (**Fig. 7.8**). The scala vestibuli begins at the base of the cochlea in the area of the oval window. At the apex of the cochlea, it is connected to the scala tympani by the *helicotrema*.

The **scala tympani** lies below the basilar membrane. It is also filled with perilymph, and stretches between the helicotrema and the *round window*.

The **organ of Corti** (spiral organ, **Fig. 7.8**) lies on the inner part of the basilar membrane facing the modiolus and contains the sensory and supporting cells. The *tectorial membrane*, an acellular structure composed of amorphous material and fibrils, covers the sensory cell region of the organ of Corti starting from the spiral lamina. The *reticular membrane* connects the ciliated surfaces of the sensory cells with one another and creates a partition between the endolymphatic

**Fig. 7.7 Axial section through the cochlea**

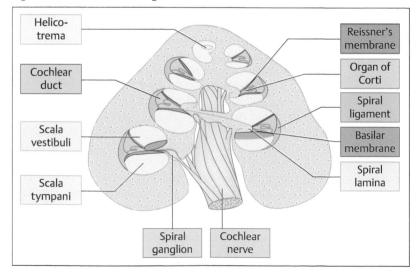

- Helico-trema
- Cochlear duct
- Scala vestibuli
- Scala tympani
- Spiral ganglion
- Cochlear nerve
- Reissner's membrane
- Organ of Corti
- Spiral ligament
- Basilar membrane
- Spiral lamina

The cochlea has been sectioned through the center of the modiolus. The cochlear nerve ends there and divides into separate nerve fibers that run in small bony canals and form the spiral ganglion near the bony spiral lamina. The scala vestibuli and scala tympani, which contain perilymph, are shown in blue. The endolymph-filled cochlear duct is shown in orange.

**Fig. 7.8  Organ of Corti**

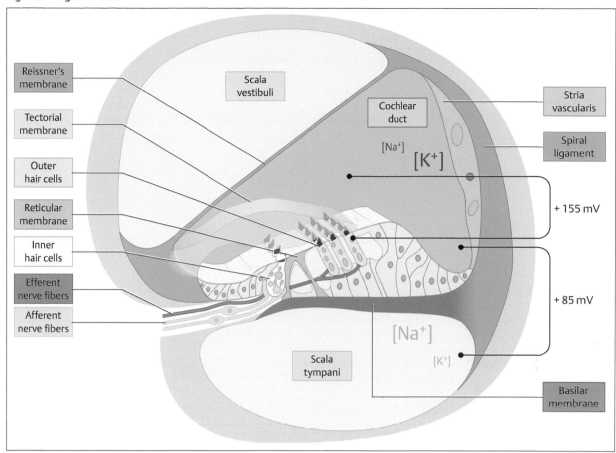

The organ of Corti rests on the basilar membrane. Tight junctions between the supporting cells form the reticular membrane, which separates the perilymphatic space (light blue) from the endolymph (dark blue). The inner hair cells form one row toward the modiolus, and the outer hair cells form three rows over the basilar membrane. The tectorial membrane is connected to the cilia of the outer hair cells.

space above the membrane, which contains the cilia and tectorial membrane, and the perilymphatic space below the reticular membrane. Because of this arrangement, the reticular membrane forms a voltage boundary.

*Hair cells* are mechanoreceptors surmounted by a bundle of stereocilia of varying length on a specialized surface. The stereocilia are arranged in longitudinal rows and packed together in hexagonal arrays. The stereocilia themselves are tiny, stiff rods that are interconnected by transverse fibrils. Any deflection of the stereocilia bundle at its base toward the longest stereocilia generates an adequate excitatory stimulus for the sensory cell. Two types of hair cells are distinguished (**Fig. 7.8**):

- *Inner hair cells:* Normally, the cochlea contains around 3,000 inner hair cells, which are arranged in a single row along the cochlea and are surrounded by supporting cells (see **Fig. 7.8**). Their stereocilia form a continuous palisade. Each inner hair cell is connected to several afferent fibers of the cochlear nerve.

The inner hair cells are the actual "hearing cells," which transform acoustic information into nerve impulses.

- *Outer hair cells:* There are three to four times more outer hair cells than inner hair cells (~12,000) in the cochlea. The outer hair cells are cylindrical, are generally arranged in three rows along the cochlea, and are anchored only at their base and apex by a complex network of supporting cells. Except from their ciliated end, which projects into the endolymphatic space, they are surrounded by perilymph (see **Fig. 7.8**). Their stereocilia are firmly attached to the tectorial membrane. The outer hair cells have few afferent connections and are supplied mainly by efferent cochlear nerve fibers. Due to unique construction of their cell wall, they undergo rhythmic contractions in the acoustic frequency range up to 30,000 Hz. Based on this ability as well as their anatomy and arrangement, the outer hair cells are viewed as the effector or "motor" of the cochlear amplifier.

**Fig. 7.9   Cochlear amplifier**

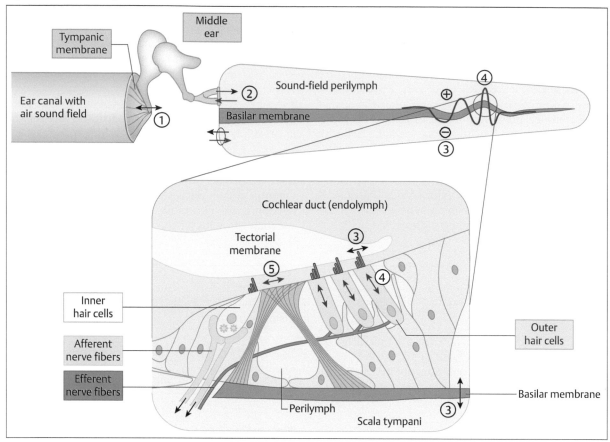

Schematic representation of the mechanic-acoustic function of the ear with the cochlear amplifier. ① The sound field of the air is transmitted by vibrations of the tympanic membrane and the ossicles to the inner ear. ② The stapes footplate creates a similar sound field within the perilymph by an instantaneous pressure wave and antiphase movements of the round window membrane. ③ The perilymphatic sound field induces pressure differences across the basilar membrane leading to the buildup of a traveling wave, leading to a shear movement between the tectorial membrane and the organ of Corti. ④ The movements of the fixed stereocilia of the outer hair cells induce an active contraction of the outer hair cells providing amplification of the basilar membrane vibrations. ⑤ The stimulation of the inner hair cells is most likely induced by subtectorial flow of the endolymph. It creates the action potential of the afferent nerve fibers.

## Function of the Cochlea

The translation of acoustic information into neural signals is basically a problem of temporal resolution, since much of the information contained in acoustic vibrations lies in their temporal structure. Vibrations in the typical range of several thousand hertz are transmitted to neural structures with a characteristic refractory period, which allows no more than several hundred impulses to be processed each second. This precludes a 1:1 temporal transduction of acoustic information into neural signals. Transduction is also hampered by noise and by very large differences in pressure levels.

The cochlea solves these complex problems with the aid of two different mechanical functions:

- **Frequency analysis:** Certain frequencies are assigned to nerve fibers at specific locations. This is the *tonotopic principle.*

- **Biomechanical amplification:** Vibrations at low amplitude are magnified with the aid of the *cochlear amplifier.*

The functions of the cochlea can be further subdivided into a macromechanical function within the fluid compartment and a *micromechanical* function at the cellular level. The macromechanical function is mainly concerned with frequency analysis, while the micromechanical function deals more with amplification. The two functions are closely interrelated, however. With its frequency analysis and amplifier functions, the cochlea is able to process vibrations at the limit of what is physically possible.

### Macromechanical Function: Compression Wave and Traveling Wave

The sound field of the air is transmitted by the middle ear and the stapes footplate to the perilymph, spreading virtually instantaneously and creating a similar sound field within the cochlea fluid. The stimulus reaches the round window in only a few tens of microseconds after its generation through the stapes footplate, leading to an antiphase movement of the round window membrane. This way of sound propagation is called compression or fast wave (**Fig. 7.9** ②).

The perilymphatic sound field within the cochlea then leads through pressure differences across the basilar membrane or between the scala vestibuli and scala tympani to a frequency-dependent vibration of the basilar membrane. This wave is called the travelling or slow wave and it takes more time to build up with a delay of the order of a few milliseconds (**Fig. 7.9** ③). Each frequency causes a maximum deflection at a different site along the membrane. Described by Bekesy in 1928, this mechanism allows for:

• Passive frequency analysis.

• Tonotopicity—i.e., the representation of certain frequencies in corresponding areas of the basilar membrane, thereby assigning the frequencies to specific nerve fibers.

High frequencies cause maximum vibration of the basilar membrane near the base of the cochlea, while low frequencies induce maximum vibrations near the apex. The resolution of these passive traveling waves is much too crude for a discriminating acoustic analysis, however.

## Micromechanical Function: Cochlear Amplifier

The micromechanical function serves to *amplify and fine-tune* the basilar membrane vibrations produced by the passive macromechanical cochlear function. This is chiefly made possible by the activity of the outer hair cells in the organ of Corti, which amplify low-amplitude vibrations. This fine tuning and amplification by the **cochlear amplifier** (**Fig. 7.9** ④) result in a sharp, detailed sound pattern at the basilar membrane. Events are as follows: The pressure waves in the perilymph induce a frequency-dependent traveling wave in the basilar membrane (**Fig. 7.9** ③). This traveling wave displaces the outer hair cells attached to the basilar membrane. Because their cilia are connected to the tectorial membrane, they are deflected radial to the cochlea, creating an excitatory stimulus. This produces an intrinsic vibration of the outer hair cells (**Fig. 7.9** ④), resulting in a positive feedback that amplifies the vibration. The motile capacity of the outer hair cells is powered by the *endocochlear potential*, which works like a battery. It generates a voltage of approximately 85 mV based on the different ionic compositions of the endolymph and perilymph (see **Fig. 7.8**).

🖉 The endocochlear potential is the *largest extracellular* potential difference in the human body.

An even greater potential difference of approximately 155 mV exists between the cytoplasm of the outer hair cells and the endolymph.

The potential gradient is maintained by active ion-exchange processes in the stria vascularis, a specialized region of the spiral ligament that borders the endolymphatic duct.

The outer hair cells are suspended in this voltage field, and any reduction in the voltage leads to a reduction or cessation of the active amplification process.

**Transduction:** The inner hair cells transform the physical stimulus of the acoustic vibration into nerve potentials. As in the case of the outer hair cells, a deflection of the cilia radial to the cochlea produces an adequate stimulus for the inner hair cells (**Fig. 7.9** ⑤). It is not yet known for certain how the deflection of the basilar membrane is transformed into this stimulus for the inner hair cells. The vibration of the basilar membrane does not stimulate the cells directly, and the stimulus is probably evoked by radial streaming of the endolymph.

## Nonlinear Function—Otoacoustic Emissions

While the passive traveling wave grows in proportion to the sound level, the cochlear amplifier does not function in a linear way and becomes saturated at approximately 60 dB SPL.

🖉 The lower the vibrational energy, the greater the amplification factor.

The proportional amplification of weak and strong vibrations would result in an unstable and nonfunctional system.

Nonlinear amplification like that in the cochlear amplifier tends to have natural modes of vibration and is subject to distortion. Because the ear transmits vibrations not only from outside to inside (antegrade) but also in retrograde fashion from the cochlea through the middle ear to the tympanic membrane, which emits the vibrations into the ear canal like the membrane of a loudspeaker, these natural vibrations of the cochlear amplifier can be detected as faint sounds by a small, sensitive microphone placed in the ear canal. These sounds emitted by the cochlea, called **spontaneous otoacoustic emissions** (**SOAEs, Fig. 7.10**), occur at certain frequencies in many normal-hearing persons as evidence of a functioning cochlear amplifier. One theory is that they result from a slightly asymmetrical arrangement of the hair cells at certain locations.

An acoustic stimulus acting on the cochlea from the outside (e.g., a click) induces **evoked emissions** that can also be recorded in the ear canal. Distortion products from the cochlear amplifier can also be detected (see 🔖8.4, Otoacoustic Emissions).

## Clinical Implications

The cochlea is constantly exposed to acoustic stimuli, keeping it in a mechanically active state. The number of sensory cells in the cochlea is relatively small, and it is unlikely that they regenerate in humans. This makes it all the more remarkable that the system generally functions flawlessly and remains stable for many decades.

**Mechanical overloading** of the cochlear amplifier is the cause of *noise-induced hearing loss* (see 12.2) and may also be a factor in *age-related hearing loss* (see 12.3, Age-Related Hearing Loss).

The highly specialized **metabolism** of the cochlear fluids, hair cells, and stria vascularis is also susceptible to dysfunction. *Drugs* can lead to cochlear hearing loss in this way. For example, aminoglycoside antibiotics can damage the metabolism of the hair cells, and loop diuretics such as furosemide can alter the metabolism of the stria vascularis, thereby affecting the endocochlear potential.

Loss of the cochlear amplifier is at least partly responsible for the phenomenon of *recruitment*, or the abnormal growth of loudness. Recruitment is a clinical sign of cochlear hearing loss caused by abnormal dynamics of sound processing. With loss of the cochlear amplifier, soft sounds are not perceived, whereas loud sound events are of undiminished loudness because an amplifier is not needed to perceive them.

**Fig. 7.10 Spontaneous otoacoustic emissions**

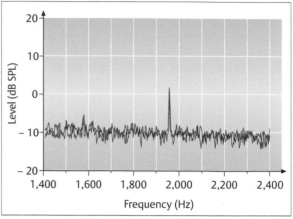

The two superimposed curves (two measurements) represent a frequency spectrum recorded spontaneously in a normal ear canal using a probe microphone. The peak at 1,952 Hz is a faint tone emitted from the inner ear—a spontaneous otoacoustic emission.

# 8    Audiology (Auditory Testing)

## 8.1    Examination of the Ear and Clinical Auditory Testing

The goal of clinical auditory testing is to acquire information on the integrity and sidedness of hearing by means of simple tests. The results of these tests can then be used to select more specific tests for the further investigation of hearing. Like other clinical examination, auditory testing consists of history taking, inspection (otoscopy), and function tests.

### History

Every patient should be questioned about the three most important symptoms of an inner ear disorder:
- Hearing loss (hypacusis).
- Tinnitus.
- Vertigo.

If the patient has specific complaints involving the ear or hearing, the examiner should ask about additional symptoms such as pain or aural discharge. Descriptions of any previous ear surgery, tympanic membrane perforation, or other ear injuries are also important.

### Inspection and Otoscopy

Examination of the ear and hearing should always start with a thorough inspection of the auricle and its surroundings. Attention should be given to:
- Changes in the shape of the auricle or ear canal.
- Surgical scars.
- Crusting in the external ear canal and discharge: cerumen, mucus, pus, blood, cerebrospinal fluid.
- Redness and swelling of the auricle or surrounding areas.

### Otoscopy

 Before performing otoscopy, the examiner should check for tragal tenderness and pull on the auricle to check for pain.

These signs indicate otitis externa (see 10.3 and 10.4). When present, they warrant a particularly careful otoscopic technique.

*Technique:* Otoscopy is performed with a hand-held otoscope (**Fig. 8.1**; see also 10.1, Examination) or with an otomicroscope. The auricle is rotated gently backward and upward for the examination, avoiding excessive traction. This maneuver straightens the external ear canal and brings the lateral cartilaginous part of the canal in line with the medial bony part. The diameter of the ear speculum should conform to anatomic constraints, keeping in mind that a broad speculum provides better exposure and illumination. The speculum is slowly introduced into the ear canal

Fig. 8.1   Otoscopy

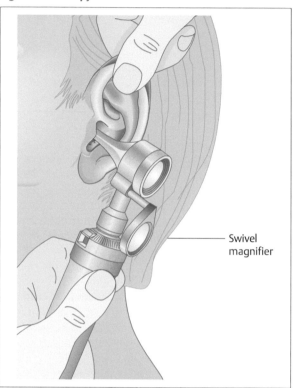

Swivel magnifier

The hand-held otoscope has a battery handle and may have two interchangeable magnifier lenses, one removable at the funnel and one swivel-mounted. The examiner gently pulls the auricle backward and upward to introduce the scope. The largest possible speculum should be used to provide good exposure and adequate illumination of the ear canal. The funnel-mounted lens can be replaced by the swivel lens for manipulation in the ear canal.

under visual guidance, inserting it past the vibrissae but without touching the bony and pain-sensitive medial portion of the ear canal. This should afford a clear view of the ear canal and tympanic membrane. Abnormalities and cleansing of the ear canal are described in 10.2.

*Clinical evaluation of the tympanic membrane:* Not infrequently, the anterior angle of the tympanic membrane cannot be seen with the otoscope, because it is obscured by the prominence of the temporo-mandibular joint. The normal tympanic membrane

**Fig. 8.2 Normal appearance of the tympanic membrane**

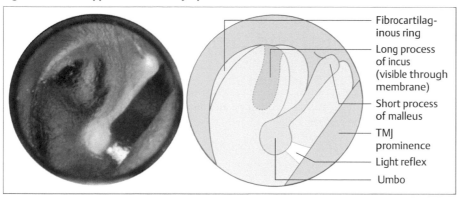

Fibrocartilag-
inous ring

Long process
of incus
(visible through
membrane)

Short process
of malleus

TMJ
prominence

Light reflex

Umbo

The normal tympanic membrane has a light reflex indicating a smooth surface and displays various anatomic landmarks. Its transparency and color are variable. The figure illustrates a right tympanic membrane.

has a grayish color and variable transparency. With a thin tympanic membrane, it is possible to identify middle ear structures such as the long process of the incus or the chorda tympani (**Fig. 8.2**, see also Chapter 11). The normal tympanic membrane exhibits the following three properties:

- **It reflects light:** The tympanic membrane is covered by smooth squamous epithelium that reflects light in a typical way. A "cone of light" is often seen in the anteroinferior quadrant, but other reflections may be seen at other sites on the normal tympanic membrane, depending on the position of the membrane. When the smooth epithelium becomes swollen due to inflammation, the normal light reflexes disappear.

- **It is differentiated:** Normal anatomic structures such as the fibrocartilaginous ring and malleus handle can be distinguished (**Fig. 8.2**). When an acute inflammation is present, these structures can no longer be identified and the tympanic membrane has an *undifferentiated* appearance.

- **It is mobile:** To perform its function, the tympanic membrane must be able to vibrate. The mobility of the tympanic membrane may be restricted by effusion in the middle ear or by scars or defects in the membrane. Its mobility can be tested by having the patient perform the Valsalva maneuver or by using Siegle's pneumatic otoscope (see ✎11.1, Examination). As a rule, the mobility of the tympanic membrane is most clearly appreciated in the posterosuperior quadrant.

## Clinical Hearing Tests

### Tuning Fork Tests

The goal of tuning fork tests is to differentiate between conductive and sensorineural hearing loss. Two tests are adequate for this purpose: Weber's test (**Fig. 8.3**) and Rinne's test (**Fig. 8.4**).
**Conductive hearing loss** is caused by disease of the external auditory canal or middle ear, whereas

**sensorineural hearing loss** has its cause in the cochlea or the neural structures of the auditory system.

✂ Hearing loss is not detected directly with tuning fork tests.

*Technique:* A tuning fork that vibrates between approximately 250 and 800 Hz is used. Lower frequencies are not suitable for auditory testing due to interference from the perception of low-frequency vibrations. The resonant frequency of the middle ear is about 1,000 Hz, and test results in this higher range are often equivocal.

The tuning fork should have a broad base with a large surface area. To test bone conduction, the base of the vibrating tuning fork must be pressed firmly against the cranial bone to transmit the vibrations to the bone and overcome dampening by the skin.

**Weber's test:**
*Technique:* The tuning fork is placed in the midline of the skull, usually on the vertex or the forehead (**Fig. 8.3a**). The vibrations are transmitted by bone conduction to the cochlea.
*Interpretation:* When hearing is normal, the vibrations are perceived as equally loud on both sides, and so the sound is heard midway between the ears. In an abnormal test, the sound will be lateralized to one side or the other.

- If the patient has sensorineural hearing loss, the tuning fork is lateralized to the better-hearing ear (**Fig. 8.3b**).

- If the patient has a conductive hearing loss, the tuning fork is lateralized to the affected ear because the vibrational energy is more poorly transmitted from the cochlea through the middle ear and it is more difficult for ambient sounds to reach the cochlea (less masking). As a result, more vibrational energy is present in the normally functioning cochlea, and the sound is perceived as louder (**Fig. 8.3c**).

**Humming test:** Lateralization can also be detected by having the patient hum, since a loud hum also induces vibration of the cranial bone.

**Fig. 8.3  Weber's test**

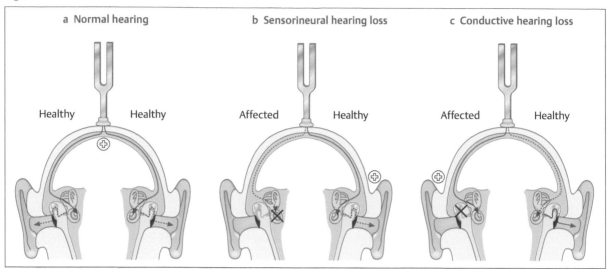

| a Normal hearing | b Sensorineural hearing loss | c Conductive hearing loss |
|---|---|---|
| Healthy   Healthy | Affected   Healthy | Affected   Healthy |

Weber's test is performed by placing a vibrating tuning fork on the midline of the skull.

**a** When hearing is symmetrical, the sound (+) is perceived with equal loudness in or between both ears.

**b** With unilateral sensorineural hearing loss, the sound (+) is lateralized to the better ear.

**c** With unilateral conductive hearing loss, the sound (+) is lateralized to the affected side.

### Rinne's test:

*Principle:* Rinne's test compares the levels of air and bone conduction in the same ear (unlike Weber's test, which compares the right and left ears).

*Technique:* To create standard conditions, air conduction is tested by holding the tuning fork just outside the ear canal without touching it, and bone conduction is tested by pressing the tuning fork firmly against the mastoid.

- The patient is told to compare the loudness in the first position (air conduction) with that in the second position (bone conduction).
- If the patient is unsure which is louder, air and bone conduction can be compared by testing for *threshold*: the tuning fork is struck and pressed to the mastoid, and the patient tells the examiner when the sound becomes inaudible. Then the tuning fork (without being struck again) is shifted to a position just outside the ear canal (see above).

*Interpretation:* In a normal (positive) test, the tuning fork vibration is transmitted to the cochlea better by air conduction than by bone conduction.

- If Rinne's test is *positive*, air-conducted sound is perceived as louder than bone-conducted sound and lasts at least 15 seconds longer (**Fig. 8.4a**).
- When conductive hearing loss is present, the sound is perceived as louder on the mastoid than outside the ear canal (**Fig. 8.4b**). Rinne's test is *negative.*
- When sensorineural hearing is better on one side than the other, it is necessary to mask the opposite ear before performing Rinne's test (see **Fig. 8.7a**). Without masking, the opposite ear may perceive the sound as louder via bone conduction than the

test ear via air conduction, leading to a *pseudonegative* Rinne's test. The opposite ear is rarely masked in routine tests, however, and the hearing threshold in this situation is usually assessed by pure-tone audiometry (see ✑8.3).

***Interpreting the tuning fork tests:*** **Fig. 8.5** shows the information that can be obtained from a combination of Weber's and Rinne's tests. Occasionally, however, these tests may yield "illogical" findings that cannot be definitively interpreted.

## Screening Speech Tests

The severity of hearing loss can be clinically assessed without instrumented test methods by having the patient listen to and repeat spoken numbers and letters. Screening speech tests and tuning fork tests can provide information about the presence of uni- or bilateral hearing loss and its nature. They supply the clinical information for selecting further appropriate audiometric test procedures.

🖉 The examiner should maintain a constant loudness level during the test and provide a standardized test environment.

### Whispered-voice test:

*Principle:* The whispered-voice test uses sets of three random numbers and letters to assess overall hearing. The examiner whispers the sets after an unforced expiration, making use of a fairly constant sound level possible. The whispered-voice test correlates well with a hearing loss in the pure-tone audiometry.

**Fig. 8.4  Rinne's test**

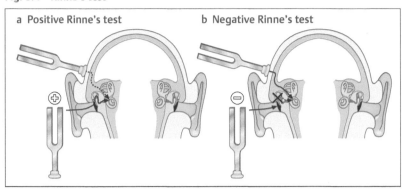

a  Positive Rinne's test

b  Negative Rinne's test

Air and bone conduction are compared in the same ear to determine the auditory threshold for the tuning fork and/or its loudness.

**a** In the absence of conductive hearing loss, air conduction (+) is perceived as being louder and/or of longer duration than bone conduction.

**b** When conductive hearing loss is present, bone conduction is perceived as being louder and/or more prolonged than air conduction (–).

**Fig. 8.5  Tuning fork tests**

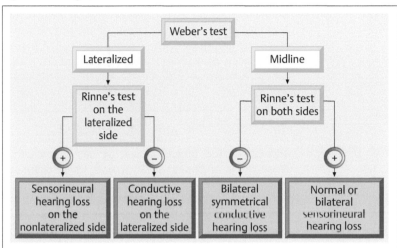

Classification of sensorineural and conductive hearing loss with the tuning fork tests. A normal result (symmetrical Weber's test and positive Rinne's test) is not substantially different from the result in patients with bilateral sensorineural hearing loss (shown at lower right).

*Technique:*
- The examiner stands an arm's length (0.6 m) behind the patient to avoid visual clues (**Fig. 8.6**).
- The examiner presents a set of three single digits and letters (e.g., "7k8") and instructs the patient to repeat the sets aloud.
- The examiner then whispers at least three sets after unforced expiration aiming at a constant sound level. The patient should repeat each set immediately.

*Interpretation:* If the patient repeats correctly at least two-thirds of the sets of digits and letters, the screening test for hearing loss is passed. The patient can be assumed to have no substantial two-sided hearing loss. If the whispered-voice test is not passed, formal audiometric examination becomes necessary.

**Test for one-sided hearing loss:**
*Principle:* The whispered-voice test assesses overall hearing; it does not discriminate between the two ears. However, the detection of asymmetrical hearing loss is of clinical importance. To detect one-sided hearing loss, crossover hearing of the other ear must be prevented. This can be achieved only by masking the non-test ear with appropriate levels of noise.

**Fig. 8.6  Whispered-voice test**

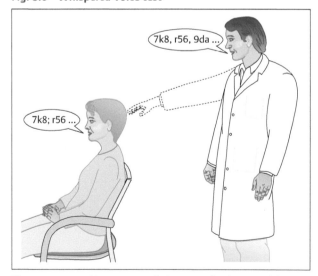

The examiner whispers sets of three single digits and letters standing at an arm's length behind the patient. Normal overall hearing can be assumed if the patient repeats the sets correctly.

*Technique:*
- The examiner stands beside the patient.
- A moist cotton wad is placed into the non-test ear canal and a masking noise is created by gently wiggling the cotton with the finger (**Fig. 8.7**).
- The examiner, with the head turned away from the test ear of the patient, whispers sets of three random numbers and letters and instructs the patient to repeat the sets aloud.
- If the patient does not understand the sets, the examiner presents them at progressively smaller distances from the test ear.
- Distances between the right and left ears are compared.
- If the sets are still not understood when whispered just outside the ear canal, the test is repeated with the sets spoken at a normal loudness level.

**Fig. 8.7   Test for one-sided hearing loss**

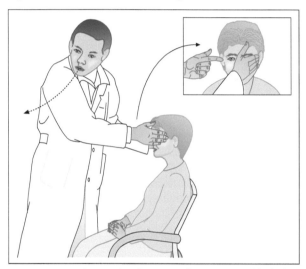

Hearing is tested on each side separately using a modified whispered-voice test. The examiner masks the non-test ear by wiggling moist cotton within the ear canal. The examiner then whispers speech items, beginning with his/her head turned away from the test ear and turning progressively closer to the ear if the items are not understood correctly. The two sides are compared.

*Interpretation:* The sets of numbers and letters whispered with the head turned away from the patient can normally be heard equally on both sides. If the numbers are unintelligible or are understood only when whispered just outside the ear canal, the patient is considered to have **severe hearing loss** at that side. If the numbers are unintelligible when spoken close to the ear at a normal or even loud level, the patient is considered to have **functional deafness** for speech in that ear.

🖌 With some practice, an examiner can reliably assess hearing with these simple tests and can recognize differences between the right and left sides.

**Range of hearing:**

*Principle:* Formerly, the degree of hearing loss was tested by determining the range at which the patient could hear spoken or whispered numbers. These measurements are imprecise and depend on many uncontrolled factors, and today the quantitative degree of hearing loss should be determined only by audiometric testing.

*Technique:* The range of hearing can be tested in meters if a large testing suite and an assistant are available (**Fig. 8.8**). The assistant masks the non-test ear and blocks the patient's view of the examiner. The patient turns the test ear toward the examiner, who whispers sets of three random numbers and letters toward the patient from a distance of 6 m. If the patient does not understand the sets, the examiner moves closer and determines the range at which the sets become intelligible. If necessary, the sets may be spoken at a normal conversational level. It is essential that constant test conditions be maintained.

*Interpretation:* Hearing loss can be stated in terms of the distance at which the sets are still intelligible. In a **normal** test, the subject can understand sets of three numbers and letters whispered from about 6 m away.

**Fig. 8.8   Hearing range test**

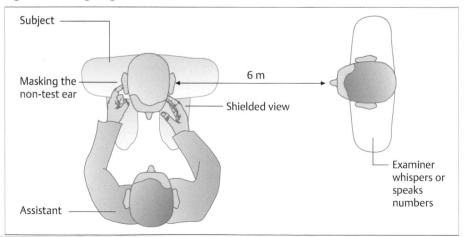

Subject

Masking the non-test ear

Shielded view

6 m

Examiner whispers or speaks numbers

Assistant

To test the hearing range, an assistant masks the non-test ear while shielding the patient's view.

# 8.2    Basic Principles of Audiometry

Audiometry is the measurement of auditory functions. Since it employs acoustic stimuli that are physically defined, we begin this unit by reviewing some of the basic physical principles of acoustics. The response to acoustic stimuli may be recorded in the form of a voluntary reaction, such as pushing a button, or an involuntary physiologic response such as contraction of the stapedius muscle. Behavioral audiometry is based on voluntary responses and is described more fully in 🔖8.3. Involuntary responses, which are measured in objective audiometry, are discussed in 🔖8.4. The goals of clinical audiometry are the following:

- Detection of a hearing disorder.
- Localization of the hearing disorder.
- Quantification of the hearing disorder.

## Basic Concepts in Acoustics

### Production and Propagation of Sound

Sound is produced by mechanical vibrations (**Fig. 8.9**) which propagate as *sound waves* in an elastic medium (air, liquid, or a solid medium such as bone). The sound waves can be described in terms of the following properties:

- Frequency.
- Sound pressure.
- Propagation velocity.

The velocity of sound ranges from 340 m/s in air to approximately 5,000 m/s in solid media.

When sound travels from one medium to another, as from air to water, it is either reflected or absorbed. As a rule, sound is partly absorbed and partly reflected, depending on its frequency.

Fig. 8.9    **Production and propagation of sound waves**

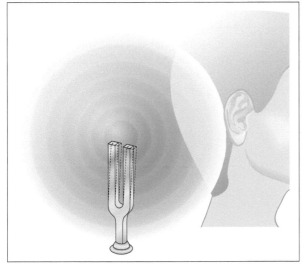

Sound is produced by a vibrating source, in this case a tuning fork. It propagates uniformly in a medium. Human hearing is specialized for the perception of sound in air.

## Sound Frequency Spectrum

Frequencies in the range of about 20 to 20,000 Hz can be perceived as an auditory stimulus by humans.

A sound is usually made up of various frequencies. All of these frequencies taken together constitute a sound event and are called the **frequency spectrum** (**Fig. 8.10**):

- A *pure tone* consists of a single sinusoidal vibration (**Fig. 8.10a**). It can be precisely described by the frequency, amplitude, and phase of the vibration. Pure tones, which rarely occur in nature, are well suited for acoustic measurements. They are used in audiology to determine the frequency-dependent sensitivity of hearing (pure-tone threshold).
- A *musical sound* consists of a fundamental frequency plus harmonic overtones, which are integral multiples of the fundamental frequency. The sound is characterized by, and can be recognized by, its harmonic overtones (**Fig. 8.10b**). Based on the different spectra of the overtones, the listener can easily distinguish a note played on a violin from the same note played on a piano.
- *Noise* consists of sound events containing multiple frequencies that are harmonically unrelated (**Fig. 8.10c**)—that is, they are not integral multiples of one another. Noise is by far the most common acoustic stimulus.

The most important sound source for humans is the voice, whose fundamental frequency of about 100 Hz in men and 200 Hz in women is produced by vibrations of the vocal cords (see 🔖18.1). The spectrum of basic frequencies is individually modulated by the resonance of the upper airways, enabling the voice to serve as a means of identification.

## Sound Pressure

Sound waves are extremely small fluctuations of atmospheric air pressure caused by the alternating condensation and rarefaction of atoms and molecules. These variations of pressure amplitude can

**Fig. 8.10   The frequency spectra of different auditory stimuli: tone, musical sound, and noise**

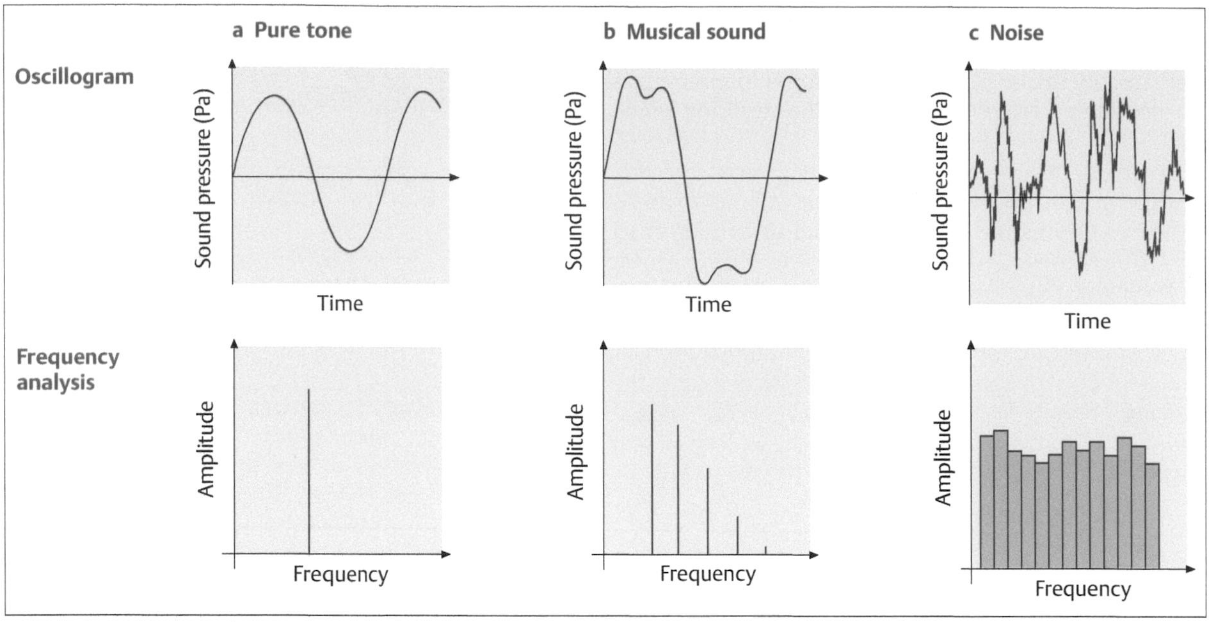

a **Pure tone**: a single frequency produces a sinusoidal waveform (e.g., a tuning fork tone).
b **Musical sound** contains a fundamental frequency plus one or more harmonics, whose frequencies are integral multiples of the fundamental frequency (e.g., violin, piano).

c **Noise** consists of numerous nonperiodic frequencies that are not integral multiples of one another. A pitch cannot be determined (e.g., the noise from a jackhammer).

be physically measured. The unit of measurement is the pascal (Pa):

$$1\ \mathrm{Pa} = 1\ \mathrm{N/m^2} = 10\ \mu\mathrm{bar}$$

A sound pressure of 1 Pa is approximately equal to the sound pressure in a discotheque. By comparison, the atmospheric pressure is of the order of $10^5$ Pa. Human hearing can just perceive sound pressure variations as small as 20 µPa ($2 \times 10^{-5}$ Pa, the hearing threshold), which is 10 orders of magnitude lower than the atmospheric pressure. The pain threshold is reached at a sound pressure of about 20 Pa, which is about 1 million times greater than the normal threshold of hearing. Examples of sound pressure values associated with common events are shown in **Fig. 8.11**.
The range over which a person can perceive an acoustic stimulus without discomfort is called the *dynamic range*.
The human ear perceives the loudness levels of different sound pressures in a logarithmic fashion, rather than on a linear scale. This logarithmic relationship between stimulus and perception, called the *Weber–Fechner law*, holds true for all sensory modalities.

🗲 This is why a logarithmic scale is used for sound pressures in acoustics and audiology.

**Fig. 8.11   Examples of various sound pressures**

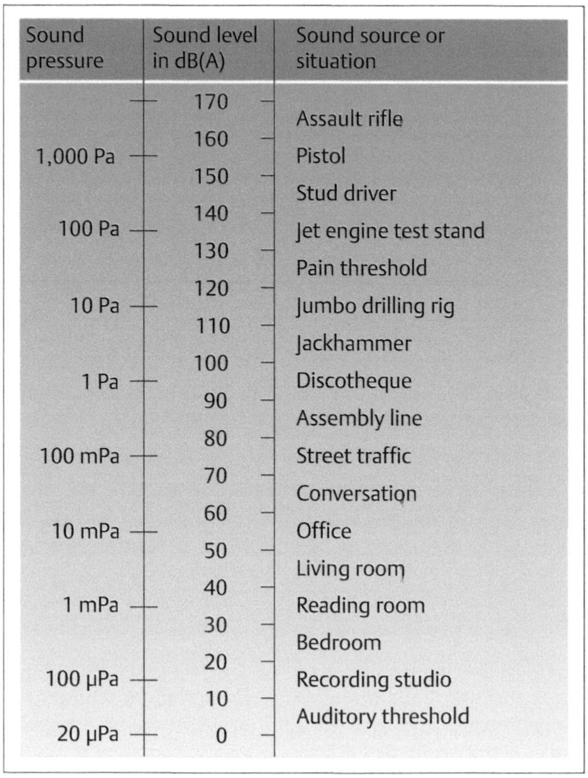

| Sound pressure | Sound level in dB(A) | Sound source or situation |
|---|---|---|
| | 170 | Assault rifle |
| 1,000 Pa | 160 | Pistol |
| | 150 | Stud driver |
| 100 Pa | 140 | Jet engine test stand |
| | 130 | Pain threshold |
| 10 Pa | 120 | Jumbo drilling rig |
| | 110 | Jackhammer |
| | 100 | |
| 1 Pa | | Discotheque |
| | 90 | Assembly line |
| | 80 | |
| 100 mPa | 70 | Street traffic |
| | 60 | Conversation |
| 10 mPa | 50 | Office |
| | 40 | Living room |
| 1 mPa | 30 | Reading room |
| | 20 | Bedroom |
| 100 µPa | 10 | Recording studio |
| | 0 | Auditory threshold |
| 20 µPa | | |

## Sound Pressure Level (dB SPL)

*Definitions:* A logarithmic sound pressure scale can be created by relating the measured sound pressure p to a designated reference value $p_0$. The resulting sound pressure ratio is called the *level.*

The International Organization for Standardization (ISO) has defined the reference value as 20 µPa. This is the sound pressure at the threshold of hearing—that is, the pressure at which a normal listener can just perceive a continuous tone between 2 and 3 kHz.

The use of logarithms enables us to bring the physical and physiologic scales closer together and to appreciate more clearly the large range of physical values. The sound pressure level is stated in decibels (dB, named for the inventor of the telephone, Alexander Graham Bell). The suffix SPL stands for sound pressure level (see Applications, below).

The formula for the sound pressure level $L_p$ is as follows:

$$L_p = 20 \times \log_{10} p/p_0 \ [\text{dB SPL}]$$

or, according to ISO 131–1979:

$$L_p = 20 \times \log_{10} p/20 \ \mu Pa \ [\text{dB SPL}]$$

*Interpretation and calculations:* Since we are dealing with a relative scale, 0 dB SPL does not correspond to absence of sound pressure and the scale can become negative. Moreover, since it is a logarithmic scale, the increase in physical values is disproportionately greater at high decibel levels than at low decibels. For example, when the sound pressure level is increased by 10 dB, from 0 to 10 dB SPL, the sound pressure increases by 44 µPa; but an increase from 100 to 110 dB SPL corresponds to a 4.4 Pa increase, which is 100,000 times greater in physical terms.

☞ Decibel values cannot be added or subtracted.

When the sound pressure is doubled, the sound pressure level rises by 6 dB! Additional examples and the relationship between sound pressure and sound power are shown in **Table 8.1** and **Fig. 8.12**.

*Applications:* The sound pressure level (dB SPL) is a physical scale that is widely used in technology, including hearing aid technology. In audiology, it is used in speech audiometry but not in pure-tone audiometry.

*Explanation:* The sensitivity of hearing is frequency-dependent. It is highest in the range of about 1 to 4 kHz and corresponds to a sound pressure level of about 0 dB SPL in young, normal-hearing individuals. Hearing becomes less sensitive at higher and lower frequencies, and considerably greater sound pressure levels are needed to achieve a normal threshold.

Table 8.1 Relationship between sound pressure level, sound pressure, and sound intensity

| Sound pressure level difference $(L_2–L_1)$ | Sound pressure ratio $(p_2:p_1)$ | Ratio of sound intensity to sound energy $(I_2:I_1)$ |
|---|---|---|
| 0 dB | 1.0:1 | 1.0:1 |
| 3 dB | 1.4:1 | 2.0:1 |
| 5 dB | 1.8:1 | 3.2:1 |
| 6 dB | 2.0:1 | 4.0:1 |
| 10 dB | 3.2:1 | 10.0:1 |
| 20 dB | 10.0:1 | 100.0:1 |

Fig. 8.12 Summation of sound sources

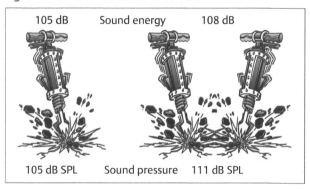

When a second jackhammer of equal loudness is operated in an area, the sound energy is doubled. The sound energy level increases by 3 dB according to **Table 8.1**, and the sound pressure level is increased by 6 dB.

Because of this, a curved line is obtained when the hearing threshold is plotted against the physical sound pressure level (dB SPL) (red curve in **Fig. 8.13**).

☞ The extension "SPL" is added to avoid confusion with the dB HL scale that is used diagnostically (e.g., in audiometry; see below).

## Decibel Scale for Hearing Levels (dB HL)

When the pure-tone threshold is measured in audiology, the physical sound pressure is of less interest than comparing the measured threshold with a normal threshold. For this reason, the values measured in dB SPL are corrected to values determined by the ISO based on the auditory thresholds of normal-hearing 18-year-olds for different frequencies (ISO 389 and 7566). The threshold at 250 Hz, for example, is approximately 25 dB SPL.

This relative decibel scale is called the dB HL ("hearing level") scale. In this type of graph, the normal hearing threshold is represented as a horizontal line at the 0 dB hearing level, making it easier to read the audiogram. However, we are still dealing with a sound pressure scale that is based on the physical pressure of the acoustic stimulus.

## 8.1 Psychoacoustics

Psychoacoustics is a branch of psychophysics that studies the relationship between the physical properties of a stimulus and the behavioral response. When a person responds to an acoustic stimulus, we call it "hearing." Psychoacoustics, then, studies the relationships between the physical properties of the acoustic stimulus and hearing, and thus forms the scientific basis for much of audiology. Concepts such as "threshold" and "loudness" are derived from psychoacoustics. Several of these concepts are briefly described in the following.

### Threshold

Threshold may refer to the smallest difference that can be perceived between two auditory stimuli that differ with regard to some physical property. This is called the *difference threshold*. In audiology, however, the term *threshold* almost always means the absolute *intensity threshold*, or the minimum sound pressure level of an acoustic stimulus that can still be perceived. In clinical pure-tone audiometry, this threshold is determined for sine-wave tones presented at different frequencies. In this test, the sound pressure level of the tone is varied and the subject indicates whether or not he or she still hears the tone.

Regardless of the method of threshold determination used in clinical audiometry, different threshold values may be determined for different test subjects even though the subjects have identical hearing from a psychoacoustic standpoint. One subject may have to detect a tone convincingly and unequivocally before signaling that it is heard, while another may respond to a much fainter signal. This will yield two different thresholds that relate less to actual hearing ability than to the internal criteria, or bias, of the persons tested.

In psychoacoustics, special methods are used to measure these criteria along with the threshold so that the actual threshold of hearing can be ascertained. These methods basically involve presenting the acoustic stimuli in random order along with equally long periods of silence. The subject responds after each period, indicating whether or not he or she has heard an acoustic signal. If the level of the stimulus is well above the auditory threshold, the differentiation is easily made. But if the stimulus level is well below the auditory threshold, the stimulus and the silent period will be detected or undetected with equal frequency. To make a threshold determination, it is necessary to determine the ratio of detected and undetected stimuli and silent periods at various levels between these extremes. The actual threshold can then be determined mathematically.

These methods are very time-consuming and are not practical for clinical audiology. When ordinary clinical methods are carefully applied in a cooperative patient, the differences that are associated with different methods are small and have no diagnostic significance, particularly since the threshold in pure-tone audiometry is determined to an accuracy of only 5 dB.

### Loudness level and loudness

The intensity of a stimulus is described physically by its level. But the sound pressure level is a poor criterion for describing the subjective perception of loudness, because this perception depends not only on the sound pressure level but also on other physical parameters such as the duration and spectrum of the stimulus.

The **loudness level** is a psychoacoustic quantity that is used to compare the subjective loudness of a sound with the loudness of a tone at 1,000 Hz. When the 1,000-Hz tone is perceived as having the same loudness as the sound, then the sound pressure level of the tone in dB SPL describes the loudness level. The unit of subjective loudness is the *phon*. Thus, a 1,000-Hz tone at 60 dB SPL has a subjective loudness of 60 phons. But a 50-Hz tone, for example, must have a sound pressure of about 80 dB SPL to reach a loudness level of 60 phons.

The values on the phon scale are often poor for describing the subjective perception of a gain in loudness as the sound intensity increases. This prompted the development of a separate scale for subjective **loudness** based on the *sone*. One sone is equivalent to 40 phons at a frequency of 1,000 Hz. Adding 10 phons doubles the sone value, and so 50 phons are equivalent to 2 sones, 60 phons to 4 sones, etc.

The subjective psychoacoustic units of measure for loudness level and loudness are not used for ordinary technical measurements. Street noise, for example, is measured using correction factors and standard filters—usually the A filter, which is matched to the auditory threshold. The measured sound level is designated by the attribute (A), written as dB (A). Again, however, the measurements are not necessarily a good indicator of subjective loudness.

### Masking

The perception of a sound event can be diminished by other simultaneous or near-simultaneous sound events. This process, called **masking**, is a general psychoacoustic phenomenon that, like loudness, cannot be accurately described using simple spectral and temporal parameters.

Masking is important in audiometry when only one ear is being tested. The non-test ear is masked with noise that prevents perception of the test stimulus.

### Adaptation and auditory fatigue

**Adaptation** is a physiologic change in the perception of an acoustic stimulus that occurs in response to constant stimulation. Neural excitation decreases over time, usually accompanied by a rapid decline in loudness perception. If adaptation exceeds a certain measure, which depends on the physical properties of the stimulus, abnormal adaptation is said to be present. Formerly, this phenomenon was applied clinically in the diagnosis of neural injury.

**Auditory fatigue** is different from adaptation; it denotes a gradual rise of the auditory threshold during or following an acoustic stress. Some degree of temporary threshold shift consistently occurs when the acoustic stress exceeds a certain level.

**Fig. 8.13 Comparison of the dB SPL and dB HL scales**

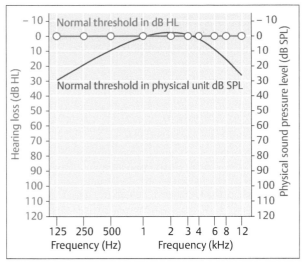

The normal auditory threshold forms a curved line when plotted against a physical sound pressure level scale (dB SPL, red curve and red scale on the right). A scale with corresponding correction factors is used clinically (dB HL, green scale on the left), and the normal auditory threshold (green) is plotted as a horizontal line. The dB HL scale directly indicates hearing loss relative to a normal population (0 dB HL).

## Audiologic Examination

### Goals of Audiologic Examination

Audiologic examination is designed to test the functions of hearing. It has the following main goals:
- Detect a hearing disorder.
- Classify a hearing disorder (diagnostic audiometry).
- Quantify a hearing disorder.

The various methods that are used in audiometry are of varying usefulness in achieving these goals. An effort must be made to address the clinical problem as efficiently as possible using the most appropriate test methods.

### Methods of Audiologic Examination

Audiometric tests may be used to *diagnose* or *screen for* hearing impairment. As a rule, the patient already has a known or presumed hearing disorder in diagnostic examinations, whereas screening is designed to detect an unrecognized hearing disorder. Audiologic screening is used to detect hearing problems in newborns, for example, or for the early detection of noise-induced hearing loss in occupationally exposed persons.

Methods in diagnostic audiometry are classified according to the nature of the tested response:
- *Behavioral audiometry* (see ♫8.3) is based on an active and usually voluntary response from the test subject.

- *Objective audiometry* tests hearing functions based on "objectively" measured parameters that represent an involuntary physiologic response (see ♫8.4).

### Site-of-Lesion Determination

The cause of a hearing disorder may lie at any level of the auditory system, from the cerumen in the external ear canal to circulatory disturbances in the auditory cortex. An important aspect of clinical and audiologic testing is site-of-lesion determination—that is, localizing the causal pathology to a particular structure or structures.

A precise clinical history and physical examination (see ♫8.1) are important for narrowing the diagnosis. The clinical examination should be able to distinguish between the following two:
- *Conductive hearing loss*, where the lesion is in the ear canal or middle ear.
- *Sensorineural hearing loss*, where the lesion involves the cochlea or the neural structures of the auditory system.

**Fig. 8.14** reviews the process of site-of-lesion determination in hearing disorders. Imaging studies can also be very useful for site-of-lesion determination.

*Retrocochlear impairment* basically refers to any hearing disorder whose cause lies central to the cochlea. However, the term is often applied strictly to an auditory nerve lesion (neural hearing loss) and is distinguished from a lesion of the central nervous system (central hearing disorder).

Hearing disorders may also be caused by *combined lesions* that involve various structures. For example, typical cases of age-related hearing loss (presbycusis) are most likely caused by cochlear dysfunction (sensory hearing loss) and by abnormalities of neural structures (neural hearing loss; see also ♫12.3, Age-Related Hearing Loss [Presbycusis]). Generally, the components are not easily distinguished by audiologic testing, and the composite term *sensorineural hearing loss* is used.

### Quantitative Classification of Hearing Impairment

Hearing disorders can be classified into various grades of severity based on audiometric findings (**Table 8.2**).

⌀ This type of classification is useful only for orientation purposes and says nothing about the actual degree of the hearing disability, which depends on many personal and social factors.

In addition, various computational methods can be used to determine the percentage of hearing loss based on the pure-tone audiogram or speech audiometry.

**Fig. 8.14   Site-of-lesion determination in hearing disorders**

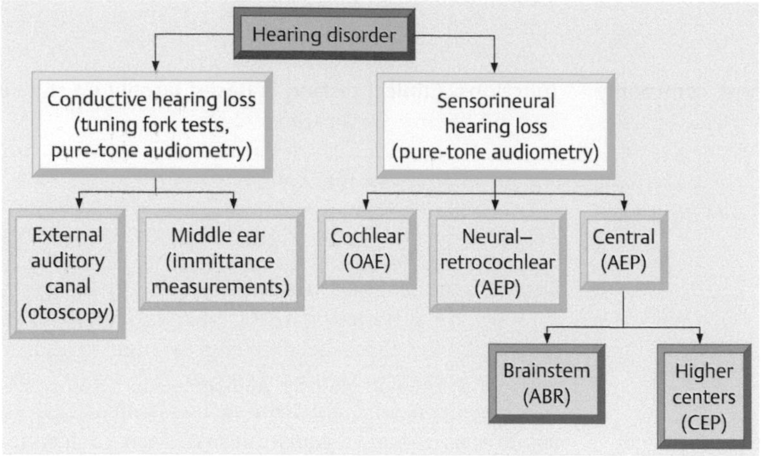

This flowchart shows the most important audiologic tests that are used in making a site-of-lesion diagnosis.

**Table 8.2   WHO Grades of hearing impairment (Grades 2, 3, and 4 are classified as disabling hearing impairment)**

| Grade of impairment | Average audiometric thresholds at 500, 1,000, 2,000, and 4,000 Hz | Performance |
|---|---|---|
| 0: No impairment | 25 dB or better | No or very slight hearing problems |
| 1: Slight impairment | 26–40 dB | Able to hear and repeat words spoken in normal voice at 1 m |
| 2: Moderate impairment | 41–60 dB | Able to hear and repeat words spoken in raised voice at 1 m |
| 3: Severe impairment | 61–80 dB | Able to hear some words when shouted into better ear |
| 4: Profound impairment including deafness | 81 dB or greater | Unable to hear and understand even a shouted voice |

These methods are important for insurance matters and in rehabilitation.

**Acquired deafness** refers to a *loss* of the sense of hearing. It is difficult to rule out the vibrational perception of low frequencies, and so deafness is often defined functionally as a complete loss of speech comprehension.

**Congenital deafness** refers to the *absence* of hearing. Hearing develops during the first years of life and is closely related to speech and language development. With congenital deafness, this development fails to occur, and the central patterns of phonation are not established. As a result, nonhearing individuals have fundamentally different speech and language concepts compared with individuals who have lost their hearing.

# 8.3    Behavioral Audiometric Testing

**Behavioral audiometric tests are the most commonly used test methods in diagnostic audiology. They are based on an active, usually voluntary response from the test subject. In principle, these methods can test the entire auditory system including higher cognitive functions. Clinical testing is based largely on the subjective auditory response to tones and speech signals:**

- **Pure-tone audiometry, which is the most common audiometric test method.**
- **Speech audiometry.**

## Pure-Tone Audiometry: Threshold Determination

In pure-tone audiometry, the sensitivity to pure sine-wave tones is measured by determining the hearing threshold (see *✐* **8.1**). The threshold is usually measured at frequencies from 125 to 8 kHz, increasing by octaves or half-octaves. This is done separately for the left and right ears, and the thresholds are tested for both air conduction and bone conduction (**Fig. 8.15**).

*Equipment:* An electronic device called an **audiometer** is used to generate pure tones of varying frequency and loudness and control their presentation. Frequencies below 125 Hz are difficult to distinguish from vibrato-tactile sensations; and with tones higher than 8 kHz, the sound pressure level cannot be accurately calibrated with ordinary headphones. Special audiometers are available for measuring thresholds from 8 to 16 kHz (**high-tone audiometry**), but these tests show greater interindividual variation than routine audiometry.

A **bone vibrator** requires considerably more energy to produce sound than headphones, which is why the threshold for bone conduction can be measured only to maximum values that are 40 to 50 dB lower than those for air conduction. More distortion occurs at higher frequencies (>4 kHz), and the measurements become less reliable.

*Technique:* The tones are first presented to one ear only by **air conduction** using headphones or special insert phones. Cross-hearing is prevented by masking the non-test ear with noise (see *✐* **8.1**).

The threshold for **bone conduction** is measured with a vibrator pressed against the mastoid or forehead. This device sets the cranial bones and cranial contents into vibration, transmitting the test sound to the inner ear.

*Interpretation:* With proper calibration and *normal sound conduction*, the thresholds for air conduction and bone conduction should be equal (**Fig. 8.16a**).

If the air conduction threshold is higher than the bone conduction threshold (i.e., if perception by air conduction requires a higher loudness level), the subject has a **conductive hearing loss** (**Fig. 8.16b**).

If **sensorineural hearing loss** is present, no significant difference is found between the thresholds for air and bone conduction. The hearing threshold is raised, often more at high frequencies than at low frequencies (**Fig. 8.16c** and **Fig. 12.1a**).

The following audiographic signs indicate a **mixed hearing loss**:

- Greater air conduction loss compared with bone conduction, indicating *impaired sound conduction*.
- An increased threshold for bone conduction (**Fig. 8.16d**).

The threshold in the pure-tone audiogram may show typical patterns that reflect the nature of the hearing disorder, such as a notch at 4 to 6 kHz pointing to noise-induced hearing loss (**Fig. 12.7**), low-frequency hearing loss at the onset of Ménière's disease (**Fig. 13.15a**), or conductive loss accompanied by a bone conduction notch at intermediate frequencies (Carhart's notch) in otosclerotic stapes fixation (see *✐* 11.4, Bone Diseases).

## Speech Audiometry

The essential functions of human hearing include the perception and recognition of speech. Consequently, the use of speech signals has a major role in audiometric testing. Speech audiometry is particularly

**Fig. 8.15    Audiometer**

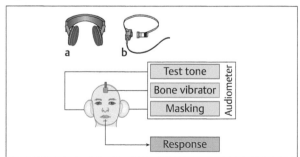

Principal function of an audiometer with the following:
**a** Headphones for air conduction testing and masking.
**b** Vibrator for bone conduction testing. The vibrator can be placed either over the mastoid behind the ear or at the forehead.

Fig. 8.16 **Pure-tone threshold audiometry**

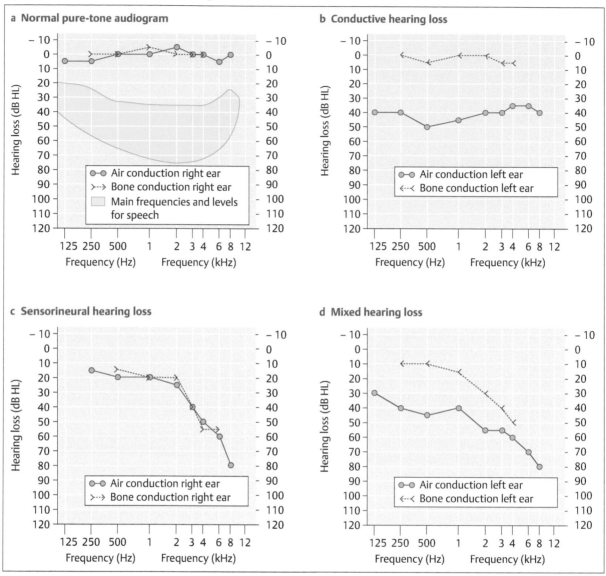

**a** Normal pure-tone audiogram for the right ear. The range of frequencies and levels that typically occur in conversational speech is shown in green.
**b** Conductive hearing loss in the left ear.

**c** Sensorineural impairment with high-tone loss on the right side.
**d** Mixed conductive and sensorineural hearing loss on the left side.

important in hearing rehabilitation and fitting patients with hearing aids.

Speech signals display typical patterns that result from a broad frequency spectrum and rapid changes of frequencies and levels in periods of milliseconds. These patterns form the basis for understanding speech. Because of the inherent variability of speech signals and their dependency on language, audiometric speech testing cannot be standardized in the same way as pure-tone audiometry. Approaches to speech audiometry are quite different in different languages. The results of speech audiometry depend not only on hearing but also on higher cognitive functions such as language comprehension, native language, vocabulary, memory, and motor speech.

## Principles of Speech Audiometry

*Threshold:* The concept of speech thresholds includes both the hearing and the recognition or understanding of words, phrases, or sentences. The threshold at which the presence of speech sounds is detected without understanding is called *speech detection threshold* or *speech awareness threshold*. It is unimportant in speech audiometry.

**Fig. 8.17 Speech audiometry: normal and abnormal performance–intensity functions**

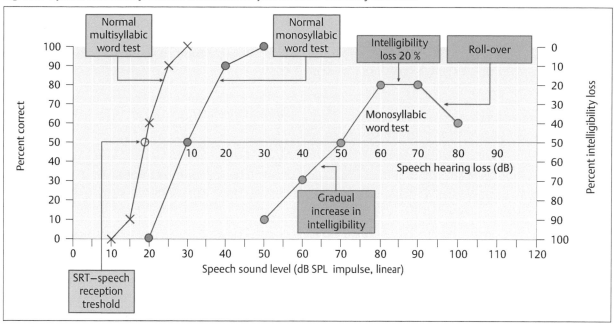

Speech audiograms with normal recognition curves for four-syllabic number words (x) and monosyllabic test words (o), and an abnormal performance–intensity function in sensorineural hearing loss.

The commonly measured threshold at which speech is understood is called the *speech reception threshold* (SRT, sometimes also called *speech recognition threshold*). It is the sound level at which 50% of the given speech test material is understood. The threshold is measured with a performance–intensity function between low levels with no speech recognition and higher levels with full understanding. The level of the function can be read most accurately at 50% recognition because it is steepest at 50% comprehension (**Fig. 8.16**).

The SRT is a common parameter in speech audiometry.

In English and in quiet, it is conventionally measured with spondees, which are disyllabic, evenly stressed words such as "pancake" or "hardware." Four-syllabic numbers are used in German for the same purpose. The SRT measured in that way corresponds highly with pure-tone thresholds, but SRT can also be measured against preset levels of background noise using other speech signals such as sentences.

**Suprathreshold speech recognition:** The percentage of understanding of speech signals is measured at either one or several predetermined levels of presentation. In English, "word recognition testing" refers to the measurement of the percentage of understanding a list of monosyllabic words at a comfortable hearing level. In German, a speech recognition curve (**Fig. 8.16**) of monosyllabic words ("Freiburger Einsilbertest") is measured. Tests with monosyllabic words are also called *speech discrimination testing*.

In patients with **conductive hearing loss**, 100% comprehension is still achieved at sufficiently high levels. **Sensorineural hearing loss** leads to a flattening of the performance–intensity function, full intelligibility is often not reached, and a decline in speech recognition at higher sound levels may occur (**Fig. 8.17**).

**Test procedures:** The speech test can be presented to one ear using headphones or insert earphones, or to both ears simultaneously using loudspeakers in the sound-field environment.

*Open-set tests* use single words or phrases, and the patient repeats what he or she is hearing. *Closed-set tests* give the patient a selection of words or phrases, and one of these items is presented. The patient chooses from the selection the item, which he or she was hearing.

Speech recognition can be measured in *quiet* or in *noise*, providing information about different auditory functions. Comprehensive clinical audiometry combines these two kinds of tests. Sentence tests are particularly useful for testing speech perception in noise. The noise presented in these tests has the same frequency content as speech and can therefore mask them. Most tests present the noise at a constant level, and the speech sound levels are varied until a prescribed degree of speech recognition is achieved, usually 50% corresponding to the SRT for sentences. The relevant parameter is then the difference between the noise and the speech level, known as the signal-to-noise ratio.

## Speech Tests

**Test material:** Speech material is generally available in the form of digital recordings and can be reproducibly presented by using an audiometer. Unlike the sound level of sustained tones or noise, the sound level of speech signals cannot be stated precisely but only as a statistical average. Speech audiometry uses specific level measuring functions in the frequency and time domains to determine the speech sound levels.

**Speech tests in quiet:** The design of speech tests is different in quiet and in noise. In quiet, routine audiometry often uses open-set tests for suprathreshold speech recognition measurements. They typically consist of several lists of monosyllabic words. Each list may have between 10 and 50 words, and the lists are usually phonetically balanced, meaning that the distribution of the various sounds in these words corresponds to that of the language in general. The *Central Institute of the Deaf W-22* (CID W-22) and the *Northwestern University Auditory Test No. 6* (NU-6) lists are examples of commonly used open-set tests in English. *Fournier's* test lists are examples in French, the *Freiburger Einsilbertest* is an example in German, and *Bocca's test* is an example in Italian.

Many different closed-set tests exist for monosyllabic words, in which a selection of words with similar sounds is presented. From these words, the patient selects the word that he or she was hearing as a stimulus. Examples are the California Consonant Test (CCT), in which the stimulus consists of one of four words, such as "pin–thin–tin–kin," or the Four Alternative Auditory Feature (FAAF) test, in which the initial or final consonant in consonant–vowel–consonant words, such as "bad–bag–bat–back" or "gab–dab–tab–cab," is varied. An example of a monosyllabic closed-set test in German is the *Reimtest of Wallenberg und Kollmeier* (WAKO).

**Speech tests in noise:** Monosyllabic word lists are not suited for speech tests in noise, because they are too short to be readily understood in noise. Sentences are the commonly used speech material in noise.

The *Matrix Sentence test* is an example of a multilingual speech test, developed first in Swedish and then in German. It is now available in many different languages and consists of 5 lists of 10 words, one list each for names, verbs, numbers, colors, and nouns. Nonsense sentences such as "Peter bought eight white ships" are randomly constructed with these lists. The SRT for sentences is typically measured with an adaptive procedure, meaning that levels of the sentences are varied up and down until the SRT can be determined reliably.

Another example in English is the *Hearing in Noise test* (HINT). It consists of 25 phonemically balanced lists of 10 sentences. Other examples are the *Synthetic Sentence Identification test* (SSI) and the *Speech Perception in Noise test* (SPIN).

## 8.2  Other behavioral audiometric tests

Besides the behavioral audiometric tests used in routine clinical audiometry (pure-tone and speech audiometry), there are several other behavioral audiometric procedures that are used for specific purposes.

### Dynamic range scaling

As noted in 7.2, Function of the Cochlea, sensorineural hearing loss is apt to produce distortion effects at suprathreshold levels. A typical distortion effect is an abnormal increase in loudness perception, called *recruitment*. Even though the hearing threshold is increased, with the result that tones at a relatively high sound level are either not heard or faintly perceived, the opposite may occur in the perception of suprathreshold sounds: tones that are well tolerated by normal-hearing individuals are perceived as louder or uncomfortable. As a result, the range of useful loudness levels, called the dynamic range, is significantly reduced in patients with sensorineural hearing impairment.

The reduction and distortion of the dynamic range play a major role in fitting patients with hearing aids and cochlear implants, because soft signals should be amplified sufficiently whereas loud signals should not. Consequently, an audiometric evaluation of the dynamic range should be performed in patients fitted for a hearing aid.

### *Technique:*

- The simplest method is to determine the *uncomfortable loudness level*. This is done by determining the level of a pure tone, or preferably noise with a narrow frequency spectrum, at which the test subject perceives the signal as uncomfortably loud.
- *Dynamic range measurement (dynamic range scaling)* evaluates how subjects perceive increasing loudness within their dynamic range. The patient rates the subjective loudness of signals presented at various loudness levels and at various frequencies (500, 1,000, 2,000, 4,000 Hz) as "very soft," "soft," "medium," "loud," "very loud," or "too loud."

### Tests for nonorganic hearing loss

Behavioral audiometric tests may elicit an intentionally or unintentionally false response indicating an increased hearing threshold. *Malingering* refers to the deliberate feigning of hearing impairment by a normal-hearing individual. Other malingerers may *exaggerate* the severity of an existing hearing problem. A far more common phenomenon, however, is self-deception by a patient who has *psychogenic hearing loss*. Objective tests (see 8.4) are available that can quickly disclose the feigning of hearing loss.

There are also several special behavioral audiometric tests that can suggest or confirm psychogenic hearing loss or malingering, but they are not widely practiced today. An experienced examiner may suspect a "false" hearing threshold based on certain behavioral cues (reaction time, changing responses).

Feigning is also suggested by a discrepancy between the pure-tone threshold and speech recognition threshold. The loudness of speech signals is more difficult to assess subjectively than the loudness of pure tones. As a result, subjects with nonorganic hearing loss may show less hearing impairment in speech audiometry than in pure-tone audiometry.

### Sound localization and directional hearing

The localization of a sound source and the separation of different sources are important central auditory functions based on binaural hearing. Directional hearing is managed chiefly by brainstem neurons of the central auditory pathway, and an asymmetry of hearing levels between the right and left ears is detrimental.

Complex sound-field setups make it possible to measure directional hearing directly (angle in degrees). Other arrangements using several sound sources for speech and noise allow measurement of the improvement gained from hearing with both ears (binaural hearing) over hearing with just one ear. The sound sources are arranged in different patterns and changes in the SRT for sentences are typically measured.

# 8.4    Objective Hearing Tests

Unlike the subjective psychoacoustic methods used in behavioral audiometry, objective audiometry makes it possible to test hearing without eliciting an active response from the patient. Objective audiometry employs tests that measure hearing functions based on involuntary physiologic responses and "objective" parameters. These responses may consist of the stapedial reflex (see Acoustic Immittance Measurements), the bioelectric potentials of neural structures (see Auditory Evoked Potentials [AEPs]), or the acoustic vibrations of the cochlea (see Otoacoustic Emissions [OAEs]).

Objective test findings aid in the interpretation of behavioral audiometric results. Objective audiometric tests are also useful in infants, small children (see 9.2, Diagnostic Methods in Pediatric Audiology), and patients with mental or cognitive impairment.

*Methods:* Three main types of response are measured clinically in objective audiometry using various techniques:

- Immittance measurements: changes in the acoustic impedance of the tympanic membrane are measured with an intra-aural probe.
- Auditory evoked potentials (AEPs): acoustically evoked bioelectric responses of the cochlea, auditory nerve, auditory tract neurons, or cerebral cortex are analyzed using surface electrodes and averaging techniques (see also Auditory Evoked Potentials [AEPs] below).
- Otoacoustic emissions (OAEs): a microphone probe is used to measure sound events in the ear canal that are produced by spontaneous or acoustically evoked active biomechanical vibrations in the cochlea (see also Otoacoustic Emissions [OAEs] below).

*Interpretation:* It cannot always be determined with complete confidence whether or not a response is present in objective audiometry. But modern, computer-assisted methods of measurement will generally establish whether a stimulus response has occurred.

 The objectivity of these methods relates to the selection of the stimulus response, not to the interpretation of the test.

## Acoustic Immittance Measurements

*Definition:* The impedance of an acoustic system is a measure of the resistance that the system (e.g., the middle ear) offers to the absorption of sound waves. A system with high acoustic impedance reflects most of the sound energy and absorbs very little. Conversely, a system with low impedance absorbs a large amount of sound energy in the form of vibrations. Sound absorption is also referred to as the **compliance** of the tympanic membrane. The middle ear transforms the sound waves in air in such a way that they can induce waves in the cochlear fluid with little resistance (impedance matching by the middle ear; see 7.1, Middle Ear).

*Principle:* The acoustic impedance of the external ear canal and tympanic membrane can be measured with an intra-aural probe. The probe emits a tone at a certain frequency, usually 220 Hz, into the ear canal. The impedance value of this probe tone depends on the overall acoustic system comprising the ear canal, tympanic membrane, middle ear, and cochlea as well as the frequency of the tone and individual factors. A freely vibrating tympanic membrane, for example, will absorb more energy and reflect less than a stiff tympanic membrane. The impedance value will be lower.

The absolute value of impedance is of less interest in audiometry than the impedance changes that are caused by specific external manipulations. Two main types of impedance testing are performed clinically (**Fig. 8.18**):

- *Tympanometry,* which provides a graphic representation of the impedance changes caused by applied air pressure in the external ear canal.
- The *stapedial reflex,* which produces an acoustically evoked change of impedance.

## Tympanometry

Selectively raising or lowering the air pressure in the external auditory canal causes a stiffening of the middle ear, thereby increasing the acoustic impedance in the ear canal. As a result of this, more sound is reflected from the tympanic membrane. Normally, the air pressures in the ear canal and middle ear are equal and correspond to the atmospheric pressure. In this condition, the tympanic membrane has the lowest impedance (resistance) and therefore absorbs sound best. The greater the positive or negative pressure in the ear canal, the greater the "acoustic stiffness" of the tympanic membrane, and the lower its sound absorption or compliance. The tympanogram is a

**Fig. 8.18   Immittance measurements**

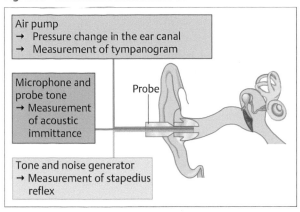

The external auditory canal is hermetically sealed with a probe that has various access ports. The acoustic impedance is measured with a probe tone (usually 220 Hz). An air pump generates a positive or negative pressure in the ear canal (tympanogram), and additional tones or noise evoke a stapedius reflex. The reflected portion of the probe tone is fed to a measuring instrument by an integrated microphone and plotted as a tympanogram.

graphic representation of compliance changes as the applied air pressure is varied over a negative-to-positive range. This requires that the intra-aural probe be hermetically sealed in the ear canal. The pressures are usually varied over a range of ±300 mm $H_2O$ or daPa. Pathologic changes in the tympanic membrane and middle ear lead to a change in compliance, which correlates clinically with various tympanogram shapes (**Fig. 8.19a–c**). With partial atrophy of the tympanic membrane or an ossicular discontinuity, the tympanogram may also exhibit multiple peaks.

## Stapedial Reflex (SR)

*Physiology (Fig. 8.20):* The stapedius muscle inserts on the stapes, and its contraction has the effect of stiffening the sound conduction apparatus. This changes the impedance of the middle ear and tympanic membrane, and the impedance change can be measured with a tone emitted by a probe placed in the ear canal. The stapedius muscle contracts as a reflex in response to additional acoustic stimuli of a certain intensity. With normal hearing, a stimulus of about 80 to 90 dB HL is sufficient to evoke the stapedial reflex. Broadband stimuli evoke the reflex at sound levels that are about 10 to 20 dB lower.

*Definitions:* When sound is delivered to only one ear, the stapedius muscles on both sides contract via the acousticofacial reflex arc. The stapedial reflex on the acoustically stimulated side is called the uncrossed or *ipsilateral stapedial reflex*. The reflex recorded on the opposite side is called the crossed or *contralateral*

**Fig. 8.19   Normal and abnormal tympanogram patterns**

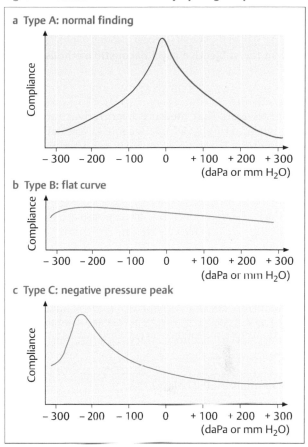

**a** The normal tympanogram has a prominent, sharp peak between +100 and –100 daPa.
**b** The type B tympanogram is flat or has a very low, rounded peak. This indicates immobility of the tympanic membrane, which may be due to fluid in the middle ear or tympanic atelectasis.
**c** The type C tympanogram has a peak in the negative pressure region below –100 daPa, consistent with impaired middle ear ventilation.

*stapedial reflex.* The *stapedial reflex threshold* is the minimum sound pressure level needed to produce a measurable change in tympanic membrane impedance.

⚑  A type A or C tympanogram must be present to test the stapedial reflex.

*Technique:*
• For **ipsilateral testing**, the "probe ear" is stimulated with tone pulses at 500 to 4,000 Hz or with broadband stimuli at incremental sound pressure levels that are 70 to 90 dB above the normal hearing threshold. The first impedance change recorded in response to the probe tone is equal to the *stapedial reflex threshold*.

**Fig. 8.20 Stapedial reflex**

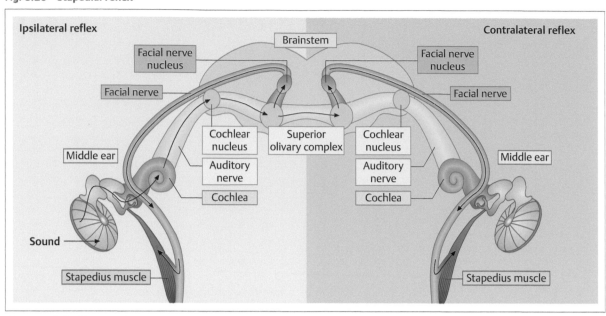

The stapedial reflex is evoked by peripheral acoustic stimulation. The reflex arc extends from the cochlear nucleus to the superior olivary complex and the facial nerve nuclei in the brainstem.

- For **contralateral testing**, which follows the same principle, the "probe ear" or "response ear" is different from the "stimulus ear."

*Interpretation: Absence of the stapedial reflex* or an *increased threshold* for the reflex may be caused by a lesion at various sites in the reflex pathway:
- *Ossicular chain* pathology (disruption or stiffening, e.g., due to otosclerosis; see ✥11.4, Bone Diseases).
- Abnormal sound reception by the *cochlea* and/or auditory *nerve* in a patient with cochlear or retrocochlear impairment (e.g., vestibular schwannoma; see ✥15.3, Tumors of the Internal Auditory Canal and Cerebellopontine Angle).
- Lesion of the *brainstem* (e.g., multiple sclerosis, hemorrhage).
- Lesion of *the facial nerve* (e.g., idiopathic facial nerve palsy; see ✥14.2, Inflammatory Changes).
- Disease of the *stapedius muscle* (e.g., myasthenia gravis).

### Applications of Immittance Measurements

*Tympanometry* is used in diagnosing middle ear pathology. It is of minor value by itself, however, and should always be interpreted in conjunction with otoscopic examination of the tympanic membrane.
*Measurement of the stapedial reflex* is always performed after tympanometry. It is useful for the investigation of numerous hearing disorders. The stapedial reflex threshold should be determined on both sides for both the crossed and uncrossed reflexes. The various stapedial reflex patterns are useful in differentiating middle ear hearing loss from cochlear and retrocochlear hearing loss. Moreover, the difference between the subjective hearing threshold and the stapedial reflex threshold provides a measure for evaluating recruitment. This difference is 60 dB or more in normal-hearing subjects. In patients with cochlear hearing loss and abnormal recruitment, it may be possible to evoke the stapedial reflex at only 10 dB above the auditory threshold ("objective" or *Metz recruitment*).

### Auditory Evoked Potentials (AEPs)

*Principle:* The physiologic process of hearing involves a great many bioelectric potential changes that take place in the cochlea, auditory nerve, and central nervous system. These potential changes can be utilized in the objective testing of auditory function.

*Technique:* AEPs are recorded from the scalp using needle or surface electrodes. As in an electroencephalogram (EEG), the potentials from many cells are recorded simultaneously by this technique. The potential changes caused by the auditory system are not detectable in an ordinary EEG trace because their amplitude is too small relative to the total activity of the central nervous system.
**Averaging** makes it possible to record very small potential changes that are buried in noise. It involves the iterative summation of a short EEG segment in a computer, making certain that a constant temporal relationship is maintained between the EEG segment

to be analyzed and a constant, repetitive acoustic stimulus. The intermittent stimulus evokes specific, uniform potentials during this time interval, which always occur at the same time and can be amplified by the repetitive summing of the EEG segment. This summation also tends to reduce unwanted, randomly timed background potentials that do not correlate with the auditory stimulus (stimulus-independent EEG activity). Since positive and negative background potentials are added together, they cancel out after a sufficiently large number of summations. When the summed entries are averaged, the displayed potentials can be assigned temporally to the acoustic stimulus as AEPs.

## Classification and Terminology of Auditory Evoked Potentials

The properties and shapes of AEPs depend partly on the time at which they occur after presentation of the acoustic stimulus, or their *latency* (in milliseconds). AEPs with a short latency occur very shortly after the stimulus and originate from structures that respond very quickly to the stimulus. Several types of electric response measurements are distinguished based on the different sites of origin and latencies of the AEPs:

- **Electrocochleography (ECochG)**: measures the potentials arising in the cochlea and auditory nerve. These potentials occur approximately 1 to 3 ms after the stimulus is presented.
- **Auditory brainstem response (ABR) audiometry** (also known as brainstem electric response audiometry): measures the potentials arising in the auditory nerve and brainstem structures, with a latency of up to approximately 10 ms.
- **Auditory middle latency response (AMLR) audiometry**: measures potentials with a latency of 10 to 100 ms that originate in the thalamus and primary auditory cortex.
- **Cortical evoked potentials (CEP)** (also known as cortical electric response audiometry): measures potentials with a latency of 100 to 1,000 ms.
- **Auditory steady state response (ASSR)**: evokes potentials not with short, transitory stimuli, but with a steady amplitude- or frequency-modulated stimulus, allowing concentration of the frequency of the stimulus to a narrow region. Various arrangements are used to measure potentials in the frequency domain, which can be generated at different levels of the auditory system.

The term *electric response audiometry* (ERA) is often used in audiology as a synonym for AEP.

## Auditory Brainstem Response (ABR)

The AEPs that are most commonly recorded for diagnostic purposes are the brainstem potentials, usually referred to as the auditory brainstem response. The ABR occurs during about the first 10 ms after an acoustic stimulus is presented. It is usually evoked by a click stimulus that lasts only a few milliseconds and has a broad frequency spectrum. To record the ABR, the stimulus must be repeated from 1,000 to 2,000 times and the EEG responses are averaged. Adhesive surface electrodes placed on the vertex and over the mastoid can record a typical waveform that is virtually unchanged even during sleep and under general anesthesia (important in small children). It is characterized by the presence of five or six waves numbered from I to VI as described by *Jewett*. With a normal brainstem response, the individual waves can be roughly assigned to specific anatomic structures (**Fig. 8.21**). This cannot be done with an abnormal ABR.

*Indications:* The main clinical applications of the ABR are in differentiating between *cochlear* and

> 🔧 **8.3 Applications of other auditory evoked potentials**
>
> **Electrocochleography** (ECochG) measures nerve potentials as well as receptor potentials and shifts in the endocochlear potential (cochlear microphonics [CM], summation potential [SP]). Electrocochleography requires that an electrode be placed as close to the cochlea as possible. Needle electrodes may be passed through the tympanic membrane to the promontory, or specially designed electrodes can be inserted into the ear canal. Auditory nerve potentials as well as cochlear potentials can be recorded with this technique. Electrocochleography is used in the diagnosis of Ménière's disease (see 🔖13.4, Ménière's Disease) and in the diagnostic evaluation of patients for cochlear implants (see 🔖9.3, Cochlear Implants).
>
> **Auditory steady state responses (ASSR)** are used mainly in pediatric audiology to make frequency-specific threshold measurements. Thresholds at several frequencies can be measured at the same time, also at low frequencies. ASSR are helpful for fitting hearing aids in children.
>
> **Auditory middle latency response (AMLR) audiometry** can be used to determine the hearing threshold in the low-frequency range. Natural sleep and general anesthesia affect these potentials, making them more difficult to interpret.
>
> **Cortical evoked potentials (CEP)** can, in principle, be elicited by any repetitive acoustic stimulus. The physical properties of the stimulus, as in auditory brainstem response (ABR) and AMLR, lead to stimulus-correlated responses that can be used for the objective, stimulus-specific determination of auditory threshold. The information content of a stimulus can also evoke typical *event-correlated potentials* (ECPs), which are useful in the evaluation of cognitive processes.

**Fig. 8.21 Auditory brainstem response**

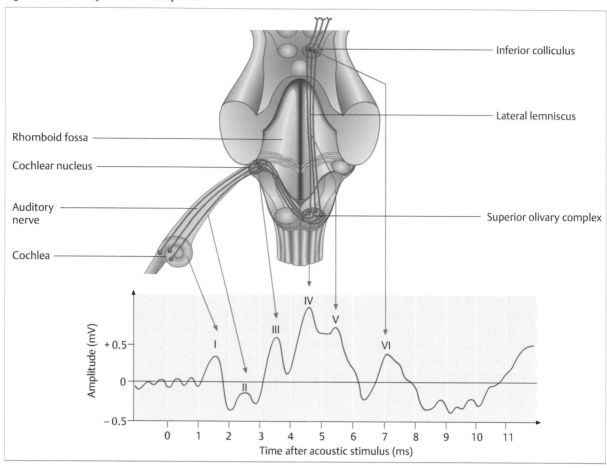

The curve shows the typical ABR waveform, which consists of five or six waves (numbered I through VI). The potentials reflect the acoustically induced activity of the auditory nerve and auditory neurons. The waves are produced by dipole generators in the various anatomic structures.

*retrocochlear hearing loss* and in the objective measurement of the *hearing threshold*.

- The ABR is important for threshold testing in pediatric audiology (see ✎9.2, Diagnostic Methods in Pediatric Audiology). Because potential thresholds are of interest in determining hearing thresholds in small children, it is important to have quiet examination conditions. While the ABR can usually be measured in adults without difficulty, infants and small children must be tested while sleeping or sedated and occasionally under general anesthesia.
- Both the shape of the curve (absence of waves, indistinct waves, etc.) and the latent period between waves I and V (normal interpeak latency is ~4.3 ms or less) are important in the diagnosis of retrocochlear hearing loss. A prolonged interpeak latency is a sign of retrocochlear hearing loss and should prompt further investigations (see ✎12.1, Retrocochlear Disorders).
- The ABR can also be important in the diagnosis of neurologic diseases (multiple sclerosis, ischemic brainstem lesions, etc.).

- Auditory evoked brainstem potentials are also tested intraoperatively to monitor hearing.

The ABR mainly tests hearing at middle and high frequencies (> 1 kHz). It is more difficult to obtain information on low-frequency hearing.

**Interpretation:** The most important parameters of the ABR are the time intervals between the waves and the threshold for the detection of wave V. Normally, wave V can be detected at only about 10 dB above the hearing threshold.

## Otoacoustic Emissions (OAEs)

The vibrations produced by the biomechanical amplifier of the cochlea (see ✎7.2, Micromechanical Function: Cochlear Amplifier), either spontaneously or in response to an acoustic stimulus, are transmitted in retrograde fashion across the ossicles to the tympanic membrane, which acts like the membrane of a loudspeaker, emitting the vibrations as sound waves into the external ear canal. A sensitive microphone probe inserted into the ear canal can detect these active cochlear vibrations, which are called otoacoustic emissions (OAEs).

OAEs are clinically important in that they can be used to test the function of the "cochlear amplifier." The emissions reflect the functional integrity of the cochlea. The outer hair cells are a particularly important source of OAEs; the auditory nerve is not involved. The detection of OAEs in the ear canal is contingent upon normal middle ear function, for otherwise the cochlear vibrations would not be transmitted to the tympanic membrane.

*Classification:* Owing to the high sensitivity of the cochlear amplifier, vibrations can arise spontaneously in the cochlea without an external stimulus (**spontaneous OAEs**). At the same time, an acoustic stimulus of low to moderate intensity will consistently induce cochlear vibrations and emissions (**evoked OAEs**). OAEs are classified into several types based on the nature of the stimulus:

- **Spontaneous otoacoustic emissions, or SOAEs:** These emissions occur without an external acoustic stimulus in approximately 50% of normal-hearing subjects and are detectable as low-level, continuous tones. They have little clinical importance.
- **Transient evoked otoacoustic emissions, or TEOAEs:** These emissions are consistently detected in response to a brief stimulus (click) in subjects with normal cochlear function. They are detected using an averaging technique similar to that described for AEPs (see above). The measurement of TEOAEs is a commonly used objective audiometric test method.
- **Distortion product otoacoustic emissions, or DPOAEs:** Acoustic distortions in the cochlear amplifier can be detected by stimulation with two continuous tones that have different but adjacent frequencies. The measurement of DPOAEs is another frequently used objective audiometric study.
- **Stimulus frequency otoacoustic emissions, or SFOAEs:** Stimulation with a sine-wave tone evokes tonal emissions of the same frequency. These emissions are more difficult to detect than TEOAEs and DPOAEs. They have little clinical significance.

## Transient Evoked Otoacoustic Emissions

TEOAEs are recorded in response to a brief stimulus (click) and reflect the spectrum of the stimulus. A microphone probe inserted into the external ear canal records the acoustic signals, which are averaged in a similar way as the bioelectric signals in AEPs (see above).

*Interpretation:* The click consistently evokes a cochlear acoustic response (TEOAE) in subjects with *normal hearing* (**Fig. 8.22**). Almost always, this confirms the functional integrity of the cochlea and middle ear. TEOAEs do not occur in patients with *middle ear disease* or a *cochlear hearing loss* with an approximately 30 dB threshold increase.

TEOAEs recorded in *normal-hearing infants* usually have a greater amplitude than those recorded in adults.

## Distortion Product Otoacoustic Emissions

DPOAEs are also used in clinical testing. The test involves measuring the OAEs that are evoked by stimulation with two continuous tones (**Fig. 8.23**). When the two stimulus frequencies are properly selected, distortion products occur as interference tones that bear a fixed relationship to the stimulus frequencies but are not identical to them.

The use of continuous tones allows for measurements within a narrower frequency range and at higher sound levels than are possible with TEOAEs. As a result, it may still be possible to detect DPOAEs even when the function of the cochlear amplifier is impaired. Automated measuring systems can be used to quickly measure the response of the cochlear amplifier in discrete frequency ranges. On the other hand, it is easier to eliminate artifacts when TEOAEs are measured. The clinical indications for DPOAEs are the same as for TEOAEs.

## Application of Otoacoustic Emissions

The most important application of OAEs is for *screening cochlear function in newborns, infants, and small children* (see ☜9.2, Screening). TEOAEs and DPOAEs provide a fast and simple way to test cochlear function without sedation or general anesthesia, thus facilitating the early detection of hearing problems.

The majority of hearing disorders in this age group have a cochlear etiology. The location of the hearing loss (middle ear or sensorineural) and its degree cannot be determined by analyzing OAEs.

▯ In the absence of OAEs, additional audiologic tests such as AEPs and behavioral audiometry must be used.

OAEs can also be used to investigate *nonorganic hearing loss*, to *objectify audiometric findings* in adults, and to *assess cochlear function* in risk groups (e.g., patients using ototoxic medications).

**Fig. 8.22    Transient evoked otoacoustic emissions (TEOAEs)**

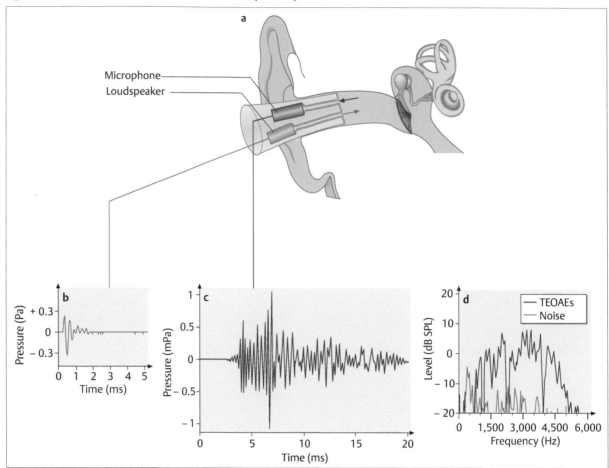

**a** Setup for measuring TEOAEs: measuring probe with microphone and loudspeaker.
**b** Waveform of the stimulus, which lasts about 2 ms. Note that the scale of the stimulus sound pressure (Pa) is 1,000 times greater than the scale for the sound pressure responses recorded in the ear canal (see **c**).

**c** The waveform recorded 2.5 ms after initiation of the stimulus reflects the time course and amplitude of the sound pressure of the TEOAEs.
**d** Spectrum of the evoked response (from **c**), indicating the frequency distribution of the TEOAEs (purple). The orange trace represents the spectrum of noise.

**Fig. 8.23 Distortion product otoacoustic emissions (DPOAEs)**

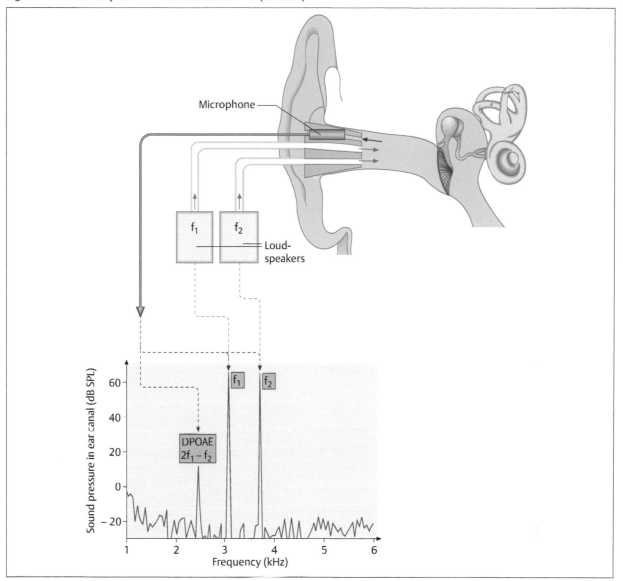

The cochlea is stimulated with two tones, $f_1$ and $f_2$, delivered by a probe. A microphone records the sound pressure in the external ear canal, detecting both the emitted sound pressure of the response and the sound pressure of both primary tones $f_1$ and $f_2$. The curve represents the frequency spectrum of the microphone signal. Besides the stimulus tones $f_1$ and $f_2$, an additional tone with a frequency of $2f_1 - f_2$ is recorded. This tone originates in the cochlea as a DPOAE.

# 8.5 Rehabilitation and Hearing Aids

The general goal of auditory rehabilitation is to restore or improve auditory communication. Specific rehabilitative measures are tailored to the degree of hearing loss, the needs of the patient, and other individual or social requirements. Hearing aids are frequently prescribed for moderate to severe hearing loss, while cochlear implants (inner ear implants) may be used in patients with profound hearing loss or deafness. Ancillary measures such as auditory training and learning to lip read are just as important as the accurate fitting of a hearing aid.

The indications and basic principles of hearing aid care in children are reviewed in 9.3.

## Indications and Possibilities of Auditory Rehabilitation

Hearing loss that is measurable by audiometry is always an "impairment"—that is, it always compromises the physical integrity of the patient. Whether hearing loss is disabling in everyday life depends on factors that include the degree of the hearing loss as well as individual auditory requirements and demands. Thus, measures to improve auditory performance should not be based entirely on audiometric hearing loss but should also take into account the individual auditory disability and the resulting impairment.

Medical treatment is an option for hearing loss only in rare cases.

If the patient with hearing loss does not experience subjective hearing impairment and is not disabled by the loss, rehabilitative measures will generally be unrewarding due to a lack of motivation.

> On the other hand, rehabilitative measures should not be long delayed in patients who are subjectively disabled by their hearing loss, because rehabilitation at an earlier age is more successful and can prevent additional disability relating to auditory deprivation.

A variety of rehabilitative options are available, depending on the nature and degree of the hearing loss and the degree of disability that it imposes.

**Surgery:** A surgical operation to improve hearing can provide functional restoration of hearing in patients with *conductive hearing loss* (e.g., stapes surgery in otosclerosis; see 11.4, Otosclerosis).

**Hearing aids:** A hearing aid selectively amplifies and modifies auditory signals (**Fig. 8.24**). The hearing aid may be worn behind the ear (BTE aid) or inside the ear canal (in-the-canal or ITC; completely-in-the-canal or CIC). Several possibilities exist to connect a BTE to the ear canal. A tube can be connected to a custom-made ear mold (**Fig. 8.24a**). Such an arrangement can amplify sound highly effectively, but the ear canal is typically occluded by the ear mold creating a hollow sound (closed-fit). Alternatively, an acoustic tube being hold in the ear canal by a soft tip delivers the amplified sound (**Fig. 8.24b**), or the BTE has a thin cable connected to a small speaker resting in the ear canal without occluding it (**Fig. 8.24c**). These fittings are called *open-fit*; they rely on strict electronic control of acoustic feedback by the hearing aid and allow less amplification than closed-fits.

ITC or CIC are usually individually fitted with a custom-made shell.

**Active middle ear implants:** An amplifier is implanted which transforms sound waves into mechanical vibrations. The vibrations are transmitted directly to the cranial bone, ossicular chain, or round window ("inverse cochlear stimulation").

**Cochlear implant:** In patients with a complete or almost complete absence of cochlear function, this surgically implanted device can transform sound waves into electric impulses that directly stimulate the auditory nerve with intracochlear electrodes.

**Vibrotactile aids:** Acoustic signals are picked up by a microphone and converted to vibrations that are transmitted to the wrist or fingers.

**Other assistive devices:** A variety of assistive devices can improve communication for hearing-impaired patients. These devices include optical or vibrating wake-up alarms, light flashers, telephone amplifiers, text telephones, television headphones, and digital communication devices such as smartphones, faxes, text messaging, and the internet.

**Training:** Hearing-impaired patients can be trained in:

- Selective hearing (hearing tactics, auditory training).
- The proper use of hearing aids and other assistive devices.
- Learning to lip read.
- Improving their speech.

> The goal of rehabilitation is to achieve a maximum restoration of aural communication, which is crucial for social functioning and patient well-being.

## Hearing Aid Fitting in Adults

The hearing aid is a special type of acoustic amplifier. Sound from the environment is received by one or

Fig. 8.24  **Hearing aids**

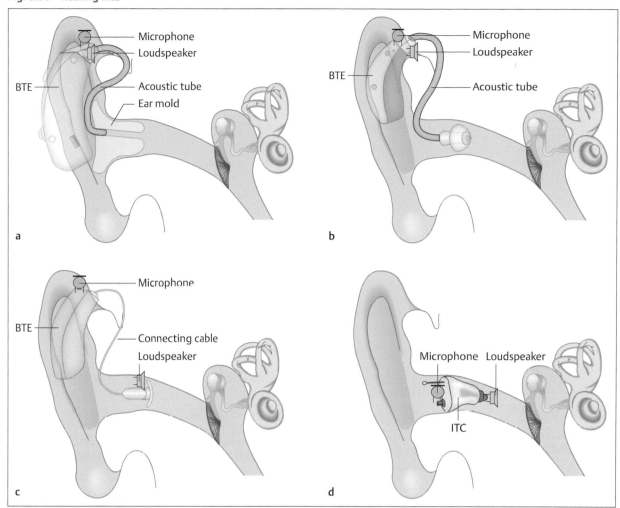

Schematic diagram of different hearing aid types:
**a** Behind the ear (BTE aid) with individually shaped ear mold.
**b** BTE with soft tip.
**c** BTE with speaker resting in the ear canal.
**d** In-the-canal (ITC) hearing aid.

The position of the microphones (⬜) and loudspeakers (🔊) are indicated by symbols. The hearing aid amplifies soft sounds more than loud ones, limits maximum loudness level (compression), and suppresses noise and feedback.

several *microphones*, *amplified*, and transmitted by a *loudspeaker* to the ear (**Fig. 8.24**). For a hearing aid to work properly, the cochlea must be able to receive the amplified and processed signal and relay it to the auditory nerve. Microchip and digital technology allows for differentiated processing of the acoustic signal and makes it possible to tailor the hearing aid to the patient's individual hearing loss and requirements.

The fitting of a hearing aid, which is an important means of aural rehabilitation for many patients with hearing impairment, involves a series of steps:

**Determining candidacy:** Before the patient is fitted with a hearing aid, candidacy must be determined on the basis of an accurate history and audiologic evaluation. Contraindications such as cholesteatoma or vestibular

schwannoma should be ruled out, and there should be no reasonable prospect of improving the patient's hearing by surgery. Moreover, the patient must be willing and able to use and maintain the hearing aid.

**Audiologic examination:** The *audiologic examination* should include pure-tone audiometry, speech audiometry, and a determination of the dynamic range—for example, by dynamic range scaling (see 🔗 **8.2**).

**Hearing aid trial:** Based on the clinical and audiologic findings and the desires of the patient, a hearing aid is selected on a trial basis. Fitting of the hearing aid is usually done by a trained specialist (audiologist or hearing aid specialist). Prefitted hearing aids sold over the counter or consumer-adjustable hearing aids are also available for slight or moderate hearing loss.

Patients with a largely symmetrical hearing loss should be fitted with binaural aids, as these will provide a significant gain (binaural summation), allow directional hearing, and improve speech recognition in background noise. Binaural fitting will also help to prevent auditory deprivation of the unaided ear.

*Final hearing aid selection:* The hearing aid specialist should offer the patient several devices to choose from. The final selection and fine-tuning of the amplifier can be done only in practical trials. *Speech audiometric testing* with and without background noise, the *subjective auditory impression* of the patient, and acoustic measurements in the ear canal (*in situ measurements*) support the final selection. After the fitting, the patient must become accustomed to the device and the auditory sensation it produces to derive optimum benefit.

*Follow-up care:* The follow-up regimen includes the points listed earlier under Training in addition to an audiologic evaluation.

🖉 Despite the sophisticated technology, a hearing aid is still a peripheral listening aid that cannot replace or substantially improve the fine frequency resolution of the cochlea or essential central auditory functions.

These limitations can be particularly noticeable in a noisy and unsteady environment. As a result, hearing aids often provide less satisfactory gain in speech recognition when *background noise* is present.

Additional technical measures can dampen background noise in hearing situations where a microphone is being used (telephone, lecture halls). For example, the microphone signal can be directly transmitted as an electromagnetic signal using an induction coil, bypassing the microphone component of the hearing aid. Induction coils of this kind are built into many lecture halls and churches. Another option is direct radio-signal transmission from the microphone to the hearing aid (audio input, FM transmitters, Bluetooth).

## Cochlear Implants in Adults

Even the best hearing aids reach their limits as the degree of hearing loss becomes more severe. When the cochlea contains few or no hair cells able to transform a vibration into bioelectric signals, even the strongest and most discriminating acoustic amplification will be unable to improve aural communication. The cochlear implant (CI) is an option for these cases.

*Principle:* The functional principle of the CI is shown in **Fig. 8.25.** An electronic receiver is implanted into the temporal bone under the skin. The receiver is connected to an electrode array inserted into the cochlea. The electrodes directly stimulate the auditory nerve and spiral ganglion, functionally bypassing the cochlear hair cells. The acoustic signal that is received by microphones worn behind the ear (**Fig. 8.25** ①) is processed by an external speech processor, which is usually worn behind the ear like a hearing aid (②). This processor extracts the useful sound components that are important for speech recognition, transmits the signal through the skin to the implanted receiver, and stimulates the various intracochlear electrodes (③). After stimulating the auditory nerve (④), the signal undergoes further central processing like any acoustic signal.

Marked individual differences occur in the position of the intracochlear electrodes and in the number of residual nerve fibers and ganglion cells that are still present. This makes it necessary to adjust the electric stimulation, and thus the processing of the speech signals by the speech processor, individually for each patient.

*Indication:* The criteria for prescribing a CI are as follows:
- *Acquired*, bilateral, predominantly cochlear deafness (postlingual deafness) with a functional auditory nerve and intact central auditory pathway. Complete loss of hearing in one ear (single-sided deafness) may also be an indication for a CI.
- *Congenital* or *early acquired* deafness in children (prelingual deafness); see 🖘9.3, Cochlear Implants.
- Lack of benefit from binaural hearing aid fitting despite optimum adjustment of the hearing aids.
- A motivated patient willing to learn the operation and maintenance of the implant.

The CI requires a partially functional auditory nerve that is responsive to stimulation by the intracochlear electrodes. The implantation surgery is a safe, standardized procedure that has relatively few side effects. Later complications, including possible malfunction, are also rare.

*Follow-up care:* Adjustment of the speech processor begins several weeks after the operation and generally lasts for several months. The follow-up program includes:
- A technical check of CI function.
- Checking and adjusting the speech processor.
- Auditory training.

**Fig. 8.25 Cochlear implant (CI)**

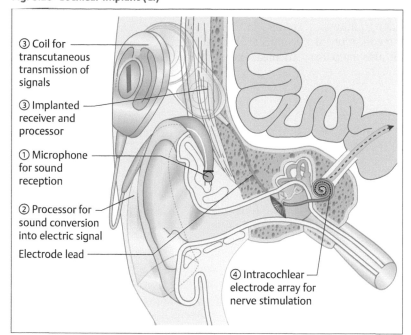

③ Coil for transcutaneous transmission of signals

③ Implanted receiver and processor

① Microphone for sound reception

② Processor for sound conversion into electric signal

Electrode lead

④ Intracochlear electrode array for nerve stimulation

The sound is received by one or several microphones worn on the ear and fed to the speech processor ①. The external speech processor converts the microphone signals into a series of electric impulses ②. An external coil with magnetic fixation transmits the impulses as radio frequencies through the skin to the implanted portion of the CI (receiving coil) ③. The necessary power supply is also transmitted; the implant itself does not require a separate power source. An electrode lead goes to an intracochlear electrode array ④, which directly stimulates the neural elements of the cochlea.

Under the guidance of speech therapists and/or hearing-impaired teachers, the patients learn to interpret the electric impulses as speech. Speech recognition may be further supported by teaching the patients to lip read.

Over 90% of patients derive definite benefit from a CI, and more than 50% can achieve *open speech compre-* hension—that is, they can understand CI-mediated speech without relying on visual cues (e.g., over the telephone or a public address system).

The success of a CI is partly influenced by the time of onset and duration of the deafness. In adults, patients with deafness of short duration derive the greatest benefit from the implant.

# 9    Hearing Disorders in Children—Pediatric Audiology

## 9.1    Causes and Effects of Pediatric Hearing Disorders

Hearing disorders in infants and small children can be difficult to recognize and may go undetected without universal screening of newborns. While hearing disorders in children can have the same causes as in adults, special perinatal causes are also encountered in infants and newborns. The frequency distribution of the causes is also different. The development of speech is closely related to hearing ability, and hearing disorders during this formative period can have specific consequences in terms of language and personality development.

*Epidemiology:* Significant hearing impairment is present at birth in approximately 1 in 500 newborns. Most of these cases involve sensorineural hearing loss due to cochlear impairment.

During the **first years of life**, the number of permanent hearing-impaired children rises by 50 to 90% and roughly 3 in 1,000 children have permanent one- or both-sided, usually sensorineural hearing loss when entering school. Hearing disorders are much more prevalent in **small children and preschoolers**, but hearing impairment in this age group is usually a temporary conductive loss secondary to otitis media, occurring in approximately 3 to 4% of children.

*Classification:* Besides the description of hearing loss by type (sensorineural, conductive, mixed, central) and degree (see **Table 8.2**), the classification of hearing impairment in relation to its onset is of great importance in pediatric audiology, particularly the relation to language and speech acquisition:
- **Prelingual hearing loss** is present before the development of normal speech. It may be **congenital** (present at birth), **perinatal** (acquired during birth), or **postnatal** (acquired in the period between birth and the first 2–3 years). Such a hearing loss will affect the normal development of language and speech.
- **Postlingual hearing loss** develops after the acquisition of normal speech or after 2 to 3 years of age.

### Causes of Pediatric Hearing Disorders

The causes of early childhood hearing loss approximate a "quarter rule." Roughly 50% are caused genetically, 25% have other known causes such as infections, and the cause is unknown in another 25%. Causes fall into several categories:
- Hereditary genetic causes:
  – Congenital.
  – Occurring postnatally or later.
- Acquired causes:
  – Acquired in utero (also congenital).
  – Acquired perinatally.
  – Acquired postnatally or later.

### Monosymptomatic, Nonsyndromic Genetic Hearing Loss

The majority of hearing disorders that are due to a genetic cause affect only hearing and are described as monosymptomatic. Except for the hearing impairment, the child is normal. About 75% of these hearing disorders are inherited as an autosomal-recessive trait, and so the family history is usually negative.

▷ The hearing impairment is not obvious in these cases and, without screening, is often detected later due to abnormal speech development.

Around 50% of the autosomal-recessive hearing losses are due to mutations of the GJB2 gene, encoding the gap junction protein connexin 26 in the organ of Corti. Two to three percent of the European population carries such heterozygous mutations. Other forms of monosymptomatic genetic hearing loss are covered in ✎ 12.2, Hereditary Sensorineural Hearing Loss, because they are not confined to the pediatric age group.

### Hearing Loss in Genetic Syndromes

Around one-quarter of genetic hearing disorders are associated with other symptoms or disorders, often including malformation of the ear. Thus, the hearing loss is one feature of a congenital syndrome. **Table 9.1** reviews several of the more than 400 known syndromes that are associated with hearing loss. They are classified according to the affected organs or tissues.

▷ The presence of hearing loss profoundly affects the further development and rehabilitation of children with these syndromes.

Aside from cases with an anomaly of the auricle or ear canal, direct signs calling attention to a hearing disorder may be missing when these children are infants. Consequently, children with syndromes must be specifically tested for hearing impairment as soon after birth as possible.

| Classification by anomalies | Syndrome | Inheritance | Typical features | Type of hearing loss | | |
|---|---|---|---|---|---|---|
| | | | | Conductive | Sensorineural | Mixed |
| Malformations of the external ear | **Mandibulofacial dysostosis** (Treacher–Collins syndrome) | Autosomal-dominant | Anomalies of the external and middle ear | X | | |
| | **BOR syndrome** (brachio-otorenal syndrome) | Autosomal-dominant | Anomalies of the external ear | X or | X or | X |
| | **CHARGE syndrome:** **c**oloboma, **h**eart defect, **a**tresia of choanae, **r**etarded growth, **g**enital hypoplasia, **e**ar anomalies | Sporadic | Anomalies of the external ear | | X | |
| Retinal degeneration and ocular anomalies | **Usher's syndrome:** sensorineural hearing loss and progressive retinitis pigmentosa | Autosomal-recessive | Type I–III, retinal degeneration, with or without vestibular dysfunction | | X (stable or progressive) | |
| Musculoskeletal disorders | Craniosynostosis: <br>• **Apert's syndrome** <br>• **Crouzon's syndrome** | Autosomal-dominant | | X <br> X | | |
| | **Osteogenesis imperfecta** (various forms) | Autosomal-dominant | | | | X |
| Renal function impairment | **Alport's syndrome** | Variable | Chronic nephritis | | X (progressive) | |
| Nervous system disorders (with ataxia) | For example, Cockayne's syndrome, Lichtenstein–Knorr syndrome, Klippel–Durante syndrome | Variable | | | X | |
| Endocrine and metabolic dysfunctions | **Pendred's syndrome** (thyroid dysfunction) | Autosomal-recessive | Association with Mondini's dysplasia or dilated vestibular aqueduct, possibly goiter | | X (severe, can be progressive) | |
| Cutaneous and pigmentary anomalies | **Waardenburg's syndrome** | Autosomal-dominant | White forelock, heterochromia iridis, telecanthus | | X | |
| Cardiac anomalies | **Jervell–Lange–Nielsen syndrome** | Autosomal-recessive | Prolonged QT interval | | X (severe) | |
| Chromosome abnormalities | **Ullrich–Turner syndrome** | Sporadic | | X (frequent) or | X or | X |
| | Trisomy 21 | Sporadic | | X or | X or | X |

## Acquired Hearing Loss

Besides genetic syndromes, congenital syndromes can be acquired in utero, such as:
• **Rubella syndrome** with cochlear hearing loss, pulmonary stenosis, intellectual disability, and microphthalmia.

• **Hyperbilirubinemia syndrome** with athetoid cerebral palsy and sensorineural hearing loss.
• **Congenital syphilis** with interstitial keratitis, Hutchinson's teeth, and sensorineural hearing loss.

Hearing loss may be acquired before birth (intrauterine, prenatally), during birth (perinatally), or after birth (postnatally). Infections from the so-called

TORCH organisms are the most frequent pre- or perinatal causes. "TORCH" stands for:

- **To**xoplasmosis,
- **R**ubella,
- **C**ytomegalic virus, and
- **H**erpes.

**Table 9.2** lists the most frequent causes of acquired hearing loss in newborns and infants.

## Hearing Impairment in Newborns

It is often difficult to distinguish between a congenital and perinatally acquired hearing loss. Because hearing loss unassociated with other disorders or malformations is not obvious in newborns, delayed speech development is the earliest sign of hearing impairment in many unscreened children. A delay in diagnosis makes it even more difficult to distinguish between congenital and perinatally acquired disorders.

Certain structures of the auditory system are particularly susceptible to harmful influences at certain times during the neonatal period. A typical example is kernicterus, in which high bilirubin levels in the blood cause damage to central structures. It is also believed that the cochlea in newborns is exceptionally vulnerable to hypoxia, toxic agents (antibiotics), and noise. The maturity of the newborn is an important factor in this regard, and premature infants are at particularly high risk. Overall, hearing impairment is present in approximately 4% of all newborns who require treatment in an intensive care unit.

## Hearing Impairment in Infants and Small Children

A hearing loss produces very few signs in infancy, regardless of its degree of severity. Even when parents notice that "something is wrong," they are often reassured that their child's development is merely delayed, and auditory tests are not performed. An opportunity is missed to refer the child for special services.

🖉 When the slightest evidence of hearing impairment is noted in an infant or small child, an audiologic evaluation should be performed. In many cases, this evidence comes from parents and is too often ignored. "The parents are always right" is a good rule to follow.

An acquired, temporary hearing loss due to otitis media is the most common type of hearing loss in small children and preschoolers. Both acute and chronic forms of middle ear effusion are common in this age group, and up to 75% of children have this condition for some period of time. The clinical features of otitis media are described in 🖉 11.2 and 🖉 11.3.

**Table 9.2 Causes of acquired hearing loss in newborns and infants**

| Timing of insult | Classification | Examples |
|---|---|---|
| Prenatal | Infectious | Rubella, toxoplasmosis, congenital syphilis |
| | Drug toxicity | Quinine, alcohol, thalidomide |
| Perinatal | Infectious | Cytomegalovirus, herpes simplex virus |
| | Metabolic | Kernicterus, asphyxia |
| | Obstetric trauma | Forceps, intracerebral and intracochlear hemorrhage |
| Postnatal | Infectious | Meningitis, labyrinthitis, otitis media, mumps, measles |
| | Drug toxicity | E.g., aminoglycoside antibiotics |
| | Traumatic | Noise (susceptible period?), head trauma |

Acute otitis media itself, the subsequent fluid collection in the middle ear, and chronic middle ear effusions lead to varying degrees of conductive hearing impairment. A chronic, bilateral middle ear effusion may be present for months or years without causing symptoms other than conductive hearing loss. In cases of this kind, or in children who have frequently recurring acute middle ear infections, a prolonged hearing impairment can cause delays in speech and language development with articulation problems, vocabulary deficits, and dysgrammatism (see 🖉 19.1 and 🖉 19.2).

## Effects of Hearing Loss in Children

### Bilateral Hearing Loss

🖉 A hearing loss in infants and small children threatens normal speech and personality development, underscoring the unique importance of hearing loss in this age group.

Hearing is crucial to the development of verbal communication. The central nervous system of the newborn and infant appears to include structures whose maturation is triggered by linguistic stimuli. It also appears that this maturation takes place only during certain critical periods. The longer the child is without auditory stimulation by speech, the more difficult it is to acquire the missed linguistic skills. The impaired speech development and altered acoustic environment have a direct influence on personality development and the relationship of the individual to society. The *severity of the disability depends on various factors. The most important, perhaps, is the degree of hearing loss* (**Table 9.3**). The effects also depend on the time of onset of the hearing disorder. When deafness occurs during the initial months after meningitis, for example, early rehabilitation can build upon previous acoustic experience. This advantage is not available in a congenitally deaf child who has never experienced speech reception through the auditory system. The earlier and more selectively auditory services are provided, the more effectively the natural developmental periods of the child can be utilized. This emphasizes the critical importance of an early diagnosis and therapy in hearing-impaired children.

## Unilateral Hearing Loss

A **mild to moderate** unilateral hearing loss in early childhood usually has little or no adverse sequelae. Often, the child is unaware that he or she has a hearing problem, and the condition is first detected by screening, audiometric testing when the child enters school, or even later.

With a **severe** unilateral hearing loss, however, it is possible that speech development may be hampered. Usually, the child experiences little disability from the disorder. Subtle deficits and impairments may arise and in some cases are reflected in poor academic performance and delayed speech development. Difficulties with unilateral hearing loss tend to arise in acoustic settings where there is a poor signal-to-noise ratio. Situations of this kind are common in classrooms and can lead to fragmentary perception of the academic material.

**Table 9.3 Effects of hearing loss in children**

| Degree of hearing loss | | Effects |
|---|---|---|
| Mild: 20–40 dB | Unvoiced consonants and sibilants are not heard clearly | Articulation problems, delay in language acquisition, dyslalia, possible difficulties in school |
| Moderate: 40–60 dB | The majority of speech sounds are not heard | Abnormal speech development with dysgrammatism, a deficient vocabulary, and poorly intelligible speech |
| Severe: 60–90 dB | | Absence of spontaneous speech development |

## 9.1 Malformations involving the ear

### Malformations of the middle ear

The embryology of the ear was reviewed in 7.1 (**Fig. 7.6**). Conspicuous malformations of the auricle and external ear canal are frequently associated with an anomaly of the middle ear. On the other hand, isolated auricular anomalies often develop without hearing impairment, and isolated changes in the ear canal often lead to conductive hearing loss. These anomalies are described in 10.1. The significance of external ear malformations in syndromic conditions is reviewed in **Table 9.1**. External malformations, unlike isolated middle ear anomalies, are easily diagnosed and should always prompt auditory testing.

**Atresia of the ear canal** necessarily causes changes in the tympanic membrane plane and malleus. The rest of the middle ear may be normally developed, but there are often concomitant anomalies of varying degree affecting other middle ear structures. Congenital aural atresia is therefore classified as a middle ear anomaly.

**Middle ear anomalies with a normal external ear** are not detectable by external inspection. They invariably cause hearing impairment, usually consisting of an isolated, significant conductive hearing loss. Middle ear malformations relevant to hearing involve the ossicular chain and particularly the stapes. Other middle ear structures such as the facial nerve, vessels, or intra-aural muscles may also show anomalies of varying significance.

Middle ear malformations are classified into various *grades of severity*. Usually, it is sufficient to distinguish between "major" and "minor" anomalies. A more precise analysis of the malformed structures can supply prognostic information that is useful in planning surgical treatment.

*Treatment:* Bilateral middle ear malformations should be treated as early as possible with special hearing aids that employ a bone-conduction vibrator. Corrective surgery is usually deferred until preschool or school age. With a unilateral anomaly, it must be determined immediately after birth whether normal hearing is present on the opposite side. If that is the case, there is no need for immediate surgery to improve hearing.

### Malformation of the inner ear

Inner ear malformations result from an arrest or abnormality of embryonic development between the third and ninth weeks of gestation (see 7.1). The division of the otocyst into two anatomically and functionally distinct parts (the utriculovestibular part and the sacculocochlear part) plays a key role in the pathogenesis of anomalies, since the division itself may be abnormal (forming a "common cavity"), or independent anomalies may develop in one or both parts after the otocyst has divided. Imaging with MRI and CT are used routinely in the evaluation of hearing loss in infants. They are helpful in recognizing and describing malformations of the inner ear, which are classified as follows (after Sennaroglu and Saatci):

- Complete labyrinthine aplasia (Michel's deformity, **Fig. 9.1a**): the formation of all cochlear and vestibular elements is missing.
- Cochlear aplasia: the formation of cochlear elements is missing.
- Common cavity (**Fig. 9.1b**): cochlea and vestibule form a cavity without separation; the formation is arrested at the fourth week.
- Cystic cochleovestibular malformation (incomplete partition type I, **Fig. 9.1c**): cochlea and vestibule form two cystic cavities without complete separation.
- Cochleovestibular hypoplasia: cochlea and vestibule are clearly separated, but either cochlea or vestibule or both are hypoplastic.
- Mondini's malformation (incomplete partition type II, **Fig. 9.1d**): the cochlea has only 1.5 turns and the interscalar septum is missing.

In addition, malformations of the vestibular elements, the vestibular aqueduct, and the internal auditory canal can occur together with cochlear malformations or in isolation.

**Fig. 9.1 Examples of cochlear malformations**

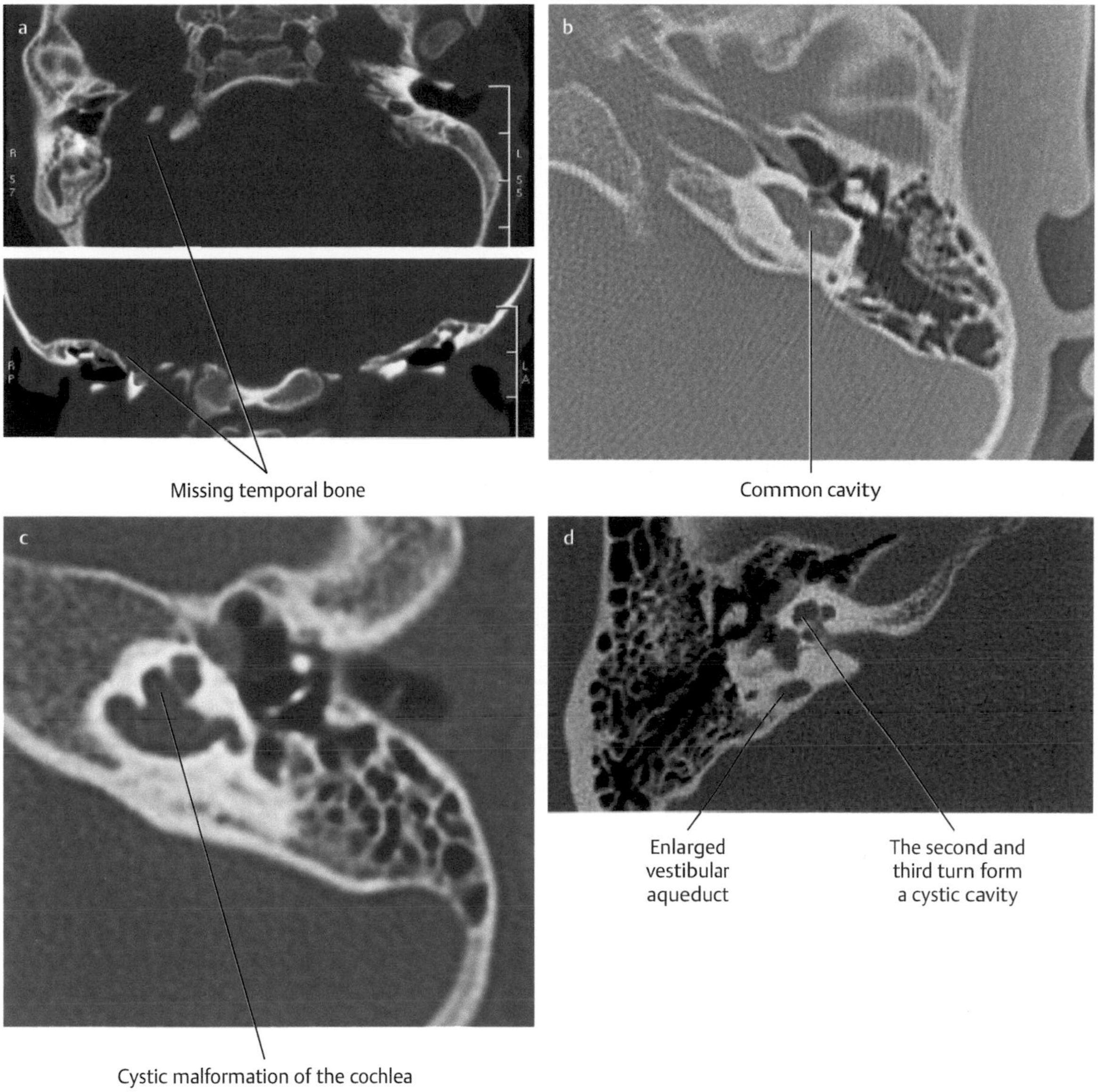

Missing temporal bone

Common cavity

Cystic malformation of the cochlea

Enlarged vestibular aqueduct

The second and third turn form a cystic cavity

**a** Aplasia of the temporal bone resulting in Michel's deformity.
**b** Common cavity: vestibule and cochlea are not separated.

**c** Incomplete partition type I or cystic cochlear malformation.
**d** Enlarged vestibular aqueduct and Mondini's malformation with cystic formation of the cochlear apex.

# 9.2 Detection and Investigation of Pediatric Hearing Disorders

Hearing disorders in newborns, infants, and small children are detected with audiometric methods that are adapted to the special difficulties inherent in detecting and quantifying a pediatric hearing problem. Screening tests are best for detecting hearing impairment in newborns. Any suspicion of a pediatric hearing disorder warrants an immediate audiologic work-up that includes objective tests and behavioral audiometric methods that are appropriate for the age of the child.

## Screening

Because hearing impairment is not an obvious condition in newborns, it must be detected by screening. If the baby does not pass the screening, a hearing loss should be confirmed and an audiologic evaluation performed during subsequent weeks.

**Risk screening:** This is a selective program that screens only children with features that are known to be associated with an increased risk of hearing loss (see below and ♠9.1, Causes of Pediatric Hearing Disorders). Newborns meeting at least one of the following criteria have a substantially increased risk for hearing loss:

- Having been in an intensive care unit for more than 48 hours.
- Having a positive family history of hearing impairment.
- Manifesting craniofacial anomalies.

The overall prevalence of a permanent, moderate to severe hearing loss in these three groups is 4%. Consequently, the hearing of all newborns in these groups should be routinely tested (methods: see below). This risk-based screening will detect approximately half of all hearing problems in infants.

**Universal screening:** The universal screening of all newborns can detect up to 80% of all hearing problems and is therefore more effective than risk screening. The best time for screening is 2 to 3 days after birth (e.g., during the second routine examination), since most babies are easily available for hearing screening at that time, depending on the health care system. Screening may have to be organized differently in health care systems in which babies may be available only during the first 24 hours after birth.

Additional screening examinations are performed when the child is older—at routine pediatric visits, for example (distraction test, see below), or when the child enters school.

## Screening Procedure

**Newborn hearing screening** is based on objective audiometric test methods that are specially adapted for screening requirements. Useful tests are otoacoustic emissions (OAEs) and the auditory brainstem response (ABR; early auditory evoked potentials), described in ♠8.4. Two-stage screening is performed in most cases, i.e., if a response is not elicited, the test is repeated 1 to 2 days later or is supplemented by an additional test (e.g., transient evoked otoacoustic emission [TEOAEs], described in ♠8.4, followed by the ABR). Children who do not pass the screening should be referred for a differentiated audiologic evaluation (see below). Approximately 1 in 10 of these babies has a permanent hearing loss.

Screening in **older children** employs the above methods in addition to behavioral tests such as the distraction test or, in preschool and school-age children, pure-tone audiometry.

## Diagnostic Methods in Pediatric Audiology

### Objective Methods

The methods of objective audiometry can be used at any age, as long as passive cooperation of the child can be achieved (by sedation if necessary). Hearing loss can be detected, and a site-of-lesion determination can be made.

**Otoacoustic emissions:**
*Indication:* OAEs provide a rapid method for assessing the function of the cochlear amplifier (see ♠7.2, Nonlinear Function—Otoacoustic Emissions). OAEs cannot be used to determine the degree of hearing loss.
*Interpretation:* If OAEs are present, it may be assumed that peripheral hearing is satisfactory.

> ♪ The presence of OAEs does not exclude a hearing disorder. Rarely, a neural or central hearing disorder may be present.

**Auditory evoked potentials:**
*Indication:* Auditory evoked potentials (AEPs) are the most important objective method for the investigation of hearing loss in infants and children. The ABR (see ♠8.4, Auditory Evoked Potentials) is most commonly

**Fig. 9.2  Visual reinforcement audiometry (VRA)**

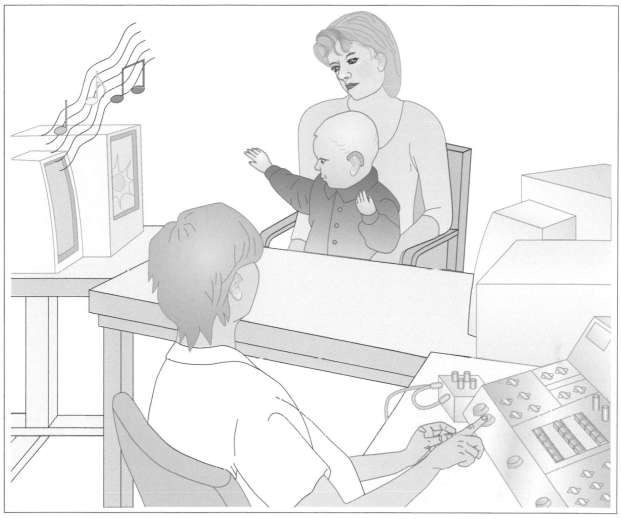

The test signal is presented by one of two loudspeakers. If the child looks to the correct side, it is rewarded with an attractive image such as a dancing teddy bear.

tested. It can be used to determine the hearing threshold, which is done more accurately at frequencies above 1 kHz than at lower frequencies.

*Interpretation:* If an ABR is not elicited, it should be concluded that severe hearing loss is present.

The latency of the ABR is significantly longer in newborns and infants than in adults. By 2 to 3 years of age, the latency values are approximately equal to those in adults. The maturation process of central auditory structures is reflected in this gradual shortening of ABR latencies.

**Immittance measurements**:

Immittance measurements play a minor role in newborns and infants because it cannot be done accurately using ordinary equipment. It is commonly used in small children, however, for the documentation and follow-up of middle ear effusions with associated conductive hearing loss (see 11.3, Otitis Media with Effusion).

## Behavioral Audiometric Methods

*Indication:* Behavioral methods are important for testing subjective auditory responses in pediatric audiology. They are also necessary in rehabilitative measures such as hearing-aid fitting.

*Prerequisites:* Behavioral audiometric tests can be performed at virtually any age. The methodology must be age-appropriate, however, and the reliability of the tests is variable.

The examiner must have experience and patience in conducting and interpreting the examination. It is necessary to gain the attention of the child, hold it for as long as possible by adapting the test situation, and correctly recognize and interpret the responses. The examiner must gather as much relevant information as possible within a short time.

**Reflex audiometry:** Nonspecific responses to auditory stimuli can be elicited in normal infants from birth on.

Sucking responses, motor responses such as the Moro reflex, or changes in respiratory pattern can be elicited. Generally, these reflexes require loud auditory stimuli of about 80 dB.

**Response audiometry:** By about 5 months of age, acoustic stimuli evoke typical response patterns in normal infants that can be used to test hearing. For example, the infant will turn its head toward a sound source that is outside the visual field. This response is initially present in the horizontal plane and later occurs in the vertical plane as well. This response is contingent upon normal maturation of directional hearing.

- *Distraction test:* This test is administered by two testers in a standardized, quiet environment using various standard acoustic stimuli.
- *Visual reinforcement audiometry (VRA;* **Fig. 9.2***):* This test again utilizes the head-turn response, aided by positive reinforcement, to obtain audiometric threshold measurements. An acoustic stimulus is combined with the activation of a moving toy, such as a dancing bear. After conditioning, the child will turn the head toward the toy when hearing the acoustic stimulus.

**Play audiometry:** This is a variant of pure-tone audiometry (see 8.3). By 1 to 2 years of age, it is possible to incorporate the tasks and responses of pure-tone audiometry into a play setting. For example, the child may stack one building block onto another as soon as a certain acoustic stimulus is withdrawn. The play situation, the tasks, and the presentation of the acoustic stimulus vary with the age of the child and the clinical problem.

*Indication:* These techniques are used for the detection of hearing impairment and for the fitting of hearing aids and cochlear implants.

**Pediatric speech audiometry:** The easiest way to test speech discrimination is by verbally instructing the child to select a certain toy or picture that is on a table along with several other toys or pictures. This technique can be used to screen for speech recognition problems by telling the child, at increasing distances, to point to objects displayed in pictures. This kind of test can be administered by 2 years of age.

By about 3 to 4 years of age, the examiner can use audiometric speech tests that have been specially designed for children—e.g., the Pediatric Speech Intelligibility (PSI) test.

By the time the child enters school, basically the same speech audiometric methods can be used as in adults, with minor modifications.

# 9.3    Treatment of Pediatric Hearing Disorders

The medical treatment of hearing disorders in children is basically the same as in adults. It is merely adapted to the special circumstances in the pediatric age group. *Hearing ability* is improved by means of hearing aids or cochlear implants whenever possible. To attain satisfactory *speech proficiency* in small children with permanent hearing loss, however, additional rehabilitative and training measures are necessary in the form of special education services, which should be instituted as early as possible.

*Indications:* There is a general consensus that children with a bilateral, moderate, permanent hearing loss should be treated to prevent significant impairment of speech and language development. More controversial are the treatment measures that are appropriate in children with a mild or unilateral hearing loss.

*Basic options:* Conductive hearing loss can often be improved by surgery. For example, malformed elements of the ossicular chain can be reconstructed, or middle ear ventilation can be surgically established in small children with recurrent effusions (see ✎ **11.2**, Reconstructive operations, and 📖 11.3, Otitis Media with Effusion). Medical treatment is rarely an option for hearing disorders.

In other cases, every effort should be made to utilize residual hearing as fully as possible while also providing appropriate services to stimulate and support the child's auditory development. **Hearing aids** should be prescribed for moderate to severe hearing loss, while **cochlear implants** are indicated for deafness or profound hearing loss that does not benefit enough from hearing aids. Other support services are also instituted with the goal of **promoting speech and language development**. These rehabilitative measures are different from communicative training in adults due to the absence or impairment of speech development in children.

## Auditory Devices

See also 📖 8.5.

### Hearing Aids

**Types of aid:** Children are generally fitted with two *behind-the-ear hearing aids*. This can be done in infants only a few months old. A special case is bilateral aural atresia, in which *bone conduction hearing aids* are fitted shortly after birth.

The **fitting** itself is considerably more difficult in children and requires a great deal of experience. Infants and small children are very limited in their ability to cooperate, and these patients lack auditory experience. Children with a hearing aid hear a spectrum of sounds that is unfamiliar to them. With greater degrees of hearing loss, this problem becomes more serious, and more time is needed to achieve a proper fitting. The task in hearing-aid fitting is to work with the child to reach both the possibilities and limitations of acoustic amplification.

**Follow-up:** After the hearing aids have been fitted, their function must be regularly tested by parents and educators because initially the child is unable to detect and report malfunctions. But if the hearing aids are of definite benefit, the child will soon ask for them him-/herself and later will make it known if the devices are not functioning properly.

### Other Assistive Devices

**FM transmitters** are used frequently and successfully in classrooms and often can be coupled to the hearing aid. Placing the microphone close to the teacher allows the teacher's voice to reach the student with significantly less interference from background noise. Another option is the use of smartphones and its direct connections to the hearing aid.

### Cochlear Implants

*Indications and advantages:* Cochlear implants are used in patients who have cochlear damage and an auditory nerve that is responsive to stimulation. They are mainly an option for two categories of hearing-impaired children (see also 📖8.5, Cochlear Implant in Adults):

**Congenital deafness or profound hearing loss:** The earlier cochlear implantation is performed in these children, the better the device can exploit the natural adaptability and receptivity of the central auditory structures. Most children treated early with a cochlear implant learn to understand speech. Many can even *understand speech without lip reading* (open speech comprehension). It is equally important to *train the child's speaking ability*. Cochlear implantation after puberty very rarely provides open speech comprehension or a significant improvement of speech.

**Bilateral acquired deafness** (e.g., after meningitis): Cochlear implantation should be performed as soon as possible so that existing auditory development is not lost and can be exploited with the cochlear implant during rehabilitation. In practice, this means that co-chlear implantation should be scheduled as soon as the child is diagnosed with bilateral deafness or profound hearing loss that is not treatable with hearing aids. As a rule, hearing aids should be tried for several months before this determination is made.

*Surgery:* Cochlear implantation surgery is a low-risk procedure even in children. It is very rarely contra-indicated for medical reasons.

*Speech processor fitting:* The speech processor is fitted to the child on an individual basis in sessions that are consistent with pedagogic and audiologic principles. Like hearing-aid fitting, it is a process that requires a great deal of patience, empathy, and experience.

## Education Services

Whenever a child is diagnosed as having a significant, permanent hearing loss, the child should receive special education services from a trained, licensed teacher. At their simplest level, these services will help children learn how to use and care for their auditory devices. Education and counseling should also be provided to parents and other family members on dealing with issues of deafness within the family. For small children, these services are generally provided in the home. Auditory perception is trained and practiced in a play setting, while parents are taught behavioral rules and assistive measures. The goal of early education services is to integrate the hearing-impaired child into public schooling and thus into the society of normal-hearing persons. Specialized kindergartens and schools are available for children who cannot be main-streamed.

Some institutions specialize in a total communication approach that combines oral communication with other modalities such as sign language.

### Rehabilitative Measures for Unilateral Hearing Loss

Audiologic and education services in children with unilateral hearing loss are generally limited to *audiometric surveillance* of the healthy side and to *counseling.*
Favorable *seating in the classroom* is essential. The child should sit as close to the teacher as possible and listen with the good ear turned toward the instructor. It is also important to instruct the teacher in maintaining *correct speech habits.* The use of an *FM system* may be necessary in some cases.

🔍 **9.2 Meningitis and cochlear implantation**

The relationship of cochlear implants (CI) and meningitis is twofold. Patients with CI have a somewhat increased risk of meningitis because the electrode array can form a lead for infections to the perilymphatic space and its connections to the cerebrospinal fluid. That is why, all patients should be vaccinated against *Streptococcus pneumoniae* before surgery for CI.

Otherwise, acute meningitis can induce hearing loss, often profound, or even deafness. Moreover, it can lead to labyrinthitis with calcification within the cochlea, making the introduction of the electrode array into the cochlea difficult and leading nearly always to deafness. This is most common in meningitis with *S. pneumoniae* in infants. Hearing loss and the beginning of cochlear calcification are not evident in such infants, leading to critical delays in diagnosis and treatment. All children with meningitis should undergo gadolinium-enhanced magnetic resonance imaging of the inner ear in the first 1 to 2 weeks with the aim to detect labyrinthitis. The hearing of these children should also be tested as soon as possible. If deafness and labyrinthitis or early signs of calcifications of the cochlea are detected (**Fig. 9.3**), a cochlear implantation may become urgent.

**Fig. 9.3    Cochlear calcification after meningitis**

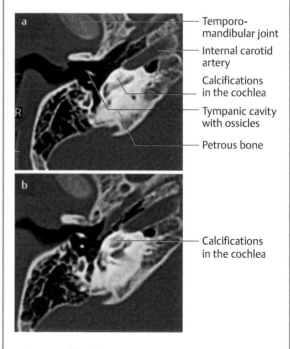

- Temporo-mandibular joint
- Internal carotid artery
- Calcifications in the cochlea
- Tympanic cavity with ossicles
- Petrous bone

- Calcifications in the cochlea

**a** Lower cochlear turn.
**b** Cochlear apex.

# 10    The External Ear

## 10.1    Special Anatomy and Examination of the External Ear

It is necessary to know the special anatomy of the external ear to understand the specific manifestations of diseases of the auricle and external auditory canal. Because this anatomy is closely linked to the examina- tion technique, this 🕮 also deals with the general technique of otoscopy and evaluation of the ear canal. Otoscopic evaluation of the tympanic membrane is covered in Chapter 11.

### Anatomy

#### Auricle

The auricle and the external auditory canal (external acoustic meatus, ear canal) form an anatomic and functional unit. The lateral cartilaginous structures of the external ear are continuous with the medial bony structures. The *medial boundary* of the external ear is the tympanic membrane. The *shape of the auricle* is defined by the elastic cartilaginous plate (**Fig. 10.1**). The perichondrium of the elastic cartilage forms a unit with the lateral dermis of the auricle; there is no actual subcutaneous tissue in this region. As a result, cutaneous changes and swelling frequently affect the perichondrium and cartilage, which can lead to severe pain, poor absorption, and cartilage destruction with permanent changes in auricular shape.

#### External Auditory Canal

The auricle and the **cartilaginous portion** of the ex- ternal auditory canal form a unit both anatomically and in many pathological aspects (**Fig. 10.2**). Diseases of the auricle often spread to the ear canal, and vice versa. The lateral two-thirds of the external auditory canal consist of a fibrocartilaginous framework that is angled downward and forward relative to the bony medial third. This is why, at otoscopy, the mobile cartilaginous part of the ear is pulled upward and backward.

The **bony portion** of the ear canal is formed by the tympanic part of the temporal bone. The skin in that region of the ear canal is very thin and directly over- lies the periosteum; this accounts for the temperature and pain sensitivity of the medial canal skin and can influence the pathogenesis and course of ear canal dis- eases such as necrotizing otitis externa (see 🕮10.4, Necrotizing Otitis Externa).

The bony ear canal grows considerably less than the cartilaginous ear canal. The cartilaginous part is short- er than the bony part in infants, but both parts are of approximately equal length by 5 to 6 years of age. The ear canal in adults is approximately 2.5 cm long.

Fig. 10.1    Normal auricle

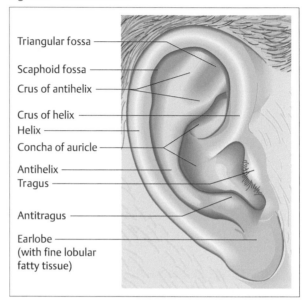

- Triangular fossa
- Scaphoid fossa
- Crus of antihelix
- Crus of helix
- Helix
- Concha of auricle
- Antihelix
- Tragus
- Antitragus
- Earlobe (with fine lobular fatty tissue)

Fig. 10.2    External auditory canal

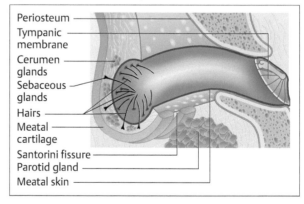

- Periosteum
- Tympanic membrane
- Cerumen glands
- Sebaceous glands
- Hairs
- Meatal cartilage
- Santorini fissure
- Parotid gland
- Meatal skin

### Innervation

Most of the external ear receives its sensory supply from branches of the great auricular nerve (from the cervical plexus) and auriculotemporal nerve (from the third division of the trigeminal). Portions of the con- cha and ear canal are supplied by the auricular branch of the vagus nerve, whose stimulation by otoscopy can induce coughing (vagal irritation). In some cases, the ear canal and concha are also supplied by the auricular branches of the facial nerve (somatosensory portion).

## Anatomic Relations

The external ear and particularly the ear canal border on the following structures, which can lead to changes in the ear canal:

- Anterior to the cartilaginous and bony ear canal is the *temporomandibular joint*. Trauma to this joint can lead to swelling and bleeding of the ear canal.
- The *parotid gland* borders the cartilaginous ear canal anteriorly and inferiorly. Inflammations and tumors can spread through Santorini's fissures from the ear canal to the parotid gland or vice versa.
- Posterior to the ear canal is the *mastoid*. The posterior bony canal wall forms part of the anterior wall of the mastoid, and the medial part of the canal wall adjoins the tympanic cavity. Inflammation of the mastoid (mastoiditis) can lead to sagging of the posterosuperior canal wall.
- The external ear is bordered superiorly by the temporalis muscle and the squamous part of the temporal bone. The superomedial portions of the bony canal wall form the floor of the epitympanum (attic) in the middle ear.

## Examination

*History and inspection:* The patient should be questioned specifically about otalgia, aural fullness, or hearing loss (currently or in the past), and particular attention should be given to aural discharge (otorrhea). The auricle is a relatively common site of injury due to its exposed location. Generally, these injuries are visible due to the absence of deeper subcutaneous structures. Examination of the ear, then, always begins with a careful inspection of the auricle, its surroundings, and the opening of the ear canal.

*Palpation:* Before the ear is examined further and before otoscopy, the tragus should be palpated. Tragal tenderness signifies an inflammation of the cartilaginous portion of the ear canal, because displacement of the rigid tragus moves and irritates the perichondrium attached to the rest of the meatal cartilage. The same effect can be achieved by pulling gently on the auricle.

▰ Otoscopy should be performed with particular care when tragal tenderness or otalgia is present.

*Otoscopy:* Examination with a hand-held otoscope or aural speculum allows inspection of the external ear canal and tympanic membrane. The technique of otoscopy and the findings in the ear canal are described in this chapter and in ▰8.1. Tympanic membrane findings are described in ▰8.1 and ▰11.1–11.4.
When otoscopy is performed with an aural speculum that is shaped such that it normally cannot reach the

**Fig. 10.3  Otoscopy**

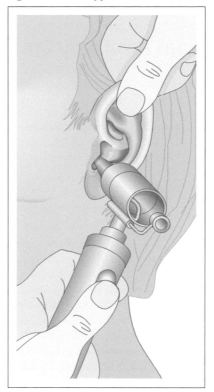

Technique: The auricle is gently rotated or pulled upward and backward to straighten the ear canal so that the otoscope can be inserted with the left hand, leaving the right hand free for manipulations. After the speculum has been introduced, it is held securely in alignment with the bony ear canal, and the auricle can be released.

tympanic membrane, the danger of tympanic membrane injury is very slight. A relatively broad speculum affords good exposure of the ear canal and tympanic membrane and provides better illumination. Narrow specula may be advanced unnecessarily far into the ear canal.

▰ Touching the medial bony portions of the ear canal with the tip of the speculum is not only painful but can injure the delicate skin of the canal wall.

The auricle is gently rotated backward and upward to align the cartilaginous ear canal with the bony canal for examination (**Fig. 10.3**). Once the otoscope has been introduced under vision and stably aligned with the bony canal, the auricle can be released.
Proceeding laterally to medially, the examiner inspects the course and appearance of the external canal as far as the tympanic membrane. Contaminants in the form of cerumen, debris, drainage, or foreign bodies are removed by suction, with a small instrument, or by irrigation of the ear canal (see ▰10.2, Foreign Bodies in the Ear Canal).
The lateral portions of the ear canal can also be examined with a rhinoscopylike **speculum**. Whenever possible, manipulations in the deeper portions of the ear canal should be done under stereoscopic vision using an **otomicroscope**.

# 10.2 Noninflammatory Diseases and Injuries to the External Ear

A common noninflammatory condition is obstruction of the ear canal by an accumulation of cerumen. Cleansing the ear canal is a common medical service that must be done carefully due to the proximity of middle ear structures and the sensitivity of the ear canal skin. Injuries, foreign bodies, and stenoses are other important medical findings in the external ear.

## Deformities and Malformations

### Prominent Ears

Prominent or protruding ears are a normal congenital variant that has no functional consequences. The normal angle between the auricle and head is approximately 20 to 30 degrees. This angle may be increased due to a deep concha or lack of development of the antihelix.

*Treatment:* Surgical correction consists of reducing the size of the concha and reconstructing the antihelix. In children, the surgery is usually performed at preschool age under general anesthesia. An ear dressing is worn for about 2 weeks after the operation.

### Hyperostoses and Exostoses of the Ear Canal

**Exostoses** of the external ear canal are true osteomas that are most commonly located near the annulus on the superomedial canal wall. They develop from ossification centers and appear otoscopically as pale, rounded bony prominences.
**Hyperostosis** is an appositional growth of the bony ear canal, usually induced by periosteal irritation such as frequent contact with cold water (synonym: swimmer's ear).

*Diagnosis:* The otoscopic appearance is characteristic (**Fig. 10.4**). The ear canal is usually narrowed in its bony portion by several smooth, pale prominences. These may form a stenosis that occludes the tympanic membrane. The narrowed site is hard and tender when probed with a small, blunt hook.

*Complications:* A stenosis causing retention of squamous debris and water can lead to recurrent otitis externa. In the absence of inflammation, only high-grade stenoses cause conductive hearing loss.

*Treatment:* If complications arise, the growths should be surgically removed.

**Fig. 10.4 Hyperostoses and exostoses of the ear canal**

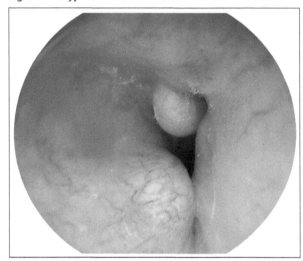

Hyperostoses and exostoses of the left auditory canal. A typical, spherical exostosis is visible superiorly, and the ear canal is markedly narrowed interiorly by hyperostoses.

## Cerumen and Cerumen Impaction

*Physiology:* Cerumen ("earwax") is produced by the cerumen and sebaceous glands in the skin of the ear canal. It forms a protective film in which fatty acids, lysozymes, and the creation of an acid milieu effectively protect the skin of the ear canal. Self-cleansing of the ear canal, with natural removal of accumulated cerumen, is normally accomplished by epithelial migration from the tympanic membrane toward the external meatus.

*Pathophysiology:* Cerumen impaction may result from a disturbance of the normal self-cleansing mechanism or from altered cerumen secretion. The cerumen plug consists mainly of secretions from the cerumen glands mixed with sebum, exfoliative debris, and contaminants. Imprudent cleaning of the ear canal (especially with cotton-tipped swabs!) can interfere with the self-cleansing mechanism and displace the cerumen toward the tympanic membrane.

### 🔎 10.1 Malformations of the external ear

A continuum exists between a normal variant of auricular shape and an anomaly (see Prominent Ears). The auricle is formed embryologically from six mesenchymal hillocks and migrates in a cranial direction with further development. Low-set ears may therefore signify an anomaly of the external auditory canal or middle ear.

#### Auricular appendages

These appendages, composed of skin and cartilage, develop from aberrant embryonic cell rests that become trapped in the area of the first branchial cleft. They are usually preauricular and have no functional importance. Rarely, they are associated with other ear malformations or hearing impairment. Treatment consists of excision for appendages that are cosmetically objectionable.

#### Congenital auricular fistulas and cysts

Aural fistulas, preauricular fistulas, and cysts develop from sites of epithelial retention in the area of the first branchial cleft. The fistulous tracts usually terminate blindly. The fistulous openings are most commonly found at preauricular sites on the helical rim. A continuum exists with high cervical fistulas located at an infra- or retroauricular site. Possible *complications* include infections. In these cases, the fistula must be completely excised, based on a knowledge of the possible course of the fistulous tracts and their relations to the facial nerve and external ear canal (**Fig. 10.5**).

#### Malformations of the auricle

Auricular dysplasia is classified into three grades:

**Grade I dysplasia (minor anomalies)**: The structural subunits of the auricle are present but malformed.
Prominent ears are an example. Other anomalies are macrotia, tubercles (darwinian tubercles), helical projections (auricular apex), and macacus ear with partial absence of the helix. These anomalies require either no correction or a relatively simple corrective procedure.

**Grade II dysplasia (mild microtia)**: The auricle is small, severely misshapen, and lacks some subunits. An anomaly of the external meatus is often present. Microtia requires meticulous corrective surgery (see 🔎 **10.2**).

**Grade III dysplasia (microtia and anotia)**: Normal auricular structures are absent, and the ear canal is almost always atretic (**Fig. 10.6**). Objective audiologic tests should be performed shortly after birth to determine whether acceptable auditory function is present on at least one side. Children with unilateral atresia should receive a bone-conduction hearing aid during the first months of life. Surgical reconstruction of the ear canal and middle ear can be performed by about 10 years of age. Auricular reconstruction is usually done later. Methods of surgical reconstruction are described in 🔎 **10.2**.

#### Stenosis and atresia of the ear canal

Stenoses and atresias of the external ear canal are frequently but not always associated with auricular anomalies. Unilateral atresia is generally not treated surgically, as this would be unlikely to significantly improve the quality of life.

**Fig. 10.5  Congenital preauricular fistula**

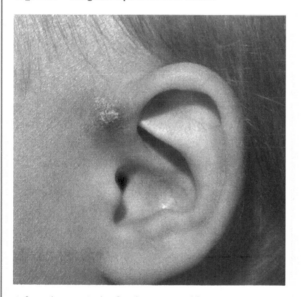

Infected preauricular fistula on typical location just anteriorly of the helix.

**Fig. 10.6  Microtia (left ear)**

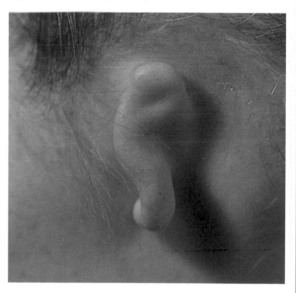

Grade III dysplasia with complete atresia of the ear canal.

Obstruction of the ear canal by cerumen may be caused by the impaction or swelling of a cerumen plug. This often occurs after contact with water. With aging, drying of the meatal skin and changes in secretions can lead to the formation of a hard cerumen that tends to be retained in the ear, especially with a narrow canal.

**Symptoms:** Cerumen impaction causes a pressure sensation in the ear with concomitant hearing loss. Some patients complain of vertigo or tinnitus.

**Diagnosis:** With a cerumen impaction, otoscopy may show obstruction of the ear canal by a yellowish-brown to black material. The consistency of the cerumen is variable. A detailed otologic history should be obtained.

🔒 Particular attention is given to tympanic membrane perforations and previous temporal bone fractures or otologic surgery.

**Differential diagnosis:** An epithelial plug or crust can result from a cholesteatoma in the external ear canal. Occasionally, the ear canal is obstructed by a thin skin flap, or cuticle. Tumors, foreign bodies, and crusted blood should also be excluded.

**Complications:** Otitis externa may develop, but generally complications are rare.

**Treatment:** Cerumen and cerumen plugs are removed with a small instrument (hook, curette), by suction, or by aural irrigation.

🔒 Instrumental cleaning of the ear canal is best done under stereoscopic vision by a specialist using an otomicroscope.

### Technique of aural irrigation

🔒 Irrigation is contraindicated in patients with a positive otologic history (see above).

- Hard cerumen can be softened by pretreatment with hydrogen peroxide, a glycerin-containing agent, or other detergents for several days.
- The ear is irrigated with bacteriologically pure water at 37°C using an ear syringe with a blunt cannula.
- The water jet is directed posterosuperiorly; it is not trained directly on the tympanic membrane (**Fig. 10.7**).
- Irrigation should be followed by otoscopy and a clinical hearing test (tuning fork test).

**Fig. 10.7 Irrigation of the ear canal**

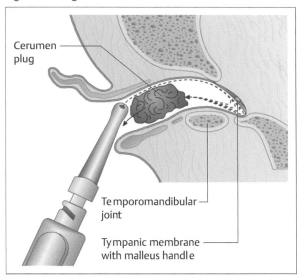

Cerumen plug

Temporomandibular joint

Tympanic membrane with malleus handle

The diagram shows a transverse section through the ear canal. The irrigation jet is directed posteriorly and superiorly.

*Contraindications* (referral to a specialist):
- Positive otologic history (see above).
- Single hearing ear affected.
- Restless, uncooperative patient.
- Foreign body.

**Prophylaxis:** The best preventive measure is to avoid improper cleaning of the ear canal, particularly the regular use of cotton-tipped swabs.

## Foreign Bodies in the Ear Canal

**Causes:** Most cases occur when small children insert small play objects such as beads or Lego pieces into the ear canal. Most foreign bodies in adults consist of noise-reducing ear plugs or objects used for manipulations in the ear canal. Insects may also become trapped in the ear canal.

**Diagnosis:** The history is usually diagnostic, and generally the foreign body is easily identified at otoscopy. Difficulties can result from secondary injuries, swelling, or inflammation.

🔒 Check for signs of associated injury to middle- or inner-ear structures such as tympanic membrane perforation, otitis media, facial nerve lesions, vertigo, nystagmus, or sensorineural hearing loss.

**Differential diagnosis:** The differential diagnosis includes cerumen impaction, dried blood, tumors of the ear canal, cholesteatoma, and otitis externa (e.g., due to fungal infection).

**Fig. 10.8 Foreign bodies in the ear canal**

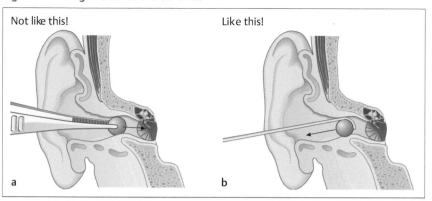

Not like this!    Like this!

a                  b

**a** A foreign body should not be extracted with tweezers or forceps, as it may slide deeper into the ear.
**b** During examination with an otomicroscope, a small blunt hook is positioned behind the foreign body and can extract the object without danger to the tympanic membrane or middle ear.

*Complications:*
A deeply penetrating foreign body can cause middle- and inner-ear damage. The prolonged retention of a foreign body in the ear generally leads to secondary otitis externa, often with a fetid discharge.

*Treatment:* The foreign body should be carefully removed with a small extraction hook or suction. Care is taken not to push the foreign body deeper into the ear canal or through the tympanic membrane (**Fig. 10.8**).

🔖 Aural irrigation should not be used on foreign bodies in the ear canal.

In children, it is often preferable to extract the foreign body under general anesthesia rather than try hazardous manipulations. Insects can be killed with a 10% lidocaine solution. Very rarely, a surgical incision may be needed to remove foreign bodies lodged tightly in the ear canal.

## Injuries and Physical Damage

### Auricular Hematoma, Auricular Seroma

*Definition:* An auricular hematoma or seroma is a collection of blood or serous fluid between the perichondrium and auricular cartilage.

*Pathogenesis:* Blunt trauma like that commonly occurring in contact and combative sports (wrestling, boxing, water polo) causes the skin and attached perichondrium to separate from the auricular cartilage. If the injury remains closed, a hematoma or seroma may form between these layers. There is little tendency for the fluid collection to be reabsorbed.

*Symptoms:* The trauma itself is painful, but typically there is no pain afterward.

**Fig. 10.9 Auricular hematoma**

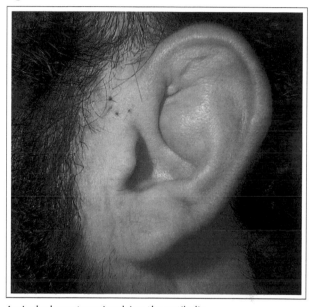

Auricular hematoma involving the antihelix.

*Diagnosis:* The findings on inspection and palpation are unequivocal (**Fig. 10.9**). The skin over the lateral auricular cartilage shows swelling and fluctuation.
The examiner should exclude associated injuries to the temporal bone, ear canal, middle ear, and temporomandibular joint and secondary infection of the hematoma.

*Differential diagnosis:* Recurrent polychondritis can give rise to a spontaneous seroma.

*Complications:* A secondary infection, often caused by needle aspiration of the hematoma, can lead to perichondritis. Poor reabsorption of the fluid collection can result in permanent deformity of the cartilaginous framework with the development of an irreversible "cauliflower ear."

**Fig. 10.10    Partial avulsion of the auricle**

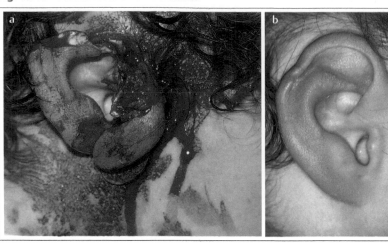

**a** Auricular injury on the right side with partial avulsion in a 9-year-old girl bitten by a dog.
**b** Appearance after surgical treatment and healing.

*Treatment:* The hematoma or seroma is surgically evacuated and the perichondrium is reattached to the cartilage. A contoured dressing (e.g., of oil-impregnated cotton) is then applied. Seromas may recur even after surgical treatment.

*Prophylaxis:* Ear protection should be worn for all contact sports.

### Sharp Auricular Injury and Auricular Avulsion

*Definition:* In an open auricular injury, the cartilage is exposed over an area of variable size. An auricular avulsion may be partial (with an intact bridge of skin; **Fig. 10.10**) or complete (part of the auricle is completely detached).

*Diagnosis:* The injured site is carefully cleaned, and the extent of the injury is determined.

🖉 Intact bridges of skin and cartilage should always be left intact.

Associated injuries to the temporal bone, ear canal, middle ear, or temporomandibular joint should be excluded.

*Complications:* A soft-tissue infection and perichondritis may develop secondarily. Crushed or severed parts may succumb to necrosis.

*Treatment:* Primary measures for an auricular avulsion:
• Cover the wound with a sterile dressing.
• Refer the patient to an ear, nose, and throat (ENT) facility right away.
• Send severed ear parts with the patient.
• Cool the part whenever possible, but do not pack it directly in ice (risk of tissue damage!). The ideal solution is to wrap the part in moist gauze, place it in a waterproof plastic bag, and immerse the bag in ice water.

The wound is closed with perichondrial and cutaneous sutures. Exposed cartilage should be covered with skin, using flap advancement if necessary (see ✍ 3.4, Soft-Tissue Injuries and Plastic Surgery). The lateral skin is reapproximated with a contoured ear dressing. With a partial auricular avulsion, the specialist should attempt a reanastomosis if an adequate skin bridge is present, the avulsed part is not too large and is not badly crushed, and the injury is no more than approximately 6 hours old. As an alternative and for most complete avulsions, the cartilage can be implanted subcutaneously at a retroauricular or cervical site and used 6 months later to perform a secondary reconstruction.

*Prognosis:* The prognosis depends on the extent of the injury. Because the tissue has a good blood supply, parts still attached by a small bridge of skin have a chance of healing, and even some small detached parts may become revascularized. The prognosis for healing tends to be poor with a complete avulsion, however.

### Burns and Frostbite Injuries

*Definition:* Thermal injuries to the auricle are graded as follows:
• Damage confined to the skin:
 – Grade I: localized erythema.
 – Grade II: blistering of the skin.
• Damage involving the entire skin–cartilage unit:
 – Grade III: deep tissue necrosis.

*Etiology:* The auricle is a frequent site of **frostbite** due to its exposed location and inadequate protection from the cold. **Burns** confined to the auricle are somewhat rare.

*Diagnosis:* A **burn** is easily diagnosed from the recent history. **Frostbite** may appear initially as a white skin discoloration that is demarcated from its surroundings. The patient typically does not notice the initial cold injury, which does not become painful until the frostbitten area is rewarmed.

Associated injuries should be excluded, especially with burns. The examiner should check for concomitant involvement of the ear canal and tympanic membrane.

***Differential diagnosis:*** Caustic chemical injuries and electrical injuries can produce similar skin changes.

***Complications:*** A deep thermal injury may give rise to cartilage necrosis and permanent deformity. Chilblains may develop on the helical rim with ulcerations and itching. Perichondritis can also occur.

***Treatment:*** Treatment follows the general principles of surgical wound care for burns and frostbite.

✒ Local treatments (dressings) should not exert pressure on the auricle to avoid further compromise of the auricular blood supply.

***Burns:*** Consistent with the general principles of burn care, superficial burns in particular should be cooled immediately and treated with other local anti-inflammatory measures. Surgical debridement may be necessary later for more severe burns.

***Frostbite:*** The frostbitten area should be gently warmed (e.g., with a heat lamp), taking care not to burn the tissue. The best strategy for injuries with bulla formation or necrosis is to provide dry treatment and await demarcation of the frostbitten area. Circulatory stimulants such as dextran or pentoxifylline can be used.

**Reconstructive surgery** is deferred until the site has completely healed, which usually takes around 6 months.

***Prognosis:*** More severe burns or frostbite injuries are often associated with permanent auricular deformity.

## Injuries to the External Auditory Canal

***Etiology:*** Isolated injuries to the external ear canal are caused mainly by foreign bodies or harmful manipulations.

🔎 **10.2 Reconstructive surgery of the auricle**

Surgical reconstruction of the auricle may be necessary after trauma, for malformations, or after a tumor resection. The extent and complexity of auricular reconstructive surgery depend on the underlying condition and on what the reconstruction can and must achieve. Total auricular reconstruction is among the most difficult and demanding procedures in plastic and reconstructive surgery.

Auricular reconstructions fall into several categories:

**Shape corrections:** These are relatively simple procedures that are used in the treatment of prominent ears, for example (see above).

**Partial reconstructions:** These may be indicated following a partial resection or for grade II dysplasia. The auricle is reconstructed using available local cartilage whenever possible. The necessary skin coverage is obtained with advancement flaps (see 🔖3.4, Soft-Tissue Injuries and Plastic Surgery) or preliminary subcutaneous expansion.

**Total reconstruction:** This is mainly necessary for congenital aplasias and severe anomalies (grade III dysplasia). A total reconstruction is very challenging and complex and is usually staged in several sittings. Missing cartilage is reconstructed with autologous cartilage grafts (costal cartilage) or replaced with synthetic prostheses.

**Epithesis:** An external prosthesis may be considered as an alternative to auricular reconstruction. The epithesis may be attached to implanted titanium screws or an eyeglass frame, or it may be glued directly to the skin.

***Diagnosis:*** The history usually indicates previous trauma to the ear. The meatal skin is tender, and there is bleeding from the ear canal. Otoscopy may reveal an epithelial injury, bleeding, a hemorrhagic bulla, or crusted blood. Associated injuries to the tympanic membrane, middle ear, temporomandibular joint, and skull base should be excluded.

***Complications:*** Ear canal injuries may be complicated by secondary infection. Later, during healing, there may be cyst formation or stenosis of the ear canal due to scarring.

***Treatment:*** Detached epithelium should be reapproximated whenever possible. For bleeding, it may be necessary to pack the ear canal with Gelfoam or synthetic sponge.

***Prognosis:*** Isolated injuries to the ear canal are usually uncomplicated and show a good healing tendency.

# 10.3 Overview: Differential Diagnosis of Inflammatory Changes in the External Ear

Inflammatory changes in the external ear are common and are often treated initially by a primary-care physician. It is important, therefore, to be familiar with the various types of external ear inflammation, their hazards, and their appropriate management. An inflammatory condition of the auricle or external auditory canal is diagnosed clinically; additional tests are rarely needed. Different inflammatory conditions of the external ear are interrelated in their pathogenesis, sometimes making it difficult to differentiate the various forms. Specific diseases are discussed in 10.4. The present unit deals with issues of differential diagnosis, reviewing pathophysiologic relationships and associated problems of differential diagnosis that must be considered in otitis externa.

## General

Inflammations of the external ear may manifest acutely with severe pain, may manifest subacutely, or may present with chronic complaints such as itching and scaly skin. Acute inflammations are often caused by bacterial infection, while chronic forms more closely resemble eczema.

The term **otitis externa** usually refers to inflammation of the external auditory canal. This cannot always be clearly differentiated from **auricular inflammation**, however, since inflammations of the external canal may spread to the auricle, and vice versa. Nevertheless, typical forms of auricular inflammation are distinguishable from inflammatory conditions of the ear canal.

Since the structure of skin is different in the lateral, cartilaginous part of the ear canal than in the medial, bony part (see 10.1, "Anatomy"), typical inflammatory conditions can be distinguished also within the ear canal, showing clearly different conditions and courses (**Fig. 10.11**). Certain forms of otitis externa are confined to parts of the ear canal, such as furunculosis to the lateral part and mycosis to the medial part, and necrotizing otitis externa tends to appear at the boundary of the two parts.

It is not always easy to **distinguish among the various inflammatory conditions** of the external ear, which are interrelated in their pathogenesis. For example, chronic eczema may give rise to an acute infection of the ear canal, or a fungal infection of the ear canal may develop from a subacute, bacterial otitis externa. Moreover, otitis media (see 11.3) may incite a concomitant inflammation of the external ear.

> A profuse, mucopurulent aural discharge often originates in the middle ear and not in the external ear canal, particularly when pulsation within the discharge can be noted.

## Pathogenesis

Inflammations of the external ear are often caused by factors that interfere with the normal defenses against infection. The normal cerumen film (acid pH, antibacterial fatty acid content) and the physiologic lateral migration of the epithelium lining the ear canal create an effective barrier to infection. Any of the following factors may disturb the self-cleansing of the ear canal and its protective mechanisms, predisposing to otitis externa:

- **Exogenous factors:** maceration of the skin by water, the creation of a warm moist chamber, pH changes caused by soaps and shampoos, manipulations with cotton-tipped swabs, insert earphones, or ear plugs.

Fig. 10.11   **Localizations of different forms of otitis externa**

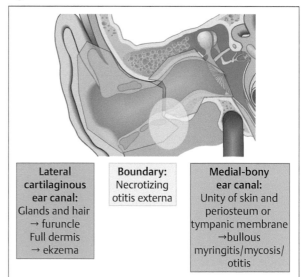

| Lateral cartilaginous ear canal: | Boundary: | Medial-bony ear canal: |
|---|---|---|
| Glands and hair → furuncle Full dermis → ekzema | Necrotizing otitis externa | Unity of skin and periosteum or tympanic membrane →bullous myringitis/mycosis/otitis |

Because of the different skin structures in the lateral and medial external ear canal, different forms of infection develop in the two parts. Necrotizing otitis externa develops typically on the floor of the boundary of the two parts.

Fig. 10.12  Differential diagnosis of acute otitis externa

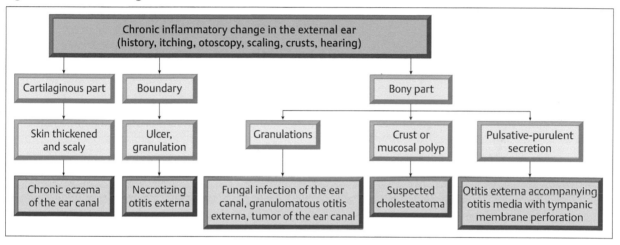

Fig. 10.13  Differential diagnosis of chronic otitis externa

- **Endogenous factors:** proneness to eczema, allergies, metabolic disorders such as diabetes mellitus.
- **Local changes:** exostoses, stenoses, anatomic variants.

It is common for several of these factors to be combined. Treatment and prophylaxis are geared toward preventing or correcting the causal factors.

## Differential Diagnosis of Acute Inflammatory Change

Acute inflammations of the auricle or external ear canal are manifested clinically by severe pain (**Fig. 10.12**). Obstruction of the ear canal by drainage or skin swelling can lead to conductive hearing loss. Generally, there is tenderness on movement of the auricle or tragus. Initial external inspection will show whether the inflammation involves the auricle. If this is the case, a pure *perichondritis* can be distinguished from a spreading *soft-tissue infection* (e.g., cellulitis) by its confinement to the cartilage. With an acute inflammation of the ear canal, careful otoscopy can usually differentiate a *furuncle* of the meatal hairs or glands from *acute dermatitis*.

If the ear canal is filled with purulent discharge, it can be difficult to distinguish between otitis externa and *suppurative otitis media* with a perforated tympanic membrane.

The Valsalva maneuver is helpful in diagnosing suppurative otitis media with a perforated tympanic membrane, as it may cause air bubbles to appear in the discharge.

The typical history of *bullous otitis externa* consists of severe otalgia with a bloody discharge. The diagnosis can often be established simply by the otoscopic detection of hemorrhagic bullae on the bony canal wall. *Herpes zoster oticus* manifests with small vesicles on the auricle and also in the ear canal.

## Differential Diagnosis of Chronic Inflammatory Change

The dominant symptom of chronic otitis externa is usually itching, not pain (**Fig. 10.13**). Inspection will generally reveal redness and scaling or crusting about the meatal orifice.

It is important first to assess the condition of the tympanic membrane and middle ear. A mobile tympanic membrane (Valsalva maneuver, pneumatic otoscopy, see 📖11.1, Examination; tympanography, see 📖8.4, Tympanometry) or the absence of conductive hearing loss (positive Rinne's test, see 📖8.1, Clinical Hearing Tests) indicates that the tympanic membrane and middle ear are intact. The skin of the ear canal shows typical changes that may consist of eczema, ulceration, or granulations. Purulent drainage in the ear canal can hamper visual inspection and may have to be carefully removed (e.g., with a fine suction tip).

When *chronic otitis media* is present, the chronic inflammatory changes in the external canal are generally caused by drainage from the middle ear. In these cases, too, the drainage in the ear canal often hampers an accurate evaluation and should be carefully removed. Conductive hearing loss is present.

The presence of mucosal polyps in the ear canal or of firmly adherent crusts in the superior part of the bony canal often signifies an *inflammatory middle ear cholesteatoma* (see 📖11.3, Chronic Otitis Media with Cholesteatoma).

# 10.4 Inflammatory Diseases of the External Ear

As described in the preceding 📖, it is common to encounter mixed inflammatory conditions of the external ear. Typical clinical manifestations can be distinguished, however. It is helpful, therefore, to consider inflammations of the auricle and ear canal separately, for at least the onset of the inflammation often presents a typical form. The various forms are described separately in this unit.

## Auricle

### Eczema and Dermatitis of the Auricle

*Definition:* An inflammatory condition of the auricle confined to the dermis. The cartilage and perichondrium are not involved.

*Pathogenesis:* The pathogenesis is the same as in other skin regions and is based on immune/allergic, toxic, or physical causes. Eczema and dermatitis of the auricle are frequently caused by:
- Jewelry items (ear rings, piercings).
- Soaps and cosmetics (shampoo, hair spray).
- Listening aids (hearing aids, earmolds, insert earphones).
- Thermal injury (sun exposure, radiotherapy, frostbite).

*Symptoms:* The cardinal symptoms are itching and occasional burning with little pain. The skin is erythematous and may be dry and scaly or moist and weeping, depending on the stage and severity of the eczema. The cartilage and perichondrium are not affected, and the contours of the auricle are unchanged. The changes may also be confined to one region such as the earlobe (jewelry) or retroauricular crease (hearing aid).

*Diagnosis:* If an allergy is suspected, skin tests should be done to identify the cause.

*Differential diagnosis:* It is necessary to exclude pyoderma, perichondritis, and cellulitis, which may occur as complications. Differentiation is also required from other dermatoses such as seborrheic dermatitis and psoriasis, which frequently occur in the retroauricular crease.

*Complications:* The cracked skin is susceptible to bacterial complications in the form of pyoderma, perichondritis, or cellulitis.

*Treatment:* The causes, if known, should be eliminated. Treatment of the skin lesions is based on dermatologic principles. Antibiotics are given only if bacterial superinfection has occurred.

### Perichondritis of the Auricle

*Definition:* Perichondritis is an acute inflammation of the skin and perichondrium that also involves the auricular cartilage. The changes are localized and do not spread beyond the auricular cartilage.

*Pathogenesis:* Most cases are caused by a bacterial infection stemming from a small injury in the conchal cavity or auricle. Bacterial infection of the lateral portions of the auricle is often associated with perichondritis due to the close attachment of the skin to the perichondrium. The predominant causative organisms are staphylococci and *Pseudomonas* species. A toxic-allergic or autoimmune etiology is less common.

*Symptoms:* The clinical picture is characterized by severe pain of rapid onset and a feeling of tension. The auricular contours are effaced, and it is common to find swelling of the concha with marked tenderness. Blisters may develop on the skin. Areas that are devoid of cartilage, like the earlobe, are spared. Regional lymph nodes may be painful and enlarged, and systemic symptoms such as fever may occur.

*Diagnosis:* The tympanic membrane appears normal at otoscopy, and hearing loss does not occur unless otitis externa is also present. Blood tests generally show leukocytosis and elevated inflammatory parameters such as C-reactive protein (CRP).

🔖 If raw, weeping skin areas are found, a smear should be taken for bacteriologic examination and sensitivity testing, as a problem organism may be present.

*Differential diagnosis*:
Perichondritis requires differentiation from an inflammation not involving the cartilage (eczema, dermatitis) and from a spreading infection (cellulitis, zoster oticus).
Recurrent autoimmune polychondritis (relapsing polychondritis, see 🔎 **10.3**) often begins in the auricle. In the absence of other symptoms caused by the destruction of bronchial, nasal, or laryngeal cartilage, it is virtually indistinguishable from bacterial perichondritis.

### Recurrent polychondritis

This is a chronic autoimmune disease directed against cartilage tissue. Auricular perichondritis is often seen as the initial manifestation. Involvement of the cartilage in the airways, larynx, and nose occurs in later stages. The disease takes a chronic course that is marked by deformities of the auricle and nose, chronic bronchitis, and occasional dyspnea resulting from cartilage damage in the trachea and larynx.

*Synonyms:* relapsing polychondritis, systemic chondromalacia, chronic atrophic panchondritis.

*Diagnosis:* The diagnosis is based on the presence of a systemic inflammatory disease, the detection of antibodies against cartilage tissue, the histologic examination of cartilage tissue, and the course.

*Treatment:* Treatment consists of oral corticosteroids. Other immune-specific agents are also used.

### Chronic chondrodermatitis nodularis helicis (Winkler's disease)

The diagnosis of chondrodermatitis is based on the presence of a painful epithelial nodule with an umbilicated center on the free border of the helix or antihelix (**Fig. 10.18a**). This is an inflammatory skin lesion of the cutaneous-perichondrial unit. Its cause is unknown. Older patients are predominantly affected. *Treatment* consists of complete excision, and subsequent histologic examination confirms the diagnosis. The *differential diagnosis* includes tumors and gouty tophi. Recurrence is not uncommon even after complete excision.

### Gouty tophi

Gouty tophi may form near the joints and on the auricular cartilage. They appear as small, pale, freely movable subcutaneous nodules on the helical rim. Generally, there is no need for local treatment.

### Benign cutaneous lymphadenosis (Bäfverstedt's disease)

This lesion appears as a firm, reddish nodule on the earlobe (**Fig. 10.18b**). The lymphadenosis represents a cutaneous manifestation of infection with *Borrelia burgdorferi*, and patients often give a prior history of tick bite. The treatment is the same as for a *Borrelia* infection.

### External auditory canal cholesteatoma

Similar to the formation of a cholesteatoma in the middle ear (see 11.3, Chronic Otitis Media with Cholesteatoma), the epithelium of the medial ear canal skin can rarely form a cholesteatoma on the floor of the bony part of the ear canal without involvement of the middle ear. Etiologic factors include recurrent microtraumas through cotton-tipped applicators or hearing aids, smoking, and radiotherapy. The *diagnosis* is established otoscopically and with computer tomography. Surgery is needed as *treatment*. The *differential diagnosis* includes necrotizing otitis externa, tumors, and Langerhans' cell histiocytosis.

### Granulating otitis externa and medial canal fibrosis

Circumscribed or diffuse granulations may form on the skin of the bony ear canal and on the tympanic membrane, occurring spontaneously or as a sequel to otitis externa or ear surgery. Often, the precipitating cause cannot be determined, and the inflammation usually takes a refractory course. The end stage is often a complete occlusion of the medial ear canal by fibrous scar tissue. The shortened ear canal ends in a blind epithelia sack, the tympanic membrane cannot be recognized, and there is conductive hearing loss. *Treatment* consists of removing the granulations followed by the topical application of antibiotics and corticosteroids in the beginning. Fibrosis can be surgically treated by excision and lining of the bony ear canal with split-thickness skin grafts. Recurrence is common. Necrotizing otitis externa and a tumor should be excluded.

### Specific otitis externa

Syphilis (mainly stage II), *Mycobacterium tuberculosis*, and atypical mycobacteria are very rare causes of otitis externa.

**Fig. 10.18    Inflammatory changes of the auricle**

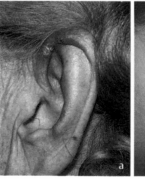 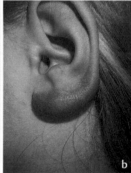

**a** Chondrodermatitis nodularis helicis (left ear) with epithelial nodule.
**b** Benign cutaneous lymphadenosis with nodule of the ear lobe.

**Fig. 10.14 Auricular cellulitis, right ear.**

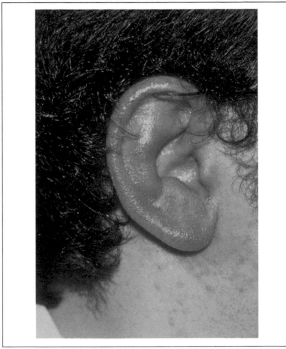

The entire auricle including the ear lobe is red and swollen. The skin around the auricle is also reddened.

*Complications:* Unless adequately treated, the inflammation will cause cartilage destruction with permanent auricular deformity.

*Treatment:* Primary treatment relies on systemic antibiotics that are active against staphylococci. The auricle and ear canal should be carefully and thoroughly cleansed. Antiseptic or antibiotic-containing ointments should be applied locally, and pain is controlled with nonsteroidal anti-inflammatory agents.

## Auricular Cellulitis

*Definition:* Auricular cellulitis is an acute streptococcal infection of the subcutaneous tissue involving the auricle and its surroundings.

*Pathogenesis:* The streptococci usually gain access to the auricle through small injuries in the concha or external meatus.

*Symptoms:* The clinical manifestations typically consist of redness, swelling, and warmth of the auricle and its surroundings. The earlobe and adjacent facial skin are also involved. Malaise is present with associated fever and otalgia. The disease progresses swiftly without treatment (**Fig. 10.14**).

*Diagnosis:* Inspection and cleansing of the ear canal, with evaluation of the tympanic membrane, are necessary to exclude a middle ear infection.

An attempt should always be made to identify the causative organism in smears and determine its antibiotic sensitivity.

*Differential diagnosis:* Differentiation is required from eczema, dermatitis, and perichondritis. Dermatitis generally does not produce systemic effects such as fever or an elevated white count. In perichondritis, the surrounding soft tissues and the earlobe usually are not affected. In zoster oticus, there is usually concomitant involvement of the inner ear or facial nerve.

*Complications:* Rare cases may be complicated by a necrotizing fasciitis or other deep neck infections (severe, intractable subcutaneous infection, often with the presence of anaerobes). In infections with group A streptococci, known systemic complications such as glomerulonephritis, rheumatic fever, or rheumatic endocarditis may develop (see ⌕ **5.3** and ⌕ **5.4**).

*Treatment:* The standard treatment is a high-dose regimen of penicillin G (e.g., 4 × 2 mega-IU), preferably by IV administration. Other antibiotics with antistreptococcal activity can also be used. Pain is adequately managed with nonsteroidal anti-inflammatory agents. The auricle and ear canal should be carefully cleansed.

## Herpes Zoster Oticus

*Pathogenesis:* This disease, also known as Ramsay Hunt syndrome, is caused by reactivation of the dormant varicella zoster virus (VZV) in ganglion cells. Zoster oticus involves cranial nerves VII and/or VIII (and occasionally IX and X).

*Symptoms:* Patients initially experience ear pain or burning on one side in the absence of physical findings. Typical vesicles erupt shortly thereafter, no more than a few days after symptom onset. This is followed by hearing loss, vestibular complaints (vertigo, disequilibrium), and often facial nerve palsy.

*Diagnosis:* **Inspection** reveals typical clustered ("herpetiform") vesicles about the meatus and concha and occasionally on the pinna (**Fig. 10.15**). There is accompanying lymphadenitis of the high cervical lymph nodes. **Clinical examination** may demonstrate as evidence of seventh and eighth cranial nerve involvement facial nerve palsy, sensorineural hearing loss, nystagmus, and unilateral hypoexcitability of the vestibular organ. These signs may occur singly or in combinations.

The diagnosis can usually be made clinically. It can be confirmed by the direct electron microscopic **detec-**

**Fig. 10.15   Herpes zoster oticus**

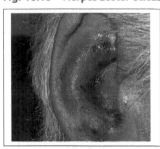

Typical bullae with acute inflammation in herpes zoster oticus. The 56-year-old man also displayed clinical signs of vestibular nerve dysfunction and facial nerve palsy.

**tion of VZV** in vesicular aspirate (costly) or later by at least a fourfold titer increase on serologic testing.

*Differential diagnosis:* In its early stage, herpes zoster oticus is important in the differential diagnosis of sudden hearing loss and acute facial nerve palsy. The disease requires differentiation from other forms of otitis, especially bullous otitis externa. Other causes of seventh and eighth cranial nerve lesions such as otitis media, mastoiditis, labyrinthitis, cholesteatoma, and tumors of the ear and lateral skull base should be excluded.

*Complications:* An important local complication is secondary bacterial infection, usually with staphylococci or *Pseudomonas* species. Zoster meningoencephalitis results from the intracranial spread of the VZV. A severe, refractory postzoster neuralgia may develop as a late complication, especially in older patients.

*Treatment:* Whenever herpes zoster oticus is suspected clinically, systemic therapy with acyclovir, valacyclovir, or famciclovir should be instituted without delay. The concurrent use of corticosteroids is recommended when facial nerve palsy is present. The lesions are also treated locally with an antiseptic solution.

*Prognosis:* Older patients in particular are apt to have residual morbidity with permanent functional deficits. The prognosis of facial nerve palsy after herpes zoster oticus is poorer than in cases of idiopathic facial paralysis.

## External Auditory Canal

### Diffuse Otitis Externa and Eczema of the Ear Canal

*Pathogenesis:* An inflammatory condition of the external auditory canal involving the canal skin (eczema, dermatitis due to mechanical injury, toxicity, or allergy) gives rise to an acute bacterial infection of the skin with a mixed flora that includes gram-negative organisms (*Pseudomonas aeruginosa*, *Proteus mirabilis*) and anaerobes. Primary or secondary fungal infections of the ear canal may also develop (see Otomycosis below). The tympanic membrane is also occasionally involved (myringitis). A warm, moist climate promotes the development of a diffuse otitis externa (swimmer's otitis).

*Symptoms:* The main initial symptom is itching. Pain is present with an acute infection. The patient may notice crusting, and a purulent aural discharge may occur. Obstruction of the ear canal can lead to conductive hearing loss.

*Diagnosis:* With eczema of the ear canal in the absence of acute infection, the canal skin appears dry, cracked, and scaly on otoscopic examination. The skin may be thickened and shows sites of desquamation. The presence of an infection is manifested by diffuse swelling of the lateral canal skin with associated discharge or crusting. A fetid discharge means that anaerobes are involved. Bacteriologic examination is necessary only in cases with persistent or recurrent infection or if the diagnosis is uncertain.

*Differential diagnosis:* Acute otitis media or chronic suppurative otitis media can lead to an accompanying otitis externa and should be excluded by otoscopic examination. A fungal infection (see Otomycosis below) or tumor of the ear canal should be considered in persistent cases, and necrotizing otitis externa should be considered if otalgia is also present.

*Complications:* The cracked skin in otitis externa can allow bacterial entry causing perichondritis, cellulitis, or abscess formation. Necrotizing otitis externa may develop in predisposed patients.

*Treatment:* The first and most important step in treatment is meticulous, repeated cleansing and drying of the ear canal followed by the instillation of antiseptic, antibiotic drops that will reduce the swelling.

⚕ Steroid- and antibiotic-containing ear drops should be used for no more than 2 weeks due to the risk of sensitization, antibiotic resistance, and the development of a fungal infection.

Steroid- and antibiotic-containing ear drops are contraindicated in patients with a fungal infection of the ear canal, antibiotic hypersensitivity, or a perforated tympanic membrane. Emphasis is placed on meticulous aural hygiene, which includes protecting the ear from shampoos, soaps, and cotton-tipped swabs.

Fig. 10.16   Localized otitis externa left ear

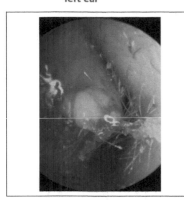

Furuncle with pus pocket at the beginning of the ear canal.

Fig. 10.17   Treatment of acute otitis externa

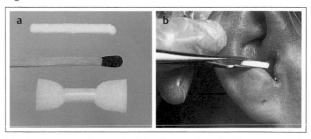

Medications can be applied to foam wicks in the ear canal, which absorb liquids and exert a gentle pressure.
**a** *Above:* compressed foam wick before use. *Below:* foam wick after fluid absorption.
**b** The foam wick is inserted into an acutely inflamed ear canal.

## Localized Otitis Externa (Furunculosis)

*Definition:* Known also as a furuncle, this is a circumscribed lesion caused by an acute bacterial infection of the cartilaginous portion of the ear canal.

*Pathogenesis:* Local mechanical trauma and contamination of the ear canal (e.g., from an ear plug, dusty environment, bath water, or attempted self-cleaning of the ear) lead to obstruction of the hair follicles or glandular ducts, followed by a staphylococcal infection of the pilosebaceous units.

*Symptoms:* A furuncle in the ear canal presents as a very painful, tender swelling that can cause mild hearing loss and rarely leads to otorrhea. Patients are generally afebrile.

*Diagnosis:*
- **Inspection and palpation:** tragal tenderness accompanied by a circumscribed, very painful swelling in the cartilaginous portion of the ear canal.
- **Otoscopy:** pronounced swelling of the ear canal with debris in the residual lumen. Frequently, the tympanic membrane cannot be seen, but it is normal (**Fig. 10.16**).
- **Simple hearing test:** The ear canal may be swollen shut, causing some degree of conductive hearing loss.
- **Bacteriologic examination:** The purulent center of the lesion (pus pocket) can be opened carefully with a small, blunt hook to obtain a smear.

Patients with recurrent furuncles should be examined for a predisposing systemic condition such as diabetes mellitus.

*Differential diagnosis:* Various disorders can produce similar clinical manifestations—for example, foreign bodies in the ear canal, otitis externa accompanying chronic suppurative otitis media, an infected retroauricular atheroma, and tumors of the ear canal.

*Complications:* In rare cases, an abscess in the ear canal with involvement of the surrounding soft tissues may spread to infra-auricular and preauricular sites. Spread to the auricular cartilage may incite perichondritis. Superinfection with *Pseudomonas* can lead to necrotizing otitis externa in predisposed patients (see below). Furuncles may take a particularly severe course in patients with diabetes mellitus.

*Treatment:* The ear canal is *meticulously cleaned* and then treated locally for 1 to 2 days with 70% *alcohol*, which is applied hourly to a self-expanding foam or gauze wick inserted into the ear canal (**Fig. 10.17**). This treatment provides disinfection, reduces local swelling by fluid absorption, and exerts a cooling action that relieves pain. Crusts can be dissolved with *antibiotic-containing ointment strips*. After the swelling has subsided, *antibiotic- and steroid-containing drops* can be instilled into the ear. *Nonsteroidal anti-inflammatory agents* are administered for pain. Abscesses should be incised after they have become clearly demarcated. *Systemic antibiotics* are used in patients with systemic symptoms and severe local signs of infection.

## Necrotizing Otitis Externa

*Pathogenesis:* Necrotizing otitis externa, also known as malignant otitis externa, is a dangerous, necrotizing form of otitis externa that occurs almost exclusively in older patients with diabetes mellitus.
Most cases begin with a simple otitis externa that becomes infected with *P. aeruginosa*, leading to ulceration and osteitis on the floor and the boundary of the cartilaginous and bony ear canal. The bone infection may subsequently spread to the middle ear, skull base, retromandibular fossa, and parotid compartment.

*Symptoms:* The initial history is that of an insidious, persistent otitis externa that does not heal. At first, there is moderate pain, which may become severe, often occurring at night as the condition takes a chronic course. A fetid aural discharge may occur but is not always present.

*Diagnosis:*
- **Inspection:** reveals signs of infection in surrounding tissues.
- **Otoscopy:** almost always shows an ulcer on the canal floor with exposed, brownish bone and a fetid discharge.
- **Smear** (with sensitivity testing!): *P. aeruginosa*.
- **Magnetic resonance imaging, computed tomography:** these studies define the extent of the infection and bone destruction.

Diabetes mellitus is almost always present. Other immune defects should be excluded.

*Differential diagnosis:* Differentiation is mainly required from simple otitis externa and cholesteatoma of the external ear canal. A biopsy should be taken if a tumor is suspected. Complications from chronic otitis media can produce similar findings.

*Complications:* The infection can lead to otitis media, mastoiditis, petrositis, and soft-tissue abscess. Cranial nerve deficits (VII, VIII, IX, X, XI), sepsis, venous sinus thrombosis, or meningitis may occur in the late stage, causing the disease to become life-threatening.

*Treatment:* The ear canal is locally debrided and cleaned at regular intervals. In cases with minimal bone involvement, high doses of an antibiotic effective against *P. aeruginosa* can be administered for 6 weeks. Diabetes mellitus should be closely monitored and adequately controlled. If there is poor response to conservative therapy or extensive involvement, or if complications arise, the affected bone should be resected. This surgery may be minor or may consist of petrosectomy, depending on the extent of disease.

*Prognosis:* The prognosis is guarded and depends on prompt, appropriate treatment. There is only a 50% chance of survival in cases that develop facial nerve palsy or venous sinus thrombosis.

## Bullous Otitis Externa

*Pathogenesis:* Bullous otitis externa (flu-related otitis, hemorrhagic otitis externa) is presumed to have a viral etiology, but the exact causal agent is unknown. The influenza virus has been isolated in sporadic cases. The infection causes toxic capillary damage in the thin epithelial layer of the medial meatal skin and on the tympanic membrane, leading to the formation of hemorrhagic epithelial bullae.

*Symptoms:* The disease begins with severe otalgia of sudden onset, often followed by a bloody discharge from the ear canal. Both conductive and sensorineural hearing loss may develop.

*Diagnosis:* **At otoscopy,** serous or hemorrhagic bulla formation is observed on the epithelium in the bony portion of the ear canal and on the tympanic membrane. Rupture of the bullae can cause spontaneous bleeding from the ear canal, which contains fresh blood that later dries to form crusts.

*Differential diagnosis:* Toxic or traumatic injury to the ear canal or middle ear (barotrauma) can produce similar findings. Differentiation is also required from herpes zoster oticus and from tumors of the ear canal.

*Complications:* Involvement of the middle ear and/or inner ear (labyrinthitis) is relatively common and may be associated with sensorineural hearing loss and vertigo. Rarely, the infection ascends along the statoacoustic nerve and may incite a life-threatening encephalitis in the brainstem.

*Treatment:* A specific antiviral therapy is not available. Pain is treated with local anesthetic ear drops and nonsteroidal anti-inflammatory drugs. If bacterial involvement of the middle and inner ear is suspected, systemic antibiotics should be administered.

## Otomycosis

*Pathogenesis:* Cerumen often harbors saprophytic fungi that have no specific pathologic significance. *Aspergillus, Candida albicans, Mucor,* and dermatophytes may, however, aggressively infect the skin of the medial ear canal if the milieu has been altered by the use of steroid- and antibiotic-containing ear drops or other factors. A warm, moist climate is conducive to fungal infections, which are most common during the summer months.

⚡ It is rare for a fungal infection of the ear canal to signify a general decline in host resistance.

*Symptoms:* Otomycosis is manifested less by pain than by severe itching and a feeling of fullness in the affected ear.

*Diagnosis:* The fungi often appear otoscopically as a white, yellow, or black membrane lining the swollen, erythematous skin of the ear canal. The bony portion of the canal is affected almost exclusively. Mycelia can be identified in direct samples. The causative organism is established by microbiologic examination.

**Differential diagnosis:**

🖉 The harmless, superficial fungal colonization of cerumen or drainage should be distinguished from an actual invasive mycosis.

Otomycosis is occasionally difficult to distinguish from other forms of otitis externa, especially diffuse otitis externa. Mixed forms commonly occur. A fungal infection may also develop in the setting of chronic suppurative otitis media.

**Course:** Otomycosis typically runs a refractory course and has a tendency to recur.

**Complications:** A fungal infection of the tympanic membrane epithelium can lead to perforation and subsequent otitis media. Spreading fungal infections with necrosis occur only in immunocompromised patients.

**Treatment:** First, it is essential that the ear canal be thoroughly cleaned and dried. Once this has been accomplished, local antimycotics can be administered. It is also necessary in many cases to soften the uppermost epithelial layer with salicylate-containing solutions to enhance the antifungal action of specific medications. Systemic antimycotic therapy is necessary only in immune-suppressed patients.

# 10.5 Tumors of the External Ear

Tumors of the auricle are relatively common, easily recognized, and treatable, whereas tumors of the ear canal are rare and are often misinterpreted. It is important to make an early diagnosis and to differentiate benign tumors from premalignant and malignant lesions of the external ear.

## Tumors of the Auricle

The auricle is heavily exposed to weathering effects due to its location. As a result, the auricle is a common site of occurrence for epithelial skin tumors that are caused by, or related to, actinic exposure. Men older than 60 years are predominantly affected. **Table 10.1** reviews the principal tumor entities, which together account for more than 90% of auricular tumors. Fibromas, histiocytomas, chondromas, ceruminomas (arising from the cerumen glands), cylindromas (Spiegler's tumor, carcinoma of the eccrine sweat glands; not to be confused with adenoid cystic carcinoma), hemangiomas, and lymphangiomas are examples of rare nonepithelial tumors that may affect the external ear. It is also important to distinguish true neoplasms from nevoid lesions, cysts, inflammatory changes such as chondrodermatitis and gouty tophi (see ⊙ 10.3), and deformities (see ✎10.2). The *diagnosis* is usually made histologically following excision of the tumor. This surgery may require reconstruction of the auricle, depending on the location and extent of the lesion. The specific reconstructive measures (see ⊙ 10.2) depend on the overall situation, including the need for postoperative radiotherapy. A suspected malignant tumor should be excised and its nature as well as its complete excision should be assessed. Extensive tumors may necessitate a complete auricular resection.

The *differential diagnosis* includes skin lesions such as cysts, keloids, otophymas, and nevoid lesions. Nevi mainly require differentiation from melanoma. The *prophylaxis* of auricular tumors consists of adequate protection from sun exposure.

## Tumors of the Ear Canal

Isolated tumors of the external auditory canal are rare. Involvement of the ear canal most commonly occurs in association with an auricular tumor. This concomitant involvement of the ear canal by an auricular malignancy generally alters the approach to treatment, as a simple excision is no longer possible in most cases. Unlike tumors of the auricle, isolated tumors of the ear canal are frequently misinterpreted and are treated for some time as otitis externa. The most common malignant tumor of the ear canal is carcinoma of the canal skin. Less common are adenoid cystic tumors, adenocarcinomas, and basal cell carcinomas. These tumors usually present as a painful, ulcerated, nonhealing lesion in the skin of the ear canal. Many cases manifest bleeding and secondary infection with chronic, purulent otorrhea.

🗡 For this reason, every nonhealing, ulcerated or granulating lesion of the ear canal should be biopsied under the operating microscope.

The *differential diagnosis* should include chronic otitis externa, especially necrotizing otitis externa, chronic otitis media with mucosal polyps, a middle ear tumor, and a penetrating parotid tumor. Further investigation relies on imaging, which can define the extent of tumor infiltration in the bone, parotid compartment, and middle ear.

*Treatment* is generally surgical, with or without postoperative irradiation. The *prognosis* depends largely on the extent of disease but tends to be unfavorable compared with auricular tumors.

**Fig. 10.19  Tumors of the auricle**

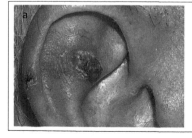 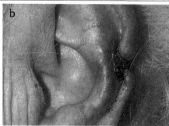 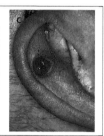

**a** Cutaneous horn.
**b** Basal cell carcinoma.
**c** Squamous cell carcinoma.

**Table 10.1 Epithelial tumors of the auricle**

| | Name of tumor | Typical sites and occurrence | Clinical features | Treatment | Prognosis | Additional features | Synonyms |
|---|---|---|---|---|---|---|---|
| Benign tumors | Kerato-acanthoma | Helix | Fast-growing reddish papule with central keratin plug | May clear spontaneously, otherwise excision | Good | Possible relationship to human papillomavirus | |
| | Seborrheic keratosis | Entire auricle, patients older than 60 years | Flat to exophytic papule, dark to light brown in color, sharply circumscribed, irregular shape and surface | Removal with a sharp curette in confirmed cases | Good, but new tumors are common | | Senile verruca, seborrheic verruca |
| | Atheroma | Retroauricular, often behind earlobe | Subcutaneous tumor, freely movable; secondary infection common | Elliptical excision, preceded by incision and drainage when infection is present | Recurs after incomplete removal | Cutaneous glandular retention cysts | Epidermal cyst |
| Premalignant lesions | Actinic keratosis | Helix or retroauricular site | Hyperkeratotic skin lesion, yellowish-brown with indistinct margins | Excision, curettage, cryosurgery, cytotoxic ointment | 10–20% show progression to squamous cell carcinoma | On a continuum with carcinoma in situ and carcinoma | Solar keratosis, senile keratosis |
| | Cutaneous horn | Lateral surface of auricle | Conical, dirty gray horny excrescence occurring on intact skin (**Fig. 10.19a**) | Excision | Good, rarely coexists with squamous cell carcinoma | May arise separately or in association with Bowen disease or carcinoma | Hypertrophic actinic keratosis |
| | Bowen's disease | Helical rim, lateral surface of auricle | Psoriaform plaque, reddish or reddish-brown, may be erosive or scaly | Complete excision | Obligate pre-malignant lesion | Carcinoma in situ of the epidermis | Intraepithelial epithelioma |
| Malignant tumors | Basal cell carcinoma | Entire auricle | Nodular-ulcerative form most common on the ear; firm tumor, reddish or pigmented, telangiectasias, possible central ulcer (**Fig. 10.19b**) | Complete excision with histologic control of margins | Good with complete excision; metastases are very rare | Cartilage invasion occurs relatively early | Basal cell epithelioma, basalioma |
| | Squamous cell carcinoma | Entire auricle, especially the borders of the helix and antihelix | Destructive, exophytic and endophytic tumor, may be hyperkeratotic or ulcerating, raised edges (**Fig. 10.19c**) | Complete excision with histologic control of margins, may require auricular resection; treatment of lymph nodes | Lymph-node metastases in 10–20% | Metastasis to regional lymph nodes (parotid, deep cervical), rarely hematogenous | Spinocellular carcinoma |
| | Malignant melanoma | Auricle and surroundings | Raised, pigmented macular lesion with irregular margins and nonuniform coloration | Complete excision, depending on depth of invasion (Clark level) | Malignant skin tumor | Various manifestations (lentigo maligna, nodular, superficial spreading lesion) | |

# 11  The Middle Ear

## 11.1  Anatomy, Physiology, and Examination of the Middle Ear

The middle ear, with its complex anatomy, occupies a central position in the temporal bone. Sound transmission by the ossicles and the ventilation of the temporal air cells via the eustachian tube are complex mechanisms, and disturbances of these mechanisms account for much of the pathology of the middle ear. This unit explores the anatomy and function of the middle ear in greater detail as a follow-up to ✎7.1 (Peripheral Auditory System, Middle Ear). Understanding these principles forms the basis for examination of the middle ear.

### Special Anatomy and Physiology of the Middle Ear

As noted in ✎7.1 (Peripheral Auditory System), the middle ear consists of three parts: the tympanic cavity bounded laterally by the tympanic membrane, the system of temporal bone air cells, and the eustachian tube. When the middle ear transmits sound waves (alternating variations in air pressure), it performs impedance matching by equalizing the differences in impedance (acoustic resistance) between the air and perilymph. The eustachian tube equalizes static differences in air pressure between the middle ear and external auditory canal.

### Tympanic Membrane

*Function:* The tympanic membrane (eardrum) has two functions: it gathers sound like the membrane of a microphone (see ✎7.1, Peripheral Auditory System), and it provides sonic shielding of the round window membrane. Sound waves that directly impinge on the round window can counteract the perilymphatic fluid displacement induced by the stapes, reducing the sensitivity of the cochlea.

*Anatomy:* The normal anatomy of the tympanic membrane is shown in **Fig. 11.1**. It consists of two portions called the *pars tensa* and *pars flaccida*. The much larger **pars tensa** is a funnel-shaped area stretched between the malleus handle and the bony ear canal. It is composed of three layers (**Fig. 11.2**):
- The outer layer of the pars tensa, called the *cutaneous layer*, consists of smooth, stratified squamous epithelium that normally reflects light.
- The inner layer bordering the tympanic cavity, called the *mucosal layer*, consists of a single layer of squamous epithelium.
- Between the outer and inner layers is the *lamina propria*. It consists of two layers of connective-tissue fibers: an outer layer of radially directed fibers (*radiate layer*) and an inner layer of circular fibers

**Fig. 11.1  Normal anatomy of the tympanic membrane**

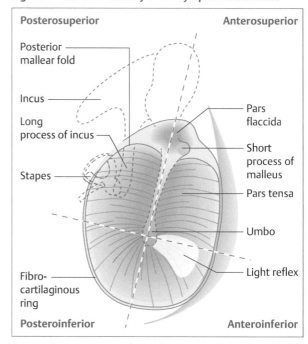

Posterosuperior — Anterosuperior
Posterior mallear fold
Incus
Long process of incus
Stapes
Fibro-cartilaginous ring
Posteroinferior — Anteroinferior
Pars flaccida
Short process of malleus
Pars tensa
Umbo
Light reflex

Otoscopic appearance of a right tympanic membrane. The longitudinal axis of the malleus handle and a line perpendicular to it divide the tympanic membrane into quadrants.

(*circular layer*). These fibers blend with the fibrocartilaginous ring at the circumference of the tympanic membrane. This ring anchors the tympanic membrane in the tympanic sulcus of the bony ear canal.

The **pars flaccida** (synonym: Shrapnell's membrane) is located superior to the malleolar folds. It cannot always be clearly identified at otoscopy and may blend with the superior canal wall. Microscopically, the pars flaccida lacks the reinforcing fibrous layers that are present in the pars tensa. As a result, this portion of the tympanic membrane often retracts first in response to negative pressure in the middle ear, creating an epithelial pocket.

## Tympanic Cavity

The aerated tympanic cavity (synonyms: middle ear space, middle ear cleft) allows for unrestricted mobility of the tympanic membrane, which is necessary for effective sound transmission. Most of the air enters the tympanic cavity through the eustachian tube, but some gases diffuse directly into the middle ear through blood vessels in the mucosa.

**Levels of the tympanic cavity:** The tympanic cavity (see **Fig. 7.1** and **Fig. 11.3**) is divided into three levels relative to the plane of the tympanic membrane:

- The portion of the tympanic cavity at the level of the tympanic membrane is called the *mesotympanum*. It contains the round window, the oval window with the stapes, and the promontory (bony prominence overlying the basal turn of the cochlea).
- Above the plane of the tympanic membrane is the *epitympanum* (synonyms: attic, epitympanic recess). The tympanic part of the facial nerve defines the boundary between the epi- and mesotympanum on the medial wall of the middle ear. The epitympanum contains the principal mass of the auditory ossicles with their associated ligaments and several mucosal folds. The epitympanum is small and contains little air, and inflammations may become encapsulated in that area. The epitympanum communicates with the mastoid antrum via the aditus ad antrum and also with the air cells of the mastoid process. The antrum contains the bony prominence of the lateral semicircular canal, which is often the first part of the labyrinth to be attacked by an osteoclastic disease process in the middle ear. A thin bony layer, the tegmen tympani, forms the roof of the epitympanum and separates it from the middle cranial fossa.
- Below the level of the tympanic membrane is the *hypotympanum* (synonym: hypotympanic recess). It borders on the bulb of the jugular vein and contains cells (tympanic cells) that communicate with the mastoid air cells.

**Auditory ossicles:** The ossicles in the middle ear have several distinctive features. They are the smallest bones in the human body and are freely suspended, being nourished entirely through their periosteal attachments. They are attached by thin tendons to the smallest muscles in the body, the intra-aural muscles (tensor tympani and stapedius).

The handle (manubrium) of the *malleus* is attached along its length to the tympanic membrane. The tip of the handle forms a central spoon-shaped depression, the umbo, which is an important landmark for evaluating the tympanic membrane.

The next bone in the ossicular chain is the *incus*, which articulates with the malleus. The head of the malleus and the body of the incus are located in the

**Fig. 11.2   Microscope structure of the tympanic membrane**

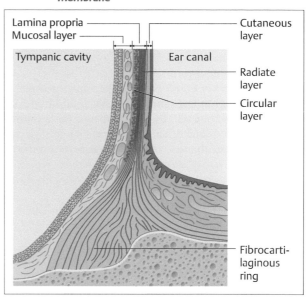

The shape and attachment of the pars tensa are determined by the radially and circularly arranged fiber layers and by the fibrocartilaginous ring (annulus).

**Fig. 11.3   Tympanic cavity**

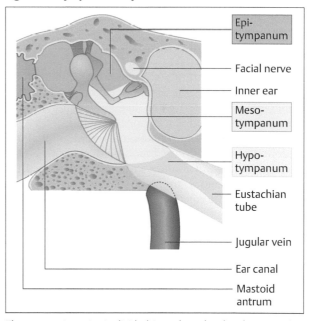

The tympanic cavity is divided into three levels relative to the plane of the tympanic membrane. Note the connection of the epitympanum (attic) to the mastoid cells and the connection of the hypotympanum to the eustachian tube.

epitympanum and comprise most of the mass of the auditory ossicles.

The long process of the incus articulates with the *stapes*. The footplate of the stapes is attached to the rim of the oval window by the elastic annular ligament, creating a movable interface between the stapes footplate and the perilymphatic space.

**Intra-aural muscles:** The *stapedius muscle* inserts onto the head of the stapes and occupies a bony canal parallel to the mastoid part of the facial nerve, which also innervates the muscle.

The *tensor tympani muscle* lies parallel to the eustachian tube and is innervated by the trigeminal nerve. It inserts onto the head of the malleus.

Reflex contractions of the intra-aural muscles (stapedial reflex, see ✏8.4, Objective Hearing Tests) may serve to moderate the internal noise level produced by mastication and speech, and it may also be a mechanism to protect the inner ear from high, sustained external noise levels.

**Anatomic relations of the tympanic cavity:** The cavity of the middle ear is surrounded by functionally and clinically important structures:

- The lateral wall is formed by the tympanic membrane and the bony ear canal.
- The medial wall borders the cochlea.
- The inferior wall borders the bulb of the jugular vein.
- The superior wall borders the dura of the middle cranial fossa.
- The anterior wall borders the internal carotid artery.
- The posterior wall borders the mastoid part of the facial nerve.

The tympanic cavity is traversed by the chorda tympani, which arises from the facial nerve and contains gustatory fibers for the anterior two-thirds of the tongue (see ✏14.1, Clinically Relevant Anatomy, Function, and Evaluation of the Facial Nerve).

**Blood supply and innervation:** The tympanic cavity receives its blood supply from various branches of the external carotid artery (middle meningeal artery, ascending pharyngeal artery, maxillary artery, and stylomastoid artery).

It derives most of its sensory innervation from the tympanic nerve, which arises from the glossopharyngeal nerve (see **Fig. 16.4**). This connection accounts for the "referred otalgia" that can occur in association with pharyngeal processes. The tympanic nerve also has connections with parasympathetic portions of the glossopharyngeal nerve, sympathetic fibers of the internal carotid plexus, and the trigeminal nerve.

### Air Cells of the Temporal Bone

The mucosa-lined air cells of the temporal bone all communicate with the tympanic cavity and, like the middle ear itself, are aerated via the eustachian tube. The *pneumatization of the mastoid* and other parts of the temporal bone develops gradually during childhood, similar to the development of the paranasal sinuses (see also ✏1.1, Paranasal Sinuses). The mastoid antrum and several adjacent air cells are generally present in infants. The degree of pneumatization that subsequently develops is variable and depends partly on the ventilation of the tympanic cavity, the function of the eustachian tube, and the inflammatory history of the middle ear. As a rule, few pneumatized cells develop in children who have a history of chronic otitis media. On the other hand, "normal" pneumatization of the temporal bone can have a broad range of appearances, analogous to the paranasal sinuses. With extensive pneumatization, the air cells may extend into the zygomatic arch, the temporal squama, and the petrous apex.

The *function* of the temporal bone air cells in humans is unknown. Perhaps, a greater air volume is better for equalizing pressure differences and thus can help to protect the middle ear. The air volume behind the tympanic membrane is unimportant for sound transmission in humans (unlike small rodents, for example, in which the air space of the tympanic cavity contributes more importantly to the physical properties of the sound-conducting apparatus in the middle ear).

### Eustachian Tube

The eustachian tube connects the tympanic cavity with the nasopharynx, where the inlet of the tube forms a funnel-shaped orifice behind the choana (see **Fig. 1.5**).

**Functions of the eustachian tube:**

- Ventilates the tympanic cavity and air cells.
- Equalizes pressure differences between the tympanic cavity and the atmosphere.
- Drains the middle ear spaces.
- Creates a barrier to ascending infection.

The eustachian tube runs more horizontally in *infants and small children* than in adults. It is considerably shorter and broader and consists of softer cartilage. Presumably, this compromises the overall function of the eustachian tube, accounting for the higher incidence of otitis media in children. By about 7 to 10 years of age, the eustachian tube closely approximates the adult tube in its anatomy and function.

**Anatomy (Fig. 11.4):** The lateral third of the eustachian tube framework consists of a bony canal that conveys the tube in addition to the tensor tympani muscle. The medial framework is a patent cartilaginous tube that is suspended from the skull base. The narrowest portion of the tube, called the *isthmus*, lies at the junction of the bony and cartilaginous parts. Inflammatory stenosis may develop at that location. The medial part of the tube is surrounded by fatty tissue, glands, veins, and muscles. It is actively opened by the tensor veli palatini muscle. Eustachian tube function in general relies on a complex balance between opening forces, such as muscle tone, middle ear pressure,

## Fig. 11.4 Eustachian tube

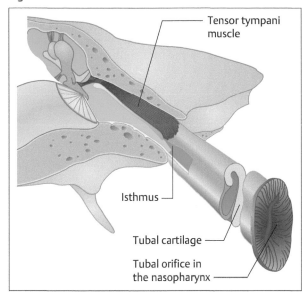

- Tensor tympani muscle
- Isthmus
- Tubal cartilage
- Tubal orifice in the nasopharynx

The eustachian tube consists of a bony part (lateral third) and a cartilaginous part (medial two-thirds). At their junction is the narrowest part of the tube, the isthmus.

and cartilage resilience, and closing forces generated by tissue pressure, mucosal surface tension, and a negative pressure in the middle ear.

## Examination

### History

There are no complaints that are specific to middle ear disease. Otalgia, aural discharge (otorrhea), a feeling of pressure, or hearing loss can occur with diseases of the external ear or inner ear. But a history of chronic inflammatory ear diseases usually signifies otitis media. This type of inflammation can lead to scarring and decreased ventilation of the middle ear. Before any otologic manipulations are performed, the patient should be asked specifically about *tympanic membrane perforation*, previous *trauma* to the ear, or any *surgery* of the middle ear. Most patients will be able to provide this information.

### Otoscopy

🗸 Otoscopy with evaluation of the tympanic membrane is the mainstay for the investigation of middle ear diseases.

The examination begins with **inspection** of the external ear and its surroundings, particularly the mastoid. The technique of otoscopy and normal tympanic membrane findings are covered in 📖8.1 and 📖10.1.

For the otologist, evaluation of the tympanic membrane with a stereoscopic microscope is essential for the diagnosis of middle ear diseases.
*Interpretation:* Normally, otoscopy will reveal nothing more of the middle ear than the lateral aspect of the tympanic membrane. A normal tympanic membrane has differentiated features, is mobile, and reflects light (see 📖8.1, Otoscopy). The mobility of the tympanic membrane provides clues to the condition and ventilation of the tympanic cavity.

**Function tests:**
Tympanic membrane mobility can be tested actively or passively during otoscopy.
*Passive mobility test:* The external ear canal is sealed with the speculum, and a positive pneumatic pressure is produced in the ear canal, causing movement of the tympanic membrane (Siegle's pneumatic otoscopy).
*Active mobility tests:* In active tests of tympanic membrane mobility, air is forced up the eustachian tube into the middle ear, inducing an outward movement of the tympanic membrane. Usually, this movement is most clearly appreciated in the posterosuperior quadrant (see **Fig. 11.1**). Since this also tests eustachian tube patency, the active mobility tests are particularly important for examination of the middle ear.
- In the Valsalva maneuver, the patient is told to swallow and then pinch the nostrils and "bear down" to produce a positive pressure in the pharynx.
- In the Politzer maneuver, air is forced into one side of the nose by squeezing an air bag while the other nostril is occluded and the soft palate is closed off.
- In the Toynbee maneuver, a negative pressure is created in the pharynx by having the patient swallow with the nostrils pinched shut. This induces an inward movement of the tympanic membrane.

🗸 None of these maneuvers should be used in patients with an acute inflammation of the middle ear or nasopharynx.

*Interpretation:* A negative Valsalva maneuver may be due to:
- Improper technique.
- A nonpatent eustachian tube.
- A thickened, scarred tympanic membrane.
- A perforated tympanic membrane.

When the tympanic membrane is perforated, there may be an audible rush of air through the opening. With drainage in the ear canal with a perforated tympanic membrane, the Valsalva maneuver may produce visible air bubbles—a strong suggestive sign of otitis media.

## Fig. 11.5 Normal computed tomography of the temporal bone

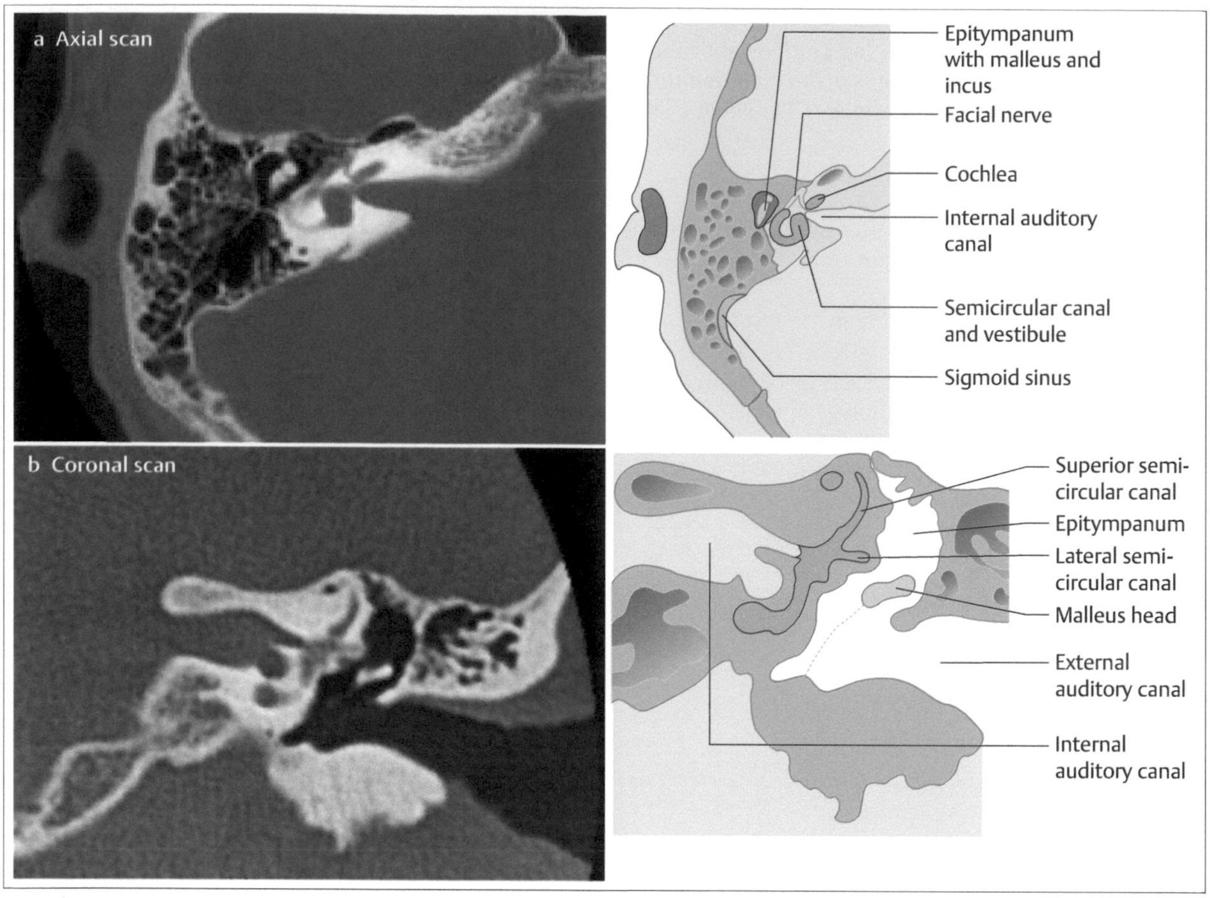

**a** Axial CT scan through a normal temporal bone. The epitympanum, containing the head of the malleus and body of the incus, is clearly defined. The ossicles resemble an ice cream cone.

**b** Coronal CT scan across the internal and external auditory canals. The middle and inner ear are clearly visualized.

## Hearing Tests

The typical clinical presentation of middle ear disease includes **conductive hearing loss**, in which Weber's test is lateralized to the affected ear and Rinne's test is negative (see ✍8.1, Clinical Hearing Tests).

*Pure-tone audiometry* shows a difference between bone conduction and air conduction thresholds (air–bone gap, see ✍8.3, Pure-Tone Audiometry: Threshold Determination).

*Tympanometry*, which can be performed only with an intact tympanic membrane, may show a flattening or shifting of the peak into the negative pressure region (type B and C tympanograms, see ✍8.4, Tympanometry). If the tympanogram is normal, the function of the ossicles can be assessed by testing the *stapedial reflex* (see ✍8.4, Stapedial Reflex).

Middle ear disease generally leads to an absence of *otoacoustic emissions* (OAEs; see ✍8.4, Otoacoustic Emissions), which cannot be transmitted laterally across the diseased middle ear.

The following findings, then, are indicative of **normal middle ear function:**
- Normal otoscopic appearance of the tympanic membrane.
- Positive Rinne's test.
- Normal tympanogram (type A) and a positive stapedial reflex.
- Detectable OAEs (assuming normal cochlear function).

## Imaging Studies

Since visual inspection of the middle ear is generally limited to the tympanic membrane, imaging studies are an important adjunct to function tests. Radiographic studies are the most rewarding due to the preponderance of bony structures.

**Standard projections** of the temporal bone will invariably superimpose numerous structures. This problem can be reduced by obtaining *special views* of the temporal bone in which fewer structures are superimposed, such as Schüller's or Stenvers' view.

Even with special views, several structures are still superimposed and essential fine details in the middle ear may be obscured. Thus, conventional radiographs are of limited value due to their relatively poor sensitivity and specificity.

**Computed tomography:** The most important modality for temporal bone imaging is *high-resolution three-dimensional computed tomography (CT)*, which is able to define specific bony structures for specific investigations (**Fig. 11.5**). Slice thickness of 0.4 to 0.6 mm provides enough details in general. Contrast administration is rarely necessary in examinations of the middle ear alone, with the important exception when complications are suspected.

**Other imaging modalities:** *Magnetic resonance imaging (MRI)* is used less frequently for middle ear imaging because it is inferior to CT for defining bony structures. It can be helpful, however, for selected indications such as tumors and suspected otitis; also, diffusion-weighted MRI (DW-MRI) can be used for the detection of cholesteatoma. Similarly, *angiography* is used specifically for investigating tumors, suspected vascular lesions, pulsatile tinnitus, etc.

*Cone-beam computed tomography (CBCT)* can be used as an alternative to CT for examination of the bony structures of the middle ear.

## Diagnostic Tympanotomy

Surgical exploration of the middle ear (tympanotomy) is also available as a diagnostic option. The tympanic cavity is opened for inspection through the ear canal under an operating microscope by incising the canal skin in front of the tympanic membrane and reflecting the skin and membrane as a flap. Endoscopes can be applied additionally and the bony canal wall may have to be taken down, depending on the pathology. In most cases, diagnostic tympanotomy is combined with the surgical correction of any abnormalities that were noted in preoperative studies.

# 11.2 Pathophysiology and Otoscopic Features of Otitis Media

This 🐟 explores the relationships between the development of chronic inflammatory middle ear diseases and the resulting chronic structural changes ("scars") that are accessible to otoscopic examination. The central elements in the pathophysiology of otitis media are impaired ventilation and mucosal inflammation in the middle ear. They lead to typical changes in the tympanic membrane, various clinical forms of chronic otitis media, and functional sequelae. It is important to distinguish between the inflammatory disease process itself and its sequelae, which often persist after the disease has resolved. The disease processes and associated clinical manifestations of otitis media are described in the next 🐟.

## Pathophysiology of Otitis Media

The most common pathologic process in the middle ear is inflammation, termed *otitis media*. Regardless of its clinical presentation, otitis media is the product of fundamental pathophysiologic processes that can produce several typical otoscopic changes (see Otoscopic Features of Otitis Media below).

### General

The pathophysiology of most chronic middle ear diseases is based largely on two functional disturbances: impaired middle ear ventilation and inflammation. These mechanisms are closely interrelated and often cannot be separated from each other in any given case. A chronic impairment of middle ear ventilation leads to inflammation of the mucosa, which in turn compromises eustachian tube function and middle ear ventilation (**Fig. 11.6**). This vicious cycle is a pivotal element in most inflammatory conditions of the middle ear.

### Causes of Impaired Ventilation

Impaired ventilation of the middle ear is almost always caused by eustachian tube dysfunction. Decreased tubal patency is more common in this regard than excessive patency. Various factors can compromise the ventilating function of the eustachian tube:

- Stenosis of the tube lumen due to inflammatory *mucosal swelling* (e.g., caused by an upper respiratory viral infection). The air in the tympanic cavity is absorbed, and a negative pressure develops that further compromises eustachian tube function.
- A *negative pressure* can also develop in a healthy middle ear due to a rapid rise of ambient air pressure, as during an aircraft landing (see 🐟 11.4, Barotrauma of the Middle Ear). The mucosa of the eustachian tube collapses, and the negative pressure itself incites mucosal swelling.
- *Extrinsic obstruction* of the tube, as by a tumor.

- *Deficient active opening* of the tube by the tensor veli palatini muscle. The special anatomy of the eustachian tube in small children (see 🐟 11.1, Eustachian Tube) hampers the function of the tensor veli palatini. Malformations of the jaw and palate can further compromise or even disable the tube-opening muscles, resulting in chronic inflammation of the middle ear.
- A congenital or acquired *bony stenosis* or *stricture* due to scarring.

Excessive patency of the eustachian tube may also cause a negative pressure to develop in certain compartments of the middle ear. The negative pressure during inspiration is transmitted through the patent tube into the tympanic cavity. This negative-pressure effect is magnified when air is forcibly inhaled through the nose (sniffing), which may be done habitually. As mucosal folds are raised in the middle ear, a chronic negative pressure may develop, especially in the epitympanum, leading to retraction of the tympanic membrane and chronic inflammation.

### Infection and Inflammation

Infections and noninfectious inflammations play another key role in the pathogenesis of otitis media.
**Adenoiditis:** Initial contact with microorganisms and environmental agents in infants and small children can induce intensive immunologic-inflammatory changes affecting the tissues in Waldeyer's ring. The adenoids (pharyngeal tonsils) are particularly important in the development of otitis media. The size of the adenoids is of relatively minor importance because the adenoids rarely, if ever, cause direct mechanical obstruction of the eustachian tube. The problem, rather, is chronic adenoiditis, which creates a reservoir for pathogenic microorganisms and induces adenoid hyperplasia. Adenoiditis is promoted in turn by obstructed nasal breathing and by rhinitis or rhinosinusitis.

**Fig. 11.6 Pathophysiology of chronic otitis media**

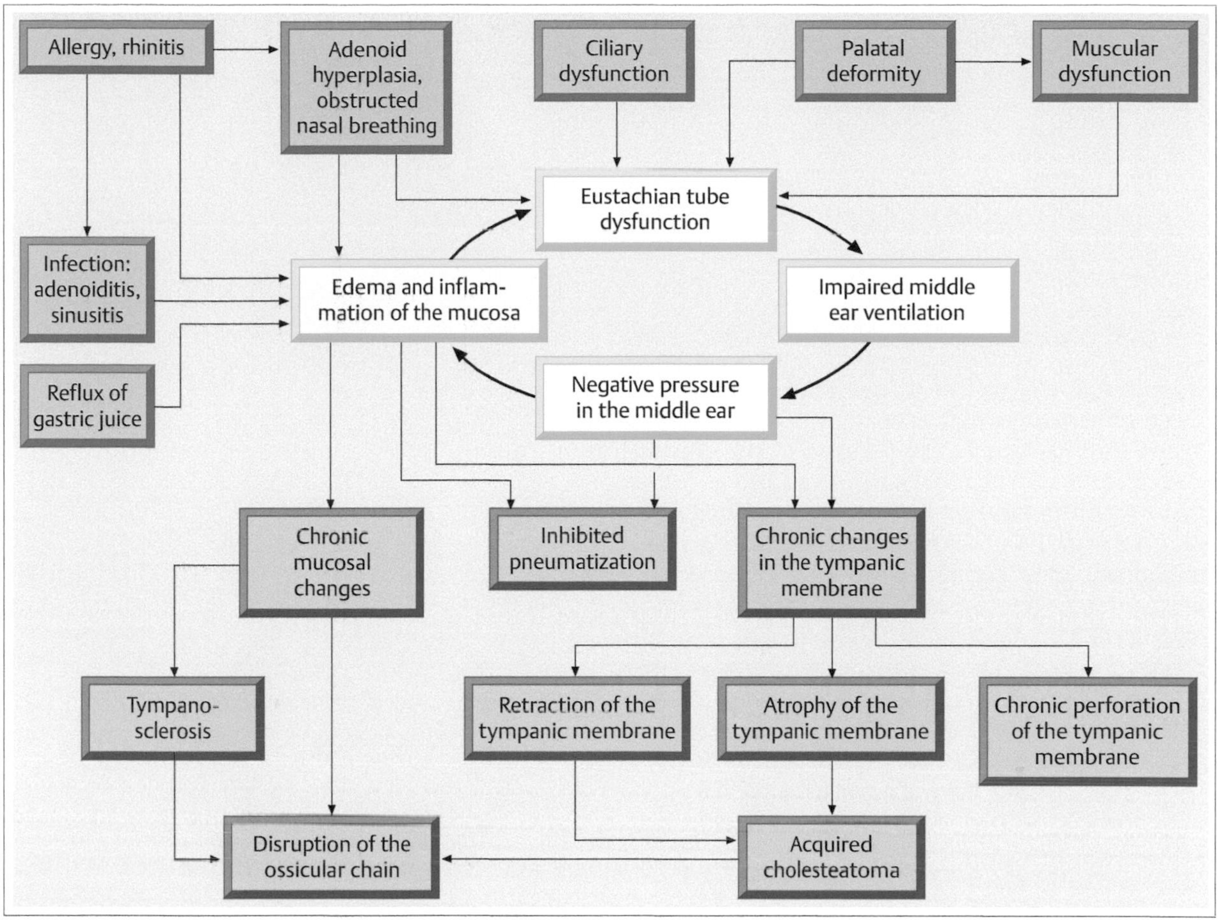

```
┌─────────────┐     ┌─────────────┐   ┌─────────────┐   ┌─────────────┐   ┌─────────────┐
│Allergy,     │────▶│Adenoid      │   │Ciliary      │   │Palatal      │   │Muscular     │
│rhinitis     │     │hyperplasia, │   │dysfunction  │   │deformity    │──▶│dysfunction  │
└─────────────┘     │obstructed   │   └─────────────┘   └─────────────┘   └─────────────┘
                    │nasal        │
                    │breathing    │
                    └─────────────┘
                           
                    ┌──────────────────────────┐
                    │Eustachian tube           │
                    │dysfunction               │
                    └──────────────────────────┘

┌─────────────┐     ┌──────────────────┐        ┌──────────────────┐
│Infection:   │────▶│Edema and inflam- │        │Impaired middle   │
│adenoiditis, │     │mation of the     │        │ear ventilation   │
│sinusitis    │     │mucosa            │        └──────────────────┘
└─────────────┘     └──────────────────┘

┌─────────────┐     ┌──────────────────┐
│Reflux of    │     │Negative pressure │
│gastric juice│     │in the middle ear │
└─────────────┘     └──────────────────┘

┌──────────┐   ┌──────────────┐   ┌──────────────┐
│Chronic   │   │Inhibited     │   │Chronic changes│
│mucosal   │   │pneumatization│   │in the tympanic│
│changes   │   └──────────────┘   │membrane      │
└──────────┘                      └──────────────┘

┌──────────┐   ┌──────────────┐   ┌──────────────┐   ┌──────────────┐
│Tympano-  │   │Retraction of │   │Atrophy of the│   │Chronic       │
│sclerosis │   │the tympanic  │   │tympanic      │   │perforation of│
└──────────┘   │membrane      │   │membrane      │   │the tympanic  │
               └──────────────┘   └──────────────┘   │membrane      │
                                                      └──────────────┘

┌──────────────┐              ┌──────────────┐
│Disruption of │              │Acquired      │
│the ossicular │              │cholesteatoma │
│chain         │              └──────────────┘
└──────────────┘
```

The central pathophysiologic process is eustachian tube dysfunction interacting with a chronic inflammation of the middle ear mucosa (shown in green). Various causal factors (red) can initiate this cycle, which in turn can have various sequelae (blue).

**Infections of the middle ear mucosa:** Viral and bacterial infections of the upper respiratory tract, which are common in children, can also directly affect the middle ear mucosa. They have a tendency to ascend through the eustachian tube into the middle ear (tubogenic infection). With a perforated tympanic membrane, gram-negative bacteria in particular can also enter the middle ear from the external canal, inciting an acute otitis media or perpetuating a chronic inflammation.

**Noninfectious inflammations:** Allergic or toxic inflammations of the upper respiratory tract contribute to adenoiditis and nasal airway obstruction or (less commonly) may spread to involve the middle ear mucosa. The reflux of gastric juice may also contribute to the inflammation. This mechanism may be particularly important in infants and small children who have a short eustachian tube that offers little protection.

## Otoscopic Features of Otitis Media

The pathophysiologic processes described above are difficult to detect directly by clinical means. They do produce typical effects, however (see **Fig. 11.6**), that can be detected by otoscopic inspection. We are dealing with a descriptive classification in which specific pathologic significance cannot be ascribed to the observed changes.

First, it is helpful to distinguish changes in the external ear canal from changes in the middle ear (see 📖 10.1, Anatomy). Both can produce similar tympanic membrane changes, and the cause is often not easy to recognize. The history and other findings generally provide an adequate basis for differentiation, however. Otoscopic changes in the middle ear are classified into *acute inflammatory, chronic inflammatory,* and *cicatricial* changes. The presence of one type of change does not exclude any of the others. For example, a cicatricial change (scar) may also be acutely or chronically inflamed.

## Acute Inflammatory Changes

An acute inflammation of the middle ear generally incites acute inflammatory changes in the tympanic membrane. The eardrum is thickened, erythematous, and less transparent than normal (**Fig. 11.7**).

🖋 The transparency of the tympanic membrane shows individual variations even when the membrane is not inflamed, and so this is not a reliable sign.

The swelling and thickening of the tympanic membrane give it an irregular surface that is no longer smooth and reflective, but *opaque*. The typical light reflex is either absent or fragmented.

When fluid collects in the middle ear, the tympanic membrane may bulge outward. This *bulging* is often first evident in the pars flaccida. As the inflammation progresses and the fluid pressure rises, the tympanic membrane may become perforated. Generally, the perforation begins in a small area of the eardrum, allowing the fluid to drain into the ear canal. If an open connection exists between the acutely inflamed middle ear mucosa and the discharge in front of the tympanic membrane, pulsations may be transmitted from the inflamed mucosa. *Pulsatile discharge* in the ear canal is therefore indicative of acute otitis media.

## Middle Ear Effusion

A *middle ear effusion* is a fluid collection in the middle ear without a perforated tympanic membrane and with no signs of acute inflammation (**Fig. 11.8**).

**Partial middle ear effusion:** Air bubbles or an air–fluid level behind the tympanic membrane signifies the entry of air, confirming at least some degree of ventilation through the eustachian tube. Generally, then, a partial effusion in the middle ear signifies a subacute, serous inflammation with a good prognosis. This type of effusion is typically found after viral infections of the upper respiratory tract.

**Complete middle ear effusions** devoid of air can be detected indirectly by noting an immobile tympanic membrane at otoscopy or by recording a flat tympanogram (see **Fig. 8.19b**). Most of these effusions are chronic and become increasingly mucoid as the mucosa forms increased numbers of goblet cells. The color of the effusion changes from amber to grayish, dark, or blue.

🖋 The color of the effusion is not a reliable criterion for assessing the duration or composition of a middle ear effusion.

**Fig. 11.7    Acute inflammation of the tympanic membrane**

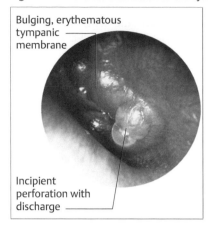

Bulging, erythematous tympanic membrane

Incipient perforation with discharge

Otoscopic findings in acute otitis media. The left tympanic membrane is bulging and erythematous. Incipient perforation with discharge is evident in the posteroinferior quadrant.

**Fig. 11.8    Partial middle ear effusion**

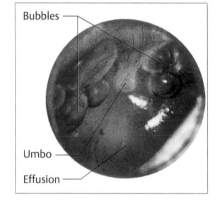

Bubbles

Umbo

Effusion

Serous effusion behind an intact, not thickened tympanic membrane, which is slightly retracted. Air bubbles are clearly visible.

## Chronic Tympanic Membrane Perforation

**Findings:** A tympanic membrane perforation without acute inflammatory changes is usually easy to detect at otoscopy (see **Fig. 11.15a**). Basically, the tympanic membrane has a strong capacity for self-healing, and even large perforations can heal spontaneously. But various cicatricial and atrophic changes in the middle ear can result in a nonhealing perforation, which is considered a hallmark *of chronic suppurative otitis media*. The tympanic cavity is visible through the perforation. The remaining tympanic membrane and the tympanic cavity can have various otoscopic appearances:

- Cicatricial, noninflammatory change.
- Chronic inflammatory changes with thickened, hyperplastic mucosa and a mucous discharge.
- Acute inflammatory change with marked erythema and a purulent discharge (see **Fig. 11.15b**).

**Sequelae of tympanic membrane perforation:** A chronic tympanic membrane perforation can contribute to the resolution of chronic otitis media, but it can also pose a hazard. The following adverse sequelae may occur:

- *Recurrent infections* of the middle ear may develop via the external canal, with associated recurrent otorrhea. This may also adversely affect the inner ear (serous labyrinthitis, see 12.2, Labyrinthitis).
- The degree of *conductive hearing loss* depends on the size and location of the perforation.
- A *cholesteatoma* may form due to the ingrowth of squamous epithelium into the middle ear. Cholesteatomas usually develop from atrophic epithelial pockets in the tympanic membrane or from a *marginal perforation*. They rarely develop with a dry, central perforation that does not reach the fibrocartilaginous ring.

A chronic tympanic membrane perforation can also have desirable effects:

- A chronic perforation can contribute to the healing of mucosal inflammation, since it provides a route for *middle ear ventilation*.
- The perforation also provides a route for fluid drainage from the middle ear, resulting in *relief of pain*.

The adverse sequelae predominate in most cases, however, and surgical closure of the perforation (especially with intact eustachian tube function) is indicated (myringoplasty or tympanoplasty, see 11.1).

## Atrophic Scars of the Tympanic Membrane

A perforated tympanic membrane may undergo incomplete healing and scarring that cover over the perforation. This is particularly likely to occur after a chronic inflammation of the tympanic membrane. The lamina propria can no longer reconstitute its normal fibrous structure, and consequently this layer is thin or absent; the tympanic membrane loses its normal strength and tension. Various conditions may ensue, depending on the size of the atrophic scar and the ventilation of the middle ear, and these conditions have varying otoscopic appearances:

**Circumscribed atrophic scar** (Fig. 11.9): Only part of the tympanic membrane is atrophic, usually an area located in the posterosuperior quadrant. With normal middle ear ventilation and eustachian tube function, the scar lies in the anatomic plane of the tympanic membrane. The atrophic area is abnormally mobile in response to pneumatic otoscopy or a Valsalva maneuver.

**Fig. 11.9 Atrophic scars of the tympanic membrane**

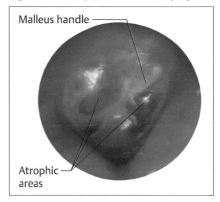

Malleus handle

Atrophic areas

Right tympanic membrane is heavily scarred but intact. Most of the scarring is atrophic.

**Fig. 11.10 Partial atelectasis of the middle ear**

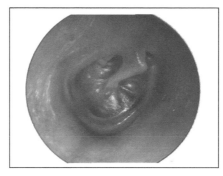

A right-sided, overall atrophic tympanic membrane is severely retracted into the tympanic cavity. The long process of the incus is clearly visible in the upper posterior quadrant.

**Retraction pocket:** A circumscribed atrophic scar in the tympanic membrane is retracted inward by a negative pressure in the tympanic cavity. A sustained negative pressure causes the pocket to expand in the middle ear. At some sites in the pocket, the epithelium can no longer migrate laterally into the ear canal. The trapped, stagnant squamous debris may then become infected, resulting in the formation of a cholesteatoma (see 11.3, Chronic Otitis Media with Cholesteatoma).

**Middle ear atelectasis (Fig. 11.10):** The entire tympanic membrane is thin and markedly retracted. The tympanic cavity is no longer aerated, and the fine squamous epithelium of the tympanic membrane lines the mesotympanum. Occasionally, it is difficult to distinguish a complete tympanic membrane perforation from middle ear atelectasis by otoscopic examination.

## Sclerosis and Fibrosis

Besides atrophic scars, fibrous and sclerotic scars can also form in the middle ear. The following types are distinguished according to the nature and location of the scars.

**Sclerotic tympanic membrane scar:** The fibrous lamina propria of the tympanic membrane shows typical calcific deposits that are clearly recognized as white areas (**Fig. 11.11**). With a normal position of the tympanic membrane and normal middle ear ventilation, sclerotic scars have no adverse sequelae and do not cause hearing impairment.

**Tympanosclerosis:** The sclerosis predominantly affects the tympanic cavity in addition to the tympanic membrane. Calcium deposits form in the middle ear mucosa and can cause ossicular fixation with associated impairment of sound conduction. Tympanosclerosis has a strong tendency to recur after surgical treatment, which often provides only a temporary improvement in hearing.

**Fibrosis:** This refers to extensive scarring of the tympanic membrane or, more commonly, the tympanic cavity in the absence of calcifications. The sequelae and otoscopic findings are similar to those in tympanosclerosis.

**Fig. 11.11    Sclerotic scar of the tympanic membrane**

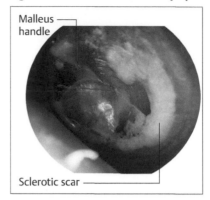

Malleus handle

Sclerotic scar

Left tympanic membrane has a sclerotic scar in its posteroinferior quadrant. Atrophic areas are also evident.

# 11.3   Otitis Media

The most common diseases of the middle ear are inflammations. Infections play a major role in these diseases. As explained in the previous section, otitis media and impaired middle ear ventilation are closely interrelated. This 📖 focuses on the various inflammatory conditions that can affect the middle ear and their immediate sequelae in the form of inflammatory complications. Chronic structural sequelae ("scars") were described in the preceding 📖.

## Classification and Terminology

The classification of otitis media (middle ear inflammation) is not standardized, and the terminology is diverse and not always logical. We showed in the previous section that the various forms of otitis media are on a continuum. For example, acute otitis media is generally followed by several weeks of middle ear effusion like that occurring in otitis media with effusion. But unlike acute otitis media, otitis media with effusion does not necessarily present with initial pain, and it may progress to acute otitis media when an acute infection supervenes.

Nevertheless, various inflammatory conditions of the middle ear or phenotypes of otitis media can be distinguished clinically, and these entities will be described separately below. The terminology in this unit is based on an international consensus of proposed and accepted terms.

## Myringitis

As the boundary between the external and middle ear, the tympanic membrane rarely develops an isolated inflammation. An inflammation of the tympanic membrane, called *myringitis*, usually develops in association with otitis externa or otitis media (see below). The principal diseases that can lead to a more or less isolated form of myringitis, such as bullous otitis, were covered in Chapter 10 (see 📖 10.4).

## Acute Otitis Media

*Epidemiology:* Acute otitis media is a common disease in infants and small children but can occur at any age. More than 50% of infants experience one or more episodes of acute otitis media during their first year of life. This increases to about 80% by 3 years of age.

*Pathogenesis:* The disease is generally caused by an infection that ascends to the middle ear through the eustachian tube. Bacteria can be isolated from the middle ear in approximately two-thirds of cases. The main causative organisms are *Streptococcus pneumoniae*, *Haemophilus influenzae*, and *Branhamella catarrhalis*. One-third of cases are probably caused by respiratory viruses. Adenoids are a frequent nidus for middle ear infections in children, even if they are not enlarged.

*Factors that increase or reduce risk:* Besides craniofacial anomalies, several risk factors for acute otitis media have been identified in children. A previous episode of acute otitis media or the presence of chronic serous otitis media will increase the risk for a recurrence of acute otitis media. Parental smoking is a proven risk factor. Siblings and the attendance of infants and small children at daycare centers are also known to increase the risk and may expose children to a more harmful microbiological flora.

On the other hand, extending the period of breast-feeding has been shown to lower the childhood risk of acute otitis media.

*Symptoms:* Acute otitis media is nearly always preceded by a viral infection of the upper respiratory tract. The initial symptom is a severe earache, which in babies may be manifested by rubbing the affected ear or by nonspecific disease symptoms. Fever is usually present during the first 24 hours. In infants, nonspecific symptoms such as irritability, vomiting, or diarrhea may be the dominant features. Perforation of the tympanic membrane is manifested by aural discharge and by an improvement or resolution of otalgia.

*Diagnosis:* On **physical examination**, the mastoid shows no swelling but may be moderately tender to pressure.

**Otoscopy** reveals an opaque, thickened, erythematous, and sometimes bulging tympanic membrane (see **Fig. 11.12** and **Fig. 11.7**). The tympanic membrane is immobile by pneumatic otoscopy; a Valsalva maneuver should not be performed. Otoscopy may be difficult in children due to cerumen in the ear canal and fussy behavior.

The typical features of **conductive hearing loss** are also present.

Generally, a **bacteriologic examination** is not performed when the tympanic membrane is intact, but it should always be done in patients with a spontaneous

**Fig. 11.12 Acute otitis media (AOM)**

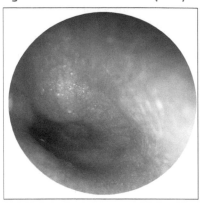

Bulging, thickened, undifferentiated left tympanic membrane in acute otitis media.

perforation or paracentesis. *Paracentesis for a bacteriologic examination* is indicated in immunocompromised patients and treatment failures, as well as if complications arise.

*Differential diagnosis:* Acute otitis media must be distinguished from other forms of otitis. It should be differentiated from otitis externa and from an acute exacerbation of chronic otitis media, particularly in a draining ear with a perforated tympanic membrane.

*Course:* Spontaneous perforation of the tympanic membrane may occur. After the acute phase of the inflammation has subsided, a residual inflammatory effusion will persist in the tympanic cavity for several weeks, with associated conductive hearing loss.

*Complications:* Complications are rare. The most common is acute mastoiditis, but any of the otogenic complications described below may occur.

*Treatment:* Nonsteroidal anti-inflammatory analgesics or acetaminophen is given for pain relief. Decongestant nose drops or irrigations may be necessary for relieving nasal airway obstruction.

ᑫ Unobstructed nasal breathing improves the drainage function of the eustachian tube.

If the diagnosis of acute otitis media is certain, if the child is younger than 2 years, if the tympanic membrane is perforated, or if serious illness is present, immediate antibiotic therapy is started. With less serious illness, recovery without antibiotic therapy can be awaited for 1 to 2 days. Antibiotics should be continued for 7 to 10 days and should be active against the main pathogens listed above. If there is no response to the antibiotic or if signs and symptoms worsen within 48 hours, a different antibiotic should be tried. If improvement is unsatisfactory, paracentesis should be performed to obtain a sample for bacteriologic examination.

*Prophylaxis:* Risk factors should be avoided whenever possible, and the breastfeeding of infants should be prolonged. Vaccination against *S. pneumoniae* seems to reduce the frequency of acute otitis media.

## Recurrent Acute Otitis Media

*Definition:* The occurrence of four or more episodes of acute otitis media in 1 year, or three episodes in 6 months, is classified as recurrent acute otitis media. The middle ear heals and effusions in the tympanic cavity clear between episodes.

*Epidemiology:* Recurrent acute otitis media is a disease of infants and small children. It occurs in approximately 10% of children who have had a previous bout of acute otitis media.

*Etiopathogenesis:* The pathogenesis of the individual episodes is basically the same as in acute otitis media (see ᑫ11.2), but with a greater prevalence of risk factors.

*Symptoms, diagnosis, and course:* The individual episodes run the same course as a single bout of acute otitis media. An allergy should be excluded if the history is suspicious for an allergic reaction. The course and complications of the episodes are basically the same as described for acute otitis media.

*Differential diagnosis:* It is difficult to distinguish recurrent acute otitis media from repeated acute infections in a setting of chronic otitis media with effusion. This differentiation can be made only by detecting a normally aerated tympanic cavity after each acute episode.
The exclusion of acquired or congenital cholesteatoma is particularly important in these cases, but is often difficult.
Chronic otitis media with a perforated tympanic membrane and recurrent flare-ups can also have a similar clinical presentation.

*Treatment:* The episodes are treated the same as an isolated bout of acute otitis media. Additionally, there are several actions that can be taken to prevent new recurrences:
• Prophylactic antibiotics are effective but controversial due to the development of resistance.
• Vaccinations against pneumococci can help to prevent new episodes.

ᑫ Otitis media is caused by different *Haemophilus* strains than meningitis and therefore is not prevented by *Haemophilus* vaccinations.

- An adenotomy can decrease the bacterial burden in the nasopharynx and improve eustachian tube function. The placement of a ventilation tube in the tympanic cavity can improve middle ear ventilation.

## Otitis Media with Effusion

Synonyms: secretory otitis media, serous otitis media, mucoid otitis media, glue ear

*Definition:* Otitis media with effusion (OME) refers to an inflammatory effusion behind an intact tympanic membrane that is not associated with acute otologic symptoms or systemic signs. The process may be classified as acute (effusion lasting up to 3 weeks), subacute (up to 3 months), or chronic (more than 3 months).

### In Children

*Epidemiology:* OME is the most common ear disease in preschool-age children and one of the most common diseases overall. Approximately 3 to 4% of children have the chronic form. Generally, both ears are affected.

*Etiopathogenesis:*
See ✑11.2.

*Symptoms:* Acute symptoms are usually absent in children. The major symptom is **hearing loss**, but the children themselves rarely report this. Speech and language developmental delay and perceptual impairment may occur, particularly in bilateral cases.

*Diagnosis:* The diagnosis is made otoscopically and by tympanometry. The tympanic membrane often appears *opaque, thickened*, and occasionally *retracted* (**Fig. 11.13**, see also **Fig. 11.10**). Its color may be pale, reddish, yellowish, or bluish, depending on the effusion. Pneumatic otoscopy showed decreased or absent mobility of the tympanic membrane.

Fig. 11.13  **Otitis media with effusion (OME)**

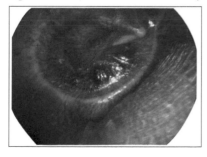

Right-sided middle ear effusion behind a thickened and retracted tympanic membrane with chronic inflammatory signs.

The tympanogram is a graphic record of tympanic membrane mobility. It may show a flat curve (type B) or occasionally a negative-pressure peak (type C) in mild and acute cases (see ✑8.4, Tympanometry). A tympanogram should be recorded to provide a baseline for follow-up.

*Differential diagnosis:* Other diagnoses are rare in children, but a cholesteatoma behind an intact tympanic membrane should be considered if the case has an unusual appearance or runs an atypical course.

*Complications:* The most frequent complication is acute otitis media, from which other otogenic complications may arise.

*Treatment:* The **acute or subacute form** is treated conservatively in an effort to improve nasal breathing and eustachian tube function. This may include the short-term use of decongestant nose drops, moisturizing and hygienic measures, or occasional topical steroids. The value of antibiotic therapy is controversial. Middle ear ventilation can also be improved by having the patient inflate balloons with the nose. Risk factors for otitis media should be curtailed or eliminated as much as possible.

The **chronic form** of OME should be treated surgically if significant hearing loss is present. *Paracentesis* (incision of the tympanic membrane) provides access for aspirating the effusion, which will immediately restore normal hearing. Ordinarily, the incision will close spontaneously in 1 to 2 weeks, allowing a new fluid collection to form. This can be prevented by inserting a ventilation tube or myringotomy tube (**Fig. 11.14**); this creates a "chronic" perforation and provides ventilation of the tympanic cavity through the external ear canal. A myringotomy tube will not impair hearing but is associated with a risk of middle ear infection from the ear canal.

Adenotomy may be performed additionally at the time of paracentesis. Various strategies can be applied using various combinations of these measures.

*Prognosis: Unilateral* OME has a good prognosis and should resolve within 3 months. Since speech hearing is less impaired, a conservative approach can often be taken in these cases. The detection of air in the middle ear (bubbles, air–fluid level) is also considered a good prognostic sign, as it confirms partial function of the eustachian tube (see also ✑11.2, Otoscopic Features of Otitis Media).

A greatly thickened tympanic membrane and a symptom duration that exceeds 3 months indicate a protracted course for most cases. A rapid cure is unlikely, and generally these cases should be managed surgically.

**Fig. 11.14  Myringotomy tube**

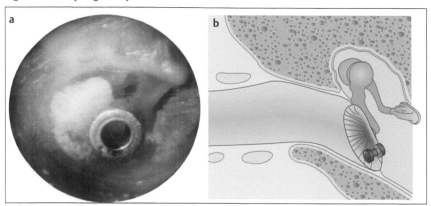

Placed in the anteroinferior quadrant of the tympanic membrane, the myringotomy tube provides ventilation of the tympanic cavity through the ear canal.

### In Adults

*Etiopathogenesis (see also ☜11.2):*
OME is basically the same disease in adults as in children. In adults, however, it is necessary to consider certain causes of eustachian tube dysfunction that are not a factor in children, such as sleep apnea syndrome and tumors of the nasopharynx. Conversely, adenoid hyperplasia and chronic adenoiditis have little importance in adults.

*Symptoms:* Patients complain of a clogged or pressure sensation in the affected ear. Pain is rarely present. Some patients complain of a popping or sloshing sound. Unlike small children, adults tend to find the hearing loss and pressure sensation very troublesome.

*Diagnosis:* A **history** of a cold often precedes the complaints.
OME is diagnosed **otoscopically** (see also ☜11.2). This examination reveals an opaque tympanic membrane with very poor mobility. A Valsalva maneuver either does not force air into the tympanic cavity or does so only with difficulty. The effusion in the tympanic cavity is easily recognized when air is present (bubbles, level) but is often difficult to appreciate with a complete middle ear effusion.
**Hearing tests** show the presence of conductive hearing loss. Weber's test is lateralized to the affected ear in unilateral cases, and Rinne's test is negative. Tympanography yields a flat curve. Pure-tone audiometry indicates an air–bone gap, and otoacoustic emissions are absent.

  ☝ If a middle ear effusion persists for more than 3 weeks, an endoscopic examination of the nose and nasopharynx should be performed to exclude a tumor.

*Differential diagnosis:* Bullous otitis externa should be considered as a special cause of middle ear effusion.

The differential diagnosis also includes other causes of conductive hearing loss with an intact tympanic membrane, such as otosclerosis and ossicular chain disruption. Effusions can also result from barotrauma, a cerebrospinal fluid (CSF) leak from the lateral skull base, or tumors of the temporal bone. A perilymphatic fistula generally leads to inner ear symptoms.
The patent eustachian tube syndrome can produce similar complaints, but conductive hearing loss is absent and the tympanic membrane is mobile.

*Complications:* A bacterial, generally ascending infection can develop leading to acute otitis media and its complications. A serous labyrinthitis may develop via the round or oval window.

*Treatment:* Acute and subacute OME are treated conservatively as in children. Emphasis is placed on relieving nasal airway obstruction and treating infections of the nose and paranasal sinuses. The patient should be instructed to perform regular Valsalva maneuvers.
If the disease persists for more than 3 months and the tympanic membrane becomes markedly thickened, there is little chance that the inflammatory effusion will resolve any time soon. Surgical treatment is recommended for these cases, and a myringotomy tube should be inserted if conductive hearing loss is present.

*Prognosis:* The prognosis is good in general and in cases with a nonspecific cause. Unilateral middle ear effusions with air bubbles or an air–fluid level almost always have a good prognosis, and the otitis media should resolve within 3 months.

## Chronic Suppurative Otitis Media

*Definition and general information:*
A tympanic membrane perforation will usually heal spontaneously in a few weeks. A nonhealing perfora-

**Fig. 11.15 Chronic suppurative otitis media**

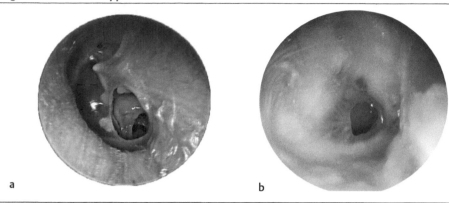

a

b

**a** Dry chronic perforation in the posterior quadrants of a left tympanic membrane. The long process of the incus, the promontory, and the round window niche are visible.
**b** Chronic perforation of the tympanic membrane with purulent discharge.

tion is almost certainly the result of chronic inflammation. Chronic otitis media, then, should be diagnosed in the presence of a **chronic tympanic membrane perforation**, even if there are no active signs of mucosal inflammation. If a specific infection or cholesteatoma can be excluded, the disease should be classified as **chronic suppurative otitis media**. This process may be **dry** (**Fig. 11.15a**), and thus without active inflammatory signs such as pain, discharge, and swelling of the mucosa. If discharge is present, it is classified as a **wet** or **draining form** (**Fig. 11.15b**). Generally, this means that bacteria have infected the middle ear through the nonintact tympanic membrane. This type of infection may occur **acutely** and resolve quickly, or it may become **chronic** (chronic mucosal suppuration). Thus, the clinical manifestations and otoscopic appearance of chronic suppurative otitis media tend to change over the course of the disease.

***Etiopathogenesis (see also ✎ 11.2):***
The pathogenesis is usually multifactorial. The following factors play a role:
- Chronic inflammation secondary to eustachian tube dysfunction.
- Genetic and constitutional factors that affect the healing capacity and resistance of the mucosa.
- Special anatomic characteristics of the middle ear spaces such as pneumatization and relative sizes.
- The nature, pathogenicity, virulence, and resistance of the infecting organisms.

***Symptoms:*** Chronic suppurative otitis media presents initially with chronic otorrhea—generally a mucopurulent discharge—through the nonintact tympanic membrane. After the infection clears, the patient has few or no symptoms other than a variable degree of hearing loss.
The recurrence of infection may cause pain, but this is not always present. Aural discharge reappears and may be creamy or mucopurulent in the presence of an acute infection. Chronic drainage may consist of odorless, stringy mucus or it may have a fetid smell due to chronic infection with *Pseudomonas* or anaerobes.

***Diagnosis:*** The diagnosis is made from the **history** and **otoscopic findings** (**Fig. 11.15**). Examination reveals a *central perforation* in the tympanic membrane that does not involve the fibrocartilaginous ring. Often, this can be appreciated only in a dry ear. The extent of the perforation can be highly variable. The tympanic membrane and middle ear may show additional features of chronic inflammation such as calcifications, atrophic areas, retractions, or ossicular destruction.

🖋 Eustachian tube patency should always be tested and documented (Valsalva maneuver).

In a *draining ear*, the external ear canal contains secretions and may also be inflamed and swollen. Occasionally, the perforation is difficult to see due to drainage or general inflammatory changes involving the ear canal and middle ear. A Valsalva maneuver may cause air bubbles to appear in the secretions. A **smear** should be taken for bacteriologic examination. **Conductive hearing loss** is more pronounced in the draining ear.

***Differential diagnosis:*** In cases with an acute infection and pronounced inflammatory changes, chronic suppurative otitis media often cannot be positively distinguished from a **cholesteatoma**. Even imaging studies such as CT are not helpful in this regard. Imaging studies are not indicated in the acute stage and are necessary only for preoperative planning or if complications arise. An expert can differentiate the conditions by otoscopic examination following treatment and resolution of the acute stage. The differential diagnosis also includes otitis externa, specific infections (e.g., with mycobacteria), inflammatory causes such as granulomatosis with polyangiitis (GPA, Wegener), and tumors of the middle ear.

***Course:*** A tympanic membrane perforation may be dry for years and cause few, if any, complaints. Other cases may present with recurrent or persistent otorrhea.

This depends in large part on the patient's diligence in protecting the ear and practicing aural hygiene.

*Complications:* The occurrence of infectious complications such as mastoiditis or abscess formation is rare and atypical in chronic suppurative otitis media. In chronic cases, conductive hearing loss is generally accompanied by the development of cochlear hearing loss, probably the result of a toxic serous labyrinthitis.

*Treatment:* Acute suppurative episodes occasionally require treatment with systemic antibiotics, but this is not consistently necessary. The selection of a specific agent should be directed by antibiotic sensitivity testing. *Otherwise*, the treatment of otitis media with drainage through the perforated tympanic membrane consists of local measures:
- Repeated, meticulous cleansing and drying of the ear is essential.
- Ear drops that contain ototoxic substances (aminoglycoside antibiotics) should be avoided.
- It is important to provide adequate ear protection while bathing or showering, for example, to keep soap and water out of the ear. This can be done by inserting petrolatum cotton wads or commercially available ear plugs. Otherwise, the ear canal should remain clear and should not be packed with cotton.

🛇 Adequate ear protection is also important in dry ears to prevent reinfection.

When the ear has been dry for about 3 months, surgical closure of the tympanic membrane can be performed (tympanoplasty, see 🔎 **11.1**). Chronic, intractable suppuration requires ablative surgery of the middle ear consisting of a simple or extended mastoidectomy.

# Chronic Otitis Media with Cholesteatoma

## Definition of Cholesteatoma

*General definition:* A cholesteatoma has two characteristic features:
- Keratinizing squamous epithelium is found in bony spaces at an abnormal location.
- Bone is destroyed through an inflammatory osteoclastic process.

Thus, chronic otitis media with cholesteatoma can be defined as an osteoclastic inflammation of the mucosal spaces in the middle ear. Often, there is a coexisting infection, usually with gram-negative and anaerobic bacteria, leading to a fetid aural discharge. Infection is not always present, however.

*Types of cholesteatoma:* Cholesteatoma may be congenital or acquired. The **congenital** or **true cholesteatoma** is very rare and is usually found behind an intact tympanic membrane. It can occur anywhere in the temporal bone and will not be discussed here further. **Acquired cholesteatoma** arises in connection with inflammations and ventilation problems of the middle ear. Two forms are distinguished:
- Primary acquired cholesteatoma, known more accurately as *pars flaccida cholesteatoma* (**Fig. 11.16**), develops from a squamous epithelial pocket in the pars flaccida and initially expands in the epitympanum, where it tends to destroy the lateral attic wall. An unfortunate synonym for this type of cholesteatoma is a "true" cholesteatoma. Other synonyms are epitympanic cholesteatoma, attic cholesteatoma, and attic retraction cholesteatoma.
- Secondary acquired cholesteatoma, known more accurately as *pars tensa cholesteatoma*, originates either from a perforation of the pars tensa with destruction of the fibrocartilaginous ring (marginal perforation) or from a retraction pocket in the pars

**Fig. 11.16   Pars flaccida cholesteatoma**

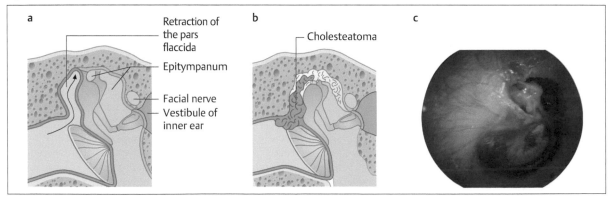

a    Retraction of the pars flaccida
     Epitympanum
     Facial nerve
     Vestibule of inner ear

b    Cholesteatoma

c

**a** The pars flaccida is retracted inward (arrow) by negative pressure in the epitympanum.
**b** Epithelial debris creates a nidus for infection and inflammation, which leads to the actual cholesteatoma.

**c** Pars flaccida cholesteatoma in the right ear with partial destruction of the bony ear canal.

Fig. 11.17 Pars tensa cholesteatoma

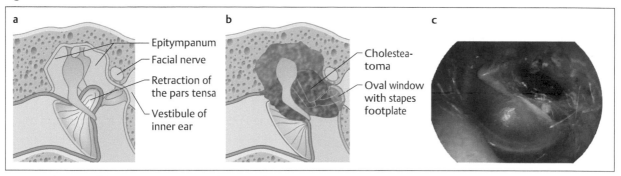

**a** An atrophic area of the pars tensa is retracted toward the mesotympanum.
**b** Epithelial debris creates a nidus for infection and inflammation, which leads to cholesteatoma and mucosal inflammation.

**c** Pars tensa cholesteatoma of the upper posterior quadrant in the left ear. The other parts of the tympanic membrane including the pars flaccida are not yet affected.

tensa, usually located in the posterosuperior quadrant (**Fig. 11.17**). This cholesteatoma initially develops in the mesotympanum but often expands from there into the epitympanum.

## Clinical Aspects of Cholesteatoma

*Epidemiology:* A cholesteatoma can occur in any age group but is rare in small children.

*Pathogenesis:* The primary cause of acquired cholesteatoma is probably an impairment of middle ear ventilation (see also ◈11.2, Pathophysiology of Otitis Media). Eustachian tube dysfunction causes a negative pressure to develop in the middle ear, which may be continuous (due to decreased tubal patency) or transient and recurrent (due to inadequate tubal closure and a negative pressure in the nasopharynx, as in sniffing). A retraction pocket forms in the tympanic membrane. The pocket is lined by squamous epithelium that tends to migrate on the tympanic membrane and in the external canal. On entering the middle ear, it causes inflammation and bone resorption. Secondary infection of the squamous debris can further intensify these effects.

*Symptoms:* Acquired cholesteatoma usually presents as chronic otitis media (see Otitis Media with Effusion above). Less commonly, it presents with complications such as perilymphatic fistula, labyrinthitis, facial nerve palsy, or intracranial infection.
A **dry, uninfected cholesteatoma** does not cause otalgia or otorrhea. It is manifested clinically by functional deficits. A common initial symptom is aural pressure signifying impaired middle ear ventilation. This is followed by hearing loss and later by potentially severe symptoms that require immediate treatment. These alarming symptoms include facial nerve palsy and signs of vestibular dysfunction such as rotary vertigo and disequilibrium.

A more common condition, however, is an **infected cholesteatoma with discharge**. It presents as chronic otitis media with otorrhea, generally fetid, and with hearing loss. Pain may supervene with an acute exacerbation, but this is somewhat rare. Again, functional deficits such as facial nerve palsy or vestibular dysfunction may eventually occur. Other possible complications are abscess formation and meningitis.

*Diagnostic work-up:*
**Establishing the diagnosis:** The diagnosis is made by otoscopy (**Fig. 11.16** and **Fig. 11.17**), which typically shows white epithelial debris in a retraction pocket in the attic or in the posterosuperior quadrant of the tympanic membrane. Occasionally, bone erosion is also noted in the posterosuperior canal wall close to the tympanic membrane. With a *dry cholesteatoma*, brownish-black crusts are usually found on the superior canal wall. When *acute inflammatory changes* are present, it may be difficult or impossible to make an accurate interpretation of the otoscopic findings. These cases should first be treated using the same regimen as for chronic suppurative otitis media so that an accurate diagnosis can be made (see Chronic Suppurative Otitis Media above).
**Screening for complications:** Hearing tests will generally indicate a conductive hearing loss. The presence of sensorineural hearing loss may mean that a complication has already developed.
*Facial nerve function* should be tested whenever a cholesteatoma is suspected (see ◈14.1). A *labyrinthine fistula* can be confirmed by eliciting the "fistula sign": a Politzer bag is used to generate a negative and positive pressure in the ear canal. Meanwhile, the eyes are observed with Frenzel glasses. If a labyrinthine fistula is present, the pressures will evoke rotary vertigo and nystagmus.
*Imaging studies:* High-resolution CT of the temporal bone can define the extent of bone destruction, detect intracranial complications, and offer presumptive evidence of a labyrinthine fistula. However, it does not

establish the diagnosis of cholesteatoma, which remains primarily a clinical diagnosis. Preoperative CT scans also provide information on the degree of pneumatization of the temporal bone. If complications are suspected, CT scans with contrast-agent administration should be obtained.

Diffusion-weighted MRI (DW-MRI) may help to detect clinically not apparent cholesteatomas, such as recurrences after surgery.

*Differential diagnosis:* Not infrequently, a **dry cholesteatoma** is mistaken for ordinary cerumen. A **cholesteatoma with discharge** mainly requires differentiation from chronic suppurative otitis media.

> Chronic postinflammatory changes in the tympanic membrane (e.g., retraction pockets) are on a continuum with an actual, acquired cholesteatoma.

*Course and complications:*
Without treatment, it is likely that the bone destruction will progress and complications will arise such as labyrinthine fistula, facial nerve palsy, or intracranial processes.

*Treatment:* Surgical treatment is necessary due to the bone destruction caused by cholesteatoma. The main goal of the surgery is to *eradicate* the destructive inflammatory process in the mastoid and tympanic cavity ("radical mastoidectomy," see ✎ **11.1**).
A second-line goal is to *improve hearing.* This can be accomplished with a tympanoplasty, which may be performed concurrently with the ablative surgery or deferred until a later time.
*Acute inflammatory changes* are treated with the same local measures recommended for chronic suppurative otitis media. Patients with generalized symptoms should receive systemic antibiotics.

## Otogenic Complications of Otitis

Otogenic complications may originate from the external ear or middle ear. If a complication arises from the ear canal or auricle, there will almost always be a prior or concomitant infection of the middle ear spaces.

> Because otogenic complications are both rare and hazardous, it is better to consider these complications too early than too late (i.e., maintain a high "index of suspicion").

Otogenic complications are otologic emergencies that should be investigated and treated by a specialist without delay. The patient should be evaluated as soon as possible by audiometry and CT; frequently, these studies will demonstrate a need for immediate surgery.

Besides acute complications, otitis can also lead to **chronic sequelae** that are more difficult to detect. The most important is sensorineural hearing loss due to an accompanying serous labyrinthitis. This section reviews the typical **acute local complications** of otitis media. They are most common in association with cholesteatoma but may also occur in the setting of an acute or chronic otitis media.

> Local acute complications are an important warning sign indicating the need for immediate (usually operative) treatment.

The earlier surgery is performed, the better the chance of curing the complication or at least preventing further functional deterioration. In rare cases, a chronically infected otitis media may also cause acute systemic complications such as endocarditis (in patients with valve defects), sepsis, or a severe local infection in immunocompromised patients.

### Mastoiditis

*Definition:* Mastoiditis is an inflammation of the air cells in the mastoid process. Involvement of the mucous membranes of these air cells consistently occurs in acute otitis media and is referred to as *associated mastoiditis.*
*Mastoiditis in the strict sense* is present when the inflammatory process is focused on the mucous membranes and bony structures of the mastoid (see also **Fig. 11.21**). When the temporal bone is well pneumatized, the inflammation may also involve the cells of the petrous bone (*petrositis*) or zygomatic arch (*zygomaticitis*).

*Etiopathogenesis:* Mastoiditis usually originates from an infection of the middle ear. It is the most frequent complication of otitis media, but its overall incidence is low. Important pathogenic factors are the degree of mastoid pneumatization, the virulence of the infecting organism, host immune status, and the treatment that has been provided for otitis media. Inadequate antibiotic treatment can predispose to mastoiditis.
Besides infection and abscess formation, an infrequent cause of mastoiditis is an inflammatory destructive process like that occurring in granulomatosis with polyangiitis (GPA, Wegener).

*Symptoms:* Patients present clinically with fever and local pain. In infants, mastoiditis or antritis may manifest with malaise, abdominal pain, and anorexia (occult mastoiditis or antritis).

*Diagnosis:* The classic clinical triad consists of:
• A prominent auricle with retroauricular swelling.
• Tenderness over the mastoid.
• Otorrhea.

## Curative middle-ear surgery

In cases of active inflammation like that associated with cholesteatoma, the middle ear must be surgically cleared of disease prior to reconstruction. This involves opening the pneumatized portions of the temporal bone in varying degrees and removing the inflammatory changes.

### Mastoidectomy

**Principle (Fig. 11.18a):** The cells of the mastoid and antrum are drilled out through a retroauricular incision. A broad communication is established between the epitympanic space of the tympanic cavity and the mastoid.
**Indication:** Chiefly mastoiditis.

### Extended mastoidectomy (modified, radical)

**Principle (Fig. 11.18b):** The epi- and mesotympanum are opened in addition to the mastoid cells. In the *closed or canal wall up technique*, the posterior bony canal wall is left intact; in the *open or canal wall down technique*, it is removed. This operation creates a broad connection between the mastoid air cells, tympanic cavity, and ear canal lumen, called a *radical cavity*. Today, the extended mastoidectomy is almost always combined with a tympanoplasty and the creation of a new tympanic cavity.
**Indication:** Definitive treatment of cholesteatoma generally requires an extended mastoidectomy.

### Subtotal petrosectomy

**Principle (Fig. 11.18c):** A radical cavity is created, and additional portions of the temporal bone are removed. The surgical cavity is then obliterated with fatty tissue from the abdominal wall. The eustachian tube is closed, and the external ear canal is permanently closed with sutures.
**Indication:** This operation is performed for inflammatory changes that cannot be surgically treated otherwise or in combination with implantation of an active hearing device such as a cochlear implant. It is also used for tumors and posttraumatic conditions (see 📖15.2 and 📖15.3). It completely disrupts sound conduction across the middle ear.

## Reconstructive operations

The permanent changes caused by otitis media can be treated by microsurgical reconstruction. The goal is to seal the tympanic cavity from the external ear canal and restore a largely physiologic mechanism of sound transmission. This type of operation is generally called a **tympanoplasty**. It usually consists of reconstructing the tympanic membrane (**myringoplasty**) and the ossicular chain (**ossiculoplasty**), but occasionally only one of these operations is necessary.

The curative surgery may be combined with a tympanoplasty in the same sitting, or the reconstruction may be staged, depending on the situation. The nature and extent of the reconstruction are tailored to the individual case.

### Repairing a tympanic membrane defect: myringoplasty

**Principle (Fig. 11.19):** The tympanic membrane is reconstructed with a free graft that is usually harvested from the auricle or its surrounding area during the same surgical procedure. The most commonly used graft materials are temporalis fascia, perichondrium from the auricle (tragus or concha), or thin cartilage slices. The tissue may adhere to the recipient site by surface tension, or it may be attached with fibrin glue.
**Indication:** A myringoplasty is necessary in most reconstructive procedures for otitis media and often must be combined with reconstruction of the ossicular chain.
**Result:** Because myringoplasty is performed with an avascular graft, postoperative healing depends on various local factors. There is an approximately 80% success rate of graft healing with permanent closure of the tympanic membrane, depending on the initial situation.

**Fig. 11.18 Curative middle ear surgery**

a Mastoidectomy

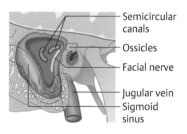

- Semicircular canals
- Ossicles
- Facial nerve
- Jugular vein
- Sigmoid sinus

b Radical mastoidectomy

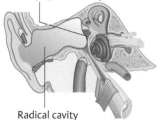

Small tympanic cavitiy

Radical cavity

c Subtotal petrosectomy

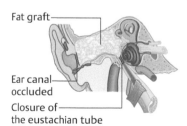

Fat graft

Ear canal occluded

Closure of the eustachian tube

**Fig. 11.19 Myringoplasty (type I)**

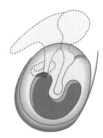
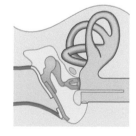

### Reconstruction of the ossicular chain: ossiculoplasty

***Principle (Fig. 11.20):*** The purpose of ossicular chain reconstruction is to restore sound-pressure transformation from the tympanic membrane to the oval window. The nature and outcome of the reconstruction depend partly on the extent of the ossicular damage. The condition of the stapes is particularly important in this regard. Three main situations are encountered:

- The stapes is intact. The reconstruction establishes a connection between the tympanic membrane (or malleus handle) and the head of the stapes, either by interposition of a remaining incus part or by using a prosthesis (**Fig. 11.20a**). A synthetic prosthesis that creates this connection is called a *partial ossicular replacement prosthesis* (PORP).
- The crura of the stapes are absent, but a mobile footplate is present. The reconstruction establishes a connection between the tympanic membrane and the footplate. The prosthesis in this case is called a *total ossicular replacement prosthesis* (TORP) (**Fig. 11.20b**).
- The footplate is absent or fixed. A new window is constructed (**Fig. 11.20c**).

***Materials:*** The ossicular chain can be reconstructed with endogenous material, allograft material, or synthetic implants made from various materials such as titanium, plastic, or ceramic. Remnants of the true ossicles are used whenever possible.

***Result:*** As a general rule, the function of the ossiculoplasty (sound transmission) is best accomplished with an intact stapes. Normal values are never achieved when a new window is constructed. Postoperative scarring and further inflammation contribute to a wide range of hearing results.

### Wullstein's classification of tympanoplasties

The microsurgical technique that is now used in many areas was first developed in 1950 for reconstructive surgery of the middle ear. Two important pioneers were the German otologists Zollner and Wullstein. In 1952, Wullstein introduced a scheme for classifying the five basic types of tympanoplasty, which is still in limited use today. It is based on the reconstruction of various functional components, i.e.:

- The tympanic membrane (type I, myringoplasty, **Fig. 11.19**).
- The lever mechanism of the ossicular chain (type II).
- Sound transmission without a lever mechanism (type III, ossicular chain reconstruction, **Fig. 11.20**).
- Sonic shielding of the round window membrane (type IV).
- Constructing a new inner ear window (type V).

Since today the lever mechanism of the ossicles is considered to have little importance in sound transmission and operations such as fenestration of the semicircular canal are no longer performed, the classification of tympanoplasties into five "classic" types is often imprecise and confusing. Only types I and III have practical clinical importance.

### Fig. 11.20   Ossiculoplasty

a Intact stapes: transposing the incus between the malleus handle and stapes head (type III)

b Mobile footplate: prosthesis between the tympanic membrane and footplate (type III)

c Absent footplate

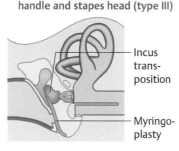

Incus transposition

Myringoplasty

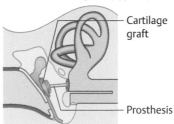

Cartilage graft

Prosthesis

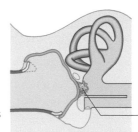

A small piece of fat assumes the function of the ossicles

Fat graft

**Fig. 11.21 Mastoiditis**

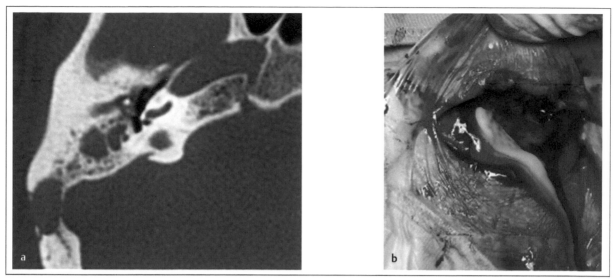

**a** CT of mastoiditis with abscess formation and destruction of the cortical bone.

**b** Intraoperative view: subperiosteal abscess with pus.

This classic presentation is somewhat unusual, however. Mastoiditis should be suspected in cases where acute otitis media fails to improve or worsens over a 2- to 3-week period.

**Otoscopy** reveals the features of acute or subacute otitis media with or without tympanic membrane perforation. The posterior wall of the external auditory canal may be erythematous and swollen ("sagging of the posterior canal wall").

The diagnosis is best established by **CT** (**Fig. 11.21a**), which can detect other complications as well. Besides clouding of the mastoid air cells and middle ear spaces, scans demonstrate erosion of the mastoid bone structure. The inflammatory parameters white blood cell (WBC) count, C-reactive protein (CRP), and erythrocyte sedimentation rate (ESR) are markedly elevated.

*Differential diagnosis:* **Otitis externa** with abscess formation behind the ear can mimic mastoiditis (pseudomastoiditis). **Inflamed retroauricular lymph nodes** can also produce tenderness and swelling over the mastoid like that seen with mastoiditis.

**Tumors** of the temporal bone such as eosinophilic granuloma, sarcoma, metastases (breast carcinoma, bronchial carcinoma, renal tumors), and lymphomas can mimic the features of mastoiditis.

*Complications:* Other otogenic complications (see below) may arise from mastoiditis, and so the risk of additional complications is increased. The potential complications of mastoiditis are reviewed in **Fig. 11.22**.

**Fig. 11.22 Complications of mastoiditis**

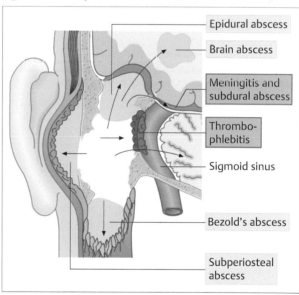

Abscesses may form beneath the skin (subperiosteal abscess), in muscle tissue (Bezold's abscess in the sternocleidomastoid muscle), or intracranially. The infection can also lead to meningitis or septic thrombosis of the sigmoid sinus.

*Treatment:* Treatment generally consists of mastoidectomy (see ✎ **11.1**), which is always combined with culture-directed intravenous antibiotics. Paracentesis and the placement of a myringotomy tube are frequently necessary to decompress the middle ear. Antibiotics without surgery are sufficient only in an early stage of mastoiditis. These cases require intravenous antibiotics and inpatient observation.

## Intracranial Complications

### Meningitis:

*Etiology:* Otogenic meningitis can result from a clinically overt otitis media, especially with cholesteatoma. It can also arise from an occult process involving the lateral skull base, which may be difficult to detect or undetectable by otoscopy.

⚕ With meningitis arising from an unknown focus, especially when the infecting organism is *S. pneumoniae*, the middle ear and lateral skull base should be considered as potential sites of origin and should be investigated by CT.

*Routes of spread:* Meningitis can result from the spread of a middle ear infection through preformed channels (blood vessels, diploic veins), through the labyrinth (tympanogenic labyrinthitis), through bone gaps caused by laterobasal fractures, or by contiguous spread from infected osteitis or cholesteatoma.

*Symptoms:* Severe headache, fever, clouding of consciousness, and nuchal stiffness become evident within a matter of hours.

The immediate *diagnostic work-up* includes CT scanning of the temporal bone with contrast agent administration and lumbar puncture.

*Treatment* with antibiotics and, if indicated, corticosteroids should be instituted without delay.

With processes involving the middle ear or lateral skull base, surgery should be performed after the patient's general condition has been stabilized. The surgery is both diagnostic to establish the cause of the infection and therapeutic to eradicate the infectious focus and eliminate its route of spread.

*Course:* Otogenic meningitis can lead to inner ear disorders or even bilateral deafness.

**Intracranial abscesses:** These lesions form via the same pathways as meningitis (see above). Otogenic abscesses are generally located in the temporal region or posterior cranial fossa (cerebellar abscess).

The following types are distinguished:

- An *epidural abscess* (between the temporal bone and dura) does not communicate with the subarachnoid space, and so it often produces few symptoms. The dominant signs are those of the underlying otitis media. Otosurgical eradication is often sufficient.
- A *subdural abscess* is located in the subarachnoid space and therefore communicates with the CSF. This lesion is on a continuum with subdural *empyema* and meningitis.
- An *intracranial abscess* leads to systemic signs such as fever, headache, nausea, and vomiting, which may be an expression of raised intracranial pressure. Focal neurologic signs depend on the location of the abscess. A temporal abscess can lead to speech disturbances, epileptic phenomena, and cranial nerve palsies (I–VIII). The effects of a cerebellar abscess may include increased intracranial pressure, cranial nerve deficits, balance disturbances, and ataxia.

Subdural (subarachnoid) and intracranial brain abscesses should be managed by a combined otosurgical and neurosurgical approach. Effective treatment generally requires the surgical eradication of middle ear disease and intracranial evacuation of the abscess.

*Complications:* All abscesses can lead to meningitis. This is particularly common with subdural abscesses.

### Inflammatory sinus thrombosis and otogenic sepsis:

Mastoiditis can lead to inflammatory thrombosis of the sigmoid sinus or jugular bulb. With an infected thrombus, dissemination and extension of the thrombus can give rise to otogenic sepsis. The thrombus may also cause intracranial venous outflow obstruction with increased intracranial pressure (especially if there is unilateral hypoplasia of the sigmoid sinus).

⚕ Septic phenomena combined with otitis should always raise suspicion of sinus thrombophlebitis.

The *diagnosis* is established by CT and MRI (**Fig. 11.23**). Treatment generally consists of mastoidectomy with surgical removal of the thrombus.

## Labyrinthitis

Tympanogenic labyrinthitis is described more fully in 📖 12.2, Labyrinthitis.

⚕ The occurrence of vestibular symptoms in otitis media (vertigo, disequilibrium, nystagmus) is a warning sign that points to labyrinthitis. An immediate otologic work-up should be performed, and appropriate treatment should be provided.

## Cranial Nerve Deficits

**Facial nerve:** Peripheral facial nerve palsy (see 📖 14.2, Inflammatory Changes) is the most frequent cranial nerve complication of otitis media. The deficit results from direct inflammatory involvement of the peripheral nerve. The tympanic segment is most commonly affected.

- Even "ordinary" otitis media can lead to facial nerve palsy, particularly in children. *Treatment* with antibiotics, combined, if necessary, with corticosteroids, may be sufficient. With concomitant mastoiditis, it is usually necessary to proceed with mastoidectomy and drainage of the middle ear spaces.
- In adults, cholesteatoma is the most common cause of otogenic facial nerve palsy. Surgery should be performed as soon as possible in these cases following an appropriate audiologic and imaging work-up.

**Fig. 11.23  Otogenic brain abscess**

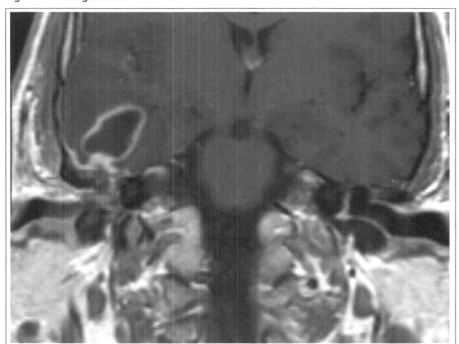

MRI scan of an otogenic brain abscess in the temporal lobe.

**Petrous apex syndrome:** The occurrence of trigeminal symptoms and abducens nerve palsy accompanied by otologic symptoms is known as *petrous apex syndrome* or *Gradenigo's syndrome*. Lesions of the petrous apex, usually inflammatory but occasionally neoplastic, cause irritation of the trigeminal nerve root with trigeminal neuralgia or hypoesthesia of the trigeminal nerve. They can also irritate the abducens nerve, causing diplopia. Associated deficits involving cranial nerves VII and VIII are often present.

**Other cranial nerve deficits:**
Almost all the cranial nerves may rarely be affected individually or in various combinations by an otogenic intracranial abscess. Deficits most commonly involve the abducens nerve, trochlear nerve, and trigeminal nerve.

# 11.4    Injuries and Noninflammatory Diseases of the Middle Ear

This 📖 deals with noninflammatory diseases that are confined to the middle ear. They may consist of injuries, ventilation problems, or bone diseases. These conditions may also compromise the function of the inner ear and cause changes involving the entire lateral skull base. There is some overlap with the material presented in Chapter 15, which deals with less localized diseases of the lateral skull base.

## Injuries

### Injuries to the Tympanic Membrane and Middle Ear

*Etiology:* Injuries to the tympanic membrane through the external auditory canal may be direct penetrating injuries from a pointed object, or they may be caused indirectly by pressure changes. **Indirect injuries** are more common. Typical cases involve slaps to the ear or sports-related injuries as in diving. **Direct injuries** are typically caused by sharp branches, self-cleaning manipulations (cotton-tipped swabs), or welder's slag burns, in which molten droplets may penetrate the ear canal and drum and enter the middle ear.
More violent trauma may affect both the middle ear and inner ear. This is more common with direct injuries.

*Pathogenesis:* Rupture of the tympanic membrane due to a rise or fall in air pressure depends basically on the rapidity of the pressure change. Atrophic scars in the tympanic membrane are sites of predilection and can perforate more easily than normal tissue in response to relatively small pressure changes.
Besides the tympanic membrane, injuries to the middle ear usually affect the ossicles in the form of fractures or dislocations. Injuries that involve the stapes often lead to involvement of the inner ear. The facial nerve is also vulnerable to direct trauma.

*Symptoms:* A traumatic perforation of the tympanic membrane causes pain of brief duration. The pain may be followed by a clogged sensation and slight bleeding from the ear canal. The patient may feel air escaping in response to a Valsalva maneuver or nose blowing.

🔲 The presence of vestibular symptoms (vertigo, disequilibrium, nausea) or facial nerve palsy signifies trauma that is not confined to the tympanic membrane.

*Diagnosis:* A tympanic membrane perforation is detectable at **otoscopy**, appearing as a slitlike or triangular opening with jagged margins and usually located in an inferior quadrant of the membrane (**Fig. 11.24**).

A **hearing test** should always be performed. With an injury confined to the tympanic membrane, hearing tests show only mild conductive hearing loss (Weber's test lateralized to the affected ear, Rinne's test weakly negative or even positive in some cases). In injuries that involve the ossicles, more pronounced conductive hearing loss is found.

🔲 Sensorineural hearing loss, nystagmus, and facial nerve palsy are signs of severe middle ear trauma with inner ear involvement. Immediate surgical exploration of the middle ear is advised.

Inner ear involvement may also occur in the form of acute noise trauma (see 📖 12.2).

*Treatment:* The tympanic membrane has a strong capacity for self-healing, and most perforations heal by themselves. They can be covered with various materials such as plastic film or cigarette paper, and any curled edges of the perforation should be straightened. The ear should be protected from water, shampoo, and soap.
Isolated tympanic membrane perforations generally heal without sequelae, but conductive hearing loss often persists when middle ear trauma has occurred. These cases require later surgical exploration of the middle ear with restoration of sound transmission.

**Fig. 11.24    Traumatic rupture of the tympanic membrane**

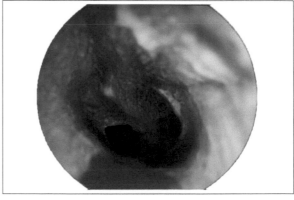

Fresh tympanic membrane rupture in the lower quadrants, left ear. Otoscopy reveals a fresh perforation with hemorrhage.

## Barotrauma of the Middle Ear

**Definition:** A rapid change in air pressure can have acute traumatic effects on the tympanic membrane and middle ear due to a negative pressure in the tympanic cavity (**Fig. 11.25**, see also 🕮 11.2, Causes of Impaired Ventilation). The Teed scale classifies barotrauma into five grades of severity based on otoscopic findings:

**I:** Erythema/retraction of the pars flaccida and/or umbo.
**II:** Erythema/retraction of the entire tympanic membrane.
**III:** Hematoma of the tympanic membrane.
**IV:** Hematotympanum.
**V:** Rupture of the tympanic membrane.

**Etiopathogenesis:** Barotrauma is caused mainly by compression events associated with airplane landings or diving. When the ambient pressure rises and there is inadequate pressure equalization through the eustachian tube, a negative pressure will develop in the tympanic cavity relative to the environment (**Fig. 11.25**). This can lead to swelling and bleeding of the middle ear mucosa. These changes, combined with a collapse of the eustachian tube walls, create a further obstacle to tubal opening. With a further rise of ambient pressure, the negative pressure in the middle ear also increases. The tympanic membrane is retracted inward, and the round window bulges into the middle ear. This can result in a perforation of the tympanic membrane or round window membrane, leading to *barotrauma of the inner ear* with sensorineural hearing loss and, less often, vestibular symptoms.

Inadequate primary opening of the eustachian tube may be caused by any kind of tubal obstruction, but simple rhinitis is the most common precipitating cause.

**Symptoms:** The initial symptom is severe ear pain that is not relieved by a Valsalva or similar maneuver. Conductive hearing loss usually goes unnoticed because of the pain. Vertigo and nystagmus may occur in some cases due to asymmetric pressure in the two middle ears (alternobaric vertigo) or inner ear barotrauma.

**Diagnosis:** The diagnosis is based on the typical history and otoscopic findings. Otoscopy may reveal tympanic membrane changes, a middle ear effusion, or a rupture of the tympanic membrane, depending on the grade of the injury.

**Differential diagnosis:** A temporal bone fracture, acute otitis media, chronic secretory otitis media, and bullous otitis externa can have similar otoscopic features. The differential diagnosis should include a perilymphatic fistula without actual barotrauma. These cases will generally require surgical exploration of the tympanic cavity. When barotrauma is related to diving, *decompression sickness of the inner ear* must be differentiated. Decompression sickness of the inner ear presents primarily with vestibular symptoms and without otoscopic findings.

**Complications:** A tympanic membrane perforation is most hazardous during diving. Cold water can enter the middle ear, causing caloric irritation of the vestibular organ with associated vertigo, loss of orientation, and possible vomiting.

Bacterial infection of the middle ear can also occur through a perforated tympanic membrane or by the tubogenic route based on mucosal swelling and discharge.

Involvement of the inner ear via the oval or round window and the formation of a perilymphatic fistula can lead to permanent cochleovestibular dysfunction.

**Treatment:** Paracentesis immediately relieves the negative pressure in the middle ear. In milder cases, an effort is made to reopen the eustachian tube by reducing swelling with medications such as nonsteroidal anti-inflammatory agents or steroids and by optimizing nasal breathing. Nonsteroidal anti-inflammatory drugs (NSAIDs) are given to control pain.

**Fig. 11.25 Barotrauma**

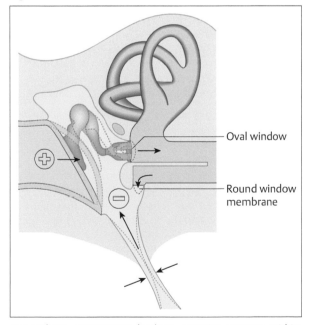

Oval window

Round window membrane

Atmospheric overpressure leads to negative pressure within the tympanic cavity with collapse of the eustachian tube. The round window membrane is displaced, and rupture can lead to inner ear barotrauma.

When there is clinical suspicion of an inner ear barotrauma due to rupture of the round window membrane, the negative pressure should be relieved (paracentesis) and the patient immobilized (bed rest). Surgical exploration of the tympanic cavity may also be required.

*Prophylaxis:* Patients with rhinitis, sinusitis, or otitis media should be prohibited from diving. Predisposed individuals making an airline flight should maintain good nasal breathing by the use of decongestants and moisturizing saline sprays. Patients should also try to equalize pressures frequently and avoid the development of a strong negative pressure in the middle ear.

## Bone Diseases

### Otosclerosis

*Definition:* Otosclerosis is a disease of the bony otic capsule in which structural changes in the bone often cause stapes fixation resulting in conductive hearing loss.

*Epidemiology:* The disease occurs predominantly between 20 and 50 years of age. It is about twice as common in women as in men, and about 10 times more common in whites than in blacks and Asians. Histologically, it is relatively common to find the structural changes described below (in up to 10% of autopsies) in the absence of clinical symptoms.

*Pathogenesis:* The cause *of the structural bone changes* is unknown. A genetic disposition with a dominant inheritance and variable penetrance and expression is presumed, leading to a positive family history in approximately half of patients. Hormonal changes in women (pregnancy) have also been implicated. Local infection with the measles virus is assumed to be also a precipitating factor. The fact that the abnormality of bone metabolism is limited to the otic capsule is probably related to the special embryonic developmental history of that structure.

The otic capsule affected by otosclerosis initially undergoes localized resorption with a spongiotic structural change. Later, the bone at the affected sites becomes sclerotic. A site of predilection is the anterior portion of the oval window niche, where involvement of the footplate and anterior crus of the stapes can cause stapes fixation.

*Symptoms:* Patients notice a slowly progressive hearing loss in one or both ears. With bilateral involvement, one ear is usually affected more than the other. Tinnitus may be present, but vestibular dysfunction due to otosclerosis is rare. The disease may cause cochlear function impairment (cochlear form).

*Diagnosis:* Typical signs of **conductive hearing loss** are accompanied by normal otoscopic findings. Weber's test is lateralized to the affected ear, Rinne's test is negative, and pure-tone audiometry shows that the air conduction threshold is considerably higher than the bone conduction threshold. The bone conduction threshold itself may also be increased in the pure-tone audiogram, especially in the range of 1 of 2 kHz (*Carhart's notch*). Acoustic immittance measurements demonstrate normal tympanogram and missing stapedial reflexes.

High-resolution CT scans can often define the otosclerotic foci in the otic capsule, demonstrating them not as sclerotic foci but as circumscribed sites of decalcification.

*Differential diagnosis:* The differential diagnosis of conductive hearing loss with an intact tympanic membrane includes the following:
- Middle ear anomalies.
- Ossicular chain disruption due to:
  - Inflammatory changes such as aseptic necrosis of the long process of the incus or tympanosclerosis; the tympanic membrane in these cases usually shows residual signs of chronic inflammation.
  - Traumatic dislocation of the ossicular chain, usually evident from the history: again, typical otoscopic findings may be noted.
- Apparent conductive hearing loss due to dehiscence of a semicircular canal (see 13.4, Peripheral Vestibular Disorders).
- Generalized disorders of bone metabolism (see below).

*Complications:* When otosclerotic foci occur at other sites in the otic capsule ("capsular sclerosis"), they can produce a variable degree of cochlear hearing loss ranging to deafness. This sensorineural hearing loss may be caused by toxic products from the bone changes that gain access to the inner ear spaces. Even in cases with stapes fixation, cochlear hearing loss may eventually develop.

*Treatment:* There is no known treatment for the structural bone changes themselves. With cochlear involvement and in other special situations, a treatment with sodium fluoride or bisphosphonates may be considered. The rehabilitation of conductive hearing loss may rely on surgical treatment or a hearing aid. Surgical treatment consists of replacing the fixed stapes with a prosthesis that can transmit acoustic vibrations to the inner ear. This requires establishing a connection with the inner ear by creating an opening in the footplate (stapedotomy, **Fig. 11.26**). The inevitable opening of the perilymphatic space carries a small degree of surgical risk. It can result in peri- or postoperative cochlear hearing loss

**Fig. 11.26 Stapedotomy**

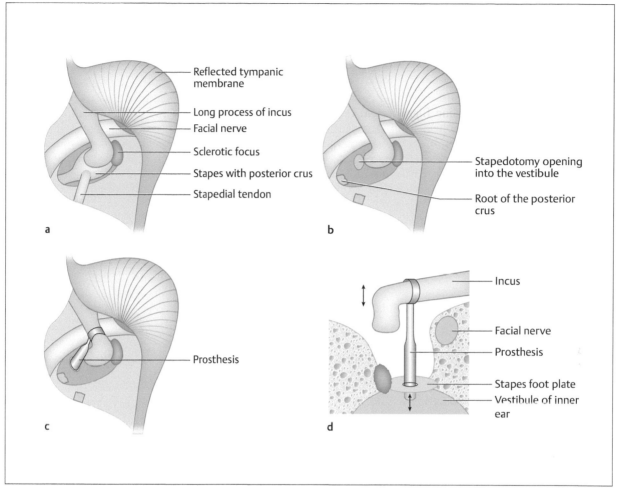

a Stapedotomy for an otosclerotic focus involving the anterior stapes crus. **b** An opening 0.5 to 0.8 mm in diameter is made in the footplate, and **c** a prosthesis is attached. **d** Vibrations of the incus are again transmitted to the perilymph.

and vestibular symptoms. While these problems can never be completely excluded, they are very rare when the stapedotomy is performed by an experienced surgeon. By and large, stapes replacement surgery is very successful and beneficial for the patient.

## Other Bone Diseases

Systemic bone diseases such as *osteogenesis imperfecta*, *Paget's disease*, and *acromegaly* can also lead to stapes fixation. Cochlear hearing loss is also common in patients with osteogenesis imperfecta.

Besides fixation of the stapes footplate, the head of the malleus may be fixed to the bony walls of the epitympanic recess (malleus head fixation). This may occur idiopathically, postoperatively, in the setting of tympanosclerosis, or in patients with anomalies. *Treatment* consists of surgically reestablishing a vibratory connection for sound transmission (see above and 🕮 **11.1**).

## Other Diseases of the Middle Ear

### Patulous Eustachian Tube

*Etiopathogenesis:* Normally, the eustachian tube is opened only by the action of the tensor veli palatini muscle. When the amount of fat and connective tissue surrounding the eustachian tube is diminished, a permanently open connection may be established between the nasopharynx and the tympanic cavity.

The cause of this may be weight reduction (decreased fat), a reduced venous pressure, or an anatomic change in the cartilage, muscles, or skull base. This type of change may occur in the postpartum period, in association with cachexia or anorexia, after radiotherapy or in acromegaly, to cite a few examples.

*Symptoms:* The history is characteristic. Women are predominantly affected and complain of aural fullness, vague hearing problems without objective hearing loss, and occasional roaring tinnitus. When questioned, many patients describe autophony, or hearing one's own voice "inside the head" with an echolike distortion. Lying down or assuming a head-down position improves or relieves the symptoms by raising the venous pressure. Physical or mental effort tends to exacerbate the symptoms. A history of weight reduction is occasionally elicited.

***Diagnosis:*** Otoscopy and hearing tests are normal. Otoscopy or immittance measurements may demonstrate movements of the tympanic membrane synchronous with respirations. Endoscopic examination of the nasopharynx and eustachian tube orifice is necessary to exclude pathology (see ✎2.1, Nasal Endoscopy).

***Treatment:*** Underlying causes should be treated whenever possible. The condition is harmless in most cases, however, and it is often sufficient to reassure the patient by explaining the cause. Regular, adequate fluid intake may be beneficial.
If the symptoms are persistent and very distressful for the patient, the submucous injection of collagen at the tubal orifice in the nasopharynx may be considered as an option. This carries a subsequent risk of decreased middle ear ventilation, however, predisposing to OME.

## Tumors

Tumors of the middle ear are rare. The most common is **paraganglioma** (synonym: glomus tumor), which presents either with typical otoscopic findings or with functional deficits of the basal cranial nerves (see ✎15.3, Tumors of the Temporal Bone). Other tumors such as meningiomas, eosinophilic granulomas, carcinomas, carcinoids, plasmacytomas, giant cell tumors, sarcomas, lymphomas, and metastases are usually manifested by nonspecific inflammatory symptoms.

🖋 Many of these tumors are misdiagnosed and treated as otitis media for a prolonged period of time.

Because the treatment of tumors often affects the entire lateral skull base, they are discussed more fully in ✎15.3.

# 12    Inner Ear and Retrocochlear Disorders

## 12.1    General Clinical Aspects of Cochlear and Retrocochlear Hearing Loss

The function of the cochlea as the basis for hearing is described in ♫7.2. This unit deals with inner ear disorders that lead exclusively or predominantly to hearing impairment in the form of sensorineural loss. The disorders that lead exclusively or predominantly to vestibular symptoms such as vertigo and disequilibrium are covered in ♫13.4. This ♫ describes the general clinical features of cochlear dysfunction and explores the distinction between cochlear and neural (retrocochlear) hearing loss.

### Introduction

The cause of sensorineural hearing loss most commonly resides in the cochlea. This condition is described as **cochlear** or **sensory hearing loss**. A similar type of impairment may be caused by an auditory nerve lesion (**neural** or **retrocochlear hearing loss**) or by a lesion of the central auditory pathway (**central hearing loss**).

> ⚐ It is often difficult clinically to distinguish between a cochlear and retrocochlear cause of hearing loss.

Pathogenic influences may act both on the cochlear sensory structures and on neural structures. Moreover, the causes of sensorineural hearing loss are frequently unknown—hence, the term *sensorineural hearing loss*, which includes disturbances of neural function at cochlear sites such as the synapses or ganglion cells. Cochlear disturbances may also be associated with disturbances of the vestibular system in patients with labyrinthine damage or systemic disease.

### Symptoms of an Inner Ear Disorder

The clinical hallmarks of an inner ear disorder are *hearing impairment, tinnitus*, and *vestibular symptoms* in the form of disequilibrium and vertigo (see ♫13.2 and 13.3). These symptoms may be isolated or combined.

### Hearing Impairment

Hearing impairment with a cochlear cause usually involves a diminished hearing ability, or *hearing loss* (synonym: hypoacusis), which is generally accompanied by a *distortion of hearing* (synonym: dysacusis). The latter type of hearing impairment is perceived as imprecise comprehension and distorted sounds. Hearing impairment due to an inner ear disorder can vary in its duration of onset and natural history:

- An abrupt, unilateral hearing impairment is also known as *sudden hearing loss*. It is described as *symptomatic* if the cause can be ascertained. Often, however, the cause of sudden hearing loss is indeterminate and the condition is described as *idiopathic sudden hearing loss* (♫12.3, Sudden Sensorineural Hearing Loss).
- More commonly, the hearing impairment takes a *slowly progressive course*, which is typical of hereditary causes, for example, and also of age-related hearing loss (presbycusis).
- *Stable hearing disorders* may occur after the cause (e.g., drugs or noise) has been eliminated.

### Tinnitus

*Definition and causes:* Tinnitus is an auditory sensation that occurs in the absence of an external acoustic or electrical stimulus and has no subjective information content. Tinnitus is a general, nonspecific symptom of an auditory system abnormality ("noise in the system") whose cause can range from an obstruction of the external auditory canal to a brain tumor. Most cases, however, are caused by a disturbance of peripheral sensorineural structures (**Table 12.1**).

Traditionally, a distinction is drawn between "objective" and "subjective" tinnitus. This distinction is flawed, however; because tinnitus is a symptom similar to pain or pruritus, it is always subjective. As a result, tinnitus cannot be measured objectively. Occasionally, however, a patient may hear vascular or muscular sounds originating in the body, and these sounds may be amplified to objectively audible levels with a stethoscope or microphone probe. This perception is then referred to as "objective" tinnitus. Tinnitus of vascular origin is often perceived as pulsatile.

Tinnitus can be assessed audiometrically by matching it to subjective pitch (frequency) and loudness by tones or noises. Frequency is determined first, then loudness. The loudness of tinnitus usually measures only about 5 to 10 dB above the hearing threshold; higher values are unusual. The reproducibility of tinnitus measurements is poor, and so they are not very useful for follow-up. Structured questionnaires are better suited for this purpose. They can also assess important associated symptoms such as hyperacusis or psychological distress.

**Table 12.1   Tinnitus: classification and causes**

| Classification | Causes | Primary diagnostic examination |
|---|---|---|
| **"Subjective" tinnitus** | | |
| Conductive tinnitus | Obstruction of the ear canal, middle ear disease | Otoscopy and hearing tests |
| Sensorineural tinnitus | Damage to the cochlea, damage to the cochlear nerve | Tone audiometry, AEP, MRI |
| Central tinnitus | Damage to the central auditory pathway | MRI |
| **"Objective" tinnitus** | | |
| Vascular tinnitus | Vascular malformations, arteriovenous fistulas, para- gangliomas | Auscultation, MRI, angiography |
| Myogenic tinnitus | Velopharyngeal myoclonus, middle ear myoclonus | Inspection, immittance measurements |

Tinnitus that adversely affects the quality of life has a prevalence of approximately 0.5% in the general population. Tinnitus is associated with sleep disturbance in about 4% of these persons, and the symptom of tinnitus can become a disease in these patients. The disease is *compensated* if it does not compromise the activities of daily living. It is *decompensated* if it causes significant disability, suffering, or suicidal ideation.
Tinnitus is classified by its duration as *acute* (3 months or less), *subacute* (4–12 months), or *chronic* (longer than 1 year).

**Treatment:** The treatment of tinnitus is challenging. Intravenous lidocaine is of temporary benefit in approximately 70% of cases, underscoring the frequent neural component of the condition.
*Acute tinnitus* can be treated similarly to sudden sensorineural hearing loss (see ✍12.3, Sudden Sensorineural Hearing Loss). Aside from anecdotal reports, the efficacy of medical treatments in general has not been positively established.

✍ Addictive treatment agents should therefore be avoided.

*Chronic tinnitus* with decompensation is best managed with a combination of behavior modification and psychotherapeutic measures. Hyperacusis that often coexists with tinnitus can be treated acoustically with noise generators that are worn like hearing aids (noisers, maskers). The goal of this sound therapy is to integrate the tinnitus into the acoustic perception of the patient in a way that is no longer disturbing or distressful.

## Diagnostic Evaluation

### History

The subjective symptoms of cochlear or auditory nerve damage described above are nonspecific and do not permit an etiologic diagnosis. Often, only a detailed history can provide evidence of **etiologic factors**. The following points in particular may have etiologic significance:
- Former and current *noise exposure* during work or leisure activities, also previous acute noise trauma.
- *Cranial trauma*, which may be associated with acute noise trauma or with a concussion of the cochlea.
- A prior history *of chronic otitis media*, which may be an indirect cause of cochlear damage.
- *Family history* of hearing disorders.
- Current or previous use of *ototoxic medications* or exposure to toxic substances.
- *General medical history* including smoking, cardiovascular disease, diabetes mellitus, dyslipidemia, immunologic disease, and psychiatric problems such as major depression or dementia.

The **actual disability** caused by a hearing disorder can be best appreciated from the patient's history, as it depends only partly on the degree of hearing impairment that can be measured by audiometry. Occupational and personal demands on hearing, the personality itself, and social behavior contribute just as much to the actual disability.

✍ It is particularly important to recognize a tendency toward social withdrawal based on the hearing disorder.

Because sensorineural hearing disorders are made noticeable by difficulties in speech recognition, especially in a noisy environment, people with hearing loss tend to avoid acoustically challenging but socially important situations such as group discussions and large gatherings to avoid misunderstandings, ridicule, and embarrassment. This can lead to social isolation and, when combined with comprehension difficulties, to mistrust.

### Clinical Examination

*Inspection* and *otoscopy* will show no abnormalities in patients with an isolated lesion of the cochlea or auditory nerve. With a moderate, symmetrical disturbance, *suprathreshold tuning fork tests* will also be normal. With a unilateral or asymmetrical disturbance, Weber's test is lateralized to the better-hearing ear and Rinne's test is normal.
The *screening speech tests* (see ✍8.1, Clinical Hearing Tests) usually show significant impairment.

## Audiometry

The following findings are noted in the typical audiometric profile of a sensorineural hearing disorder:

- The hearing threshold in the pure-tone audiogram is increased for air and bone conduction. This generally occurs first and most conspicuously in the high-frequency range ("high-tone loss," **Fig. 12.1**).
- Sound conduction is not impaired—the air and bone conduction thresholds are equal in the pure-tone audiogram, and immittance measurements are normal.

**Fig. 12.1   Pure-tone audiometry of inner ear disorders**

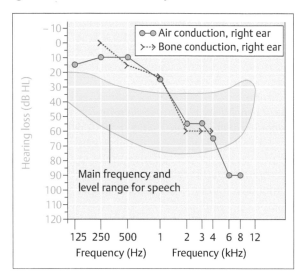

High frequencies are typically more affected than low frequencies. The thresholds for air and bone conduction are equal.

- Otoacoustic emissions are absent because the function of the cochlear amplifier is impaired.
- Speech recognition is abnormal, particularly in background noise, full intelligibility is often not reached, and a decline in speech recognition at higher sound levels may occur (see **Fig. 8.17**). Speech is heard, but it is misunderstood or not understood. In monosyllabic word tests (see ☞8.3 and **Fig. 8.17**), the performance–intensity function is flat, all of the words are not understood even at highly amplified levels, and higher levels may even be associated with poorer comprehension.

All of these findings cannot reliably distinguish between a cochlear and retrocochlear hearing disorder. Also, the suprathreshold audiometric tests that were once widely used are not effective for this purpose (see ☞8.3, Pure-Tone Audiometry: Threshold Determination). A reliable differentiation can be made audiometrically by eliciting the auditory brainstem response (ABR; see ☞8.4, Auditory Evoked Potentials). This test is of limited value for greater degrees of hearing loss, however, and imaging procedures (magnetic resonance imaging [MRI]) should be used.

### Imaging Studies

The primary imaging modality to assess sensorineural hearing loss is MRI. It can detect structural changes in the fluid compartments of the labyrinth, in the auditory nerve, and in the auditory pathways of the brainstem. Inflammation or bleeding within the inner ear, hydrops of the endolymphatic system, or tumors can be demonstrated (**Fig. 12.2**).

**Fig. 12.2   MRI of the inner ear in autoimmune inner ear disease**

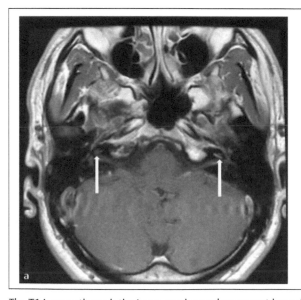
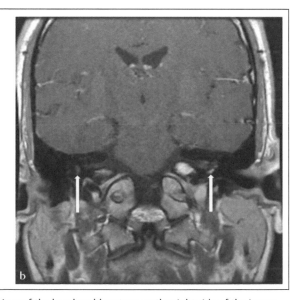

The T1 images through the inner ear show enhancement by gadolinium of the basal cochlear turn on the right side of the image.
**a** Axial section through the internal auditory meatus.          **b** Coronal section.

**Fig. 12.3 CT of the inner ear in cochlear otosclerosis**

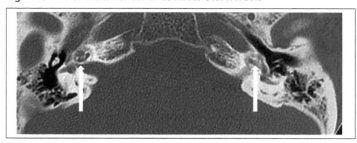

High-resolution axial CT slice of the petrous bone demonstrates the rarefied bone structure around the cochlea. A proper cochlea can no longer be recognized; the patient is deaf in both ears (compare with normal cochlea in **Fig. 7.4**).

**Computed tomography (CT) scans of the temporal bone** can additionally detect changes in the bony labyrinth such as those associated with malformations, trauma, or bone diseases such as osteogenesis imperfecta, Paget's disease, or cochlear otosclerosis (**Fig. 12.3**).

## Retrocochlear Disorders

*Etiology:* The main known causes of retrocochlear hearing impairment are tumors of the internal auditory canal and cerebellopontine angle, compression of the auditory nerve by vascular loops, and changes in the auditory nerve or its entry zone due to inflammatory processes such as viral infection or multiple sclerosis. Cerebellopontine angle tumors are discussed in ⏍15.3.

*Diagnosis:* In many cases, a sensory cochlear disorder cannot be distinguished from a retrocochlear neural disturbance of inner ear function on the basis of clinical findings. Moreover, combined lesions are not uncommon. Generally speaking, however, cochlear disturbances are predominant. It is difficult to detect a bilateral retrocochlear component of sensorineural hearing loss, but a unilateral retrocochlear disorder is of particular clinical importance.

⚕ In patients with unilateral sensorineural hearing loss, anatomic findings for a retrocochlear disorder should be excluded by MRI (**Fig. 12.4**) or ABR testing (**Fig. 12.5**).

The **subjective complaints** associated with a retrocochlear disorder are basically the same as those of a cochlear disorder (*hearing impairment, tinnitus,* and possible *vestibular symptoms*). The patient may exhibit particularly *poor speech recognition*, although this is a nonspecific sign and may be subtle when the symptoms are unilateral.

**Audiometry** exhibits the typical features of *sensorineural hearing loss*. A *speech hearing loss* that is quite pronounced in relation to the pure-tone audiogram may direct attention to a retrocochlear disorder. Because lesions of the auditory nerve cause a change in nerve conduction velocity, a disturbance of auditory temporal resolution is often noted as an early sign of a retrocochlear disorder. Pure-tone audiometry is performed using tones of longer duration, which are still clearly audible even if temporal resolution is impaired. Temporal resolution is essential for speech recognition, however, which involves the perception of rapid spectral changes.

Since the conduction velocity of the auditory nerve is abnormal, the measurement of *ABR latencies* is the most sensitive and useful audiometric test for detecting a retrocochlear disorder (**Fig. 12.5**; see also ⏍8.4, Auditory Brainstem Response and **Fig. 8.21**).

Most of the lesions mentioned above can be detected by **MRI**, and therefore this study is most important in the work-up of retrocochlear impairment (**Fig. 12.4**).

**Fig. 12.4** Retrocochlear hearing loss because of a meningioma at the porus of the internal auditory meatus

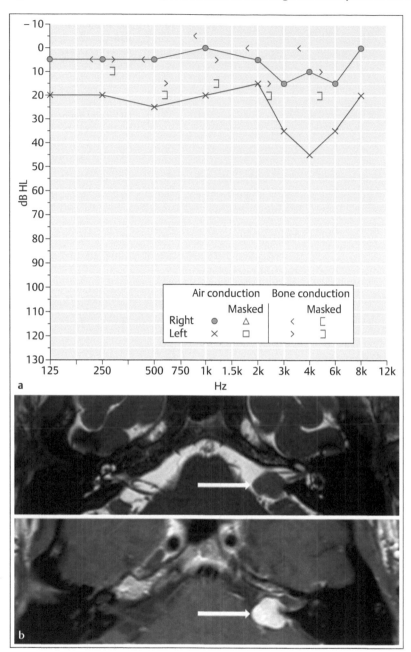

**a** Hearing loss on the left side affecting all frequencies in the tone audiometry.
**b** Axial MRI of the cerebellopontine angle. The tumor is at the posterior rim of the left porus, contacting cranial nerve VIII. Top image: T1; bottom image: T2 with gadolinium.

**Fig. 12.5 Auditory brainstem response in retrocochlear disorders**

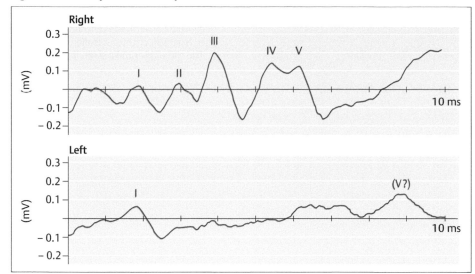

Auditory evoked brainstem potentials in a patient with a left-sided retrocochlear hearing disorder. The *right side* shows normal ABR potentials with normal latencies. On the *left side*, only potential I is clearly defined. The potentials were evoked with a brief click stimulus ~90 dB above the hearing threshold.

# 12.2    Cochlear Hearing Loss with a Known Cause

The cause of an inner ear disorder often remains un-known. Some etiologic factors such as inheritance, noise exposure, inflammations, and toxic substances are well known, however. Even so, it can be difficult clinically to relate specific causal factors to sensori-neural hearing loss. This ✍ deals with forms of co-chlear hearing loss that occur predominantly in adults and have a known etiology. The forms and effects of congenital and early childhood cochlear hearing loss were reviewed in ✍9.1.

## Hereditary Sensorineural Hearing Loss

*Classification:* Hereditary inner ear disorders are clinically and genetically diverse. A basic distinction is drawn between syndromic and nonsyndromic here-ditary inner ear disorders. **Syndromic hereditary hearing loss** is usually present at birth and is described in ✍9.1, Causes of Pediatric Hearing Disorders.
**Hereditary, nonsyndromic inner ear disorders** are classified into two forms based on the time of onset of the hearing loss:
- A congenital form: see ✍9.1.
- A later-onset form: the inner ear disorder is mani-fested after birth (occasionally not until adulthood).

*Incidence:*
Hereditary inner ear disorders are a frequent cause of cochlear hearing loss. It is estimated that approxi-mately one-third of all cases of sensorineural hearing loss have a genetic cause or a contributing genetic cause. The later-onset forms are significantly more common than the congenital forms.

*Inheritance:* Hereditary inner ear disorders may have a dominant, recessive, sex-linked, or mitochondrial mode of inheritance. Gene loci for nonsyndromic deafness are designated DFN (for DeaFNess) and DFNA refers to autosomal dominant, DFNB to autosomal recessive, and DFNX to X-linked inheritance. Whereas sensorineural hearing loss that is already present at birth usually has an **autosomal-recessive** inheritance, the later-onset forms tend to be **autosomal-dominant. X-linked** hearing disorders predominantly affect males, often begin at puberty, and may present as a mixed sensorineural and conductive hearing loss. Hearing disorders that are transmitted by **mitochon-drial** inheritance are progressive and are often asso-ciated with muscular diseases or other symptoms of mitochondrial pathology.

*Symptoms:* Nonsyndromic, hereditary hearing disorders are reasonably symmetrical: the hearing loss affects both ears to an approximately equal degree and over the same range of frequencies. Hereditary hearing loss of later onset may progress intermittently with recur-rent attacks of sudden hearing loss (especially in children), or there may be a gradual progression of hearing loss over time (most common in adolescents and adults).

*Diagnosis:* A positive family history can be elicited in cases with a dominant mode of inheritance. Audio-metry exhibits the typical features of cochlear hearing loss (see ✍12.1, Audiometry). The pure-tone audio-gram is nonspecific. A saucer-shaped curve with greater hearing loss at the middle frequencies does suggest hereditary hearing loss, but the audiogram may also show other configurations such as a low-tone or high-tone loss. More than 100 gene loci are known, many with variable penetrance, phenotypes, and several mutations. In principle, these mutations can be confirmed by laboratory tests.

*Treatment:* Treatment is limited to the prevention of further acquired damage and to rehabilitation with hearing aids and other assistive devices. Genetic counseling may be advised and should be part of laboratory tests of specific gene mutations.

## Noise-Induced Hearing Loss

*Pathogenesis and classification:* Excessive noise exposure can cause direct mechanical trauma to the delicate structures of the cochlea. When the exposure is prolonged, metabolic injury is added to the traumatic changes. The nature and extent of the damage depend on the acoustic energy of the injurious noise and the duration of exposure. The higher the energy (i.e., the level or loudness level) and the steeper the initial upslope of the energy, the greater the likelihood that mechanical trauma will occur.
Several types of noise-induced hearing loss are distin-guished on the basis of exposure time. They are not separate and distinct entities but are on a continuum:
**Acute acoustic trauma:** The ear is exposed to a sud-den, intense sound event of short duration. The loud-ness level exceeds 140 dB SPL, and the duration of the pressure rise is very short—less than 1.5 milliseconds. The most frequent noise source is a gunshot, but acute acoustic trauma may also be caused by burst tires, air-bags, firecrackers, or aerial fireworks.

**Blast injury:** In this type of injury, the ear and body are subjected to the pressure wave from an explosive blast, consisting of overpressurization followed by negative pressurization. Again, the loudness level exceeds 140 dB SPL, but the duration of the initial pressure rise is longer than with gunshot trauma (>2 milliseconds) and the frequency spectrum is lower. The pressure wave ruptures the tympanic membrane, and associated injuries are often present.

 ✒ The distinction between an acute acoustic trauma and a blast injury can usually not be made on physical grounds. The presence of a ruptured tympanic membrane signifies a blast injury.

**Acute noise-induced hearing loss:** The ear is exposed to high levels of continuous or intermittent (pulsed or impact) noise lasting from a period of seconds (e.g., jet engine) to hours (e.g., rock concert). The higher the sound pressure level, the shorter the exposure time needed to produce injury.

Acute noise-induced hearing loss is often reversible or partially reversible. Little attention may be given to the symptoms of slight deafness and tinnitus. The most frequent sources are loud power tools, musical performances, or engine noise.

**Chronic noise-induced hearing loss:** This is an irreversible cochlear hearing loss whose severity depends on the noise level, exposure time, and individual factors. Exposure to levels below 85 dB(A) for 8 hours per workday is considered safe (**Fig. 12.6**).

While potentially harmful noise exposure once occurred mainly in the workplace, noise-induced hearing loss is now a greater hazard in young people exposed to music and other noises that are associated with leisure activities (socioacusis).

**Symptoms:** The typical symptoms of noise-induced inner ear damage are a muffled sensation and tinnitus. These symptoms occur immediately in *acute events* and develop more gradually in response to less intense noise exposure. The symptoms improve after the noise is withdrawn and may disappear completely after less intense exposure.

*Irreversible, chronic noise-induced hearing loss* presents with the typical features of sensorineural hearing loss:

loss of speech discrimination, especially in background noise, and tinnitus. The tinnitus is constant, and the annoyance factor is variable and does not correlate with the degree of hearing loss.

**Diagnosis:** The audiometric hallmark of noise-induced hearing loss is a drop-off in the hearing threshold between 3 and 6 kHz (**Fig. 12.7**). Initially, a notch appears in this frequency range, indicating that the hearing threshold is better at 8 kHz than at 4 kHz.

In cases of *acute noise exposure*, the threshold curve declines over a relatively broad frequency range immediately after the exposure, but the effect is still most pronounced in the 3- to 6-kHz range. This disturbance, called a *temporary threshold shift* (TTS), generally resolves within a few hours.

With *sustained noise exposure*, hearing undergoes a permanent threshold shift (PTS) without recovery. Over time, the patient develops an irreversible, progressive high-tone hearing loss that may also affect the middle frequencies around 1 to 2 kHz.

The pitch of the tinnitus is often perceived at the frequencies of the declining pure-tone threshold curve.

**Complications:** The tinnitus may become decompensated, resulting in significant psychological distress.

**Treatment:** There is no known effective treatment for noise-induced hearing loss. It is important to avoid further damage to the inner ear from noise or other influences. Acute exposure can be treated with measures to improve metabolic conditions, the microcirculation, and the oxygen supply to the inner ear. Corticosteroids are also recommended.

**Prophylaxis:** The lack of an effective treatment for noise-induced hearing loss underscores the importance of prevention.

The most effective **primary prophylaxis** is the reduction of noise emissions, which is an engineering and legislative concern. Hearing protection should be consistently worn in situations where there is exposure or potential exposure to injurious noise. The physician should support prophylaxis by recommending the use of hearing protection and the reasonable control of noise levels in the home (e.g., music).

**Fig. 12.6 Safe weekly exposure times to noise**

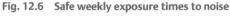
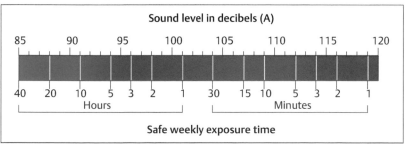

Relationship between noise exposure measured in dB (A) and the exposure time that can cause measurable hearing loss in less than 5% of normal-hearing subjects. Because the sound level is measured logarithmically, an increase of 3 dB corresponds to a 50% reduction of exposure time.

**Fig. 12.7 Pure-tone audiogram in noise-induced hearing loss**

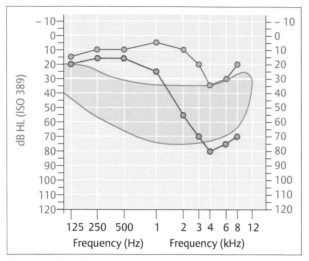

Pure-tone threshold curves in noise-induced hearing loss. A notch is typically seen at 3–6 kHz, meaning that the hearing threshold is better at 8 kHz than at 6 or 4 kHz. The hearing thresholds at an "early" stage are shown in light red, and the later configuration with a flatter notch is shown in darker red.

For **secondary prophylaxis**, people with occupational noise exposure should be regularly screened so that any noise-induced hearing loss can be detected at an early stage and appropriate measures can be taken such as hearing protection or a change of workplace.

### Traumatic Injury to the Inner Ear

Synonyms: labyrinthine concussion and contusion, labyrinthine trauma.

*Etiology and pathogenesis:* The inner ear is vulnerable to direct or indirect trauma, with most injuries occurring in association with acoustic trauma. The damage to the inner ear may be functional (labyrinthine concussion) or structural (labyrinthine contusion):
- Temporal bone fracture (see ☞15.2): the labyrinth may lie within the fracture zone.
- An impact to the skull that does not directly injure the temporal bone can still cause strong accelerating and decelerating forces to act on the labyrinth, causing bleeding or other structural and functional changes.
- Barotrauma (perilymphatic fistula, see ☞13.4, Other Causes of Peripheral Vestibular Disorders): the inner ear is damaged by pressure changes acting through the round or oval window.

*Symptoms:* Initially, there are nonspecific vertiginous complaints and hearing impairment that are often obscured by the associated symptoms of craniocerebral trauma or other injuries. Later testing often indicates only a hearing disorder, which may be more pronounced in one ear than the other. Tinnitus may be present.

*Diagnosis:* The diagnosis is based on the history and associated clinical and audiometric findings. Generally, a shallow notch appears in the 3- to 4-kHz range as a manifestation of additional acute acoustic trauma. Vestibular findings (see ☞13.2 and ☞13.3) can also help to advance the diagnosis. MRI may demonstrate specific findings of former bleeding in the inner ear or irregularities of the inner ear fluid compartments.

☞ Structural injuries to the labyrinth often cannot be detected directly: they may have to be presumed on the basis of functional disturbances.

*Differential diagnosis:* In patients with concomitant vertiginous symptoms, it is difficult to distinguish traumatic lesions of the inner ear from central vestibular and auditory lesions like those associated with a brain contusion.

*Treatment:* No specific treatment is available. The ear must be protected from additional harmful influences such as noise and ototoxic antibiotics.

### Labyrinthitis

*Pathogenesis and classification:* Labyrinthitis can result from an infection or other inflammatory process affecting either the inner ear itself or its surroundings. There are three routes by which an infection or inflammation can spread to the inner ear:
**Tympanogenic labyrinthitis:** An infection or inflammation of the middle ear may be transmitted through the round or oval window:
- *Acute toxic form (serous labyrinthitis):* The inner ear itself is not infected; presumably it becomes inflamed by substances that are released in the middle ear (e.g., inflammatory mediators or bacterial toxins). This pathogenic mechanism is probably also involved in viral tympanogenic infections (e.g., in bullous otitis externa).
- *Acute suppurative form:* A bacterial infection of the middle ear spreads to involve the inner ear.

☞ This form is rare but very dangerous and often results in permanent loss of hearing and vestibular function. It can lead to meningitis.

- *Chronic labyrinthitis:* This may eventually be manifested as inner ear damage. Chronic otitis media is among the possible causes.

**Meningeal labyrinthitis:** The inner ear may be infected bilaterally (often with *Streptococcus pneumoniae*) from the intracranial space, possibly through a patent cochlear aqueduct. In these cases, the labyrinthitis develops as an accompanying feature of meningitis, predominantly affecting infants and small children but also occurring in adults. The process may lead to complete deafness and calcification of the labyrinth.

**Hematogenous labyrinthitis:** Viruses and bacteria can infect the inner ear by the hematogenous route, resulting in hearing loss and disequilibrium. Typical causative organisms are mumps and measles viruses, human immunodeficiency virus (HIV), cytomegalovirus (perinatally), and spirochetes (syphilis, borreliosis). Other hematogenous bacterial infections of the labyrinth are rare.

***Symptoms and diagnosis:*** Labyrinthitis is manifested clinically by cochlear hearing loss, tinnitus, and vestibular symptoms (vertigo, disequilibrium, nystagmus).

☟ The appearance of vestibular symptoms in a patient with otitis media is a warning sign of labyrinthitis and necessitates an immediate otologic work-up and appropriate treatment.

Audiometry shows signs of sensorineural hearing loss. MRI can usually demonstrate inflammatory changes within the inner ear (**Fig. 12.2**). With tympanogenic labyrinthitis, high-resolution CT scans of the temporal bone are generally necessary to exclude a perilymphatic fistula.

Cerebrospinal fluid (CSF) sampling should be performed if there is the least suspicion of meningitis. Laboratory tests for syphilis, borreliosis, and labyrinthogenic viruses should be performed in all patients with suspected labyrinthitis due to an unknown cause.

***Treatment:*** Tympanogenic labyrinthitis in acute otitis media requires careful decompression of the middle ear with a myringotomy tube, either alone or combined with a mastoidectomy (see 🥄 11.2). A labyrinthine fistula also warrants immediate surgical treatment (see 🥄13.4, Other Causes of Peripheral Vestibular Disorders).

A bacterial infection is treated with high doses of antibiotics, usually administered intravenously. An antibiotic should be used that will enter the subarachnoid space. Corticosteroids are probably beneficial in cases with a viral or toxic etiology.

***Prognosis:*** Some recovery of inner ear function is possible, but most patients are left with permanent residual damage. Recovery from severe functional deficits is rare.

# Ototoxicity

***Etiology and pathogenesis:*** Toxic damage to the inner ear may affect both cochlear and vestibular functions, or each of the functions may be affected more or less in isolation. The toxic effect may be reversible or irreversible.

The causative agents of ototoxic effects may be **endogenous** (see Metabolic Disorders below) or **exogenous**. Principal exogenous toxins are listed in **Table 12.2**. A great many drugs have been named in isolated reports as producing ototoxic effects.

☟ Ototoxic effects are generally symmetrical.

An exception to symmetrical ototoxicity is the local toxic effect produced by substances in the tympanic cavity. Examples are the local application of ototoxic medications like those contained in ear drops

**Table 12.2  Ototoxic substances**

| Classification | Substances |
| --- | --- |
| **Drugs** | |
| Aminoglycosides | Streptomycin |
| | Gentamicin |
| | Tobramycin |
| | Netilmicin |
| | Amikacin |
| | Neomycin |
| Other antibiotics | Vancomycin |
| | Erythromycin |
| | Azithromycin |
| Diuretics | Furosemide |
| | Ethacrynic acid |
| Cytostatic drugs | Cisplatin |
| | Carboplatin |
| | Cyclophosphamide |
| Others | Salicylates |
| | Quinine |
| **Industrial toxins** | |
| Solvents | Aminobenzenes |
| | Nitrobenzene compounds |
| Heavy metal compounds | Lead |
| | Mercury |
| | Arsenic |
| Others | Fluorine compounds |
| | Carbon disulfide |
| | Carbon tetrachloride |
| | Organic phosphate compounds |
| | Carbon monoxide |
| Recreational drugs | Alcohol |
| | Heroin |
| | Tobacco |
| | Cocaine |

(exogenous toxin) and effects from the local endogenous toxins that form in chronic otitis media.

*Symptoms and diagnosis:* The **cochlear disorder** is frequently accompanied by tinnitus, which may be the initial presenting symptom. Generally, the degree of hearing loss is similar on both sides. Audiometry displays the typical features of cochlear hearing loss (see ✐12.1, Audiometry). Since **vestibular input is symmetrical**, there is no labyrinthine imbalance and consequently no nystagmus. The typical vestibular symptoms consist of oscillopsia and disequilibrium (see ✐13.2, History).

*Differential diagnosis:* Neurotoxicity requires differentiation from labyrinthine toxicity. Neurotoxic damage to cranial nerve VIII produces symptoms similar to those of a labyrinthine disorder. Many ototoxic substances are also neurotoxic, often making it difficult to distinguish specific inner ear damage from diffuse neurologic injury. For example, the central neurotoxic effect of alcohol is usually predominant, but alcohol also has a specific effect on the labyrinth.

## Ototoxic Drugs

**Aminoglycosides** damage the cochlear hair cells. Streptomycin and gentamicin are more likely to affect the *vestibular* system, whereas amikacin tends to affect the *cochlea*.

Ǥ The critical factor in terms of ototoxicity is the concentration of the agent in the perilymph and endolymph, which correlates only indirectly with the serum concentration.

Several other factors, some genetic and metabolic, appear to influence the ototoxicity of aminoglycosides. Impaired renal function is of particular significance. Many ear drops for otitis externa contain aminoglycosides as antibiotics, and consequently these products should not be used in patients with a perforated tympanic membrane. Applied locally in the middle ear, they can exert a toxic effect on the inner ear by way of the round or oval window. This effect is applied therapeutically in the treatment of Ménière's disease through instillation into the tympanic cavity. Patients often notice a high-pitched tinnitus as the initial subjective symptom. Tests reveal the typical signs of cochlear hearing loss, which affects the higher frequencies first, followed by the lower frequencies.

**Platin complex drugs:** The ototoxic effect of these drugs such as the cytostatic drug cisplatin is directed mainly against the hair cells. Cisplatin also has neurotoxic properties. The hearing loss associated with the use of these drugs is a typical *cochlear high-tone loss* (**Fig. 12.8**), which may be reversible to some degree.

Deafness is rare. Particular attention should be given to renal function impairment.

**Loop diuretics** such as furosemide have an ototoxic effect on the stria vascularis at high doses and cause a decrease in the endocochlear potential. This leads to a *hearing loss at all frequencies*, which is generally reversible.

**Quinine:** The use of quinine has long been linked to the development of *tinnitus, hearing loss,* and *disequilibrium.* The ototoxic effect, consisting of a hearing loss *at all frequencies,* is generally reversible. Other antimalarial drugs such as quinidine, chloroquine, and mefloquine can produce similar adverse effects, but less frequently than quinine.

**Salicylates:** Salicylic acid derivatives produce an obligate, dose-dependent ototoxic effect that is always reversible. The results are a roaring tinnitus and a mild to moderate *impairment of cochlear function for all frequencies.*

*Prophylaxis:* If the use of potentially irreversible ototoxic medications is planned, the patient's cochlear function should first be tested if at all possible. Useful tests are pure-tone audiometry, high-tone audiometry, and otoacoustic emissions.

Ǥ Inner ears that have preexisting damage are generally more susceptible to ototoxic effects. Strict selection criteria should be applied for using ototoxic medications in these patients.

During treatment with ototoxic medications, special attention should be given to dosage, renal function, and adequate hydration. Regular measurements of serum levels are helpful.

**Fig. 12.8   Ototoxic effects of cisplatin**

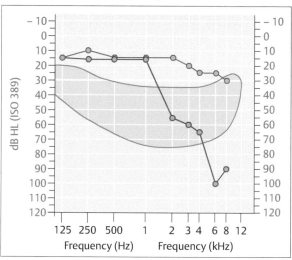

Pure-tone audiogram of the right ear in a 67-year-old woman before (light red curve) and after treatment with cisplatin (dark red curve).

For secondary prophylaxis (= early detection of disease), inner ear function should be tested by high-tone audiometry, otoacoustic emissions, or pure-tone audiometry. At the latest, these tests should be conducted when the patient first complains of tinnitus, vestibular problems such as disequilibrium, or subjective hearing difficulties.

## Other Acquired Inner Ear Disorders

### Immunologic Causes of Inner Ear Disease

Recognized autoimmune syndromes can lead to inner ear disease (**Fig. 12.2**). These disorders present clinically with bilateral, often asymmetrical cochlear hearing loss that may have a different time of onset in each ear and generally takes a rapidly progressive, occasionally fluctuating course. There may be accompanying symptoms of vestibular dysfunction.

**Cogan's syndrome** is a systemic autoimmune disorder invariably associated with a bilateral, progressive loss of cochleovestibular function along with interstitial keratitis. The disease is rare, occurring predominantly in young adults. Therapy consists of immediate treatment with high-dose corticosteroids, which may be supported with immunosuppressants such as cyclophosphamide or biological modifiers such as adalimumab or rituximab.

**Granulomatosis with polyangiitis (Wegener's disease)** and other forms of vasculitis can also lead to immune-mediated inner ear disorders. **Recurrent polychondritis** can affect inner ear function in addition to the auricle.

**Primary, organ-specific autoimmune diseases** arising in the inner ear itself are presumed to occur, but at present they cannot be confirmed clinically or by specific laboratory tests. A trial of high-dose corticosteroids is recommended in clinically suspected cases.

### Decreased Blood Flow

An acute blood flow deficit in the vertebrobasilar territory (**labyrinthine infarction**) can lead to acute, severe, usually unilateral disturbances of inner ear function. A selective decrease of blood flow may occur in the cochlear branch or labyrinthine artery. These cases may have no associated brainstem symptoms.

Whether a **chronic reduction of blood flow** such as that associated with abnormal blood pressure regulation, generalized atherosclerosis, diabetes mellitus, or nicotine abuse is causative of a functional impairment of the inner ear is difficult to establish in individual cases. Epidemiologically, statistical correlations have been found between cochlear disorders and the factors cited above.

### Metabolic Disorders

Like chronic circulatory insufficiency, metabolic changes are known to be associated with hearing loss and other labyrinthine pathology. The link to **hyperlipidemia** is well established. For this reason, the correction of such disorders is definitely advised in patients who present with unexplained chronic hearing loss. It is also believed that **uremia** can be a direct cause of labyrinthine damage.

### Cochlear Otosclerosis

Otosclerosis can lead to progressive cochlear hearing loss when it involves the labyrinthine capsule (**Fig. 12.3**) outside the oval window niche (see 11.4, Otosclerosis). The damage is most likely caused by toxic metabolic products from the diseased bone.

# 12.3 Cochlear Hearing Loss with Complex or Unknown Causes

An effort should always be made to establish a specific cause of sensorineural hearing loss. The known causes were discussed in the preceding ✍. In the majority of cases, however, even a thorough diagnostic work-up will be unable to establish a definitive or single cause for sensorineural hearing loss. The hearing loss in these cases is often assigned to a typical clinical presentation that serves as a diagnostic label. These presentations are the subject of the present ✍. It should be kept in mind that these "diagnoses" can have various known and unknown causes and are generally made by a process of exclusion. Age-related hearing loss, sudden sensorineural hearing loss, and chronic progressive idiopathic hearing loss are examples of such diagnoses.

## Age-Related Hearing Loss (Presbycusis)

*Definition:* Aging is invariably associated with sensorineural hearing loss, albeit with wide individual variations. If such a hearing loss surpasses a defined threshold, it is termed *age-related hearing loss* (ARHL) or presbycusis. Age-related hearing loss is an apparently idiopathic and symmetrical sensorineural hearing loss that affects persons older than 50 years. High frequencies are affected more than low frequencies, and speech recognition is impaired more than pure-tone hearing, especially in a noisy environment.

*Occurrence and incidence:* Initial signs of age-related hearing loss may appear as early as the fourth decade. Approximately 30% of men and 20% of women older than 70 years show significant hearing loss averaging 30 dB or more by pure-tone audiometry. The prevalence increases to 55% in men and 45% in women by age 80 years.

*Etiology and pathogenesis*:
Age-related hearing loss is a collective term that encompasses various disorders of the auditory system (peripheral and central) and various etiologic influences (multifactorial etiology). Because the hearing loss is nonspecific, a purely age-related, endogenous hearing loss is virtually indistinguishable from hearing loss that has contributory exogenous causes:

- *Aging processes* at the cellular level (hair cells and neurons) and organ level (basilar membrane, organ of Corti, stria vascularis) can have various manifestations. Postulated changes include autointoxication by metabolic products, a loss of elasticity due to connective-tissue changes, and an increase in mass due to nondegradable deposits in the cells and organs.
- An endogenous *genetic predisposition* is probably also a factor in many patients. Age-related hearing loss in these cases is on a continuum with hereditary sensorineural hearing loss of late onset.
- A *cumulative* exposure to exogenous *factors that can damage hearing* also has causal significance with aging. These factors include noise, middle ear diseases, toxic substances, and tobacco use (socioacusis).

One feature of age-related hearing loss is a **disturbance of the sensory elements** in the cochlea. This is unlike primary age-related visual deterioration, or presbyopia, which mainly involves a disturbance of the transmission system (decreasing elasticity of the lens). A more valid ophthalmologic counterpart to age-related hearing loss is age-related macular degeneration.

*Symptoms:* Patients initially complain less of hearing loss than of problems with recognizing speech in background noise. Tinnitus may also be present.

*Diagnosis:* Otoscopy and immittance audiometry yield normal findings. **Pure-tone audiometry** reveals a symmetrical sensorineural hearing loss that exceeds the normal degree of age-related hearing loss, which is defined in the pure-tone audiogram by international standards (ISO 1999, **Fig. 12.9**). Pure-tone audiometry mainly indicates a high-tone loss.
The **speech audiogram** often shows greater impairment of speech recognition than would be expected based on the pure-tone audiogram.

*Differential diagnosis:* The differential diagnosis includes virtually all known factors that lead to gradual, bilateral hearing loss (see ✍12.2). The most important of these are hereditary sensorineural hearing loss, chronic noise-induced hearing loss, cardiovascular factors including diabetes, smoking and hypertension, and hearing loss with an ototoxic or metabolic cause.

*Course:* Generally, the hearing loss is progressive, but its degree and time course are highly variable and cannot be predicted.

**Fig. 12.9    Normal age-related hearing loss**

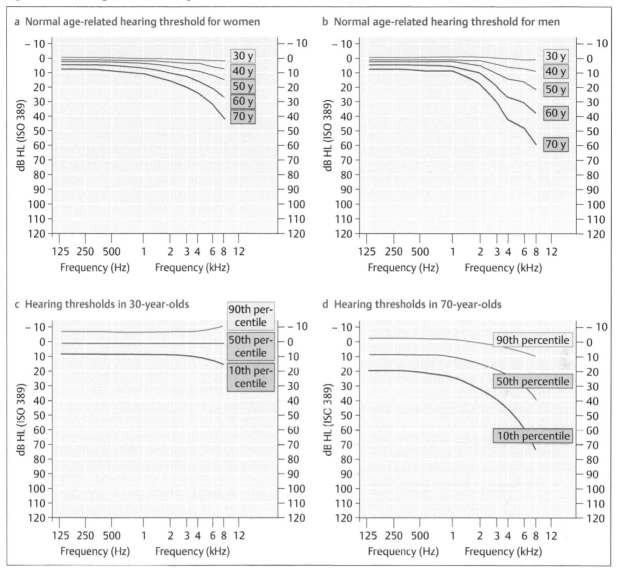

a  Normal age-related hearing threshold for women

b  Normal age-related hearing threshold for men

c  Hearing thresholds in 30-year-olds

d  Hearing thresholds in 70-year-olds

Normal age-related hearing loss is most conspicuous at high frequencies. It is defined by international standards (ISO 1999) and is less pronounced in women (**a**) than in men (**b**). The range of variation of normal values also becomes greater with aging (**c, d**).

**a** Normal age-related hearing threshold for women.
**b** Normal age-related hearing threshold for men.
**c** Hearing thresholds in 30-year-olds.
**d** Hearing thresholds in 70-year-olds.

***Treatment:*** No specific medical or surgical treatment is available. Bilateral hearing-aid fitting and other rehabilitative measures to improve communication may be necessary, depending on the auditory impairment (see ✍8.5).

## Sudden Sensorineural Hearing Loss

***Definition:*** Sudden sensorineural hearing loss refers to an immediate, unilateral hearing loss of sensorineural origin that has no apparent external cause.

There are several known causes of sudden hearing loss. If a cause is identified and a specific diagnosis can be made, the condition is described as **symptomatic sudden hearing loss**. Often, the cause remains unknown, however, and diagnostic labeling of **idiopathic sudden hearing loss** is made, when the hearing loss is 30 dB HL or more over at least three sequential audiometric frequencies.

This section deals mainly with idiopathic sudden hearing loss, since the management of symptomatic hearing loss is dependent on the cause.

*Etiology and pathogenesis:* **Idiopathic sudden hearing loss** is believed to have a viral, vascular, or autoimmune cause. A disturbance in the homeostasis of the inner ear is probably present, and psychosomatic factors may occasionally play a role.

*Symptoms:* The symptoms appear within seconds to hours, but in less than 3 days. The hearing loss is variable in its affected frequencies and degree, ranging from a mild loss to sudden deafness. Tinnitus is often present as an associated feature. Vestibular symptoms are less common; they are usually associated to high degrees of hearing loss and a bad prognostic sign.

*Diagnosis:* The clinical diagnosis of "sudden sensorineural hearing loss" is made in patients who present with sudden, unilateral hearing loss of sensorineural origin. The **history** rules out an external causal event. **Otoscopy** is normal, and **Weber's test** is lateralized to the healthy ear.
**Examination by a specialist** should not be delayed and should include *inspection* of the external ear canal and tympanic membrane with an otomicroscope, tests of *vestibular functions*, and *pure-tone audiometry* (**Fig. 12.10**). The work-up may also include *otoacoustic emissions* and *immittance audiometry*. All of these tests are intended to exclude specific causes of a symptomatic sudden hearing loss. This process can be aided by additional tests for arterial hypertension, hyperlipidemia, borreliosis, syphilis, toxoplasmosis, and neurotropic viruses such as mumps, herpes zoster, and HIV. A *neurologic or immunologic work-up* should be completed in patients who also have neurologic or inflammatory symptoms. *MRI or ABR testing* should be scheduled at a later date to exclude a retrocochlear lesion, especially a cerebellopontine angle tumor. These tests subject the inner ear to an acoustic stress, and therefore they should be done following a recovery period of at least 1 week.

*Differential diagnosis:* Because idiopathic sudden hearing loss is a diagnosis of exclusion, the differential diagnosis basically includes all causes of symptomatic sudden hearing loss, which are listed in **Table 12.3**. It is particularly important to detect a perilymphatic fistula after microtrauma, infections such as borreliosis and herpes zoster, and vestibular schwannoma (see 15.3, Vestibular Schwannoma), as these conditions require specific therapies.

The possibility of a psychogenic hearing disorder should always be considered as well.

*Treatment:* Causal treatment for **symptomatic sudden hearing loss** should be initiated as soon as possible. This particularly applies to cases caused by labyrinthitis (see 12.2, Labyrinthitis), herpes zoster oticus, or perilymphatic fistula (see 13.4, Other Causes of Peripheral Vestibular Disorders).
**Idiopathic sudden hearing loss** is usually treated with steroids, either systemically or locally by transtympanic instillation into the middle ear. Measures aimed at improving the microcirculation and oxygenation of the inner ear are also applied, but no proven effectiveness exists for any therapy.

*Prognosis:* More than 50% of patients with idiopathic sudden hearing loss show a spontaneous improvement or resolution of complaints, regardless of treatment. This usually occurs during the first few weeks.

## Chronic Progressive, Idiopathic Sensorineural Hearing Loss

Synonym: idiopathic bilateral sensorineural hearing loss.

*Definition:* Chronic progressive idiopathic hearing loss is a **bilateral** sensorineural hearing loss that usually begins between 30 and 50 years of age.

The disease is defined as having its onset before age 50 to distinguish it from age-related hearing loss.

*Etiology:* The cause of the hearing loss is unknown—there is no clinical evidence of toxic, metabolic, genetic, infectious, or other intrinsic or extrinsic causes. Nevertheless, causes such as a recessive genetic defect cannot be definitely excluded.

**Fig. 12.10   Pure-tone audiogram after sudden sensorineural hearing loss**

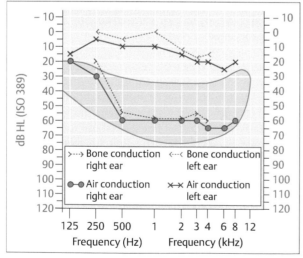

Pure-tone audiogram after sudden hearing loss in the right ear with no apparent cause. Sensorineural hearing loss is detected on the right side.

**Table 12.3  Principal causes of symptomatic sudden sensorineural hearing loss**

| Classification | Disease | Primary findings and diagnostic examination |
|---|---|---|
| **Cochlear disorders** | Perilymphatic fistula | History of pressure trauma, vestibular findings |
| | Ménière's disease and other forms of cochlear hydrops | Tinnitus, vertigo attacks, low-frequency hearing loss |
| | Acute acoustic trauma | History, tinnitus |
| | Labyrinthitis | Cochlear hearing loss, tinnitus, vestibular findings, laboratory findings |
| | Ototoxicity | History, tinnitus, both ears affected |
| | Immune-mediated hearing disorders | Both ears affected, progressive hearing loss |
| | Trauma | History, other concomitant injuries |
| **Retrocochlear hearing disorders** | Herpes zoster oticus | Eruptions of the outer ear, vestibular findings, facial palsy |
| | Cerebellopontine angle tumor (vestibular schwannoma) | Tinnitus, MRI |
| | Neural infection (borreliosis, syphilis, toxoplasmosis, viruses) | MRI, laboratory findings |
| | Multiple sclerosis | Often young patients, MRI |
| | Vasogenic hearing disorder (vertebral artery, basilar artery) | Often older patients, other concomitant neurological findings and vascular disease, MRI |
| | Migraine equivalent | History |
| **Central hearing disorders** | Psychogenic hearing loss | Objective hearing tests normal |
| | Focal, central processes | Other concomitant neurological findings, MRI |

**Symptoms:** Both sides are affected, but the course is variable and usually not symmetrical. The disease may begin with sudden hearing loss or may progress gradually. The progression of the hearing loss is variable but often culminates in severe bilateral hearing loss or deafness over a period of years or decades.

Hearing impairment is the dominant finding and is frequently accompanied by tinnitus. Vestibular symptoms are generally absent, however.

**Diagnosis:** The audiometric detection of typical cochlear hearing loss, together with the progression of symptoms and the exclusion of other etiologic factors, confirms the diagnosis.

**Differential diagnosis:** Chronic progressive idiopathic hearing loss is a diagnosis of exclusion, and therefore the differential diagnosis includes all known causes of chronic sensorineural hearing loss: metabolic, genetic, autoimmune, infectious, physical, and toxic. A retrocochlear, psychogenic, or central hearing loss should also be excluded.

**Treatment and prognosis:** Specific treatment cannot be offered in cases with an unknown cause. Rehabilitative measures in patients with an auditory disability should be instituted early, given the progressive nature of the disease. Since bilateral disease may culminate in severe hearing loss or even complete deafness, these patients should be promptly referred for comprehensive rehabilitation that may include training in lip reading. A cochlear implant is often beneficial in cases in which hearing aids no longer give acceptable improvement.

# 13 Vestibular Disorders

## 13.1 Clinically Relevant Anatomy and Function of the Vestibular System

The clinical anatomy of the petrous bone and inner ear-labyrinthine complex was covered in 🕮7.1. This unit provides additional specific and clinically impor-

tant details on the anatomy and physiology of the vestibular system.

### Vestibular End Organ

The vestibular labyrinth is part of the inner ear (see also 🕮7.1, Inner Ear). It consists of the semicircular canals, which are sensitive to angular acceleration, and the otolithic apparatus, which is sensitive to linear acceleration (**Fig. 13.1**).

### Semicircular Canals

The three semicircular canals occupy three spatial planes that lie at right angles to one other (**Fig. 13.1**). The **posterior semicircular canal** is directed along the axis of the petrous bone (~45 degrees to the sagittal and coronal plane; **Fig. 13.1a**) and is roughly vertical. The **lateral (horizontal) semicircular canal** is tilted approximately 30 degrees upward from the horizontal plane at its anterior end when the head is in a normal upright position. When caloric testing is done in the supine position, the head must be elevated by approximately 30 degrees so that the lateral canal lies vertically.

A rotational stimulus is amplified in the vestibular nuclei by a *push–pull mechanism* resulting from the mirror-image arrangement of the right and left semicircular canal systems. The inhibition of neural discharges in the semicircular canals on one side ("push") is accompanied by an increased discharge rate on the opposite side ("pull").

Each semicircular canal has a dilation at its utricular end called the **ampulla** (**Fig. 13.2**). The ampulla contains the sensory cell system of the associated semicircular canal, consisting of the crista and cupula. Due to the inertial lag of the endolymph, angular acceleration of the head causes a deflection of the cupula that displaces the sensory cilia within it. The cupular motion is a bowing rather than a swinging-door type of movement, and it is this deflection that stimulates the vestibular sensory cells.

### Otolithic Apparatus

The vestibular apparatus contains two additional sensory cell regions called the static maculae (**Fig. 13.3**). The hair-cell cilia in these regions are embedded in a gelatinous material called the otolithic membrane. This membrane is studded with otoliths (synonyms:

### Fig. 13.1 Vestibular end organ

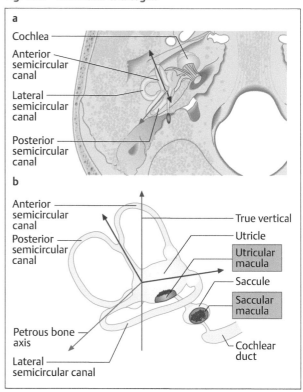

Orientation of the vestibular end organ in space:
**a** Axial view from above within the temporal bone.
**b** Sagittal view from the side.

The axis of the posterior semicircular canal (green) is aligned with the axis of the petrous bone. The "vertical" axis (purple) is tiled ~30 degrees toward the occiput. The red arrow indicates the vertical axis, so it appears only as a point in (**a**).

### Fig. 13.2 Ampulla of a semicircular canal

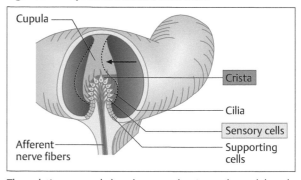

The gelatinous cupula has the same density as the endolymph. It is attached on both sides and recesses with endolymph movements transmitting this motion to the sensory cells.

otoconia, statoliths), which are calcium carbonate crystals ranging from 0.1 to 30 μm in size. With the head in an upright position, the macula of the utricle (see **Fig. 7.3**) is roughly horizontal, while the macula of the saccule is approximately perpendicular to it (see **Fig. 13.1b**).

The otolithic organs are sensitive to linear accelerations. These forces cause the relatively inert otolithic membrane to shift in relation to the layer of sensory cells. Because the gravitational force produces a static linear acceleration and because the two maculae are at approximately right angles to each other, at least one macula is stimulated at all times. Moreover, because the surfaces of the maculae are bent and the stereocilia of the macular hair cells are arranged in different directions, linear acceleration can be detected sensitively in virtually all direction. In this way, the otolithic apparatus senses the *position of the head in space*. If normal gravitation is absent (as during space flight), this function is lost and severe vestibular disturbances may arise. Translations and other dynamic linear accelerations are registered equally on both sides, resulting in a summation effect at the central level as opposed to the push–pull effect occurring in the semicircular canals.

## Central Vestibular Structures

The **vestibular nerve** is part of the eighth cranial nerve that connects the sensory cells of the end organ to the vestibular nuclei in the brainstem. It consists of two parts, a *superior part* with sensory connections to the anterior and lateral semicircular canals and the utricular macula, and an *inferior part* with sensory connections to the posterior semicircular canal and the saccular macula. The ganglion cells of the vestibular nerve are located in the distal third of the internal auditory canal (vestibular ganglia, synonym: Scarpa's ganglia).

The vestibular nuclei process and integrate both vestibular and nonvestibular information, thereby influencing the function of the oculomotor and spinal motor systems. The left and right nuclei are interconnected by functionally important commissures that play a key role in the maintenance of equilibrium. The central vestibular motor system is shown schematically in **Fig. 13.4**. The principal nonvestibular afferent projections of the vestibular nuclei are as follows:

- *Visual afferents:* Information on the movement of visual images across the retina ("retinal slip") is conveyed directly to the vestibular nuclei. This explains how a purely visual stimulus can induce a sensation of rotary vertigo (optokinetic reflex). This response is helpful in stabilizing the visual field and is evoked, for example, by looking out the window of a moving train ("train nystagmus").
- *Spinal afferents:* These are mostly afferent fibers arising from muscle and joint receptors in the neck.

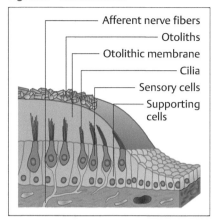

Fig. 13.3 **Static macula**

Afferent nerve fibers
Otoliths
Otolithic membrane
Cilia
Sensory cells
Supporting cells

The otoliths and the gelatinous otolithic membrane together form a mass of greater density than the endolymph. It is responsive to gravity, therefore, and transmits this motion to the cilia of the sensory cells.

They provide a pathway for conveying information on head and eye position to the vestibular nuclei. There is disagreement as to whether these afferents can induce dizziness in humans.
- *Cerebellar afferents:* A significant part of the cerebellum (the "vestibulocerebellum") is connected to the vestibular nuclei. The cerebellum functions as a control and storage center.

## Vestibular Functions

Normal vestibular function cannot be perceived or described in isolation. This is because the vestibular organ is at least tonically active at all times and is constantly interacting with other sensory systems, especially the visual and proprioceptive systems. The major functions of the vestibular system include the following:
- Fixation of the visual field for spatial orientation during rapid head movements. This function relies on direct interaction with the visual system.
- Maintenance of posture and equilibrium. This function relies mainly on interaction with the proprioceptive and motor systems.

### Vestibulo-Ocular Reflex

Some of the most important efferents of the vestibular nuclei are projected to the motor nuclei of the eye muscles. Reflex corrections in the movement and position of the eyes by the vestibular organ help to maintain spatial visual orientation through a compensatory adjustment of the visual field, allowing stabilizing a fixated object. With the rapid, small-amplitude head movements that occur during many activities, corrections by the visual system alone would be too slow for stable fixation. To make the corrections more rapidly, the vestibular signals are relayed to the eye muscles by direct efferent projections from the vestibular nuclei to the oculomotor nuclei. The vestibulo-ocular reflex (VOR, **Fig. 13.5**) is a reflex that involves three

**Fig. 13.4    Central vestibular system**

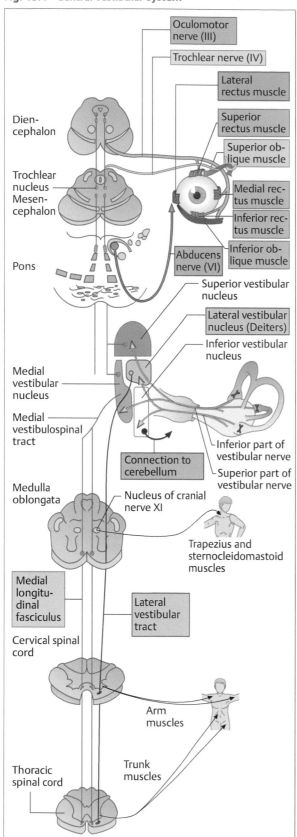

**Fig. 13.5    Vestibulo-ocular reflex (VOR)**

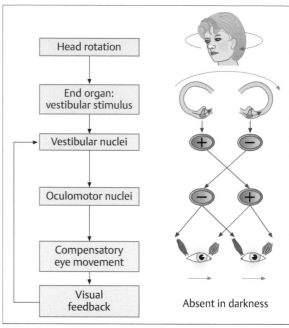

When a person looks straight ahead and fixes on an object, then turns the head to the right, the eyes must make a compensatory movement to the left to maintain the visual fixation. In this example, the movement is registered mainly by the lateral (horizontal) semicircular canals. The utriculopetal deflection of the right cupula stimulates the associated vestibular nucleus, while the utriculofugal deflection of the left cupula inhibits the opposite nucleus. Because the projections to the oculomotor nuclei are crossed, the left lateral eye muscles contract, and the gaze moves to the left.

neurons and has no direct feedback. The vestibular nuclei can receive feedback from retinal receptors for fine control, but this feedback is absent in darkness or when the eyes are closed. In this case, the VOR is an "open-loop reflex" and the corrective response is generally smaller than the actual movement.

The stimuli for the VOR come mainly from the semicircular canals. The otolithic organs, however, have also connections to the eye muscles. In particular, reflex connections between the sacculus and the contralateral inferior eye muscles are examined by the ocular vestibular myogenic potentials (oVEMP, see 🔎 **13.1**). The VOR is also influenced by polysynaptic connections between the two vestibular nuclei (e.g., convergent neurons) and by connections with the cerebellum.

## Vestibulospinal Reflexes

The vestibular nuclei can affect spinal motor activity (head position, postural stability, upright gait) directly via the *lateral and medial vestibulospinal tracts* and indirectly via the *reticulospinal tract*. The vestibulocervical reflex (VCR, also called the vestibulocollicular reflex) is particularly important for stabilizing the head position and thus for maintaining visual orientation. Reflex connections between the utriculus and the sternocleidomastoid muscle on the same side are tested with the cervical vestibular myogenic potentials (cVEMP, see ⌕ **13.1**). Spinal motor function is controlled by proprioceptive, visual, and vestibular reflexes. These three sensory systems are mutually complementary and are subject to mutual controls. An upright gait is generally possible when two of the systems are functioning. If two of the systems are damaged, upright posture and movement are impaired.

In the clinical testing of spinal motor function, the vestibular influences cannot be tested in isolation. Other sensory systems must always be tested as well.

# 13.2    Examination of the Vestibular System

**Vestibular function tests are used in the investigation of vertigo and dysequilibrium. A detailed history is of key importance and is supplemented by simple clinical tests. Based on this information, the physician can** then select further instrumented diagnostic procedures. The history and differential diagnosis in patients with vertigo are covered in ✎13.3.

The most common symptoms of vestibular dysfunction are vertigo and balance disorders, such as unsteadiness when standing or walking. Vertigo may occur in the absence of dysequilibrium and vice versa. Both are ambiguous symptoms that cover a broad range of possible diagnoses and are not necessarily of vestibular origin (see ✎13.3).

## History

A detailed history will often allow for a preliminary diagnostic classification of dizziness or dysequilibrium. The following information should be elicited:
**Nature:** systematic complaints such as vertigo or loss of balance with directional components (see ✎13.3, Differential Diagnosis of Vestibular Symptoms for details)?
**Onset:** acute or gradual onset?
**Duration:** spells lasting for seconds, minutes, or hours, or more prolonged occurrences lasting for days or more?
**Course:** diminishing, constant, or increasing?
**Provocative factors:** are complaints brought on by certain positions or movements (position-dependent or posture-dependent)?
Acoustic stimulation, usually with sound at low frequencies and high levels, may provoke vestibular symptoms (*Tullio's phenomenon*). The cause of the Tullio phenomenon is usually a perilymphatic fistula such as a dehiscent superior semicircular canal.
**Accompanying symptoms**:
- *Otologic* complaints such as hearing loss, tinnitus, or otorrhea?
- *Neurologic* complaints such as headache, loss of consciousness, or dysarthria?
- *Visual* complaints such as visual impairment, diplopia, or oscillopsia? Oscillopsia is caused by loss of the VOR, and it is a classic sign of a bilateral vestibular lesion. Rapid head movements induce instability of visual fixation and patients complain of blurred vision, an inability to read signs, or recognize other people while walking.
- *Autonomic* complaints such as nausea or vomiting?

The history should also cover the following:
- Use of drugs and medications.
- Trauma to the skull or cervical spine.
- Diseases of the cardiovascular system.
- Neurologic diseases.

## Spinal Motor Function and Coordination

The evaluation of spinal motor function should test the spontaneous coordination of the body as a whole and of the upper extremities. It should precede provocative vestibular testing, therefore. A multitude of simple clinical tests exist, but they do not test specific motor or sensory functions and provide little help for specific diagnosis. Because of their simplicity, the standard vestibular test battery may include a short selection of these tests such as:
*Romberg's test:* The patient stands upright with the eyes closed and the feet parallel and close together (to reduce the stance area). A subject with a normal vestibular system can stand in this position for 30 seconds without significant body sway.
*Romberg's test on foam:* The patient stands on a foam pad (a compliant surface) to reduce proprioceptive control. The test becomes more difficult and falls are more likely.
*Unterberger's stepping test:* With eyes closed, the patient takes 50 steps in place, bringing the thighs up to a horizontal position with each step. A tonus discrepancy due to a vestibular lesion will cause the patient to rotate toward the side of the affected labyrinth (up to 45 degrees of rotation is normal).
*Finger-to-nose test:* With eyes closed and the arm extended forward, the patient slowly brings the forefinger to the tip of the nose. Ataxia, intention tremor, and action myoclonus indicate a cerebellar lesion.
*Diadochokinesis:* Both hands are rapidly pronated and supinated to test cerebellar function and fine motor skills.
These tests always evoke a cumulative response that is only partly influenced by the vestibular system (see ✎13.1, Central Vestibular Structures). The results should be interpreted accordingly, taking into account the overall situation.

🖋 As a general rule of thumb, a vestibular disorder leads to directional instability, usually toward the side of the affected vestibular organ, while other neurologic or psychologic disorders lead to nondirectional instability or ataxia.

## Eye Movements

Abnormalities of eye movements, especially oculomotor palsies, should be distinguished from nystagmus (see below). Simple clinical tests are helpful in making this differentiation:

**Ocular motility:** The patient tracks the tester's forefinger or some other target moving in an **H**-shaped pattern (**Fig. 13.6**). Observing the eye movements provides a cumulative test for all the eye muscles. Normal motility is reflected in a complete, bilateral freedom of eye movements, which are coordinated (equal on both sides).

**Smooth pursuit** (**Fig. 13.7**): Smooth pursuit is a voluntary ocular movement following an object. A target is slowly moved back and forth at a comfortable fixation distance from the patient's eyes. The tester should not move the target more than 30 degrees to either side. A normal response consists of a smooth, coordinated tracking movement of both eyes to both sides to maintain foveal fixation of the target. The examiner watches for any corrective movements or catch-up saccades. One function of this test is to detect nystagmus. Vestibular nystagmus may induce saccadic movement in one direction only, gaze induced nystagmus to both sides, and the occurrence of conspicuous saccades to both sides indicates a central oculomotor disorder.

**Ocular tilt reaction** (**Fig. 13.8**): Asymmetry of the otholithic functions or in the processing of their central connections between left and right can cause a

### Fig. 13.6  Summary testing of ocular motility

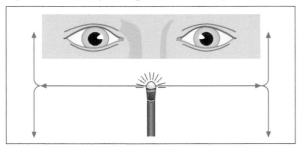

The summary integrity of ocular movements can be tested with a figure **H**, presented by a clear target. Normally, both eyes can track the moving target in all directions in a coordinated fashion.

### Fig. 13.7  Testing slow tracking eye movements

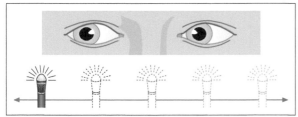

With normal oculomotor function, both eyes can track the target smoothly without catch-up saccades.

### Fig. 13.8  Alternate eye cover test for skew deviation ("test of skew")

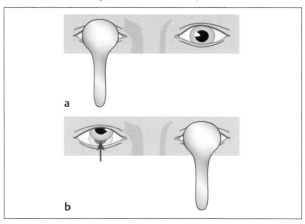

The patient fixes a stationary point in at least 1 m distance and the examiner covers one eye (a) and then the other (b). A saccadic vertical correction of the eye position indicates a skew deviation.

rotation of the eyes along the visual axis leading to a skewed visual horizon. A *tilted position of the head* should be noted, because some patients correct this skewness of the visual field by tilting their head to the other side when upright. In contrast, a rotational deviation of the eyes themselves cannot be recognized directly, but vertical misalignment of the two eye positions can be detected by the *alternate eye cover test for skew deviation* ("**test of skew**"). The patient fixes a stationary point in at least 1-m distance and the examiner covers alternately one eye and then the other. A saccadic vertical correction of the eye position indicates a skew deviation.

**Head impulse test** (HIT, **Fig. 13.9**): The patient and examiner sit opposite each other, approximately 1 m apart. The examiner moves the patient's head rapidly over about a 30-degree arc to one side while the patient keeps the gaze fixed on the examiner's nose. If the VOR in this particular direction is damaged, the patient is unable to maintain fixation and a corrective catch-up saccade will be noted. The head impulses may be performed in all directions of the semicircular planes (**Fig. 13.10**).

## Nystagmus: Definition, Classification, and Testing

*Definitions:* **Nystagmus in the broad sense** refers to any rhythmical eye movement, which may be spontaneous, provoked, or induced. The eye movement may be physiologic or may be symptomatic of an abnormal condition.

**Nystagmus in the strict sense** (**Fig. 13.11**) refers to a conjugated, coordinated eye movement about a certain axis, which can be subdivided into rhythmically

**Fig. 13.9 Head impulse test (HIT)**

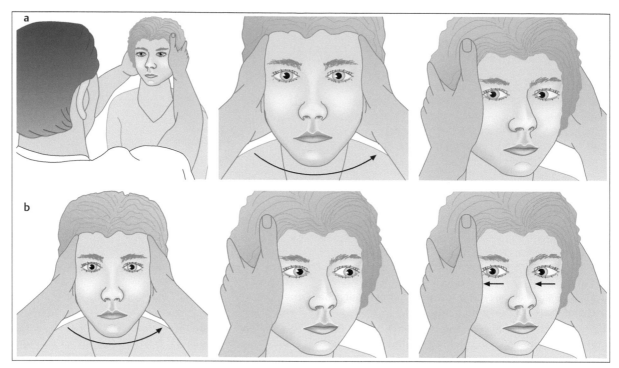

As a sign of a dysfunctioning VOR, the patient cannot steadily fix a target during rapid head movements. Catch-up saccades occur.

**a** Normal reaction; the VOR allows steady fixation of the target during head impulse testing.

**b** Positive finding during head impulse testing: the eyes deviate with the head impulse to the left, and the patient corrects his fixation with a catch-up saccade to the right (dysfunction of the left lateral semicircular canal).

**Fig. 13.10 Video head impulse test (video-HIT)**

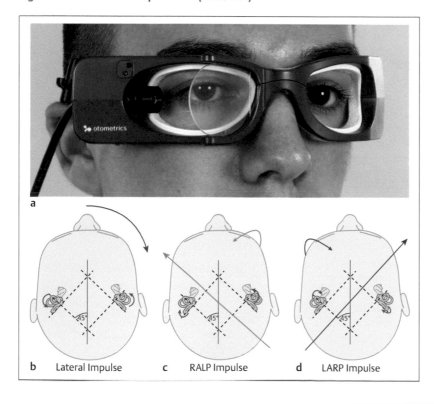

**b** Lateral Impulse  **c** RALP Impulse  **d** LARP Impulse

**a** Objective recording of the head impulse test with a high-speed video infrared camera attached to light goggles. The device allows testing of VOR in all planes.

**b** Rotation in the vertical axis tests both lateral semicircular canals. Here, a rotation to the right induces endolymphatic flows to the left (blue arrows).

**c** Rotation in the **RALP** axis tests both the **right anterior** and the **left posterior** canals. Here, an upward rotation induces a forward endolymphatic flow in the **RA** direction, and an upward endolymphatic flow in the **LP** direction (blue arrows).

**d** Rotation in the **LARP** axis tests both the **left anterior** and the **right posterior** canals. Here, an upward rotation induces a forward endolymphatic flow in the **LA** direction, and an upward endolymphatic flow in the **RP** direction (blue arrows).

**Fig. 13.11   Nystagmus**

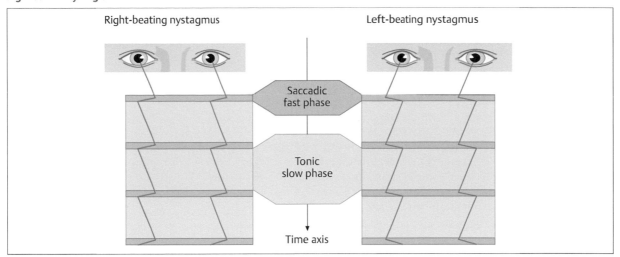

alternating slow and fast phases. The *slow phase* is the drifting eye movement induced physiologically or pathologically by a vestibular stimulus.

The opposing *fast phase* is a saccadelike refixation movement induced by the central oculomotor system. Visual perception is suppressed during the refixation movement, producing the constant rotatory sensation that is characteristic of nystagmus.

The *direction* of the nystagmus is defined by the more easily observed fast component.

Nystagmus that is present at rest within a 30-degree visual field is called **spontaneous nystagmus** (see "Types of spontaneous nystagmus" below). It has pathologic significance.

**Provoked nystagmus** is a pathologic nystagmus that can be produced by certain maneuvers. It generally has a vestibular cause and may be transient (lasting less than 60 seconds) or persistent (lasting more than 60 seconds) in response to a provocative maneuver. This differs from **induced nystagmus**, which is a physiologic phenomenon (e.g., "train nystagmus").

***Diagnosis:*** Frenzel glasses are a helpful aid in the diagnosis of nystagmus. The patient's eyes are illuminated, and glasses with a power of 20 diopters eliminate visual fixation. Generally, a minimum of three beats are needed to detect nystagmus.

## Spontaneous Nystagmus

***Screening for spontaneous nystagmus:*** First, the patient fixates on a well-defined target approximately 1 m away that is presented straight ahead and also at a 30-degree angle to the left and right. The patient may additionally be tested at 15-degree upward and downward gaze. The eyes are observed while the targets are presented.

Next, Frenzel glasses are put on to suppress visual fixation, and the same gaze directions are tested as before.

Any regular, rhythmical eye movement is classified as spontaneous nystagmus, but not the nondirectional, irregular, jerky movements ("square waves") that often occur when fixation is suppressed.

***Types of spontaneous nystagmus:*** Three main types can be distinguished:

**Vestibular spontaneous nystagmus:** Any directional nystagmus that always beats toward the same side and can be abolished or markedly suppressed by visual fixation is classified as vestibular spontaneous nystagmus.

It is caused by a peripheral or central vestibular lesion and generally beats toward the healthy side. Horizontal nystagmus can be graded according to its spontaneous presence (Alexander grading scheme):

- *First-degree nystagmus* is present only during gaze in the direction of the nystagmus.
- *Second-degree nystagmus* is also present on central gaze.
- *Third-degree nystagmus* is present in all gaze positions.

**Gaze-evoked nystagmus:** The fast phase of the nystagmus is always in the direction of gaze—i.e., to the right during gaze toward the right side, and to the left during gaze toward the left side.

This condition is a central gaze disturbance that causes a slow drift of gaze toward the center of the visual field. The gaze intention produces the recentering movement, and so the nystagmus generally becomes more intense as the deviation increases. Gaze-evoked nystagmus can also result from toxicity such as barbiturate, phenytoin, or alcohol poisoning.

Differentiation is required from the physiologic phenomenon of *end-point nystagmus*, which occurs through muscular action when the gaze deviates by approximately 40 degrees.

**Congenital nystagmus** (pendular nystagmus, fixation nystagmus) is defined as nystagmus that is most pronounced in the central position and during fixation. Usually, it displays a high frequency with no clearly distinguishable fast and slow components (hence the name "pendular nystagmus") and is present during binocular fixation. Congenital nystagmus is due to a congenital abnormality of the oculomotor centers and causes no subjective complaints. Acquired fixation nystagmus with similar lesions is a less frequent form. Fixation nystagmus may also occur in association with visual disorders (amblyopic nystagmus) and a rare variant occurs only during monocular fixation beating toward the side of the fixation (latent fixation nystagmus).

### Provocation of Nystagmus

As before, the nystagmus is observed through Frenzel glasses and can be positively identified after a minimum of three beats.

**Common provocative maneuvers are listed below**:
- *Head shaking:* Gentle, passive, horizontal shaking of the patient's head may "unleash" a spontaneous nystagmus.
- *Positional testing (static):* This involves the slow-motion assumption of various body positions (supine, lateral decubitus, head hanging). The vestibular apparatus and especially the otolithic organs are exposed to various gravitational stimuli in the different positions.
- *Hallpike–Dix maneuver:* The patient is moved swiftly from an upright sitting position to a head-hanging position and then back up again. This maneuver is done with the head forward, turned to the right, and turned to the left. It is a useful test for diagnosing benign paroxysmal positional vertigo (see 13.4, Benign Paroxysmal Positional Vertigo, and **Fig. 13.12**).

### Induction of Nystagmus

*Vestibular nystagmus* can be induced in two ways: caloric stimulation and rotational stimulation.

**Caloric stimulation:** The patient lies with the head elevated 30 degrees (so that the lateral semicircular canal is vertical, see 13.1, Semicircular Canals), and the external auditory canals are irrigated with warm (44°C) or cold water (30°C) for 30 seconds.

⚠ Make sure that the tympanic membrane is intact before performing this test.

If the tympanic membrane is perforated, warm or cold air can be used for caloric stimulation.

A difference of 7°C between the irrigating water and body temperature will induce endolymphatic movement

**Fig. 13.12   Hallpike–Dix maneuver**

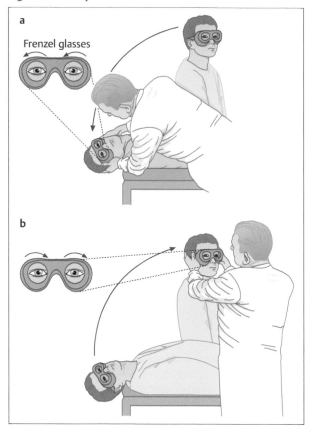

**a** From an upright sitting position, the patient is moved backward swiftly with the head hanging.

**b** After a brief pause, the patient is brought back to the upright position. When benign paroxysmal positional vertigo is present, typical nystagmus will be observed in the direction of the movement. The maneuver is done first with the head turned to the right, then to the left, and finally with the head in a neutral position. The affected side can be determined from the side of the greater response; the "down" ear is affected.

through conduction. This causes a unilateral stimulation of the vestibular labyrinth and induces a typical vestibular nystagmus, which generally lasts approximately 2 to 3 minutes.

⚠ Warm-water irrigation induces nystagmus toward the same side: h**o**t = h**o**molateral or w**a**rm = s**a**me. Cold irrigation induces nystagmus toward the opposite side: c**o**ld = c**o**ntralateral or c**o**ld = **o**pposite.

In a normal test, both labyrinths react equally. If the test is performed using Frenzel glasses, the examiner waits 30 seconds after the irrigation and then counts the number of beats for an additional 30 seconds.

**Rotational stimulation:** The rotational stimulus represents the physiologic stimulus for the VOR (see 13.1, Vestibulo-Ocular Reflex). Rotation about an axis passing through the head stimulates one or more semicircular canals on each side, depending on the head position. The left and right sides are stimulated in an opposing

🔎 13.1 Oculography and instrumental vestibular tests

**Oculography** is a procedure for recording eye position and movements. It can evaluate spontaneous or induced nystagmus also in darkness (without visual fixation) and during movements. It is used to document and calculate quantitative parameters for diagnostic and follow-up purposes.

*Technique:* **Electronystagmography** (ENG) utilizes the dipole properties of the eye to record ocular movements with electrodes affixed to the skin.
A more commonly used technique is **video-oculography**, in which the eyes are observed with an infrared camera and pupillary movements are automatically tracked and recorded.

*Interpretation:* The recorded eye movements such as spontaneous or induced nystagmus can be automatically analyzed with a computer, the slow-phase velocity being the most important parameter for further quantitative study. Standard oculographic recording may include tests for spontaneous nystagmus, analysis of smooth pursuit, and optokinetic, rotational, and caloric testing.

Many specialized **instrumental tests** are available for further investigation of the vestibular system:
- **Video head impulse test (video-HIT)**: This is an instrumental version of the clinically used HIT (see Eye Movements in this 🔖). The patient wears light goggles containing a high-speed infrared camera system, and the examiner induces the same type of head movements as in the clinical version of the test. Catch-up saccades can be detected by the system and the VOR can be tested for all semicircular canals (see **Fig. 13.10**).

- **Cervical vestibular evoked myogenic potentials (cVEMP)**: Stimulation of the sacculus by acoustic bursts and registration of ipsilateral evoked muscle potentials of the sternocleidomastoideus.
- **Ocular vestibular evoked myogenic potentials (oVEMP)**: Stimulation of the utriculus by fast and short linear accelerations (vibrations, tone bursts) and registration by surface electrodes of contralateral evoked potentials of the inferior eye muscles.
- **Dynamic visual acuity (DVA)**: Visual acuity is measured during head impulses in relation to static acuity. Visual acuity during rapid head impulses depends mainly on the VOR and its function can be measured by changes in DVA.
- Determining the **subjective vertical**: The patient sets a bar to the subjective vertical position. Otolithic asymmetry may induce deviation to one side.
- **Fundus photography**: Ocular torsion can be documented by photographic measurement of the relationship between the optic disc and fovea.
- **Posturography**: Objective recording and analysis of spinal motor function and coordination on stationary or moving (dynamic) platforms or by acceleration recordings during motor tasks.
- **Saccadic analysis**: Induction and oculographic analysis of saccades (fast eye movements).
- **Neck rotation test**: tests for nystagmus induced by rotating the body while the head remains stationary.

The different sensory elements of the vestibular system can be tested specifically and on one side only with the help of these instrumental tests. **Table 13.1** gives an overview on which test relates to which sensory element.

Table 13.1 Sensory elements of the vestibular system tested by instrumental tests

| Diagnostic test | Sensory element |
|---|---|
| Caloric stimulation | Ipsilateral lateral semicircular canal |
| Rotational stimulation | Bilateral semicircular canals vertical to the rotational axis (most often lateral canals) |
| Video head impulse test (video-HIT) | Semicircular canal vertical to the rotational axis and on the side toward the impulse (see **Fig. 13.10**) |
| Cervical vestibular evoked myogenic potentials (cVEMP) | Ipsilateral sacculus |
| Ocular vestibular evoked myogenic potentials (oVEMP) | Contralateral utriculus |

fashion: Rotating the head in one direction (e.g., to the right) induces a nystagmus toward the same side (to the right; rotatory nystagmus). When the rotation ceases, the nystagmus reverses to the opposite side (in this example, to the left; postrotatory nystagmus).
The test is conducted in darkness using nystagmography (🔎 **13.1**). Rotational testing is useful for quantitative analysis of the VOR and is therefore used in follow-ups.

In contrast to this vestibular nystagmus, rotation of the visual field while the head remains stationary induces an *optokinetic nystagmus*. The patient observes a striped pattern that preferably fills the entire visual field and is alternately rotated to the left and right, in each case inducing a nystagmus in the opposite direction.

# 13.3    Diagnosis and Differential Diagnosis of Vestibular Symptoms

Dizziness, vertigo, and postural unsteadiness are common ambiguous symptoms that can be clarified by taking a systematic history and applying targeted diagnostic procedures. The present ✍ explores options for this type of approach. Postural balance symptoms generally take precedence over vertiginous complaints. Dizziness or vertigo may well be present in the absence of postural balance symptoms, or a balance disorder may occur without vertigo, as in patients with predominantly proprioceptive or motor disturbances.

## Definition of Vestibular Symptoms

Dizziness and vertigo are frequent complains that are often difficult to relate to a specific diagnosis. This may be due partly to ambiguities in the term "dizziness" and "vertigo," which patients use to describe a multitude of complaints that can range from a vague queasy feeling to "blacking out" due to circulatory problems.

Dizziness should be differentiated from vertigo as diagnostic symptoms by the element of self-motion (**Fig. 13.13**).

**Vertigo** is defined as containing a sensation of false or distorted self-motion, which is lacking in dizziness. The false self-motion can be spinning or nonspinning such as swaying, rocking, or lifting. It can occur spontaneously or triggered by motions, positions, sound, or other events.

**Dizziness** is a broader sensation of disturbed or impaired spatial orientation without a false or distorted sense of motion. It may also occur spontaneously or triggered by events such as positions, motions, or visual surroundings.

**Postural symptoms** may include general unsteadiness, directional pulsions, falls, or near-falls.

It is assumed that these symptoms reflect disturbances of subjective spatial integrity and orientation caused by contradictory sensory information processing. There are two different ways in which dizziness or vertigo can occur:

- *The function of a sensory system is impaired:* Spatial integrity and orientation depend on proper interactions of the vestibular, visual, and proprioceptive sensory systems. Contradictory and unusual information can occur if the function of one or several of these peripheral sensory systems is disrupted (see also ✍13.1, Central Vestibular Structures). For example, the unilateral loss of a peripheral vestibular system creates an imbalance between the two vestibular systems, leading to rotary vertigo. With a constant or insidious disorder, the central nervous system (CNS) is usually able to compensate for the deficit over time, with the result that vertigo disappears or does not occur at all.
- *Central processing is impaired:* The information supplied by the normally functioning sensory systems is incorrectly processed or interpreted. This results

**Fig. 13.13    History-taking in vertigo patients**

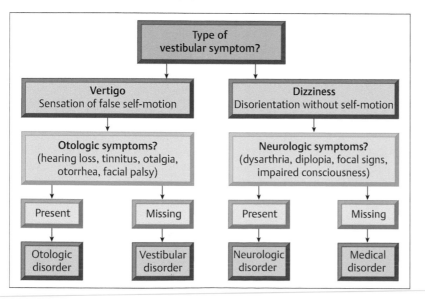

An initial history is taken to advance the differential diagnosis of vertiginous complaints. The algorithm provides clues that are helpful in directing further tests. Especially when a vestibular cause is suspected, the time course of the vertigo and associated symptoms can further narrow the differential diagnosis.

in conflicting sensory impressions and a feeling of dizziness. The processing disorder may be caused by diffuse changes such as metabolic or circulatory abnormalities, infection, trauma, or intoxication. Local CNS changes such as vascular occlusions, tumors, and inflammations may also be causative.

A combination of peripheral and central processing disorders may occur. These *multisensory dizziness or vertigo syndromes* are particularly common in elderly patients.

Contradictory sensory processing is a concept that can also explain the vestibular and spatial sensory disturbances that occur in normal individuals, such as *height vertigo* and *motion sickness*. Height vertigo is caused by a conflict between the unaccustomed visual horizon, which signals "depth" and "danger of falling," and the vestibular and proprioceptive systems, which perceive normal circumstances and no instability. In *motion sickness* (see also 🔎 **13.2**), cumulative conflicts arise between habituated patterns of interaction and the patterns that are experienced in the mode of travel. The moving vehicle repeatedly generates unaccustomed combinations of vestibular, visual, and proprioceptive stimuli that ultimately lead to motion sickness.

## Differential Diagnosis of Vestibular Symptoms

The history is important in the differential diagnosis of vestibular symptoms. First, an effort should be made to distinguish between **vertigo** with the sensation of false self-motion and **dizziness**. The next questions should be directed to otologic symptoms if vertigo is present and to neurologic symptoms if dizziness is present. These questions can narrow the differential diagnosis to a most likely group of disorders. The algorithm in **Fig. 13.13** outlines a simple approach, and **Fig. 13.14** provides another algorithm for the differentiation of vertigo based on its duration.

## Differential Diagnosis in Acute Vestibular Syndrome

Vestibular disorders are classified in different syndromes in relation to the duration of vertigo:

- **Acute vestibular syndrome (AVS)**: defined sudden onset of vertigo and nystagmus continuing for more than 24 hours with nausea, vomiting, intolerance to head movements, and unsteadiness.
- **Episodic vestibular syndrome (EVS)**: defined by episodes of vertigo, nystagmus, nausea, vomiting, and unsteadiness of less than 24 hours. The episodes may occur spontaneously, or they may be triggered by movements or positions (position-dependent vestibular syndrome [PVS]).
- **Chronic vestibular syndrome (CVS)**: defined by continuous dizziness or vertigo over weeks or months together with unsteadiness. Oscillopsia or nystagmus may be present.

Fig. 13.14 **Differential diagnosis of vestibular vertigo based on duration**

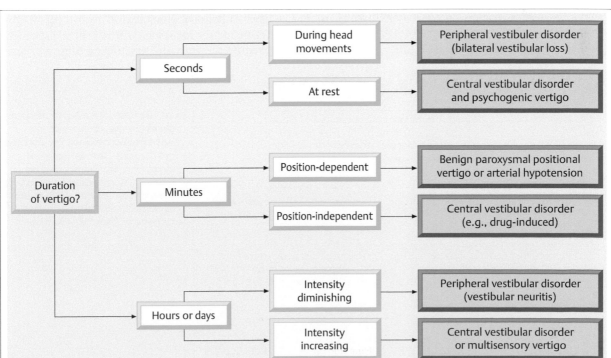

Acute vestibular syndrome is often an emergency and the main differentiation is between a peripheral acute vestibular disorder such as vestibular neuritis and vertebrobasilar stroke. Additional neurologic symptoms are often present in stroke patients, but they can be absent. Imaging may also be negative when performed early.

Clinical examination of nystagmus, VOR, and ocular tilt reaction has been shown to be highly sensitive to diagnose stroke. The acronym HINTS has been coined for this examination:

- **HI** stands for **h**ead **i**mpulse testing. Normal function of the VOR is highly predictive for stroke.
- **N** stands for **n**ystagmus. Gaze-evoked nystagmus with changing directions is also highly predictive for stroke.
- **TS** stands for **t**est of **s**kew. Corrective vertical saccades in the alternate eye cover test are again highly predictive for stroke.

Stroke rather than a pure peripheral vestibular disorder should be assumed if any of these three signs are present. One-sided acute hearing loss in acute vestibular syndrome is also pointing to a stroke. Additional signs for central vestibular disorder are:

- Severe ataxia with relatively little vertigo.
- Nystagmus with pure vertical direction (upbeat and downbeat nystagmus).
- Nystagmus not suppressible by visual fixation.
- Disturbances of the optokinetic reflex.

# 13.4   Vestibular Disorders

Peripheral dysfunction and diseases of the vestibular system are more common than central vestibular disorders. The most common clinical entities based on an isolated peripheral vestibular disorder are unilateral vestibular loss and benign paroxysmal positional vertigo.

Less common entities are Ménière's disease and bilateral vestibular loss. Central or combined vestibular disorders include vestibular migraine, stroke, and multiple sclerosis. These cases are investigated further by a neurologist.

## Peripheral Vestibular Disorders

### Acute Unilateral Vestibular Loss

Synonyms: vestibular neuronitis, vestibular neuritis.

*Definition:* Analogous to sudden sensorineural hearing loss, this disease is characterized by a sudden impairment of peripheral vestibular function on one side.

*Epidemiology:* Middle-aged individuals are affected predominantly but not exclusively. The disease often appears about 2 weeks after a viral upper respiratory infection.

*Etiopathogenesis:* The site of the lesion is probably mostly the superior part of the vestibular nerve, but the inferior part and/or the end organ may also be affected. The etiology is unknown. Viral ("neuritis"), vascular, metabolic, and mechanical causes have been proposed.

*Symptoms:* The onset is marked by a sudden, severe attack of rotary vertigo with no apparent cause. Generally, a continuous vertigo develops and persists for several days. Nausea, vomiting, and dysequilibrium cause severe subjective distress, and many patients are rushed to the emergency room with suspicion of an acute neurologic disease. There are no other otologic symptoms such as pain, hearing loss, or tinnitus, and there is no impairment of consciousness or other neurologic symptoms.

*Diagnosis:* A horizontal or rotary spontaneous nystagmus to one side can always be detected in the acute stage and is increased by suppression of visual fixation with Frenzel glasses. The head impulse test provokes catch-up saccades when the head is turned to the side of the lesion.
Caloric stimulation demonstrates non- or hypoexcitability of the affected labyrinth, which is on the side *opposite to the direction of the nystagmus.* The audiogram is normal.

*Differential diagnosis:* Differentiation is mainly required from central vestibular disorders such as vascular insufficiency and mass lesions, particularly a cerebellar infarction (see HINTS in 13.3, Differential Diagnosis in Acute Vestibular Syndrome).

*Treatment:* Treatment in the acute stage consists of bed rest in a darkened room, corticosteroids, fluid intake (infusion), and antivertiginous drugs of the antihistamine-type administered IV or by suppositories. Antivertiginous drugs of the 5-HT3 receptor antagonist type are less effective. After the acute phase and nausea have passed, medication should be stopped and the patient should be mobilized from bed as soon as possible, as this will promote central compensation. Specific balance training programs may be applied.

*Course:* The symptoms subside in a few days with spontaneous recovery of equilibrium (vestibular compensation). Younger patients tend to recover more quickly than older patients. Catch-up saccades or caloric hypoexcitability of the affected labyrinth often persists, but recovery of the VOR may occur.

*Prognosis:* The prognosis is favorable, and most patients recover completely. Latent dysequilibrium with a falling risk may persist in older patients and some patients may develop somatoform vestibular symptoms. Balance training is recommended in these cases.

### Benign Paroxysmal Positional Vertigo

Synonyms: canalolithiasis, cupulolithiasis.

*Epidemiology:* Benign paroxysmal positional vertigo (BPPV) is a frequent cause of sudden and short episodes of vertigo. Women predominate over men by a ratio of about 2:1.

*Etiology:* Possible causative factors include head trauma, a prior history of vestibular neuronitis, otologic or dental surgery, and inner ear disorders (e.g., labyrinthitis).

*Pathogenesis:* BPPV is a peripheral disorder based on a lesion of the end organ. The vertigo is believed to be incited by particles floating in the endolymph of a semicircular canal (canalolithiasis) or attaching themselves to the cupula (cupulolithiasis). The particles are probably most often otoconia that have become separated from the macula. The cupula becomes an unphysiologic gravitational and positional sensor. The increased mass of the cupula causes unphysiologic deflections during certain movements, which produce the typical symptoms.

At rest, the particles are deposited mainly in the posterior semicircular canal and BPPV of this canal is by far most common, but BPPV of the other canals are also recognized.

**Symptoms:** The patient complaints of severe, recurrent attacks of rotary vertigo lasting about 1 minute. The attacks are provoked by certain movements such as sitting up, turning in bed, or looking up. Nausea may occur, but there are no other associated symptoms. Often the symptoms are more intense following rest, and the patient may be awakened at night by vertiginous attacks. The attacks are fatigable and may disappear during the daily activities.

**Diagnosis:** The diagnosis is based on the typical history and established by positional maneuvers. The Hallpike maneuver (position change with head hanging, see **Fig. 13.12**) establishes BPPV of the posterior canal. Placing the head over the end of the table typically evokes a rotary nystagmus to one side after a latent period of approximately 10 seconds. The nystagmus increases for approximately 30 seconds, then diminishes (crescendo–decrescendo nystagmus). When the patient is brought back to an upright position, a similar nystagmus occurs in the opposite direction. This positional nystagmus is fatigable and disappears after several repetitions of the maneuver.

**Differential diagnosis:** The variant of BPPV of canalolithiasis of the lateral (horizontal) semicircular canal is found in approximately 10% of cases (vertigo when turning in bed). The anterior semicircular canal is seldom, if ever, affected.

Positional nystagmus can also occur in the setting of central or neural vestibular disorders. These cases, however, generally do not manifest the typical clinical complaints and diagnostic findings described above.

**Treatment:** Initial treatment consists of therapeutic positioning maneuvers, either brisk maneuvers such as the side-lying maneuver (Semont) or a defined sequence of head positions designed to displace and reposition the canaliths such as the Epley maneuver. In rare cases, it may be necessary to surgically block the posterior semicircular canal.

**Course:** As the name indicates, the vertigo is benign and generally resolves spontaneously in a matter of days or weeks. Occasionally, the symptoms recur after a variable period of time. It is rare for the complaints to persist for a prolonged period.

## Ménière's Disease

**Definition:** Ménière's disease is a clinically defined syndrome.

International consensus statements define the diagnostic criteria for Ménière's disease (American Academy of Otolaryngology-Head and Neck Surgery [AAO-HNS]; International Classification of Vestibular Disorders [ICVD]). The disease is mostly unilateral and the ear must present the following classic triad to make a definite diagnosis of Ménière's disease:

- Two or more spontaneous **episodes of vertigo**, each lasting 20 minutes to 12 hours.
- Documented low- to medium-frequency **sensorineural hearing loss**.
- Fluctuating aural symptoms such as **tinnitus** or fullness in the affected ear.

Terms such as "Ménière's complaints" or "atypical Ménière's disease" should be avoided, as they may refer to any type of rotary vertigo.

**Epidemiology:** Ménière's disease is rare. It can be diagnosed in only approximately 5 to 10% of patients with rotary vertigo and is certainly overdiagnosed. The typical age of onset is between the third and fifth decades, but Ménière's disease also occurs in younger and older individuals. Bilateral involvement, which is usually metachronous, occurs in approximately 20% of cases.

**Etiology:** The etiology of Ménière's disease is poorly understood. Some patients have a positive family history, suggesting that Ménière's disease is a multifactorial disorder with genetic and environmental influences. In rare cases, Ménière's symptoms can also result from previous inner ear damage, usually due to trauma (posttraumatic cochlear hydrops).

**Pathogenesis:** Endolymphatic cochlear hydrops has been identified as a morphologic correlate of Ménière's disease. It involves a relative overproduction of endolymph with distention of the endolymphatic space including the cochlear duct and the vestibular endolymphatic structures. The hydrops probably results from an inadequate reabsorption of endolymph in the endolymphatic sac rather than a true overproduction.

The hydrops of the cochlear duct causes displacement of the basilar membrane, creating an unfavorable mechanical environment for the hair cells that can lead to low-frequency sensorineural hearing loss. It has been theorized that attacks of vertigo may be caused by a rupture of the endolymphatic space, which would allow the mixing of perilymph and endolymph leading to potassium intoxication in the perilymphatic space. As yet, however, there is no proof that this type of rupture is linked to vertiginous attacks.

*Symptoms:* Ménière's disease is characterized by a typical history with the following symptoms:

- Fluctuating hearing loss and dysacusis.
- Tinnitus, which is continuous but of varying intensity and low frequency (roaring).
- Sensation of aural fullness.
- Attacks of rotary vertigo, nausea, and vomiting, which last for hours. Unsteadiness and dizziness may be present shortly before and long after the attacks.

The tinnitus and hearing loss may change before or during the attack. Most commonly, the tinnitus becomes louder, while hearing becomes poorer. Hearing generally improves again following the attack. A marked improvement of hearing during the attack itself is called the *Lermoyez phenomenon*. Sudden falls from an upright position to the ground with undisturbed consciousness may occur, usually late in the disease process. These falls are also called *drop attack or Tumarkin's otolithic crisis* and they are probably linked to a sudden disturbance of the otolithic organs with loss of vestibulospinal reflexes.

*Diagnosis:* The diagnosis is based on the typical **history** described above. **Otoscopic findings** are normal in idiopathic Ménière's disease, but late signs of previous inflammation or trauma may be found in symptomatic forms.

**Pure-tone audiometry** demonstrates a sensorineural hearing loss that mainly affects low frequencies in the initial stage of the disease (**Fig. 13.15**) and later affects all frequencies (pantonal hearing loss). **Speech audio-**

**metry** typically shows a disproportionate hearing loss for speech compared with the pure-tone audiogram. This is attributed to mechanical distortions within the cochlea.

**Auditory brainstem response (ABR) testing** is normal, and **electrocochleography** usually shows an elevation of the summation potential. Glycerin therapy (1.5 g glycerin/kg body weight) can improve the hearing threshold or reduce the summation potential in approximately two-thirds of patients (glycerol test). Endolymphatic hydrops can also be visualized by special contrast-enhanced **magnetic resonance imaging (MRI)** examination.

The **vestibular findings** in Ménière's disease are variable initially and may reflect hypofunction or hyperfunction of the labyrinth. With progression of the disease, however, peripheral vestibular hypofunction will invariably develop on the affected side. Vestibular nystagmus is detectable during the attacks and generally beats toward the unaffected side. It may also beat toward the affected side, however, and it may even change direction during an attack.

*Differential diagnosis:* The main differential diagnosis is vestibular migraine with some overlap of these two clinically defined diagnoses. Other vestibulocochlear disorders (e.g., vestibular schwannoma, sudden sensorineural hearing loss) should be excluded as well as other causes of cochlear hydrops such as syphilitic labyrinthitis.

*Treatment:*

**Acute attack:** Treatment consists of bed rest and antivertiginous or antiemetic medications administered orally, rectally, or intravenously (e.g., thiethylperazine, dimenhydrinate, metoclopramide HCl). Patients with profuse vomiting should receive infusions for fluid and electrolyte replacement.

**Fig. 13.15    Pure-tone audiograms in Ménière's disease**

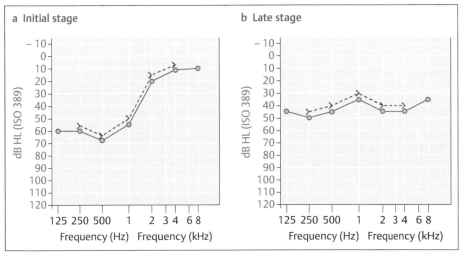

a Initial stage

b Late stage

**a** Typical low-frequency hearing loss in the initial stage of Ménière's disease. **b** Pantonal hearing loss in the late stage (flat curve). Bone conduction (broken line) is equal to air conduction (solid line) as a sign of sensorineural hearing loss.

**Prevention of attacks:** *Medical therapy between attacks* is usually tried initially in patients who experience frequent attacks. Salt restriction, betahistine, the intratympanic instillation of corticosteroids, tympanostomy tubes, pulsed pressure treatment of the middle ear, or surgery of the endolymphatic sac may be tried between attacks, although the efficacy of these therapies is uncertain. If symptoms do not improve, measures should be taken to *eliminate portions of the labyrinth.* This carries a risk of hearing loss or even deafness, and surgery may rarely lead to facial nerve paralysis. The following options are available:

- Intratympanic gentamicin: The drug is instilled into the middle ear directly through the tympanic membrane. The primarily vestibulotoxic gentamicin diffuses through the round and oval window niche, causing partial ablation of the labyrinth. Response is monitored audiometrically and by watching for nystagmus. Applications may be repeated, but only after a delay of a few weeks.
- Vestibular neurotomy: The vestibular nerve is surgically divided through a transtemporal approach (through the middle cranial fossa), translabyrinthine approach (always associated with deafness), or retrosigmoid approach (through the posterior cranial fossa).
- Labyrinthectomy: Since surgical ablation of the labyrinth sacrifices hearing, this procedure should be considered only in patients who are already deaf.

**Course:** A characteristic feature of Ménière's disease is its unpredictable course. Besides rare abortive forms in which the symptoms cease to occur after several attacks, periods of frequent attacks alternate with periods with few or no vertiginous complaints. The most distressing aspect for patients is the sudden, unpredictable attacks of vertigo. When such attacks are frequent, the patient may be incapacitated by the vertigo itself and by the fear of new attacks. Often, however, periods of frequent attacks are followed by months or years of remission in which the dominant findings are hearing loss and tinnitus. In typical cases, Ménière's disease runs a progressive course for years with gradually diminishing attacks of vertigo but increasing hearing loss that culminates in deafness ("burned-out Ménière's disease"). Cochlear implants are an option to restore hearing in these cases.

## Bilateral Vestibular Loss

**Pathogenesis:** Bilateral vestibular loss is a balance disorder caused by severe, bilateral hypofunction or failure of the peripheral vestibular apparatus. It usually has a systemic cause but may also result from bilateral disease of the vestibular apparatus. Examples of **systemic causes** are ototoxic drugs (aminoglycosides, diuretics, cisplatin), industrial toxins (aromatic hydrocarbons, heavy metals), and endogenous lesions (renal failure). Examples of **local diseases** that may occur bilaterally are bacterial, viral or autoimmune labyrinthitis, congenital or acquired labyrinthine disorders (anomalies, otosclerosis, acute vestibular loss, or Ménière's disease on both sides), temporal bone fractures, and diseases of the vestibular nerves (polyneuropathy, type 2 neurofibromatosis). About 30% of the cases are idiopathic.

**Symptoms:** Bilateral vestibular loss does not produce nystagmus because there is no asymmetry of vestibular response. There is, however, a destabilization of visual fixation with typical oscillopsia (see 🔖13.2, History). The patient describes a balance disturbance or "drunken" feeling, with an inability to recognize faces or read street signs while walking. The complaints are exacerbated in darkness.
The disorder is commonly associated with a variable degree of bilateral sensorineural hearing loss.

**Diagnosis:** The head impulse test shows catch-up saccades to both sides (see 🔖13.2, Eye Movements). Caloric and rotational stimulation of the labyrinths elicit either no response or a very weak response. Auditory testing is also indicated and will often demonstrate at least a high-frequency hearing loss.

**Differential diagnosis:** A central vestibular disorder can produce similar complaints.

**Treatment:** Physical therapy with specific balance training may be helpful, as it can enhance the compensation of vestibular function by nonvestibular systems. Technical systems providing additional nonvestibular feedbacks are available. Generally, however, patients are left with some degree of residual dysequilibrium.

## Other Causes of Peripheral Vestibular Disorders

A viral, bacterial, or autoimmune labyrinthitis generally leads to vertigo in addition to hearing impairment. Tests disclose the typical signs of peripheral vestibular dysfunction with unsteadiness, vestibular nystagmus toward the opposite side, and catch-up saccades in the head impulse test.
**Otogenic inflammatory vestibular disorders:** An acute or chronic inflammatory process in the middle ear can lead to vertigo and dysequilibrium. The associated labyrinthitis is described in 🔖12.2, Labyrinthitis. When the cause is *acute otitis media* with an intact tympanic membrane, paracentesis should be performed at once to decompress the middle ear and windows. In patients with *chronic otitis media*, a cholesteatoma with a perilymphatic fistula should be considered whenever vestibular symptoms appear. The lateral semicircular canal is affected most often.

**Dehiscence of the superior semicircular canal (SSCD):**
Patients with the syndrome of dehiscence of the superior semicircular canal complain either of vestibular symptoms such as general unsteadiness or vertigo produced by loud sounds (*Tullio's phenomenon*), or they complain of auditory symptoms such as hearing loss together with hyperacusis toward internal sounds such as eating crunchy food.

The symptoms are induced by a fistula of the superior semicircular canal toward the middle cranial fossa. The bony shell of the canal is missing (**Fig. 13.16**) leading to direct contact between the canal and the dura. The fistula leads to mechanical disturbance of the inner ear function triggering the symptoms. Typical clinical findings are nystagmus induced by sound or by increasing the air pressure of the external ear canal (*positive fistula sign*), mild conductive hearing loss in the tone audiogram with hypersensitive bone conduction, and large amplitudes in cervical vestibular evoked myogenic potentials (cVEMP, see 𝒫 **13.1**).

The condition usually develops spontaneously in adults, peaking in the fourth decade. Reasons for the dehiscence are not known.

Similar symptoms and findings can be evoked by a direct contact of a congenitally enlarged vestibular aqueduct with the dura (*syndrome of enlarged vestibular aqueduct*).

*Treatment* is surgical in cases with disabling symptoms. The dehiscence can be covered surgically ("resurfacing"), or the semicircular canal can be blocked ("plugging").

**Perilymphatic fistula:** This is a pathologic opening of the bony shell of the perilymphatic space. The opening can either be covered by tissue such as the dura in the above-described dehiscence of the superior semicircular canal or it can represent a direct connection to the middle ear space. Such direct connections occur mostly at the round and oval windows by direct trauma including surgery, or barotrauma to the middle ear (see 🗐 11.4, Barotrauma of the Middle Ear). Covered perilymphatic fistulas open either to the intracranial space or to the middle ear, most often covered by inflammatory tissue, which has resorbed the bony shell. The typical example is a perilymphatic fistula of the lateral semicircular canal in cholesteatoma of the middle ear mentioned above.

Perilymphatic fistulas are a danger to inner ear function and they can lead to vestibular symptoms and hearing disorders. Permanent damage is usually induced by either massive loss of perilymph with entrance of air into the labyrinth (pneumolabyrinth), or septic or aseptic inflammation (see 🗐 12.2, Labyrinthitis). These cases need immediate surgical repair.

*Treatment* of other cases of proven or suspected perilymphatic fistula depends on symptoms and clinical findings. It can range from bed rest with the head elevated to surgical exploration and repair.

**Posttraumatic vestibular disorders:** Vestibular symptoms may be provoked by blunt head trauma with a labyrinthine concussion or contusion, a temporal bone fracture (see 🗐 15.2), trauma to the cervical spine, or a surgical operation. Most cases involve a peripheral,

**Fig. 13.16   Dehiscence of the superior semicircular canal**

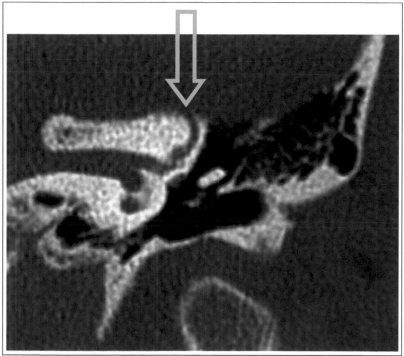

CT in the plane of the superior semicircular canal showing clearly the missing bony shell toward the middle cranial fossa (arrow).

unilateral, cochleovestibular disorder. Central vestibular disorders can also occur in patients with a brainstem contusion or cerebral contusion. It can be difficult to differentiate among peripheral, central, and combined vestibular disorders. Central compensation of the peripheral disorders may be delayed. Also, a peripheral paroxysmal positional vertigo (BPPV) may develop several weeks after the trauma (see above). Psychogenic factors also play a role in prolonged cases of posttraumatic vertigo.

# Neural and Central Vestibular Disorders

## Vestibular Disorders with a Neural Cause

**Cerebellopontine angle tumors:** Cerebellopontine angle tumors are a relatively infrequent cause of vestibular disorders, as they are usually slow-growing and symptoms are easily compensated over time. The symptoms associated with these tumors are described in ✍ 15.3.

---

### 🔎 13.2 Other vestibular disorders

#### Motion sickness
Motion sickness is related to the function of the labyrinth and, as such, is a "physiologic" response. Motion sickness does not occur in patients with nonfunctioning peripheral vestibular organs. It probably results from a shift in accustomed patterns of sensory processing (sensory conflict or mismatch). The major conflicts are between the visual and vestibular systems, bringing about the typical symptoms of malaise, fatigue, yawning, increased salivation, nausea, and finally vomiting.
*Prevention* relies on anticipating and visually perceiving the motion with as much of the visual field as possible. Motion with a limited visual field (porthole, rear seat) predisposes to motion sickness. Training can induce the development of central patterns that reduce susceptibility to motion sickness. The condition can be treated medically with antivertiginous drugs, which should be taken before travel whenever possible (scopolamine transdermal patch, dimenhydrinate, cinnarizine). These drugs may induce fatigue and therefore should not be taken before operating a motor vehicle.

#### Vestibular migraine
Similar to Ménière's disease, vestibular migraine is a clinical diagnosis defined by a set of symptoms. These are:
- Five or more episodes with vestibular symptoms of moderate or severe intensity, lasting from a few minutes to up to 3 days.
- Current or previous history of migraine with or without aura.
- One or more migraine features with at least 50% of the vestibular episodes, such as one-sided or pulsating headache, photophobia, phonophobia, or visual aura.

Vestibular symptoms include usually vertigo, but they are unspecific and mostly transient. Fluctuating hearing loss and tinnitus may occur during attacks, but permanent hearing loss is not a feature.
*Treatment* is the same as for other forms of migraine and success may help to establish the diagnosis.
Vestibular migraine has to be differentiated from *basilar-type migraine*, which is associated in many cases with central vestibular symptoms including vertigo.

#### Vestibular disorders in children
The most common type of vestibular dysfunction in small children is *benign paroxysmal vertigo of childhood*. This condition is not related to benign paroxysmal positional vertigo in adults (see Benign Paroxysmal Positional Vertigo above). It is characterized by brief attacks of vertigo lasting seconds or minutes that occur when the child is feeling well and are associated with dysequilibrium and nystagmus. The child recovers completely within a short time. The attacks are most common between 1 and 4 years of age. They progress often to migraine attacks, suggesting a link between this type of vertigo and vestibular migraines.

#### Somatoform (psychosomatic) vertigo or dizziness
Two different forms of somatoform vestibular disorders can be differentiated. Psychiatric disorders such as depression, anxiety neuroses, hyperventilation, and phobic disorders may be associated with a sensation of subjective dizziness. Patients complain of constant, vague dizziness or of brief, recurring dizzy spells. Alternatively, up to 30% of patients with organic vestibular disorders such as Ménière's disease or vestibular schwannoma develop additional somatoform vertigo. It is important to recognize somatoform vestibular disorders and treat it correctly.
The *history* provides the best information, and either no evidence of a vestibular disorder can be detected or the findings do not match the complaints.
*Treatment* is geared toward the underlying disorder. Antivertiginous drugs are of no benefit.

#### Vestibular disorders with a cervical cause
Proprioceptors located in the deep muscles of the neck and cervical vertebral joints are linked to vestibular and oculomotor centers and can evoke the cervicovestibular reflex (CVR) and cervico-ocular reflex (COR). The relationship between disturbances of these reflexes and vertiginous complaints is uncertain, however, as there is no reliable test for evaluating these reflexes. This makes it difficult to interpret the frequent concomitant complaints involving the nuchal region and the vestibular or cochlear system (tinnitus). These combinations of complaints may occur spontaneously in association with nuchal degenerative changes or may follow a whiplash injury. With whiplash trauma, interpretation is also hampered by a possible brain contusion or direct labyrinthine injury (otoliths).

A cerebellopontine angle tumor should be included in the differential diagnosis of a unilateral cochleo-vestibular disorder. Vestibular signs consist of various forms of vestibular spontaneous or provoked nystagmus and caloric hypoexcitability of the labyrinth. Large tumors may exert pressure on the brainstem leading to central vestibular signs such as impaired smooth pursuit tracking or altered optokinetic nystagmus.

**Vestibular paroxysmia:** Vestibular paroxysmia is the vestibular analogue of trigeminal neuralgia induced by neurovascular conflicts. Vascular compression of the vestibular nerve can lead to short attacks of vertigo, lasting a few seconds only and occurring in clusters many times per day. The diagnosis rests on the typical history, the demonstration of a vestibular neurovascular conflict in the MRI, and successful treatment with carbamazepine. Surgical decompression by a retrosigmoid approach is an option in cases otherwise difficult to treat.

**Vestibular neuritis:** Isolated neuritis of the vestibular nerve is recognized as one cause of acute unilateral vestibular loss (see Acute Unilateral Vestibular Loss above). This form of the disease is described under that heading.

Vestibular nerve disorders may occur in the setting of cranial polyneuritis or polyneuropathy. It is particularly important to detect or exclude treatable causes such as *herpes zoster*, *borreliosis*, and *toxoplasmosis*.

## Central Vestibular Disorders

The most frequent cause of a central vestibular disorder is circulatory disturbance in the brainstem region. The lesions may consist of transient or permanent, small or larger ischemic areas or hemorrhages. Other possible causes of central vestibular disorders are inflammation (e.g., multiple sclerosis), infection (e.g., viral encephalitis), tumors (e.g., gliomas), metabolic disorders (e.g., Wernicke–Korsakoff syndrome), and trauma (e.g., brainstem contusion). The investigation and treatment of central vestibular disorders fall within the neurologic specialty.

**Vertebrobasilar Insufficiency:** Vertebrobasilar insufficiency is a rare cause of vertiginous complaints. A transient blood-flow disturbance in the vertebrobasilar territory can lead to attacks of rotary vertigo, which usually have a central cause. But since the labyrinth derives its blood supply from the same territory (labyrinthine artery), decreased blood flow to the peripheral vestibular organs cannot be excluded. Vertebrobasilar insufficiency is also accompanied by other neurologic symptoms: visual disturbances, diplopia, drop attacks, loss of consciousness, speech disorders, or paralysis. Direct compression of the vertebral artery by a cervical spinal lesion or extreme head movements is rare, but blood flow may be reduced in a setting of transient ischemic attacks (TIAs)

or as a steal effect associated with a general decrease in cerebral blood flow.

The *diagnostic work-up* includes the assessment of cardiovascular risk factors and an ultrasound evaluation of the cranial vessels. Occasionally, vertigo and nystagmus can be provoked by a certain head position. Further investigation and treatment are directed by the findings.

*Differentiation* is required from positional vertigo and cervical vertigo.

**Vertebrobasilar stroke:** Vertebrobasilar stroke leads to symptoms with a duration of more than 24 hours, and thus to an acute vestibular syndrome. The differentiation of the acute vestibular syndrome in peripheral and central causes is essential and discussed in ✍ 13.3, Differential Diagnosis in Acute Vestibular Syndrome. Some typical syndromes can be recognized:

*Wallenberg's syndrome:* The onset of this syndrome is manifested by sudden, severe rotary vertigo, nausea, vomiting, severe ataxia, and additional brainstem signs such as dysphagia and dysphonia. There is ischemia of the lateral medulla oblongata (vertebral artery or posterior inferior cerebellar artery, PICA), leading to crossed signs. The nuclei of cranial nerves V–X are affected ipsilaterally and temperature sensation is affected contralaterally, sparing the face (spinothalamic tract).

*Cerebellar infarction (PICA infarction):* An infarction in the territory of the PICA can lead to a typical acute vestibular syndrome. Gait and stance ataxia are frequently more pronounced. MRI can confirm the presence of a cerebellar infarction, but it can be negative in the first few hours.

> ✍ Patients with a cerebellar infarction require particularly close surveillance due to the potential for an intracranial herniation (mass effect) involving the brainstem.

**Multiple sclerosis:** Vertigo and dysequilibrium occur as the initial manifestations of multiple sclerosis in approximately 5% of cases. The typical signs of a central vestibular disorder are found, often in relatively young patients. A retrocochlear hearing disorder can also be detected in most cases. MRI can demonstrate demyelinated areas in the brainstem, which require further investigation and treatment by a neurologist.

**Other causes of central vestibular disorders:** Other possible causes of central vestibular symptoms are *malformations* (basilar impression, Arnold–Chiari malformation), *degenerative CNS diseases* (Friedreich's ataxia, cerebellar degeneration, Parkinson's disease, Alzheimer's disease), *intoxication* (alcohol, barbiturates, antiepileptics), and *systemic diseases* (diabetes mellitus, renal failure, acquired immune deficiency syndrome). Very rarely, vestibular symptoms may be precipitated in a setting of epilepsy (vestibular epilepsy).

# 14 Facial Nerve

## 14.1 Clinically Relevant Anatomy, Function, and Evaluation of the Facial Nerve

The facial nerve travels an anatomically complex course through the temporal bone, middle ear, and parotid gland. Knowledge of the anatomy, relations, and various physiologic functions of the facial nerve is essential for understanding and diagnosing functional disorders.

### Anatomy

The course and various fiber components of the facial nerve are shown schematically in **Fig. 14.1**. The facial nerve can be divided into *six segments*:

**Intracranial:** The frontal branch components of the facial nucleus, unlike the other motor components, are innervated by the left and right corticonuclear tract. Before the facial nerve leaves the brainstem, its motor fibers wind around the abducens nucleus and form the "internal genu" of the nerve. After leaving the brainstem, the facial nerve enters the internal porus acusticus along with the vestibulocochlear nerve.

**Intrameatal:** Accompanied by cranial nerve VIII, the facial nerve travels through the internal auditory canal to the fundus; there, it passes anterosuperiorly through the meatal foramen, leaving the meatus. This is the narrowest point in the bony *fallopian canal* (facial canal) and is the site where the nerve is most likely to become entrapped due to inflammatory swelling.

**Labyrinthine:** After running a short distance anteriorly, the facial nerve gives off the greater petrosal nerve with its secretory fibers to the lacrimal glands and nasal mucosal glands. The facial nerve turns sharply downward and posteriorly at the geniculate ganglion, forming the first genu.

**Tympanic:** This segment of the facial nerve runs horizontally through the middle ear, passing above the stapes, to the aditus ad antrum near the lateral semicircular canal. The tympanic nerve segment is usually covered by a thin bony sheath.

**Mastoid:** The mastoid segment of the facial nerve forms the second genu by the aditus ad antrum, turning vertically downward at an angle of approximately 90 degrees. It courses through the mastoid and leaves its bony canal at the *stylomastoid foramen*; just before exiting at this foramen, the facial nerve gives off the *chorda tympani*, which runs back to the middle ear and passes through it. It contains sensory gustatory fibers.

**Extracranial:** After emerging from the stylomastoid foramen, the facial nerve enters the parotid gland (see ✎6.1, Parotid Gland), where it branches at the *pes anserinus*. The individual branching pattern within the gland is variable.

### Function

The predominant and most important function of the facial nerve is supplying motor innervation to the mimetic muscles of the face. It has secretory and sensory functions as well, however (see **Fig. 14.1**).

### Evaluation

#### Clinical Examination

**History:** The onset and course of facial nerve paralysis should be documented. The patient should be questioned about:
- Otologic symptoms and diseases or previous ear surgery.
- Trauma.
- Neurologic disease.
- Tick bites (borreliosis) or evidence of other infections.
- Systemic diseases such as diabetes mellitus, cancer, autoimmune diseases, or sarcoidosis.

The symptoms of a facial nerve lesion may also include hyperacusis (paralysis of the stapedius muscle), otalgia (irritation of the sensory fibers), gustatory disturbances, and disturbances of lacrimation (dryness, crocodile tears = gustatory lacrimation due to faulty neural regulation).

**Inspection:** A *general otolaryngologic status* should be obtained, giving particular attention to *otologic findings* and the *function of the other cranial nerves*. The presence of other cranial nerve deficits will generally exclude idiopathic facial paralysis. Any changes in the *parotid gland* should be noted. Testing the *motor function of the facial nerve* should include the following:
- *Frontal branch:* wrinkling the forehead or looking upward. Intact function of the frontal branch compared with the other facial nerve branches indicates a *central* or *supranuclear lesion* (see **Fig. 14.1**).

The cardinal symptom of a facial nerve lesion is paralysis of the mimetic facial muscles, which is the primary focus of the examination. A distinction is drawn between complete paralysis and paresis (incomplete paralysis). A detailed history and clinical examination can often establish the cause of facial nerve paralysis.

Fig. 14.1 Facial nerve: course, segments, and functions

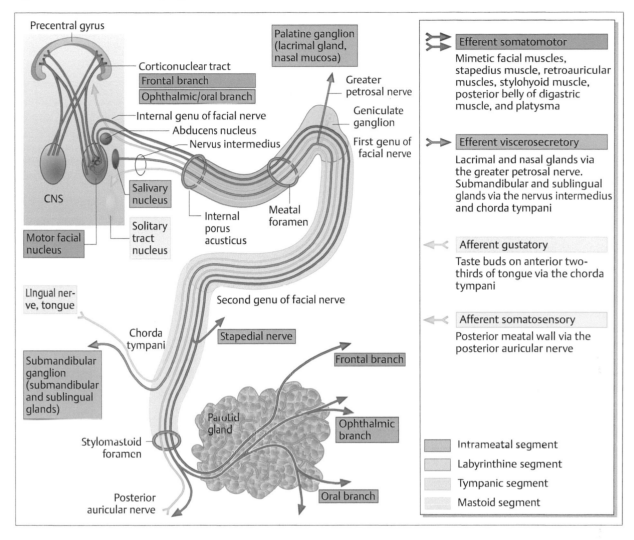

- *Ophthalmic branch:* rapid blinking (slowed in mild paresis): eyelid closure, spontaneous or against a resistance (weakened in mild paresis): or incomplete lid closure (deficit measured in millimeters, seen in severe paresis or paralysis; **Fig. 14.2**).
- *Oral branch:* baring the teeth, whistling, and inflating the cheeks; air will escape even with mild paresis.

The examiner should also watch for *synkinesis*—an involuntary associated movement of mimetic muscles accompanying the voluntary movement of other muscles, such as an unintended movement of the oral commissure induced by closing the eyes. This type of synkinesis generally persists as a residual defect following the complete degeneration of nerve fibers (neurotmesis).

*Lacrimal secretion* can be tested by placing strips of filter paper in the lower eyelid and comparing the sides (Schirmer's test, see *⌀* **14.1**). The amount of tears produced can be helpful in planning corneoprotective therapy.

Fig. 14.2 Bell's palsy

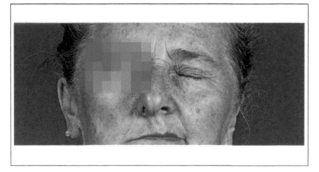

Incomplete eyelid closure due to idiopathic facial paralysis on the right side.

**Additional tests:** Patients with facial paralysis should undergo laboratory tests to screen for infectious diseases (borreliosis, herpes zoster, syphilis, human immunodeficiency virus [HIV], mononucleosis, toxoplasmosis). *Audiometric testing* (pure-tone, speech and immittance measurements) is necessary due to

Various function tests can provide limited information on the site of a facial nerve lesion. It is assumed, for example, that if Schirmer's test shows intact lacrimal gland function, the lesion must be distal to the geniculate ganglion (see **Fig. 14.1**). Due to the different sensitivities of different-sized nerve fibers, retrograde degeneration, and measurement inaccuracies, however, the tests are often imprecise for site-of-lesion determination. Imaging studies are more accurate in this regard. Function tests are considered to have only limited prognostic importance and are seldom performed today. The most important functions are:

**Stapedial reflex testing** (see 🔍8.4, Stapedial Reflex): If the reflex is absent, the lesion must be proximal to the mastoid segment. The reflex is lost even with mild degrees of nerve damage, as it is mediated by delicate fibers.

**Schirmer's test:** Lacrimation is measured with a 5-cm-long strip of litmus paper placed into the conjunctival sac. A 30% reduction in lacrimal secretion relative to the opposite side is considered abnormal.

**Gustometry:** Taste sensation is evaluated (e.g., by electrogustometry, see 🔍4.2, Taste Testing) and compared between the sides. This tests the fibers of the chorda tympani. A right–left discrepancy means that the lesion is proximal to the stylomastoid foramen.

**Sialometry:** This is a technically demanding test that is rarely practiced. The Wharton duct is catheterized on each side to measure salivary production by the submandibular glands. A discrepancy between the sides means that the lesion is proximal to the origin of the chorda tympani.

stapedius muscle involvement and the close proximity of cranial nerve VIII.

## Site-of-Lesion Determination and Imaging Studies

Today, the best and most widely used topodiagnostic tests are computed tomography (CT) and magnetic resonance imaging (MRI). Inflammatory facial nerve lesions can be demonstrated by MRI after gadolinium contrast administration. Otogenic and traumatic facial paralysis should always be evaluated by high-resolution bone-window CT scanning of the temporal bone in several planes.

## Electrical and Magnetic Testing

The importance of electrical and magnetic testing lies in the objective detection and quantification of facial paralysis. Repeated tests are useful for defining the degree of facial nerve damage and assessing the prognosis for recovery. From a pathophysiologic standpoint, three degrees of facial nerve fiber injury are distinguished:
1. *Neurapraxia:* disruption of axonal transport without degeneration.
2. *Axonotmesis:* wallerian degeneration of the myelin sheath with an intact perineurium. There is complete paralysis of the affected fibers, but regeneration of the axon is also complete.
3. *Neurotmesis:* wallerian degeneration and loss of the perineural sheath with complete paralysis of the affected fibers. Regeneration is unpredictable. The outcome is residual dysfunction with synkinesis and persistent palsy.

**Electroneurography (ENoG):** This test involves supramaximal stimulation of the nerve trunk and measuring the muscular response with surface electrodes. The degree of degeneration is expressed as a percentage relative to the healthy side (=100%). More than 90% degeneration of the nerve fibers is a poor prognostic sign in terms of complete recovery, but repeatability of test results is variable.

**Electromyography (EMG):** The electrical potentials of the mimetic muscles are measured with needle electrodes. Recordings are made during spontaneous and voluntary muscular activity for the objective detection *of paralysis* and *reinnervation*. EMG is also used for the *intraoperative monitoring* of facial nerve function during parotid and otologic surgery and intracranial operations.

**Magnetic stimulation:** The intracranial portion of the facial nerve can be stimulated with a magnetic coil to test function over the entire course of the nerve. If the nerve is responsive to stimulation when facial paralysis is present, there is a good prognosis for recovery. If the nerve is unresponsive, a prognostic assessment cannot be made.

## Diagnosis and Management of Facial Paralysis

Motor paralysis is the most important and by far the most common symptom of facial nerve pathology. Generally, it is easily determined from the history whether the paralysis is traumatic or nontraumatic. With nontraumatic paralysis, the function of the frontal branch can be tested to determine whether the lesion is central (i.e., supranuclear) or peripheral. This is followed by various diagnostic steps and considerations that are outlined in **Fig. 14.3**. It is particularly important to differentiate between complete paralysis and incomplete paralysis (paresis).

Before instrumented tests are performed, the cause of facial paralysis can almost always be determined from a detailed history and clinical examination of the external ear, middle ear, hearing, vestibular function, other cranial nerve functions, and the parotid gland. The most frequent causes of peripheral facial paralysis are listed in **Table 14.1**.

**Fig. 14.3 Algorithm for the differential diagnosis of facial paresis**

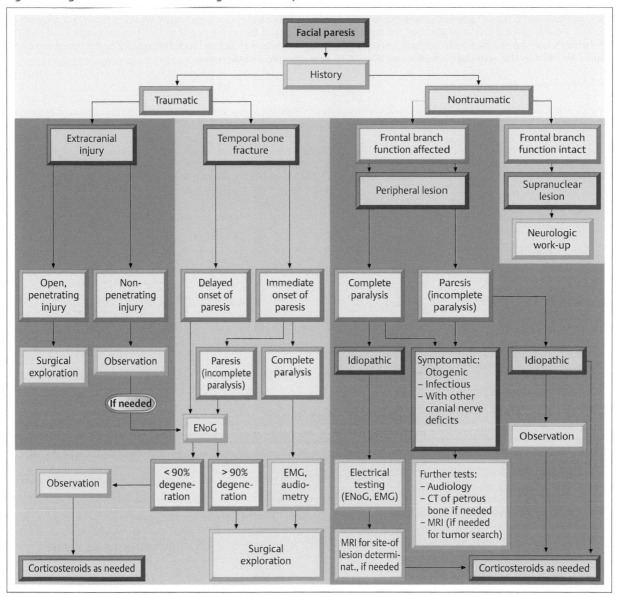

**Table 14.1** Differential diagnosis of peripheral facial paralysis

| Classification | Causes | Primary findings/diagnostic examination |
|---|---|---|
| **Idiopathic** | Bell's palsy | Diagnosis by exclusion |
| | Melkersson–Rosenthal syndrome | Recurrent swelling of face, fissured tongue |
| **Inflammatory** | Cholesteatoma | Otoscopic finding |
| | Sarcoidosis (Heerfordt's syndrome) | Parotitis, ophthalmological symptoms |
| | Guillain–Barré syndrome | Other motor paralysis |
| **Infectious** | Borreliosis | Tick bite, laboratory tests |
| | Herpes zoster oticus | Vesicles of the outer ear, disturbances of cochlear and vestibular functions |
| | Acute otitis media, mastoiditis | History, otoscopic findings |
| | Necrotizing otitis externa | History, otoscopic findings |
| | Human immunodeficiency virus | Laboratory tests |
| | Tuberculosis | Laboratory tests |
| | Mononucleosis | Laboratory tests |
| **Traumatic** | Temporal bone fracture | History, clinical findings, CT |
| | Facial injury, mandibular fracture | History, clinical findings, CT |
| | Surgical trauma (middle ear, parotid gland) | History, clinical findings |
| | Obstetric trauma | History of delivery |
| **Neoplastic** | Paraganglioma | Otoscopic findings, MRI |
| | Facial neurinoma | MRI |
| | Schwannoma of cranial nerves | MRI |
| | Meningioma | MRI |
| | Malignant tumor of the temporal bone (e.g., middle ear carcinoma, rhabdomyosarcoma, lymphoma) | CT and MRI |
| | Malignant tumor of the parotid gland | MRI, cytological findings |
| | Metastasis (breast cancer, hypernephroma) | History, MRI, cytological findings |
| **Metabolic** | Diabetes mellitus | Laboratory tests |
| | Pregnancy | Laboratory test |

# 14.2    Clinical Aspects of the Facial Nerve

The most common type of facial nerve paralysis is idiopathic or Bell's palsy, followed by traumatic and inflammatory otogenic forms. Traumatic causes can usually be established by the history, giving particular attention to possible infectious and inflammatory otogenic causes. Idiopathic facial paralysis is a diagnosis of exclusion.

## Inflammatory Changes

### Idiopathic Facial Paralysis (Bell's Palsy)

Synonyms: cryptogenic, rheumatic, or ischemic facial paralysis.

*Definition:* Bell's palsy is a unilateral, peripheral facial paralysis of acute onset that has no discernible cause and does not involve any other cranial nerves.

*Occurrence:* Bell's palsy is the most common form of facial paralysis. The incidence is approximately 20 per 100,000 population.

*Pathogenesis:* The pathogenesis is unknown. Theories include infection and inflammation (viral, autoimmune), vascular ischemia, and constitutional factors. Idiopathic facial paralysis is more common in diabetic patients and in pregnancy (third trimester).

*Symptoms:* Often, the initial symptom is retroauricular pain, followed by unilateral peripheral facial paralysis in which the frontal branch is equally affected. The paralysis is partial in 30% of cases and complete in 70% of cases. It develops within a few days (2–5 days) and has no systemic manifestations. The clinical features may include hyperacusis (stapedius muscle paralysis), dysgeusia, and decreased lacrimation.

*Diagnosis:* The diagnosis is one of *exclusion* based on the typical clinical course and the absence of an identifiable cause of the paralysis.

*Differential diagnosis:* Otogenic and infectious causes of peripheral facial paralysis should be excluded (see **Table 14.1**). Bell's palsy requires differentiation from *Melkersson–Rosenthal syndrome* (peripheral facial paralysis with recurrent swelling of the face and lips and a fissured tongue).

*Course and prognosis:* Partial paralysis always resolves completely within a few weeks. Recovery from complete paralysis takes longer (months) and is complete in only approximately 60 to 70% of cases. Approximately 15% of patients are left with troublesome residual palsy and/or synkinesis.

Progressive paralysis over more than a few days is not idiopathic and causes such as tumors of the parotid gland or the temporal bone must be searched by MRI.

*Complications:* The most serious complication is corneal damage due to lagophthalmos, ectropion, and/or decreased lacrimation. The best preventive measures are moisturization and ophthalmologic follow-up.

*Treatment:* Treatment with corticosteroids is recommended and efficacy has been confirmed. They are combined occasionally with antiviral agents. Surgical decompression of the facial nerve is of unproven benefit and carries a considerably higher risk.
It is important to protect the cornea with a watch-glass eye dressing, moisturizing eye drops and ointments, and if necessary by tarsorrhaphy or by placing a gold or titanium weight in the upper eyelid.

### Inflammatory Otogenic Facial Paralysis

*Definition:* This is a type of facial paralysis caused by the spread of an infectious or other inflammatory process from the ear and temporal bone to the facial nerve.

*Occurrence:* Facial paralysis can occur as a relatively rare complication in all forms of otitis and osteitis/osteomyelitis of the temporal bone, particularly in cases with cholesteatoma, subacute mastoiditis in pediatric patients, and advanced necrotizing otitis externa (see 10.4, Necrotizing Otitis Externa).

*Etiology:* The functional damage is caused by a direct toxic insult, inflammatory epineural edema and pressure, and, in some cases, osteitis.

*Symptoms:* Otologic symptoms are usually the dominant findings, and facial paralysis occurs as a complication. A chronic process (cholesteatoma) may have an insidious onset.

*Diagnosis:* The otoscopic findings suggest the correct diagnosis. Further investigation requires an audiologic examination and CT scans of the temporal bone.

**Differential diagnosis:** Differentiation is required from infectious diseases, especially herpes zoster oticus, and from tumors of the lateral skull base, temporal bone, and parotid gland.

**Complications:** The complications depend largely on the underlying disease.

**Treatment:** Except for facial paralysis in the setting of acute otitis media (antibiotics), treatment consists of prompt surgical exposure of the nerve and appropriate antibiotic therapy. Corticosteroids are also administered to reduce edema.

**Course and prognosis:** These depend on the degree of paralysis, the underlying disease, and the timing of treatment. The less complete and more acute the paralysis and the earlier treatment is initiated, the better the prognosis.

## Facial Paralysis Secondary to Infection

It should be determined whether facial paralysis has an infectious etiology, since infections are often amenable to specific treatment. The most frequent causes of infectious facial paralysis are herpes zoster oticus and borreliosis. A history of tick bite can usually be elicited in patients with borreliosis. This infection can be detected by proper laboratory tests and can be treated with antibiotic. Other infections that may be associated with peripheral facial paralysis are meningitis, Guillain–Barré syndrome, poliomyelitis, and HIV infection.

## Traumatic Facial Paralysis

**Definition:** A complete or partial facial nerve injury may result from a traumatic rupture or stretch injury, nerve compression (by hematoma or bone fragments), trauma-induced swelling, or thermal injury (from a drill during otosurgery). The paralysis may be *immediate* (a complete, instantaneous traumatic lesion) or *delayed* (progresses over several days following the trauma).

**Pathogenesis:** Facial paralysis may be caused by a temporal bone fracture, facial trauma (sharp or blunt), surgical trauma (surgery of the petrous bone or parotid gland), or obstetric trauma. Depending on the degree of the trauma, the effects can range from a transient conduction block (neurapraxia) or nerve damage with an intact perineurium (axonotmesis) to a complete nerve transection (neurotmesis).

**Symptoms:** Traumatic facial paralysis does not occur in isolation but is accompanied by other symptoms relating to the trauma.

**Diagnosis:** A history of trauma usually suggests the cause of the facial nerve paralysis. The paralysis may be difficult to detect in patients who are comatose. In patients who have sustained a temporal bone fracture, facial nerve function should always be tested and documented so that immediate paralysis can be distinguished from paralysis of delayed onset. Thereafter, the course is monitored by electrodiagnostic testing (neurography and EMG).
It is also important to determine the site of the lesion. This requires MRI and high-resolution CT scanning, especially in patients with a temporal bone fracture (see 15.1, Imaging Studies).

**Course:** The course depends on the extent of the injury. A nerve rupture causes immediate and complete paralysis that does not tend to resolve over time. With milder injuries, the paralysis often increases over a period of several days and then tends to resolve spontaneously. It is important, therefore, to document the course of traumatic facial paralysis clinically and by electrodiagnostic testing.

⚡ The indication for surgical decompression of traumatic facial paralysis depends on the course. For this reason, the function of the facial nerve and the course of the paralysis should always be carefully documented in patients with temporal bone fractures.

**Complications:** Complications may consist of corneal damage, residual palsy, and complications relating to the primary trauma.

**Treatment:** Every case of *immediate paralysis* should be surgically explored. The timing depends on clinical circumstances. A severed or badly damaged nerve is either directly reapproximated or microsurgically repaired with an interposed nerve graft (great auricular nerve or sural nerve).
*Delayed paralysis* is treated initially with corticosteroids to reduce edema. If neurography indicates more than 90% degeneration or if CT indicates compression by bone fragments, the nerve may be surgically explored. This is also done if other indications for temporal bone surgery exist (cerebrospinal fluid leak, ossicular chain disruption). It is usually sufficient to decompress the nerve.

# 15  Lateral Skull Base

## 15.1  Anatomy, Evaluation, and Surgery of the Lateral Skull Base

Both in the region of the paranasal sinuses (the anterior skull base) and the mucosa-lined cells of the temporal bone (the lateral skull base), the base of the skull borders on air-filled cavities that communicate with the external environment. While the anterior skull base is discussed in the chapters on the paranasal sinuses (Chapters 1–3), this chapter takes a more detailed look at the lateral skull base. This 🕮 focuses on the anatomy, symptomatology, evaluation, and treatment of this anatomic region.

### Anatomy of the Lateral Skull Base

#### Topography

The close proximity of the intracranial cerebrospinal fluid (CSF) space to the temporal bone air cells, and thus to the outside world, accounts for the special clinical features and management of diseases and injuries in this region (**Fig. 15.1**). The complex, variable anatomy of a great many vitally and functionally important structures can lead to serious sequelae and can hamper surgical treatment.

Depending on the pneumatization of the temporal bone, there are places where only a paper-thin layer of bone separates the dura mater from the mucosa of the temporal bone air cells. Venous connections exist between the dura and the mucosa, particularly at the roof of the mastoid (tegmen) and in the epitympanum, both of which border on the middle cranial fossa and thus on the temporal lobe of the brain. The posterior surface of the mastoid borders on the posterior cranial fossa and cerebellum.

#### Neurovascular Connections

In the lateral skull base region, there are many neural and vascular connections between the cranial interior on the one hand and the neck and face on the other (**Fig. 15.2**). The principal sites at which neurovascular structures pass through the bony skull base are as follows:

- The *internal auditory canal* with the facial nerve (cranial nerve VII), which reemerges from the temporal bone at the stylomastoid foramen (see 🕮 14.1, Anatomy), the vestibulocochlear nerve (cranial nerve VIII), and the labyrinthine artery.
- The *jugular foramen* with the internal jugular vein, where the sigmoid sinus drains in a siphonlike termination to form the jugular bulb. The foramen is traversed anteriorly by the basal cranial nerves, the glossopharyngeal nerve (cranial nerve IX), the vagus nerve (cranial nerve X), and the accessory nerve (cranial nerve XI). The hypoglossal nerve (cranial

**Fig. 15.1   Anatomy of the lateral skull base**

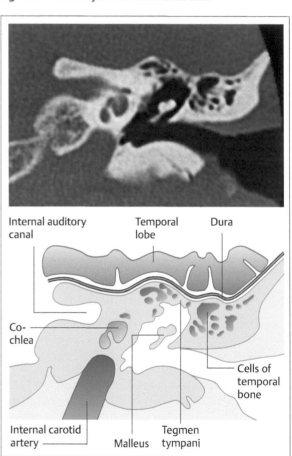

Coronal CT scan of the left internal and external auditory canals and correlative diagram. The close proximity of the brain to the cells of the temporal bone is clearly demonstrated.

nerve XII) lies in an adjacent bony canal (hypoglossal canal).

- The *foramen lacerum* with the internal carotid artery, which runs horizontally forward along the anterior border of the tympanic cavity and enters the skull by the sphenoid sinus.
- The *foramen ovale* with the mandibular nerve (third branch of cranial nerve V).

**Fig. 15.2** Neurovascular structures in the lateral skull base region

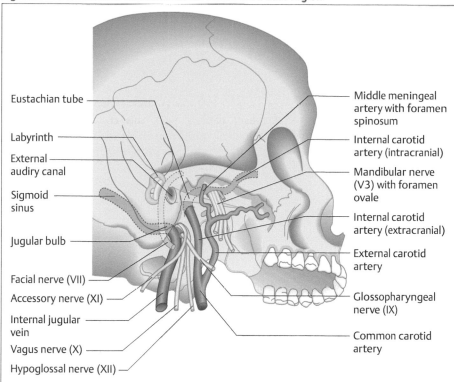

Eustachian tube

Labyrinth

External audiry canal

Sigmoid sinus

Jugular bulb

Facial nerve (VII)

Accessory nerve (XI)

Internal jugular vein

Vagus nerve (X)

Hypoglossal nerve (XII)

Middle meningeal artery with foramen spinosum

Internal carotid artery (intracranial)

Mandibular nerve (V3) with foramen ovale

Internal carotid artery (extracranial)

External carotid artery

Glossopharyngeal nerve (IX)

Common carotid artery

Course of major blood vessels and nerves in the lateral skull base region, viewed with the mandible removed.

- The *foramen spinosum* with the middle meningeal artery, a branch of the external carotid artery.

## Symptoms and Evaluation

### Clinical Examination

The symptoms of injuries and diseases of the lateral skull base are variable and diverse due to the specific anatomy of this region.

The dominant features are functional disorders of cranial nerves VII–XII, and therefore the testing of these nerves is an essential part of the clinical examination of the lateral skull base. A complete ear, nose, and throat status should always be established. For example, examination of the oral cavity (see 📖4.2) is useful for assessing the functional status of the hypoglossal and glossopharyngeal nerves, and indirect laryngoscopy (see 📖17.2, Indirect Laryngoscopy) can assess the function of the recurrent laryngeal nerve, which arises from cranial nerve X.

The clinical findings provide a basis for identifying various characteristic syndromes, which can vary considerably in their severity.

**Cochleovestibular syndrome:** The hallmarks of the cochleovestibular syndrome are sensorineural hearing loss, tinnitus, and vestibular symptoms such as disequilibrium and vertigo. Vestibular nystagmus may be present. It is often difficult to distinguish clinically between a cochlear and retrocochlear disorder, making

it necessary to rely on further audiologic testing (see 📖12.1, Retrocochlear Disorders) and imaging studies.

**Jugular foramen syndrome:** Cranial nerves IX, X, and XII are affected in various combinations. Vagus nerve involvement, manifested by unilateral vocal cord paralysis and dysphagia, is the dominant clinical finding in many cases. The history often raises suspicion of aspiration. Glossopharyngeal nerve involvement causes velum paralysis with deviation of the soft palate toward the healthy side ("backdrop sign," see **Fig. 4.8b**). Hypoglossal nerve involvement leads to paralysis of the tongue, which deviates toward the affected side (see **Fig. 4.8a**), in addition to lingual atrophy. Fasciculations of the lingual muscles on the side of the paralysis are also common.

**Petrous apex syndrome:** Gradenigo described the classic triad of purulent otorrhea, stabbing ipsilateral facial pain (trigeminal nerve irritation), and diplopia due to abducens nerve palsy in the setting of a petrous apex abscess (petrous apicitis). Today, the petrous apex syndrome is very rarely encountered in its classic form.

🗝 The combination of trigeminal nerve irritation with paralysis of the abducens nerve and occasionally of the oculomotor nerve should raise suspicion of a petrous apex lesion and requires immediate investigation by computed tomography (CT) and magnetic resonance imaging (MRI).

**Fig. 15.3    Petrous bone cholesteatoma of the apex (retrolabyrinthine cholesteatoma, epidermoid)**

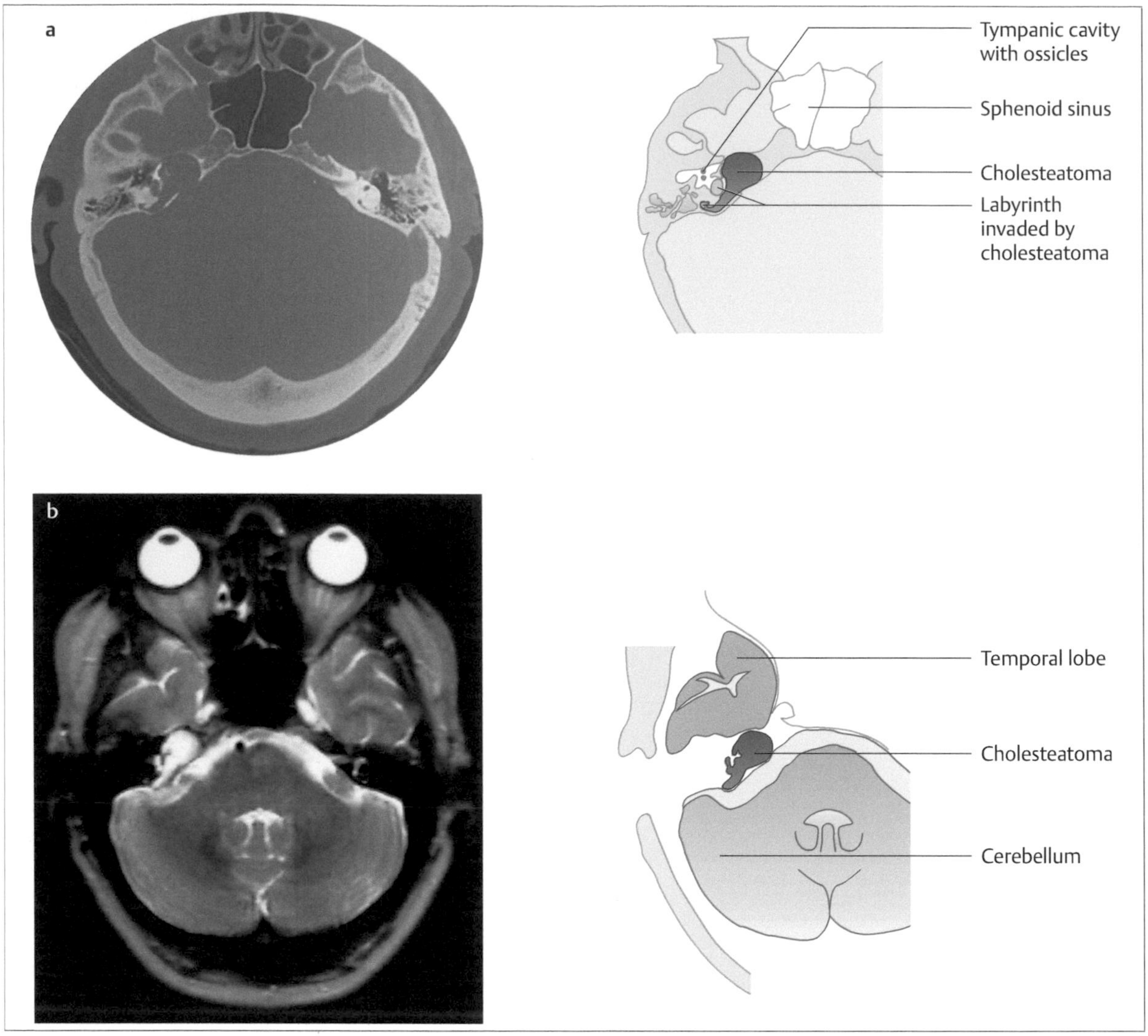

**a** Axial CT scan through the temporal bone shows cystic changes at the petrous apex.

**b** MR image of the same case demonstrates fluid in the tumor.

Most patients also complain of a deep headache, and other symptoms such as cochleovestibular disorders, facial paralysis, or meningitic signs are often present as well. The cause may be a suppurative inflammatory process (e.g., a petrous apex abscess or osteomyelitis), a congenital cholesteatoma of the petrous apex, or infiltrative lesions such as lymphomas or metastases.

## Imaging Studies

Every combined functional disorder of the laterobasal cranial nerves that cannot be diagnosed clinically requires further investigation by imaging procedures, primarily CT and MRI.

Both CT and MRI are often necessary for the precise delineation and differentiation of findings (**Fig. 15.3**). CT is best for defining the infiltration and destruction of *bony structures*. CT scans are of major importance in making a differential diagnosis and also in therapeutic and preoperative planning.

**MRI** is often better for defining and differentiating the lesion itself, which is usually a tumor or inflammatory process.

Because the disease process may be in very close proximity to major vessels, conventional **angiography** is also occasionally required. Angiography can also be used therapeutically (e.g., embolization) and therefore should be appropriately planned and coordinated.

**Fig. 15.4 Surgical approaches to the lateral skull base**

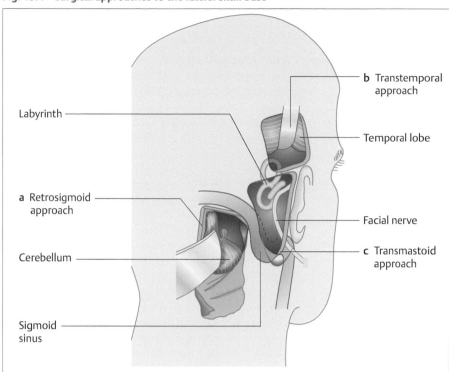

Labyrinth

b Transtemporal
approach

Temporal lobe

a Retrosigmoid
approach

Facial nerve

Cerebellum

c Transmastoid
approach

Sigmoid
sinus

The lateral skull base is
accessible by various
approaches.
**a** The retrosigmoid approach
is intracranial and intradural.
**b** The transtemporal
approach is intracranial and
extradural.
**c** The transmastoid approach
is extracranial and
extradural.

## Surgery of the Lateral Skull Base

### General

Because symptoms are influenced not just by the
nature of the disease but to a large extent also by its location, and even imaging studies cannot reliably distinguish tumors from inflammatory processes in all cases,
often a definitive diagnosis can be made only intraoperatively. Interdisciplinary approaches are the rule.
Three main routes of approach are available for surgery of the lateral skull base (**Fig. 15.4**):
* **Intracranial-intradural:** These are neurosurgical
  approaches, of which the suboccipital or retrosigmoid approach to the cerebellopontine angle is
  most commonly used.
* **Intracranial-extradural** (*transtemporal*): This is an
  otosurgical approach for exposing the surface of the
  petrous pyramid through a temporal craniotomy.
  The dura is separated from the surface of the petrous pyramid and elevated away from it with the
  temporal lobe. This approach is used, for example, in
  the surgical treatment of temporal bone fractures or
  tumors of the internal auditory canal (intrameatal
  vestibular schwannomas; see 🔖 15.3, Tumors of the
  Internal Auditory Canal and Cerebellopontine Angle).
* **Extracranial-extradural** (*transmastoid and infratemporal*): This is an otosurgical approach that is
  directed through the mastoid and/or other portions
  of the temporal bone.

### Extracranial-Extradural Approaches

**Transmastoid operation:** The mastoid air cells can be
completely excavated to gain access to broad portions
of the lateral skull base including the sigmoid sinus
and the dura of the posterior and middle cranial fossa.
The vestibular labyrinth can also be ablated (= trans-
mastoid-translabyrinthine operation) to access the internal auditory canal and cerebellopontine angle. This
approach is used to remove vestibular schwannomas
that have already caused deafness.
**Infratemporal operation:** The basis of this operation
is a subtotal petrosectomy (see 🔖 11.2). In this approach, the bony external auditory canal is removed in
addition to the mastoid, and the tympanic cavity is
broadly opened along with the mastoid cells. Both the
cutaneous ear canal and the eustachian tube are permanently occluded. In most cases, the facial nerve is exposed from the geniculate ganglion to the stylomastoid
foramen and it may be transposed anteriorly, providing
better access to the jugular bulb, the jugular foramen,
and, farther anteriorly, the internal carotid artery.
The operation can be extended anteriorly into the
deep infratemporal regions, to retromaxillary structures, and to the orbit by removing the zygomatic
arch and disarticulating the temporomandibular joint.
The postoperative cavity is usually obliterated with
abdominal fat.

# 15.2   Trauma to the Lateral Skull Base

Injuries are a frequent and important cause of latero-basal pathology, along with inflammations and (usually benign) neoplasms (see ☞15.3). Fractures of the lateral skull base consist mainly of indirect burst fractures caused by blunt head trauma. Direct trauma, as from a gunshot injury, is much less common. Latero-basal fractures generally involve the middle ear and less commonly the inner ear (see ☞12.2, Traumatic Injury to the Inner Ear). They are usually easy to differentiate from isolated middle ear trauma (see ☞11.4, Injuries to the Tympanic Membrane and Middle Ear) based on the history and clinical findings.

## Laterobasal Fractures

Synonym: temporal bone fractures.

☞ The primary examination and the initial findings and diagnosis can be very important in dealing with complications that may arise later. The accurate documentation of findings is essential, therefore.

### General

The lateral skull base is a frequent site of occurrence of basal skull fractures. The stresses generated by the deformation of the skull can lead to characteristic burst fractures of the petrous pyramids and neighboring bones. The trauma is commonly associated with fractures of the calvaria and also with brain injury.

Below, we shall review the complications that may arise in all types of laterobasal fractures. Then, we shall consider specific fracture types and their associated features, diagnosis, and management.

**Cerebrospinal fluid leak:**

*Pathogenesis:* As long as the dura mater is intact and the injuries are confined to bony structures and the mucosa of the pneumatized cavities, the interior of the skull will remain sealed and protected. But because the dura is firmly attached to the bone in some places, it may become torn when injuries are sustained, allowing CSF to leak into the cells of the temporal bone. With extensive injuries to the lateral skull base, both dura and brain tissue may prolapse into the air cells of the temporal bone.

*Symptoms:* A CSF leak is manifested by the following clinical signs:

- Air in the intracranial cavity (pneumoencephalos).
- CSF dripping as a watery discharge from the ear (CSF otorrhea) or nose (CSF rhinorrhea, see also ☞3.6).
- Infection, which may be acute (meningitis) or chronic (brain abscess).

*Diagnosis:* The clinical discovery of a CSF leak can be confirmed by laboratory tests, imaging studies, or intraoperatively.

- CSF leak can be diagnosed by sampling the watery discharge and sending it for laboratory analysis. Glucose test strips can be used to make a quick assessment of the sugar content of the fluid. A more accurate test involves the assay of CSF-specific enzymes such as $\beta_2$-transferrin, which can also be detected by inserting a foam wick into the nose or ear to collect discharge that is not clinically apparent.
- If CT demonstrates pneumoencephalos (intracranial air), this indicates at least a transient CSF leak.
- A profuse CSF leak is easily detected at operation, but this can be difficult with a smaller leak. In these cases, the leaking fluid can be visualized endoscopically with a blue filter following the intrathecal injection of sodium fluorescein.

*Treatment:* A CSF leak in the lateral skull base is associated with a relatively low risk of acute infection (meningitis) or chronic infection (brain abscess). In many cases, moreover, the leak will stop spontaneously and the fistula will become sealed. Generally, then, a CSF leak requires surgical treatment only if it persists for 5 to 7 days, or if complications such as meningitis occur. General antibiotic prophylaxis is controversial when a CSF leak is present, as it cannot reliably prevent meningitis and could promote the selection of resistant strains.

**Cochleovestibular symptoms:** Hearing loss following a laterobasal fracture may be a *conductive* hearing loss caused by fluid (blood or CSF) in the tympanic cavity or by ossicular dislocation, or it may be a *sensorineural* hearing loss or deafness caused by a fracture of the labyrinth. The latter is associated with failure of the vestibular organ and its clinical manifestations such as severe vertigo, nausea, and vomiting.

The mechanism of the injury may also cause a labyrinthine concussion or contusion, which usually occurs in association with acute noise trauma (see ☞12.2, Noise-Induced Hearing Loss).

**Facial nerve function:** With a fracture of the lateral skull base, facial nerve function is commonly affected along with cochleovestibular function (see ☞14.2, Traumatic Facial Paralysis).

☞ When a temporal bone fracture has occurred, facial nerve function should be tested and carefully documented during the initial days and weeks following the injury.

The *treatment* of traumatic facial nerve paralysis, and especially the indication for surgical repair, depends mainly on the course and degree of the paralysis. If the facial paralysis is present immediately after the injury (early paralysis), it is likely that the nerve has sustained direct trauma and the prognosis is poor. Surgical treatment is often necessary. Paralysis that occurs 24 hours or more after the trauma (late paralysis) very often resolves spontaneously, especially when the paralysis is incomplete.

⚡ Since the detection of early paralysis has major prognostic significance, the initial emergency examination should be conducted with meticulous care.

It is difficult to test facial nerve function in the unconscious trauma patient, but occasionally a grimace can be elicited in response to a painful stimulus. The results of the examination should be documented along with any uncertainties regarding the findings. Facial paralysis that is diagnosed later should be interpreted with particular care (late paralysis or undiagnosed early paralysis).

## Classification of Temporal Bone Fractures

Typical burst fractures involving the petrous pyramid are also known as *pyramid fractures*. There are also isolated fractures of the temporal squama and various combinations that include other calvarial fractures. The diagnosis and classification of a temporal bone fracture can often be accomplished clinically. CT can at least partially define the course of the fracture lines. Several different types of temporal bone burst fracture may be encountered:

**Squama–mastoid fractures:** The fracture is confined to the temporal squama and mastoid air cells. The auditory canal and tympanic cavity may also be involved.

**Longitudinal temporal bone fracture:** The fracture runs along the petrous bone and petrous pyramid (see **Fig. 15.5**, left). The typical fracture line runs along the auditory canal, continues across the mastoid roof and tegmen tympani to the carotid canal, and terminates in the sphenoid sinus.

**Transverse temporal bone fracture:** The fracture line runs transversely across the petrous bone or petrous pyramid (see **Fig. 15.5**, right) along the internal auditory canal and/or through the labyrinth.

**Isolated meatal fracture:** This fracture is most often caused by a posterior displacement of the mandibular condyle. The typical mechanism of the injury is a fall onto the chin. The fracture penetrates the posterior wall of the glenoid fossa and the anterior wall of the ear canal and is often associated with a condylar neck fracture.

**Fig. 15.5 Temporal bone fractures**

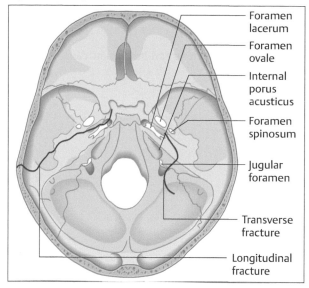

Typical longitudinal temporal bone fracture (left) and transverse temporal bone fracture (right).

Besides these more or less typical temporal bone fractures, there are also atypical fracture patterns involving other bony structures of the lateral skull base such as the occipital bone (lateral or clivus) and sphenoid bone. These patterns are particularly common with direct or high-energy trauma.

## Longitudinal Temporal Bone Fracture

**Definition:** This fracture runs along the external auditory canal and the anterior border of the petrous pyramid (**Fig. 15.6**).

**Epidemiology:** The longitudinal temporal bone fracture is the most common burst fracture affecting the lateral skull base.

**Pathogenesis:** The fracture is caused by a diffuse, lateral traumatizing force. It may result from a fall in which the head is struck without any other injuries, but it is associated with brain trauma in many cases.

**Symptoms:** Aural discharge is present and may consist of pure blood or blood mixed with CSF (CSF otorrhea). Hearing loss is also present. Occasionally, a slightly bloody rhinorrhea may also occur due to involvement of the sphenoid sinus. Approximately 10 to 20% of cases exhibit facial paralysis, which is usually of delayed onset (see above).

**Diagnosis:** The **otoscopic findings** usually establish the diagnosis when combined with the history and auditory tests. Otoscopy shows tearing of the meatal

**Fig. 15.6 Longitudinal temporal bone fracture**

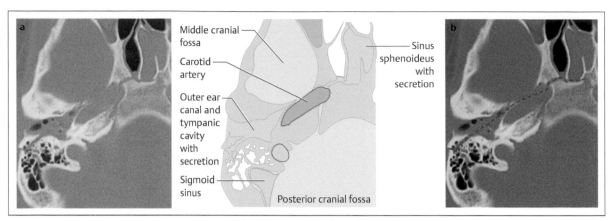

**a** Axial CT scans of a longitudinal fracture of the right temporal bone with anatomic sketch.
**b** Indication of the fracture line in the CT with typical course through the mastoid and outer ear canal, along the horizontal internal carotid artery, ending in the sphenoid sinus.

skin and tympanic membrane, with bleeding into the ear canal. Generally, the posterosuperior quadrant of the tympanic membrane and superior wall of the ear canal are affected. Blood and cerumen can hamper the examination. Cleansing of the ear canal should be left to a specialist.

⚕ The examiner who suspects a temporal bone fracture should not perform any manipulations in the ear canal and should particularly avoid irrigating the ear.

On **clinical auditory testing**, Weber's test is lateralized to the affected ear and Rinne's test is usually but not always negative.
Further evaluation consists of detecting or excluding CSF otorrhea (see above), defining the fracture line by **high-resolution CT scanning** of the temporal bone, the objective testing of facial nerve function by **neurography**, and auditory testing by **pure-tone audiometry**. All of these tests are useful in specific cases, but they are mandatory only in cases that require surgical exploration.

*Differential diagnosis:* A longitudinal temporal bone fracture mainly requires differentiation from an isolated fracture of the ear canal when otorrhea is present.
The latter type of injury mainly involves the anterior wall of the ear canal, leaving the superior wall intact. Occasionally, blood from a head wound that has flowed into the ear canal is mistaken for evidence of a temporal bone fracture.

*Complications:* Possible **early complications** are meningitis in the presence of a CSF leak, otitis media in the presence of a tympanic membrane perforation, and facial nerve paralysis.

Facial nerve damage or a perforated tympanic membrane rarely leads to **permanent sequelae**. A more frequent complication is conductive hearing loss caused by fracture or dislocation of the auditory ossicles; the incus is most commonly affected. Surgical exploration of the tympanic cavity with an ossiculoplasty is indicated in patients with permanent conductive hearing loss. Rare **late complications** are stenosis of the ear canal due to scarring or a posttraumatic cholesteatoma caused by the ingrowth of meatal skin into the middle ear through a fracture.

*Treatment:* Whenever possible, the ear should be covered with a sterile dressing and left alone. Facial paralysis is treated with corticosteroids. Surgical exploration is necessary in patients with infectious complications or a persistent CSF leak and in selected cases of facial paralysis.

## Transverse Temporal Bone Fracture

*Definition:* A transverse temporal bone fracture runs across the petrous pyramid along the internal auditory canal and/or through the labyrinth (**Fig. 15.7**).

*Epidemiology:* Transverse temporal bone fractures are much less common than longitudinal fractures.

*Pathogenesis:* This burst fracture is caused by a traumatizing force in the frontal plane. It may occur in isolation without associated injuries. The fracture line runs medial to the external auditory canal and tympanic membrane plane, with the result that these structures are not directly affected and there is no blood or CSF discharge from the ear canal.

**Fig. 15.7  Transverse temporal bone fracture**

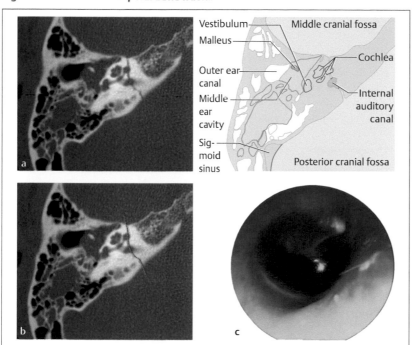

Vestibulum
Malleus
Outer ear canal
Middle ear cavity
Sigmoid sinus
Middle cranial fossa
Cochlea
Internal auditory canal
Posterior cranial fossa

**a** Axial CT of a right temporal bone with anatomic sketch.
**b** Indication of the fracture line in the CT with typical course through the cochlea and the fundus of the internal auditory canal.
**c** Typical otoscopic finding of an intact tympanic membrane with hematotympanum.

*Symptoms:* The foremost symptom is acute vestibular dysfunction with severe vertigo, generally accompanied by nausea and vomiting. Severe hearing loss or even deafness along with tinnitus occurs acutely on the affected side but often goes unnoticed. Otorrhea is absent, but there may be CSF rhinorrhea through the eustachian tube. Facial paralysis occurs in up to 50% of cases.

*Diagnosis:* On **clinical examination**, Weber's test is lateralized to the healthy ear and there is spontaneous nystagmus toward the healthy side (due to vestibular loss). **Otoscopy** typically shows signs of hemotympanum (**Fig. 15.7c**).
The fracture line is defined by **high-resolution CT scans** of the temporal bone.

*Differential diagnosis:* Autonomic symptoms caused by the vestibular disorder are often misinterpreted as central nervous system signs of craniocerebral trauma. If CSF rhinorrhea is present, the differential diagnosis should include a frontobasal fracture. Hemotympanum can also occur in this injury because blood from epistaxis may enter the tympanic cavity through the eustachian tube.

*Course and complications:* The risk of meningitis is greater with a transverse temporal bone fracture, and there is less likelihood that the fistula will close spontaneously. It is extremely unlikely that hearing or

vestibular function will be recovered. In most patients, the loss of vestibular function is well compensated by central mechanisms over time. Facial paralysis associated with a transverse fracture also has a poorer prognosis than in patients with a longitudinal fracture.

*Treatment:* A CSF leak associated with a transverse fracture may be a more urgent indication for surgical closure than a leak caused by a longitudinal fracture, because the fracture line is often gaping, and it is less likely that the leak will close spontaneously. Immediate facial paralysis may also require surgical repair. Otherwise, treatment is conservative, with emphasis placed on mobilizing the patient and restoring vestibular functions.

## Direct Trauma to the Lateral Skull Base

Direct injuries to the lateral skull base are less common than burst fractures, although both types may be combined. A depressed fracture of the temporal squama or mastoid generally leads to associated external injuries such as lacerations or injuries to the external ear or a squama–mastoid fracture.
Gunshot injuries to the lateral skull base and other direct traumas generally require surgical exploration. The first priority is the repair of injured vascular structures. After that, an effort is made to preserve the function of the cranial nerves, external ear, and middle ear.

# 15.3    Inflammations and Tumors of the Lateral Skull Base

Inflammations involving the lateral skull base most commonly originate from the middle ear. Tumors of the lateral skull base are generally rare and most are benign. Both inflammations and tumors are often manifested by varied and nonspecific signs relating to the various functional structures of the lateral skull base. As a result, the diagnosis of tumors in particular is often delayed, and the process may spread to neighboring structures. Accordingly, a continuum exists between severe inflammations and tumors of the ear canal, middle ear, intracranial cavity, and lateral skull base. The surgical treatment of these processes is challenging and often requires an interdisciplinary approach with neurosurgical consultation.

## Inflammations

**Otitis media** is usually a tubogenic condition. It is among the most common inflammations and infections that affect the lateral skull base region (see ✐ 11.3). Otogenic complications with potential extensive involvement of the lateral skull base have become rare in developed countries. The most frequent cause of an inflammatory process arising from the middle ear and spreading to the lateral skull base in these countries is *cholesteatoma* (see ✐ 11.3, Chronic Otitis Media with Cholesteatoma).

A specific form of cholesteatoma of the lateral skull base is called **petrous bone cholesteatoma**, also called **retrolabyrinthine cholesteatoma** or **epidermoid** (**Fig. 15.3**). As a rule, it is a congenital rather than an acquired cholesteatoma and grows primarily in the temporal bone and not in the middle ear cavity. Clinical presentations of petrous bone cholesteatomas match more those of tumors than inflammations leading to deficits of the inner ear and the facial nerve. They are identified by imaging and treated surgically.

**Necrotizing otitis externa** may also lead to widespread infection of the lateral skull base in its later stages, making extensive surgical therapy necessary. Other, less common local or systemic diseases such as **granulomatosis with polyangiitis** (GPA, Wegener) also play a role.

Infections can also occur as a **sequel to injuries**. The most hazardous is meningitis, which may be manifested during the initial days or weeks following an injury (early meningitis). In other cases, months or even years may elapse between the trauma and the development of an infectious complication (delayed meningitis).

## Tumors of the Temporal Bone

Virtually any structure can serve as a nidus for tumor growth. Some of the more common tumors of the temporal bone are discussed below in greater detail. The diagnosis of temporal bone tumors relies almost exclusively on imaging procedures, especially neuroradiologic studies.

## Paraganglioma

Synonyms: glomus tumor, chemodectoma, nonchromaffin paraganglioma.

*Sites of occurrence:* This tumor arises from the paraganglia of the temporal region, most commonly in the area of the jugular bulb and along the neural plexus of the tympanic cavity (tympanic plexus). Paragangliomas may be located in the middle ear (**glomus tympanicum**) or on the jugular bulb (**glomus jugulare**). They can also develop outside the temporal bone region from paraganglia at the carotid bifurcation (**glomus caroticum**) and along the vagus nerve (**glomus vagale**). These tumors often extend toward the temporal bone region. Once they have reached a certain size, their site of origin may become difficult to determine.

*Epidemiology:* Paragangliomas are the most common tumors of the middle ear and adjacent lateral skull base. Their overall incidence is low, however. They occur seldom multiple, familial, or in connection with various syndromes. About 5% of the temporal bone paragangliomas secrete catecholamines.

*Symptoms:* Paragangliomas in the tympanic cavity are sometimes manifested early by a pulsatile tinnitus and conductive hearing loss. By contrast, paragangliomas of the jugular bulb often become symptomatic at a later stage due to the development of basal cranial nerve deficits.

*Diagnosis:* Both MRI and CT can demonstrate paragangliomas. CT is necessary for the detection of bone destruction in the tympanic cavity or about the jugular foramen (**Fig. 15.8**).

On **audiologic testing**, unilateral conductive hearing loss is detected at an early stage in patients with a glomus tympanicum tumor. This is seen later with a glomus jugulare tumor. Sensorineural hearing loss may also occur due to infiltration of the inner ear.

**Otoscopy (Fig. 15.8)** may demonstrate the typical finding of a bluish mass in the lower part of the

**Fig. 15.8** Paraganglioma of the jugular bulb

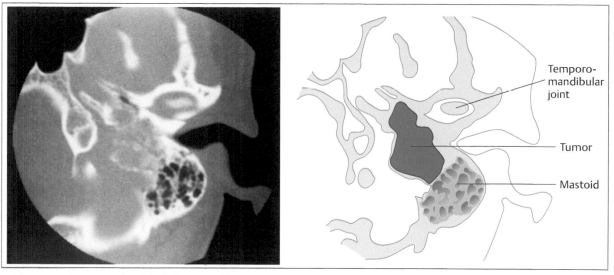

Temporo-mandibular joint

Tumor

Mastoid

Axial computed tomography of the left temporal bone.

tympanic cavity. This occurs only if the tumor has reached the mesotympanum.

**Angiography** is helpful in determining both the etiology and extent of the lesion. It should be done as an immediate preoperative study and should include embolization.

*Treatment:*

☝ The preoperative angiographic embolization of a tumor can reduce intraoperative blood loss.

**Paragangliomas** of the tympanic cavity are relatively easy to remove in their early stage by a middle ear operation.

The surgical treatment of a **glomus jugulare tumor** is challenging and generally requires a subtotal petrosectomy (see ✏ **11.2**). Embolization, radiotherapy, therapy with special radionuclides, and octreotide are other forms of therapy, which are used alone or in combinations.

## Other Tumors of the Lateral Skull Base

The symptoms and findings that are associated with tumors depend on their growth rate, invasive potential, and location. Generally, a tumor can be diagnosed with imaging procedures, but often its etiology can only be determined histologically by biopsy or operative exposure.

**Tumors of the endolymphatic sac** are specific tumor of the temporal bone. They are locally invasive and evoke cochleovestibular dysfunctions. They are associated most often with von Hippel–Lindau disease, but they also occur sporadically.

**Fig. 15.9** Otoscopic finding in paraganglioma

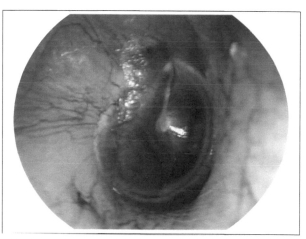

Right tympanic membrane with bulging tumor in the posterior quadrants.

Possible **benign tumors** include mucosal tumors (such as *papilloma* and *adenoma*), tumors of connective tissue and bone (such as *meningioma* and *fibrous dysplasia*), neural tumors (such as *facial neurinoma*), and *eosinophilic granuloma* in the setting of Langerhans cell histiocytosis.

**Primary malignant tumors** are *carcinomas* of the mucosa, *sarcomas*, and *lymphomas*. The lateral skull base may also be affected by *skeletal metastases* from various other tumors such as breast cancer and bronchial or renal carcinoma.

# Tumors of the Internal Auditory Canal and Cerebellopontine Angle

The most common identifiable cause of a retrocochlear hearing disorder (see ☞12.1, Retrocochlear Disorders) is a tumor of the internal auditory canal or cerebellopontine angle. These lesions can produce a unilateral cochleovestibular syndrome by exerting pressure on cranial nerve VIII and the labyrinthine artery. The most common of these tumors is vestibular schwannoma, also known as acoustic neurinoma (~80% of cases), followed by cerebellopontine angle meningioma (see **Fig. 12.4**).

## Vestibular Schwannoma

Synonym: acoustic neurinoma.

*Definition and forms:* Vestibular schwannoma is a generally slow-growing, benign tumor that arises from the Schwann cells of cranial nerve VIII. The vestibular nerve is most commonly affected. Rarely, the tumor may arise from the cochlear nerve or may form within the labyrinth.

Two forms are distinguished clinically: medial and lateral. *Medial tumors* arise from the intracranial part of cranial nerve VIII, i.e., in the actual cerebellopontine angle, while *lateral tumors* are located in the internal auditory canal.

*Epidemiology:* Though it is the most common tumor of the posterior cranial fossa, vestibular schwannoma has a low overall incidence. It seems to become more common with aging, and there are probably a considerably greater number of vestibular schwannomas that are asymptomatic and therefore undiagnosed.

Rarely, these tumors occur in the setting of neurofibromatosis type 2 (☞15.1).

*Symptoms:* The clinical hallmark of vestibular schwannoma is a unilateral hearing disorder, which may consist of tinnitus, hearing loss, or dysacusis.

 Medial tumors may reach a considerable size before becoming symptomatic. Lateral tumors evoke hearing disorders at an earlier stage.

The hearing disorder has a sudden onset (sudden sensorineural hearing loss) in approximately 20%, or the onset is gradual and may show improvement, which is usually transitory.

 Recovery from sudden sensorineural hearing loss does not exclude vestibular schwannoma. This tumor should always be included in the differential diagnosis of a unilateral hearing disorder.

Vestibular symptoms such as acute vertigo or disequilibrium are less common. Impairment of facial nerve function is unusual, even with very large tumors.

Medial schwannomas can produce trigeminal nerve symptoms such as facial pain or numbness in the jaw. Large tumors also produce signs of brainstem compression and/or hydrocephalus with ataxia, nausea, and vomiting.

*Diagnosis:* **Clinical examination** reveals the typical signs of a unilateral cochleovestibular disorder. Spontaneous nystagmus is rarely present. **Audiometry** usually demonstrates retrocochlear impairment with a lengthening of auditory brainstem response latencies (see ☞8.4, Auditory Brainstem Response).

The diagnosis is established by **MRI** (**Fig. 15.10**). The tumor enhances after gadolinium administration, but even without contrast medium it can be detected in thin-slice sequences of the posterior fossa with three-dimensional data acquisition.

*Treatment:* **Large tumors** that exceed 2.5 to 3.0 cm in diameter constitute a possibly vital indication for surgical removal. **Smaller tumors** may be managed by a "wait-and-see" approach with regular follow-ups, or the lesion may be treated by stereotactic radiosurgery or open surgery. The indication depends on the quality of hearing, vestibular symptoms, and the age and wishes of the patient. Tumors showing clear growth in the follow-up should generally be treated by open surgery or radiotherapy.

## Other Tumors of the Cerebellopontine Angle

The second most common cerebellopontine angle tumor is meningioma, which arises either from the posterior surface of the petrous pyramid or from the tentorium. Less common lesions include hemangiomas and lipomas. The clinical presentation and treatment are basically the same as for vestibular schwannomas. Postoperative function depends critically on the location of the tumor and its relation to the cranial nerves.

## Fig. 15.10 Vestibular schwannomas

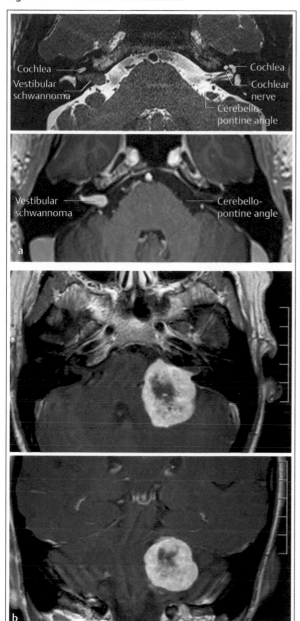

**a** Lateral vestibular schwannoma in the internal auditory canal on the right side with typical enhancement post gadolinium in the lower MRI. Normal findings on the left side.
**b** Post–gadolinium MRI showing a large, medial vestibular schwannoma in the cerebellopontine angle with compression of the cerebellum and brainstem (top: axial view; bottom: coronal view).

## 15.1 Neurofibromatosis 2

A rare special form of vestibular schwannomas is **neurofibromatosis 2** (synonym: central neurofibromatosis), an inherited autosomal-dominant disease with a genetic defect in chromosome 22, characterized by bilateral vestibular schwannomas (**Fig. 15.11**) and other tumors in the cranial cavity and spinal canal. Differentiation is required from **neurofibromatosis 1** (synonym: von Recklinghausen's disease), which involves a defect on chromosome 17 and is mainly characterized by neurofibromas of the skin and café au lait spots.

The *management* of neurofibromatosis 2 is difficult and must be tailored to the situation to preserve auditory function for as long as possible. Cases with complete bilateral deafness can sometimes be rehabilitated by direct electrical stimulation of the cochlear nucleus (brainstem implant).

### Fig. 15.11 Bilateral vestibular schwannomas

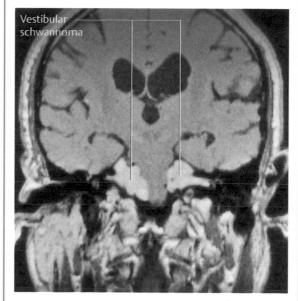

Coronal MRI. The finding of vestibular schwannomas on both sides is diagnostic for neurofibromatosis 2.

# IV Neck

# 16   External Neck

## 16.1   Anatomy of the External Neck

As the connecting link between the head and trunk, the neck contains several vitally important neurovascular structures (arteries, veins, nerves, lymphatics) within a very confined space. Its musculoskeletal system must protect the neck while also allowing maximum mobility of the head and the coordinatedprocesses of ventilation, deglutition, and speech. The neck also contains numerous lymph nodes and a high density of lymphatic vessels.

A precise knowledge of the anatomical relations in the neck is an essential prerequisite for diagnosis and surgical treatment.

### Topographic Anatomy

The neck is bounded above by the inferior border of the mandible, the tip of the mastoid process, and the external occipital protuberance. The lateral contours of the neck are defined by the palpable sternocleidomastoid muscles and the borders of the trapezius muscles. Palpable medial structures are the hyoid bone, thyroid cartilage, cricoid cartilage, and, when enlarged, the thyroid gland (**Fig. 16.1**).

The neck muscles, the cervical viscera (larynx, trachea, pharynx, esophagus, etc.), and the neurovascular structures in the neck are encased by sheets of connective tissue, the fascial planes. These fasciae are comprised of superficial, middle, and deep layers (see ⟋ **16.1**).

### Blood Supply

**Arterial blood supply:** The common carotid artery divides into its two main branches, the internal and external carotid arteries, at the level of the superior border of the thyroid cartilage (roughly the level of the C4 vertebral body). The common carotid artery arises from the aortic arch on the left side and from the brachiocephalic trunk on the right side. The lower part of the neck receives most of its blood supply from the thyrocervical trunk, which arises from the subclavian artery. Branches from the external carotid artery supply the neck and face; the internal carotid artery gives off no branches in the neck.

**Venous drainage** from the head and neck is received by the superficial cutaneous veins that open directly into the subclavian vein (external jugular vein and anterior jugular vein) and particularly by the internal jugular vein, which has a much larger lumen. The vertebral veins and the venous plexuses in the cervical spinal canal normally handle approximately 30% of the cerebral venous return.

### Lymphatic Drainage

Tributary areas in tissues are drained by lymphatic channels that lead to regional lymph nodes or groups of lymph nodes. The lymph nodes in the neck are

Fig. 16.1   Topographic anatomy of the neck

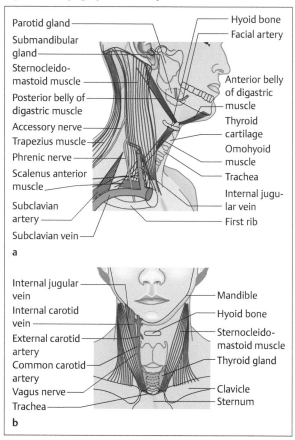

integrated as biological "filtering stations" into this network of lymphatic capillaries and vessels. Of the approximately 1,000 lymph nodes in the human body, some 300 are located in the head and neck region. The most important of these are found between the middle and deep layers of cervical fascia. Based on the arrangement of the lymphatic channels, the lymph nodes at the junction of the facial and internal jugular veins (see ⟋ **16.3**) receive drainage from almost all parts of the head and neck region and are a site of predilection for lymphogenous metastases in a large percentage of malignant head and neck tumors (**Fig. 16.2**).

On the left side of the neck, lymph drains into the junction of the left subclavian and internal jugular veins at the termination of the left thoracic duct.

## 16.1 Facial compartments in the neck

### Fascial planes

The fascial planes subdivide the neck into compartments that can easily shift in relation to one another. The **superficial cervical fascia** (synonym: superior layer of cervical fascia, **Fig. 16.3, yellow**) underlies the platysma and subcutaneous fat, invests the entire neck, and encases the sternocleidomastoid and trapezius muscles. This fascial layer is attached to the hyoid bone and stretches superiorly to the mandibular border and inferiorly to the manubrium sterni and clavicle. It is fused at the midline to the **middle cervical fascia** (synonym: pretracheal layer of cervical fascia; **Fig. 16.3, green**). This fascial layer stretches between the hyoid bone, the posterior surface of the manubrium sterni, and the clavicle and extends laterally to the omohyoid muscle and scapula. It encases the infrahyoid muscles and forms a general anterior boundary for the cervical viscera. The **deep cervical fascia** (synonym: prevertebral layer of cervical fascia; **Fig. 16.3, blue**) arises from the spinous processes of the cervical vertebrae and forms a rigid tube around the deep neck muscles that is adherent posteriorly to the superficial cervical fascia encasing the trapezius muscle. This prevertebral layer is part of a fascial system that extends continuously from the skull base to the lower end of the spinal column (prevertebral gravitation abscesses).

### Neurovascular sheath

The carotid artery, internal jugular vein, and vagus nerve are invested by their own connective-tissue sheath (**Fig. 16.3a, red**) that is attached to the middle cervical fascia at the tendon between the inferior and superior bellies of the omohyoid muscle, so that contractions of this muscle place tension on the "neurovascular sheath" and especially on the internal jugular vein.

### Neck spaces

While the space between the superficial and middle layers of the cervical fascia is closed inferiorly (common insertion on the manubrium sterni and clavicle), the visceral compartment of the neck has an open connection with the mediastinum between the middle and deep fascial layers. This allows abscesses in the cervical soft tissues and other disease processes to spread freely into the chest.

### Fig. 16.3 Topographical anatomy of the fascial compartments of the neck

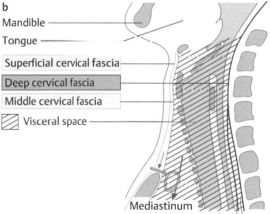

a Axillary view. b Sagittal view.

## 16.2 Carotid sinus and carotid body

The bifurcation of the common carotid artery marks the location of the **carotid sinus**. This dilatation of the carotid wall contains mechanoreceptors that are sensitive to blood pressure increases based on changes in vessel wall tension, and they can evoke an antihypertensive response in the reticular formation via the glossopharyngeal nerve.

Also located at the carotid bifurcation is the **carotid body**, composed of nonchromaffin paraganglia and measuring a few millimeters in size. It contains chemoreceptors that can modulate respiration in the reticular formation, also via the glossopharyngeal nerve, in response to changes in the arterial $Po_2$, $Pco_2$, and pH.

## 16.3 Jugular vein and its junctions with the facial and subclavian veins

The internal jugular vein arises at the confluence of the sigmoid sinus and inferior petrosal sinus and expands at the jugular foramen to form the jugular bulb.

Two venous junctions are important because they receive drainage from major groups of lymph nodes: the **jugulofacial venous junction**, formed by the termination of the facial vein at the internal jugular vein, and the larger **jugulosubclavian venous junction**, formed by the union of the internal jugular and subclavian veins at the brachiocephalic vein behind the sternoclavicular joint.

**Fig. 16.2   Cervical lymphatic system**

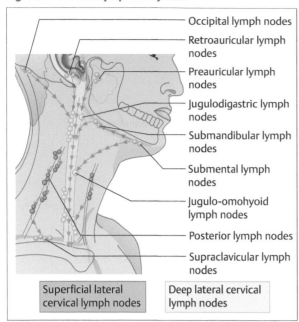

Occipital lymph nodes

Retroauricular lymph nodes

Preauricular lymph nodes

Jugulodigastric lymph nodes

Submandibular lymph nodes

Submental lymph nodes

Jugulo-omohyoid lymph nodes

Posterior lymph nodes

Supraclavicular lymph nodes

| Superficial lateral cervical lymph nodes | Deep lateral cervical lymph nodes |
|---|---|

Topographic anatomy of the cervical lymph nodes (see also **Fig. 16.7**). The deep lateral group of cervical lymph nodes is shown in dark green. The superficial lateral cervical lymph nodes are shown in blue.

Lymph on the right side drains into the junction of the right subclavian and internal jugular veins at the termination of the right thoracic duct. Included among the portals of entry to this system are the lymphatic organs of the nasopharynx and oropharynx (Waldeyer's ring).

> Normal cervical lymph nodes are neither visible nor palpable.

With a normal configuration of the neck, lymph nodes that enlarge to a diameter of 1 cm or more can be palpated.

## Innervation

The external neck receives a nonmetameric*sensory* supply from the **cervical plexus** (C1–C4),which emerges at the posterior border of the sternocleidomastoid muscle (Erb's point).
*Motor components* of the cervical plexus (inferior root) unite with motor fibers of the cervical plexus, some of which have hitchhiked with the hypoglossal nerve (superior root), to form the ansa cervicalis and supply the infrahyoid muscles and geniohyoid muscle. The hypoglossal nerve exits the skull through the hypoglossal canal and crosses over the branches of the external carotid artery.

### 16.4   Course of the glossopharyngeal, vagus, and accessory nerves

**Glossopharyngeal nerve (cranial nerve IX)**
The glossopharyngeal nerve forms the smaller **superior ganglion** in the jugular foramen and the larger **inferior ganglion** below the jugular foramen, runs between the internal carotid artery and internal jugular vein to the stylopharyngeus muscle, and passes to the tongue and lateral pharyngeal wall. The **tympanic nerve** runs from the inferior ganglion into the tympanic cavity (sensory innervation of the middle ear mucosa and eustachian tube). There, it unites with branches of the intermediate nerve (facial nerve, see 14.1) and sympathetic fibers of the internal cervical plexus to form the **lesser petrosal nerve** and passes to the **otic ganglion** (Jacobson's anastomosis) to supply parasympathetic innervation to the parotid gland. The glossopharyngeal nerve also supplies sensory fibers to the posterior third of the tongue; sensory fibers to the tongue base, tonsillar region, and large portions of the pharynx; and motor fibers to the palatal arch muscles and parts of the pharyngeal muscles.

**Accessory nerve (cranial nerve XI)**
The accessory nerve is unusual in that it contains both spinal and cranial nerve root components. After passing through the jugular foramen, the **cranial root components** have special visceromotor fibers that hitchhike with the vagus nerve. The purely motor **spinal root fibers** pass behind the internal jugular vein and in front of the transverse process of the atlas to the sternocleidomastoid muscle. They become very superficial at the upper third of the posterior border of the

sternocleidomastoid muscle (where they are vulnerable during neck surgery!), cross the posterior triangle of the neck, and reach the trapezius muscle.

**Vagus nerve (cranial nerve X)**
The vagus nerve forms a **superior (jugular) ganglion** caudal to the jugular foramen and an **inferior (nodose) ganglion** at the level of the hyoid bone. Further on in its course, it receives fibers from the cranial part of the accessory nerve and descends in the posterior part of the vascular sheath between the internal jugular vein and the internal and common carotid arteries. In its cervical portion, it distributes branches to the pharynx, larynx (**superior laryngeal nerve**), and heart (**superior and inferior cervical cardiac branches**). The **inferior (recurrent) laryngeal nerve**, which is crucial for laryngeal innervation, runs the same course between the esophagus and trachea on both sides of the neck, but after arising from the vagus nerve it winds around the brachiocephalic trunk on the right side and around the aortic arch on the left side. The vagus nerve provides *sensory* innervation to portions of the external auditory canal (the auricular branch is responsible for the vagally mediated cough reflex in ear examinations), the lower part of the pharynx, the larynx, and the upper portions of the trachea and esophagus.
The vagus nerve supplies *motor* input to large portions of the palatal and pharyngeal muscles and to the larynx. Is also provides *parasympathetic* innervation to the thoracic and abdominal viscera.

Fig. 16.4 Course of the glossopharyngeal nerve (cranial nerve IX)

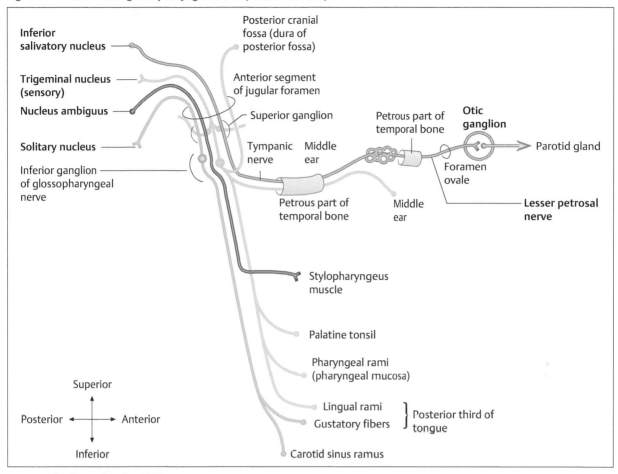

Source: Whitaker and Borley 1997.

The glossopharyngeal nerve, vagus nerve, and accessory nerve pass jointly through the jugular foramen to enter the neck (𝒫 16.4, **Figs. 16.4–16.7**).
The cervical part of the **sympathetic trunk** lies behind the neurovascular sheath between the layers of the deep cervical fascia on the prevertebral muscles. The location of the three associated ganglia is described in **Table 16.1**.

🖊 Interruption of the sympathetic trunk by drugs, tumor invasion, or trauma leads to the Horner symptom complex of miosis, ptosis, and enophthalmos.

Table 16.1 Ganglia of the sympathetic trunk

| Ganglion | Location | Segments |
|---|---|---|
| Superior cervical ganglion | Behind the internal carotid artery | C1–C4 |
| Middle cervical ganglion (inconstant) | At the bend of the inferior thyroid artery | C5–C6 |
| Inferior cervical ganglion | Between the transverse process of C7 and the head of the first rib | C7–C8; usually fused with the cervicothoracic ganglion (synonym: stellate ganglion) |

Fig. 16.5 Course of the vagus nerve (cranial nerve X)

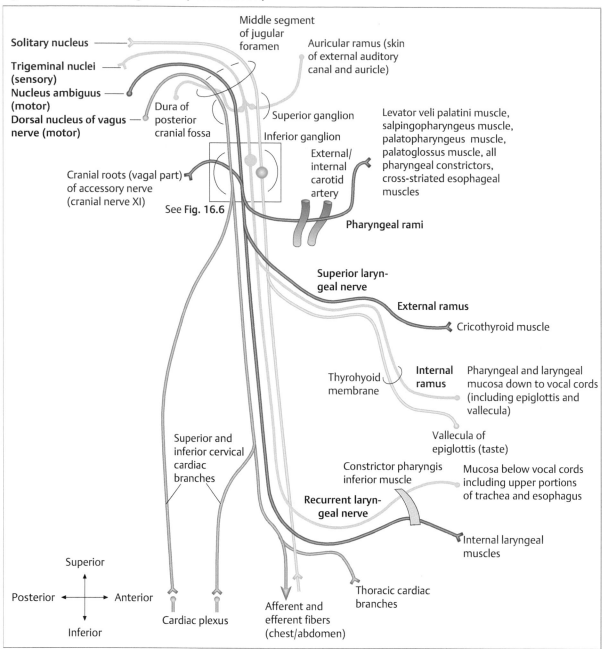

Solitary nucleus

Trigeminal nuclei (sensory)

Nucleus ambiguus (motor)

Dorsal nucleus of vagus nerve (motor)

Middle segment of jugular foramen

Auricular ramus (skin of external auditory canal and auricle)

Dura of posterior cranial fossa

Superior ganglion

Inferior ganglion

Cranial roots (vagal part) of accessory nerve (cranial nerve XI)

See Fig. 16.6

External/ internal carotid artery

Levator veli palatini muscle, salpingopharyngeus muscle, palatopharyngeus muscle, palatoglossus muscle, all pharyngeal constrictors, cross-striated esophageal muscles

Pharyngeal rami

Superior laryn-geal nerve

External ramus

Cricothyroid muscle

Thyrohyoid membrane

Internal ramus

Pharyngeal and laryngeal mucosa down to vocal cords (including epiglottis and vallecula)

Vallecula of epiglottis (taste)

Superior and inferior cervical cardiac branches

Constrictor pharyngis inferior muscle

Mucosa below vocal cords including upper portions of trachea and esophagus

Recurrent laryn-geal nerve

Internal laryngeal muscles

Superior

Posterior ← → Anterior

Inferior

Cardiac plexus

Afferent and efferent fibers (chest/abdomen)

Thoracic cardiac branches

Source: Whitaker and Borley 1997.

**Fig. 16.6  Course of the accessory nerve (cranial nerve XI)**

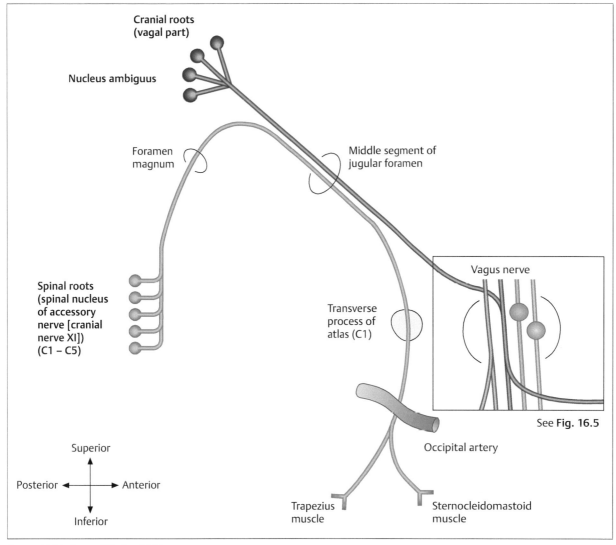

Source: Whitaker and Borley 1997.

**Fig. 16.7  Course of the hypoglossal nerve (cranial nerve XII)**

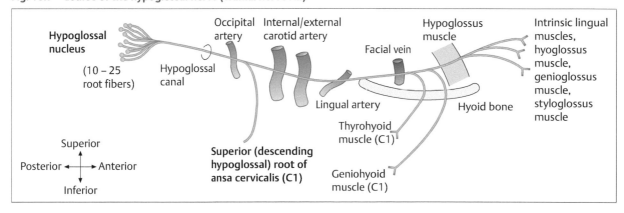

# 16.2 Symptomatology and Examination of the External Neck

Many lesions in the neck are palpable owing to the topographic anatomy of that region. Palpation of the neck is an essential part of every physical examination, therefore. Modern imaging procedures can significantly narrow the differential diagnosis and direct the planning of treatment. Diagnostic surgical exploration of the neck is still necessary in some cases, however.

## Cardinal Symptoms

Patients with diseases of the **external neck** very often complain of *shape changes* in the neck due to circumscribed or diffuse swellings or masses. Other common symptoms are *pain*, which may change with head movements, and *limitation of neck motion*. These symptoms require differentiation from *dysphagic complaints*, which are projected into the swallowing tract and are usually caused by disease in that region.

## Methods of Examination

### History

The history should focus on the duration, presentation, and time course of the symptoms (acute or chronic); the degree of pain or tenderness; constant, increasing, or fluctuant swellings; diseases involving the upper aerodigestivetract; other enlarged lymph nodes elsewhere in the body; and any prior history of similar complaints. The patient should also be questioned about possible contact with animals, travel abroad, and eating habits.

### Inspection

The history is followed by visual inspection, which focuses on the contour-defining structures of the neck and any external changes in the overlying skin such as vascular markings, venous stasis, radiodermatitis, and skin tumors. The examiner should also look for fistulous openings that might indicate a brachial fistula, thyroglossal fistula, or actinomycosis and for sites of swelling and induration (lymph nodes, abscesses). Attention is also given to the position and mobility of the head and neck (e.g., a guarded head position due to an abscess or torticollis).

### Palpation

The cervical soft tissues are palpated bimanually from the front or preferably from behind in the seated patient, alternating from right to left and comparing the sides. The patient's head should be tilted slightly forward to relax the soft tissues of the neck. It is best to palpate the various **lymph-node groups** by following a routine sequence, as illustrated in **Fig. 16.8**.

The rest of the neck should be palpated as well, giving attention to the number of any **palpable masses**, their size (in centimeters), tenderness, mobility relative to the skin and underlying tissues, consistency, and especially their relationship to surrounding neck structures.

> Both sides of the neck should never be deeply palpated at the same time, especially in older patients, due to the risk of evoking a carotid sinus reflex with vasovagal syncope.

**Pulsating masses** in the neck (paraganglia, vascular aneurysms) should be evaluated by *auscultation* as well as palpation.

The examiner should also test the mobility of the cervical spine in all planes and the mobility of the shoulder girdle.

### Imaging Studies

**Two-dimensional B-mode ultrasonography** is considered the standard method for investigating soft-tissue lesions in the neck. The ultrasound examination can supply information useful in establishing the identity of specific lesions based on sonomorphologic criteria.

**Fig. 16.8 Palpation of the cervical lymph nodes**

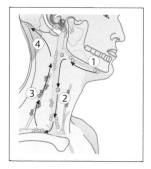

The arrows show a recommended routine for palpating the cervical nodes: from submental to submandibular, then along the sternocleidomastoid muscle and vascular sheath to the supraclavicular nodes, then back up along the course of the accessory nerve toward the nuchal region.

⚕ Ultrasound cannot positively distinguish between benign and malignant masses, however.

Ultrasound scanning of the cervical soft tissues is particularly important for the follow-up of malignant upper aerodigestive lesions to detect a possible recurrence. For physical reasons, however (the strong reflection of sound waves at air and bone interfaces), ultrasound has only limited value in evaluating lesions that are adjacent to bone, the pharynx, or the larynx. Ultrasound, especially **Doppler ultrasound**, is excellent for evaluating the extracranial cerebral arteries (stenoses, tumor invasion) and (very) vascular tumors (paraganglioma, hemangioma).

Axial **computed tomography (CT)** can provide a detailed view of inflammatory, space-occupying, infiltrating, or destructive cervical mass lesions. Scans can be obtained before and after contrast administration if required.

⚕ Iodinated contrast media should not be used in patients with a suspected thyroid disease, as they would interfere with subsequent tests.

Within limits, CT can provide a "radiologic tissue diagnosis." CT is particularly indicated in cases with suspected involvement of cartilaginous or bony structures (larynx, cervical spine, mandible), which are demonstrated less clearly by magnetic resonance imaging (MRI).

**MRI** provides better soft-tissue discrimination than CT and can aid in the differentiation of neoplastic, cicatricial, and inflammatory lesions, aided, if necessary, by paramagnetic contrast administration. Coronal and sagittal images are excellent for defining the location and relations of soft-tissue lesions.

**Plain radiographs** in the anteroposterior or lateral projection are rarely obtained in routine evaluations of the cervical soft tissues and have been largely superseded by the imaging modalities described above. Plain radiographs can detect prevertebral soft-tissue swellings, calcifications (e.g., tuberculous lymph nodes), emphysema following an upper airway injury, and radiopaque foreign bodies. They continue to have an important role in evaluating the cervical spine and, in some cases, detecting laryngeal fractures.

**Positron emission tomography (PET)**, which can demonstrate the increased uptake of injected fluorodeoxyglucose (FDG) in metabolically active tissue (tumor, inflammation), is the latest imaging modality and is applied mainly in tumor diagnosis.

In addition to metaiodobenzylguanidine ($^{123}$MIBG) scintigraphy, fluorine 18-dopa positron emission tomography ($^{18}$F-DOPA PET) CT is particularly appropriate for the diagnosis of paragangliomas, whereby the focus of the whole-body examination is on further manifestations.

In tumors with neuroendocrine differentiation, a gallium ($^{68}$Ga)-DODATATE PET scan can be helpful in detecting the primary tumor or metastases.

**Cervical lymphography** and **lymphoscintigraphy** no longer have a significant clinical role in evaluating the cervical lymphatic system.

## Cytologic and Histologic Examination

Equivocal and suspicious neck masses should always be sampled so that a histologic tissue diagnosis can be made. With cystic masses, percutaneous needle aspiration can furnish material for cytologic and/or microbiologic examination. This diagnostic puncture is separate from a possible subsequent therapeutic incision, which may be done to treat a suppurative process.

⚕ Pulsating neck masses (paraganglioma, vascular aneurysms) should not be punctured!

With solid masses, **fine-needle aspiration biopsy** can be performed (under ultrasound guidance if needed) to obtain material for cytologic analysis. This diagnostic procedure requires considerable experience in obtaining and evaluating the sample and is definitive only when positive due to the risk of false-negative findings. A negative result should be interpreted with caution.

In a **core biopsy**, the needle has a larger bore that provides a sample ("tissue core") for histologic evaluation. As in fine-needle aspiration, however, only a positive result is definitive.

The most reliable method for establishing the identity of a longstanding neck mass unresponsive to conservative therapy is **open biopsy**, in which part of the tumor or preferably the entire "lump" is excised for histologic scrutiny and possible further analysis. A prescalene biopsy (synonym: Daniel's biopsy) involves the removal of lymph nodes at the jugulosubclavian venous junction, which represents the final collecting point for lymphatic drainage in the body.

# 16.3 Malformations of the Neck

Malformations of the neck include branchial and thyroglossal duct cysts and fistulas, vascular malformations such as hemangiomas and lymphangiomas, musculoskeletal anomalies, and dysontogenetic tumors.

*Definitions:* A **cyst** is an epithelium-lined cavity that does not have an internal or external opening. A **sinus** is an epithelium-lined cavity that opens either internally (common but incorrect synonym: incomplete internal fistula) or externally (synonym: incomplete external fistula). A **fistula** is an epithelium-lined tract that has both an internal and external opening (**Fig. 16.9**).

## Branchial Cleft Cysts and Fistulas

*Etiology and pathogenesis:* The basic embryology of branchial cleft cysts and fistulas is reviewed in ℘ **16.5**. The classic theory holds that branchial cleft cysts and fistulas result from a persistence or incomplete regression of the cervical sinus (cervical sinus theory). Sinuses that open internally (incomplete internal fistulas) are viewed as a remnant of the second branchial pouch, and those that open externally (incomplete external fistulas) are a remnant of the second branchial cleft, each having a connection with the cervical sinus. (Complete) fistulas can develop only if both the entoderm of the branchial pouch and the ectoderm of the branchial cleft communicate with the cervical sinus, rupturing the pharyngeal membrane.

Fig. 16.9  Differences between a cyst, sinus, and fistula

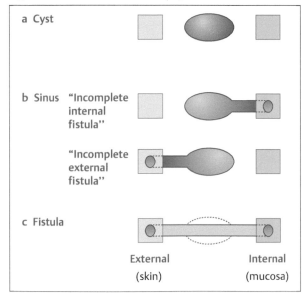

All of the lesions are lined by epithelium.

Fig. 16.10  Branchial cleft cyst at the border of the second branchial arch

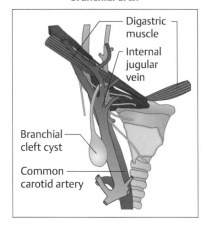

The structure in the diagram illustrates the most common site of occurrence of a branchial cleft cyst (actually a lateral internal sinus), arising from the border of the second branchial arch. The tract opens internally into the supratonsillar fossa.

*Topography:* Cervical fistulas and cysts occur predominantly at the border of the second branchial arch, because it is the largest of the arches and persists for the longest time during embryonic development. The cervical fistulas and cysts that develop there are very closely related to the carotid bifurcation. An internal sinus in this area opens into the supratonsillar fossa. The sac of a branchial cleft cyst is always located lateral to the internal jugular vein and caudal to the posterior belly of the digastric muscle (**Fig.16.10**).

Malformations of the third and fourth branchial arches (see ℘ **16.6** for location) are considerably less common.

*Epidemiology:* Branchial cleft cysts and sinuses generally manifest between 15 and 25 years of age, whereas branchial fistulas are usually noted immediately after birth. Both sexes are affected equally. Branchial cleft cysts are approximately four times more prevalent than branchial fistulas; hence, they are relatively common and one of the main causes of neck swelling in children. It is extremely rare for branchial cleft cysts to undergo malignant transformation.

*Symptoms and diagnosis:* Branchial cleft cysts generally have a short history. Patients notice a painless, tense swelling in the carotid triangle between the hyoid bone and sternocleidomastoid muscle (**Fig. 16.11a**). It is not unusual for an acute inflammation, which can

### 16.5 Embryology and malformations of the branchial apparatus

#### Embryology

The branchial apparatus is composed of six mesodermal *branchial arches* (pharyngeal arches; the fifth and sixth arches are rudimentary in humans), five entodermal *branchial pouches* (pharyngeal pouches), and four ectodermal *branchial clefts* (branchial grooves). In mammals, entodermal and ectodermal duplications of epithelium that are devoid of mesenchyma, called the *pharyngeal membranes*, separate the internal branchial pouches from the external branchial clefts at the borders of the branchial arches. (In fish, these membranes rupture to form the gills.) Each branchial arch has an artery, cartilage bar, muscular element, and nerve.

#### Theories of pathogenesis

The two main theories on the pathogenesis of branchial anomalies are presented below:

*Classic theory*: According to the classic theory, the second branchial arch enlarges disproportionately during the fifth week of development and overlaps the third and fourth arches, forming an ectodermal cavity called the *cervical sinus* (of His), which is surrounded by the operculum (**Fig. 16.12a**). Afterward, the cervical sinus becomes progressively smaller, finally closing to form an ectodermal inclusion in the mesoderm, the *cervical vesicle*, which disappears with further development (**Fig. 16.12b**). But this classic theory, which regards branchial cleft cysts and fistulas as a failure of regression of the cervical sinus and vesicle, has certain deficiencies that have been addressed in the current model proposed by Otto.

*Otto theory*: This theory disputes the notion that the cervical sinus closes to form the cervical vesicle, followed by complete resorption of the enclosed epithelium (viewing this instead as a sectioning or preparation artifact), claiming that all of the ectodermal epithelium in the cervical sinus migrates back to the surface. According to this theory, the *pharyngeal membrane stage* (separating the branchial clefts and pouches; **Fig. 16.12c**) is followed developmentally by a *stage of internal and external connecting lamellae*, with the external and internal lamellae eventually migrating back, respectively, to the external and internal body surface (**Fig. 16.12d**). Otto theorizes that a **local interepithelial adhesion (LIAD)**, represented by desmosomes and interdigitations, forms at the site of a pharyngeal membrane or connecting lamella, where a gap exists in the mesenchyma (**Fig. 16.12d**). If mesodermal fusion fails to take place at this LIAD at the proper time, epithelial retention and proliferation can occur as a *redundancy anomaly*.

**Pathogenesis of branchial cleft cysts and fistulas**: When this LIAD theory, which is valid for embryonic development in general, is applied to branchial cleft cysts and fistulas, it means that a persistent LIAD is formed in the area of the second, third, or fourth pharyngeal membrane. Further growth leads to a displacement of the ectodermal or entodermal epithelial elements in which the LIAD becomes elongated and is "dragged along" to form a fistulous tract (**Fig. 16.12e**).

If the LIAD persists in its entirety, a (complete) fistula develops (**Fig. 16.12f**). If the fistulous tract is torn from one of the two surface aggregates of epithelial cells, an internal or external sinus is formed. And if the fistulous tract is separated from both epithelia, a branchial cleft cyst will form.

The pathogenesis of thyroglossal duct cysts and thyroid anomalies is reviewed in 🔖 **16.7**.

**Fig. 16.12 Embryological development and malformations of the branchial apparatus**

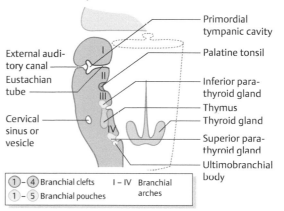

**a Early 5th embryonic week**

Maxillary process
Mandibular process
Four branchial clefts
Operculum
Future cervical sinus
Cardiac prominence
Five branchial pouches

**b Late 5th embryonic week**

External auditory canal
Eustachian tube
Cervical sinus or vesicle
Primordial tympanic cavity
Palatine tonsil
Inferior parathyroid gland
Thymus
Thyroid gland
Superior parathyroid gland
Ultimobranchial body

①–④ Branchial clefts   I–IV Branchial arches
①–⑤ Branchial pouches

**c Day 20**

3rd branchial arch
2nd branchial cleft
2nd branchial pouch
2nd pharyngeal membrane
1st branchial pouch
1st branchial cleft
1st pharyngeal membrane
1st branchial arch
2nd branchial arch

**d Day 35**

3rd branchial arch
2nd inner connecting lamella
2nd outer connecting lamella
2nd branchial arch
Hyomandibular border
Entoderm
1st inner connecting lamella
LIAD
1st outer connecting lamella
Ectoderm
1st branchial arch

**e LIAD**

Entoderm
Ectoderm

**f Fistula due to persistent LIAD**

Internal carotid artery
External carotid artery
Internal fistula opening
Fistulous tract
Common carotid artery
External fistula opening

Source **c–f**: Otto 1994.

**Fig. 16.11 Branchial cleft cyst**

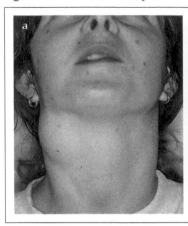 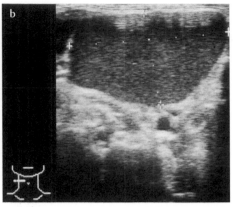

Lateral neck swelling (**a**) in a 17-year-old girl appears at ultrasound (**b**, transverse B-mode image) as a sharply circumscribed mass with homogeneous contents and distal acoustic enhancement. A fistulous opening could not be identified.

---

🔎 **16.6 Malformations of the third and fourth branchial arches**

Malformations of the third branchial arch open internally in the lateral wall of the piriform recess anterior to the plica of the superior laryngeal nerve at the level of the cricoid cartilage. The very rare malformations of the fourth branchial arch open at the tip of the piriform recess, the fistulous tract imitating the course of the recurrent nerves.

---

be difficult to distinguish from a cervical abscess, to direct attention to a branchial cleft cyst.

Besides *palpation, B-mode ultrasound* is the diagnostic method of choice, demonstrating branchial cleft cysts as homogeneous, echo-free masses with smooth margins located at a typical site (**Fig. 16.11b**). Acutely infected cysts may contain a viscous, purulent material that appears echogenic.

**Sinuses** ("incomplete fistulas") that open internally are more common than complete fistulas and can produce the same symptoms as branchial cleft cysts.

**Branchial fistulas** always open externally at the anterior border of the sternocleidomastoid muscle (usually one to two finger widths above the sternoclavicular joint) and may be marked by a clear, amber-colored discharge. Acute infections with the typical signs of pain, redness, and purulent drainage are common. Accessory cartilage may occur at the fistula opening. The tract itself can be defined by *contrast radiography*. An effort should be made to locate the pharyngeal opening of the fistula, which may be in the supratonsillar fossa, faucial pillar, lateral pharyngeal wall, or piriform recess.

*Differential diagnosis:* The differential diagnosis of **cervical cysts** includes all other cervical masses. With **fistulas**, the possible presence of lymph-node tuberculosis or actinomycosis should be considered.

*Treatment:* Surgical treatment is generally indicated.

🗡 To prevent a recurrence, no residual epithelium should be left behind.

**Fistulas** are identified intraoperatively with patent blue and excised. The close relationship of the fistulous tracts to the cervical vessels and nerves, as well as inflammatory adhesions, often makes the surgery difficult.

Even in the excision of presumed **cysts**, a careful search should be made for a tract to the supratonsillar fossa. When present, the tract should be traced and excised to prevent a recurrence. For this reason, the operation should always include a tonsillectomy. Peritonsillar abscesses following tonsillectomy may result from the presence of entodermal duct remnants (the "duct of His") in the supratonsillar fossa.

**Acutely inflamed cysts** or **fistulas** should first be treated conservatively with antibiotics to facilitate subsequent surgery.

🗡 Puncture or incision of branchial cleft cysts is indicated only in exceptional cases with severe pain.

## Thyroglossal Duct Cysts and Fistulas

*Etiology and pathogenesis:* The pathogenesis of thyroglossal duct cysts and fistulas is closely linked to the embryonic development of the thyroid gland (🔎 **16.7**).

*Epidemiology:* Approximately 75% of thyroglossal duct cysts are manifested before 5 years of age, and most are diagnosed before 12 months. The malignant transformation of thyroglossal duct cysts is rare.

*Symptoms:* Parents often notice a tense, firm swelling in the midline of the neck between the chin and thyroid gland (or very rarely at the suprasternal level).

## 16.7 Embryology and malformations of the thyroid gland

### Embryology (Fig. 16.13a)

On day 24 of embryonic development, a median epithelial thickening appears in the floor of the ectodermal pharyngeal gut, dorsal to the future tuberculum impar. It develops into the thyroglossal duct, on which the thyroid primordium descends into the neck. The thyroid gland reaches its pretracheal position by the end of the seventh week, and the thyroglossal duct is obliterated or resorbed. The foramen cecum in the midline of the tongue and the pyramidal lobe of the thyroid gland are viewed as the remnants (ends) of the thyroglossal duct. The hyoid bone develops later and has a variable relationship to the thyroglossal duct.

### Pathogenesis

#### Thyroglossal duct cysts and malformations of the thyroid gland

**Classic theory**: The classic theory attributes the formation of thyroglossal duct cysts to incomplete obliteration or resorption of the thyroglossal duct.

**Otto theory**: More recent studies call the descent of the thyroid gland into question, instead suggesting that the thyroid primordium develops near the heart with the subsequent formation of a connecting tract between the thyroid gland and the epithelium of the oral floor (thyroglossal duct); this results in an ascent of the head, taking the thyroid gland with it. According to this theory, the thyroglossal duct contains two types of epithelium: the oral floor epithelium superiorly and the thyroid epithelium inferiorly. The differentiating boundary between the two epithelial types (**local interepithelial adhesion, LIAD**; see also 🔎 **16.5**) ruptures by the middle of the sixth week (**Fig. 16.13a**).

All malformations of the thyroid gland can be explained on the basis of this theory:

If the thyroglossal duct does not rupture at the level of the differentiating boundary but at a lower level (in the thyroid epithelium), thyroid tissue will remain at the cranial end of the thyroglossal duct during the subsequent ascent of the head. Ectopic thyroid tissue or a lingual goiter may develop as a result of this mechanism (**Fig. 16.13b**). If the thyroglossal duct ruptures at a higher level (in the oral floor epithelium), nonthyroid epithelial tissue will persist between the base of the tongue and thyroid gland and may form a nidus for the development of an epithelial cyst (= thyroglossal duct cyst). These epithelial cysts may also contain thyroid tissue (**Fig. 16.13c**). The *prevalence* of thyroid anomalies is approximately 7%, the most frequent anomaly being a persistent pyramidal lobe.

**Thyroglossal duct fistulas**, which are more aptly called sinuses, are not primary lesions; they are secondary to the (inflammatory) external perforation of a thyroglossal duct cyst or to iatrogenic measures (e.g., needle aspiration).

Fig. 16.13   **Embryological development of the thyroid gland**

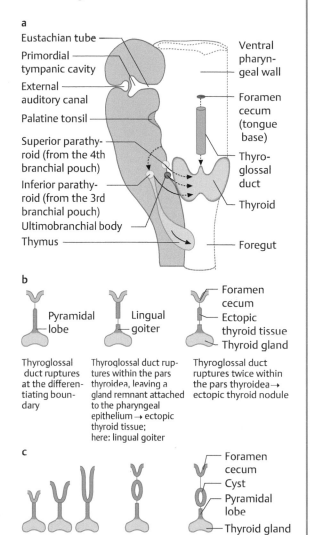

**a** Overview.
**b** Formation of lingual goiter and ectopic thyroid tissue.
**c** Formation of thyroglossal duct cysts.

Not infrequently, an inflammatory process may first draw attention to a thyroglossal duct cyst. The swelling may be intermittent or continuous. Swallowing difficulties are uncommon.

Thyroglossal fistulas are usually recognized by their external opening (typically located at the level of the thyroid notch) and the associated discharge. Inflammations with retention of secretions and abscess formation may occur.

***Diagnosis:*** The diagnosis is suggested by inspection and palpation (**Fig. 16.14a, Fig. 16.15**). A thyroglossal

**Fig. 16.14** Thyroglossal duct cyst

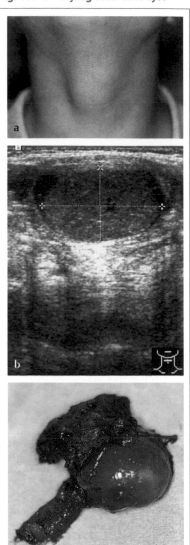

**a, b** The swelling in the neck (**a**) appears sonographically (**b**, transverse B-mode image) as a sharply circumscribed mass with homogeneous contents and distal acoustic enhancement. **c** Surgical specimen of a thyroglossal duct cyst with attached midportion of hyoid bone. Diagnostic needle aspiration is contraindicated. A thyroglossal fistula can be confirmed by radiographic contrast examination.

**Fig. 16.15** Thyroglossal duct fistula in an 11-year-old boy

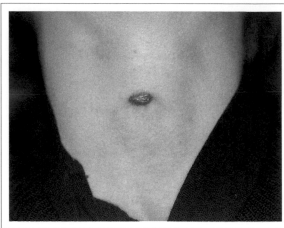

Whenever possible, the surgery should be done during an inflammation-free interval, if necessary after preliminary antibiotic therapy.

A **thyroglossal duct cyst** is typically removed through a transverse suprahyoid incision. It is important to look for remnants of the thyroglossal duct and, if necessary, trace them to the foramen cecum and excise them, since leaving behind epithelial remnants predisposes to a recurrence (recurrent cyst or fistula). For the same reason, the resection should always include the body of the hyoid bone since epithelial remnants are frequently present in or on the bone. Failure to resect the midportion of the hyoid bone is associated with up to a 50% recurrence rate, which otherwise is less than 5%. Resecting the body of the hyoid bone has no functional sequelae. It will not impair swallowing because the functionally significant hyoid muscles are attached to the cornua of the hyoid bone.

**Thyroglossal fistulas** are outlined with an elliptical excision and removed in toto. This surgery is aided by intraoperative staining of the fistulous tract with blue dye.

duct cyst will invariably move when the patient swallows.

Ultrasound may support the presumptive diagnosis by showing a well-circumscribed, elliptical, hypoechoic or echo-free mass with distal acoustic enhancement (**Fig. 16.14b**).

 It should always be confirmed that a normally developed thyroid gland is present.

Diagnostic needle aspiration is contraindicated. A thyroglossal fistula can be confirmed by radiographic contrast examination.

***Treatment:*** The only treatment option is surgical removal. The sclerotherapy of fistulas and the incision of cysts in a noninflamed condition are contraindicated.

## Vascular Malformations

### Lymphangioma

Synonym: cystic hygroma.

Lymphangiomas develop from sequestered portions of the primordial lymphatics that begin to sprout in the sixth week of embryonic development. These sequestra do not establish connections with the venous system, and they degenerate to form cystic cavities. They tend to grow by expansion and infiltration.

Ninety percent of lymphangioma are manifested during the first 2 years of life. Many are already present at birth and may cause obstruction of labor. Lymphangiomas are typically located in the lateral part of the neck (**Fig. 16.16**).

Fig. 16.16   Lymphangioma in an infant

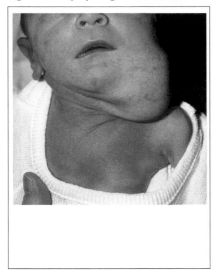

Fig. 16.17   Hemangioma

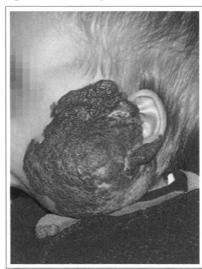

Extensive hemangioma of the cheek and neck in a 9-month-old girl.

The tumor is *palpable* as a soft, doughy mass. Generally, the true extent of the mass is underestimated by palpation due to its infiltrative growth. B-mode ultrasound provides a more accurate assessment. Local expansile growth can cause *symptoms* such as dyspnea and stridor.

*Treatment:* Unlike hemangiomas, lymphangiomas very rarely undergo spontaneous regression. Therefore, a wait-and-see approach is generally not justified and surgical treatment is required. Lymphangiomas can also be locally treated, i.e., sclerosed, using infiltration with Picibanil (OK-432, a lyophilized strain of Group A *Streptococcus pyogenes* treated with penicillin G and hydrogen peroxide). Repeated treatments are usually necessary. The local injection of a crystalline corticosteroid solution may be tried as an alternative to surgery.

## Hemangioma

Hemangiomas are growing vascular lesions (ectasias) that belong to the group of hamartomas (= dysontogenetic growth of normally formed tissue).

*Epidemiology:* Hemangiomas have a reported incidence of 10% during the first year of life. Premature infants are predominantly affected. Superficial hemangiomas are more common in females.

*Symptoms:* Hemangiomas can occur anywhere on the body appearing clinically as a soft, reddish-purple swelling (**Fig. 16.17**). Large hemangiomas may be hemodynamically significant.

*Course:* Unlike lymphangiomas, hemangiomas regress spontaneously in up to 80% of cases. The natural history proceeds in phases—a two-part proliferative phase is followed at approximately 1 year of age by a stable plateau in which the lesion ceases to grow. The involutional phase then occurs during the first or second year of life or may be delayed until puberty.

*Diagnosis:* Besides **B-mode ultrasound**, which can define the overall extent of the lesion, **color duplex ultrasound** has proved to be a particularly useful diagnostic tool.

▯ The patient should always be screened for additional hemangiomas of the internal organs (lung, liver, etc.).

*Treatment: In the past*,the high rate of spontaneous involution justified a wait-and-see approach, unless the hemangioma was growing rapidly or was causing symptoms due to its location or extent. Pediatric hemangiomas respond well to systemic β-blocker therapy (e.g., propranolol), which is nowadays therefore considered first-line therapy. With regard to effective b-blocker treatment, a wait-and-see strategy is only viable for uncomplicated hemangiomas at noncritical sites.

Further treatment options depend on the individual case and consist of systemic corticosteroid therapy (anti-inflammatory and angiostatic effect), local sclerotherapy or embolization, magnesium spiking, laser treatment—dye laser, argon laser, neodymium: yttrium aluminum garnet (Nd:YAG)—and surgical excision. Radiotherapy is used only in highly selected cases due to the risk of late sequelae.

The **Kasabach–Merritt sequence** (synonym: thrombocytopenia–hemangioma syndrome) is characterized by the presence of typically large ("giant") hemangiomas in which thrombotic processes lead to disseminated intravascular coagulation with consumption coagulopathy. The syndrome affects small infants almost exclusively.

Another rare entity is **blue rubber bleb nevus syndrome**, which has an autosomal-dominant mode of inheritance. Multiple, deep blue hemangiomas with a rubbery consistency form on the integument and persist without involution. Gastrointestinal manifestations can lead to recurrent episodes of bleeding.

## Paraganglioma

Synonym: chemodectoma.

Nonchromaffin (🔎 **16.9**) paraganglia, which function as chemoreceptors, are located at various sites in the neck: the carotid bifurcation (carotid paraganglion), the vagus nerve (vagal paraganglion), the internal jugular vein (jugular paraganglion), and the larynx (laryngeal paraganglion). Neoplasms that are derived from the chemoreceptor tissue in paraganglia are called paragangliomas. "Glomus tumor" is an archaic and also incorrect term that should no longer be used. The hereditary paraganglioma-pheochromocytoma syndrome derives from a mutation in the SDHB, SDHC, or SDHD genes of the mitochondrial respiratory chain enzyme succinate dehydrogenase. The range of this syndrome can also include clear-cell renal cell carcinomas, papillary thyroid carcinomas, and gastrointestinal stromal tumors.

*Epidemiology:* Paragangliomas are mostly solitary and benign. Malignant transformation occurs in up to 10 to 20% of cases. Paragangliomas are believed to occur more frequently in persons living at higher altitudes.

### Carotid Paraganglioma

*Symptoms:* This tumor presents as a painless, sometimes pulsatile mass in the neck. It may be accompanied by a dry cough (due to vagus nerve irritation), hoarseness (vagus or recurrent nerve lesion), and Horner's syndrome (sympathetic trunk irritation). A painful sensation is sometimes present.

*Diagnosis:* **Palpation** reveals a soft or tense, sometimes pulsatile mass at the level of the carotid bifurcation. In typical cases, the mass is mobile in the lateromedial direction but not craniocaudally. A bruit is usually heard at **auscultation**. When imaged by **B-mode ultrasound**, the paraganglioma appears as a hypoechoic mass splaying the carotid bifurcation.

The term *nonchromaffin* stems from the historical observation that the cells of the paraganglia do not take up the chromaffin stain that is used in the detection of catecholamines.

Paragangliomas cannot always be distinguished from branchial cleft cysts or enlarged lymph nodes. This differentiation is aided by **color duplex sonography**, which can clearly demonstrate the rich vascularity of paragangliomas (**Fig. 16.18**). **MRI** and **somatostatin receptor scintigraphy** can generally furnish a definitive diagnosis. Any surgical measures should be preceded by **angiography**.

⚕ Needle aspiration is contraindicated due to the rich vascularity of the tumor.

*Treatment:* The treatment of choice for paragangliomas of the carotid bifurcation is surgical removal. Most tumors infiltrate the adventitia of the carotid artery, making removal difficult. Generally, the surgery requires autologous blood donation and/or the intraoperative use of a cell saver. Preoperative embolization is not indicated.

## Torticollis

Synonym: wryneck.
Torticollis may be congenital or acquired. The possible causes are listed in **Table 16.2**. Diagnosis and treatment are usually handled by a neonatologist or orthopaedist.

## Dysontogenetic Tumors

**Embryonal tumors** are derived from immature, primitive tissue, and malignant forms are common due to the pluripotency of the cells. A particularly common representative in the neck is *embryonal rhabdomyosarcoma*, which is derived from the primordia of striated skeletal muscle. Treatment follows established protocols for soft-tissue sarcomas in pediatric oncology. Surgical treatment should be provided in collaboration with a pediatric oncologic center.

**Teratomas** are characterized by the presence of cellular elements from all three germ layers (ectoderm, mesoderm, entoderm) and show varying degrees of differentiation from immature embryonic tissue to fully formed elements (e.g., cartilage, bone, teeth). Cervical teratomas account for approximately 5% of congenital teratomas and are usually manifested before 12 months of age. Differential diagnosis is aided by plain radiographs of the neck, which often show inclusions of calcific density. Given their potential for malignant transformation, teratomas should be surgically removed. This particularly applies to teratomas

**Fig. 16.18 Carotid paraganglioma**

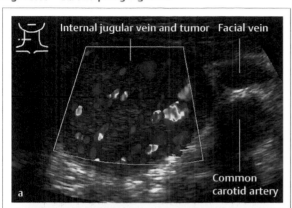
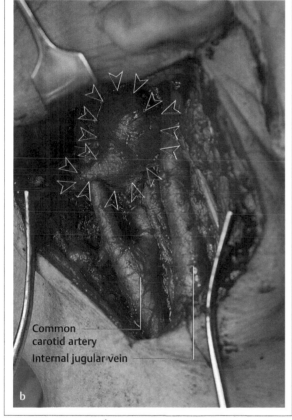

The paraganglia of the vagus nerve are usually directly adjacent to the ganglia of this cranial nerve that lie below the jugular foramen. Tumors of the vagal paraganglion are relatively rare (~3% of paragangliomas).

The **cardinal symptom** is vagus nerve palsy with hoarseness and aspiration. Extensive tumors may cause a jugular foramen syndrome (synonym: Avellis' syndrome). Intracranial extension (dumbbell tumor) is particularly common with paragangliomas close to the superior vagal ganglion.

As with carotid paragangliomas, the **diagnosis** is established by B-mode ultrasound, color Doppler ultrasound, computed tomography, magnetic resonance imaging, and in some cases angiography. The **differential diagnosis** consists mainly of vagus neurinoma.

As complete resection of a vagal paraganglioma is usually accompanied by a lesion of the vagus nerve (results: hoarseness, dysphagia), partial resection—preserving cerebral nerve function—is now the preferred **surgical treatment**, with postoperative radiotherapy.

**Table 16.2 Causes of torticollis**

| Congenital | Acquired |
| --- | --- |
| **Muscular** | • Radical neck dissection with removal of the sternocleidomastoid muscle |
| • Common: obstetric trauma with tearing and hematoma formation in the sternocleidomastoid muscle | • Trauma to the cervical spine |
| • Less common: congenital fibrous transformation of muscle tissue | • Functional disorders of the ocular muscles (ocular torticollis) |
| • Muscular dystrophies | • Analgesic guarding due to cervical abscess or pronounced lymphadenitis |
| **Bony** | • Rheumatoid disease |
| • *Klippel–Feil syndrome* with synostoses in the cervical spine | • Accessory nerve palsy |
| • *Goldenhar's syndrome* with fusion and/or absence of cervical vertebrae | • Atlantoaxial torticollis following inflammatory disease, surgery, or radiotherapy to the nasopharynx (synonym: Grisel's syndrome) |

**a** Doppler ultrasound scan of an extensive paraganglioma that has grown into the internal jugular vein. The color flow signals clearly demonstrate the vascularity of the tumor.
**b** Paraganglioma in the left side of the neck above the carotid bifurcation (arrows). The tumor does not involve the internal jugular vein.

in adults, which show a strong propensity for malignant degeneration ("teratocarcinoma").

**Dermoids**, unlike teratomas, are composed mainly of ectodermal elements with a complete absence of endodermal elements.

Dermoids are formed by the encapsulation of ectodermal epithelial elements during development and thus represent dystopic epithelium within the mesenchyme. Given the ectodermal origin of the tissue, histologic examination often reveals dermal appendages (hair follicles, sebaceous glands, sweat glands) and desquamated amorphous material.

Treatment consists of surgical removal.

**Hamartomas** result from the circumscribed, neoplastic overgrowth of tissue that is normally differentiated in most cases and is normally present in that part of the body. The most common example of a hamartoma in the neck is *hemangioma* (see above).

# 16.4   Inflammations of the Neck

For differential diagnostic and therapeutic reasons, it is necessary to distinguish inflammatory reactions of the *cervical lymph nodes* (lymphadenitis) from deep-inflammations of the *cervical soft tissues*, which may be circumscribed (abscess) or diffuse (cellulitis). This topic does not include cutaneous inflammations.

## Inflammations of the Cervical Lymph Nodes

The cervical lymph nodes are affected by (infectious) inflammations with remarkable frequency. One reason for this is that the topographic anatomy of the neck makes it easy to detect even small masses; another reason is that the upper aerodigestive tract is a frequent portal of entry for infectious microorganisms.

The **cardinal symptom** is almost always a palpable neck mass (**Fig. 16.19**). "Healthy" lymph nodes are neither palpable nor detectable by ultrasound. Constant pain and tenderness are typical signs of a (usually acute) inflammation but may be absent. Additional symptoms and findings such as neck pain, dental pain, otalgia, fever, malaise, swollen salivary glands, and skin changes can help to narrow the differential diagnosis. Possible methods of **classification** are shown in **Table 16.3**.

**Fig. 16.19   Enlarged cervical lymph nodes**

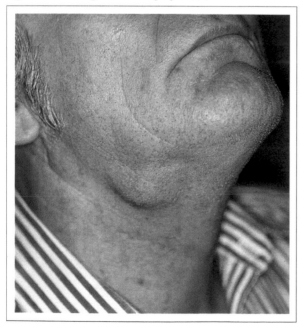

Important considerations in differential diagnosis are the rate of enlargement, consistency, and mobility of the mass and the patient's general state of health.

## Acute Cervical Lymphadenitis

*Etiology and pathogenesis:* Acute lymphadenitis in the neck is usually a reactive lymphadenopathy that develops in response to an infection of the upper respiratory tract (viral or bacterial rhinitis, sinusitis, pharyngitis, tonsillitis), the teeth and periodontal structures, the salivary glands, or the facial and neck skin (e.g., erysipelas, impetigo contagiosa). Thus, it presents few difficulties in terms of differential diagnosis.

The most frequent cause of acute cervical lymphadenitis in children is a streptococcal infection of the palatine tonsils. Other potential causes are the rubella virus and cytomegalovirus (CMV), and mycobacteria have increasingly been implicated in recent years. Infectious mononucleosis is an acute disease of the lymphatic system caused by the Epstein–Barr virus, a DNA virus that belongs to the Herpesviridae family.

*Symptoms:* Patients typically experience a systemic inflammatory reaction with fever and malaise. The cervical masses have a soft consistency and are usually painful. Multiple lymph nodes are typically affected and may be unilateral or bilateral, depending on the site of the underlying organic infection. *Infectious mononucleosis* is characterized by tonsillitis and a usually pronounced (voluminous), painful cervical lymphadenitis (see ✍ 5.4, Acute Inflammations).

In a *primary infection with the human immunodeficiency virus (HIV)*, an incubation period of 1 to 3 weeks is followed by an "acute" stage marked by flu-like symptoms, an itchy skin rash, and generalized lymphadenitis.

---

🔎 **16.11   Kawasaki's syndrome**

Kawasaki syndrome (synonym: mucocutaneous lymph node syndrome) is a diffuse vasculitis that occurs in children and presents with fever, mucocutaneous changes, and swollen cervical lymph nodes. A feared complication, occurring in one-fourth of cases, is cardiac involvement in the form of myocarditis, coronary arteritis, or both. A bacterial etiology is presumed, but it has not been possible to isolate a causative organism. Whenever the syndrome is suspected, a pediatric examination should be scheduled without delay.

*Diagnosis:* When acute cervical lymphadenitis is present, it is first necessary to look for the precipitating cause, i.e., an organic infection (mirror examination by an otolaryngologist, dental consultation if needed). B-mode ultrasound examination of the neck is helpful in detecting or excluding lymphadenitis with abscess formation (central echo = liquefaction) and can better quantify the extent of lymphadenitis in relation to palpable findings (for follow-up and monitoring therapeutic response).

*Differential diagnosis:* An acutely inflamed thyroglossal duct cyst or branchial cleft cyst should be considered when acute lymphadenitis is present, as these lesions are usually associated with an accompanying (reactive) lymphadenitis.

With repeated episodes of cervical lymphadenitis, it is not uncommon for palpable lymph nodes to persist beyond the stage of the acute inflammation. This is attributable to inflammatory fibrosis and may lead to problems of differential diagnosis.

*Treatment:* Treatment is directed mainly toward the underlying organic infection. For example, penicillin is the agent of choice for a streptococcal infection. The parenteral administration of antibiotics should be considered in patients with systemic symptoms or suppurative lymphadenitis. The latter condition requires close-interval follow-up and may require an incision for abscess drainage.

## Chronic Cervical Lymphadenitis

*Etiology:* **Table 16.3** lists diseases that may be associated with lymphadenitis.

Various medications may also cause lymphadenopathy, including antiepileptic drugs, tuberculostatics, heparin, phenacetin, salicylates and other nonsteroidal anti-inflammatory drugs (NSAIDs), allopurinol, antibiotics, gold, and methyldopa.

*Diagnosis and treatment:*

☝ Chronic cervical lymph-node enlargement (present for more than 4 weeks) often leads to diagnostic problems because it requires differentiation from a malignant disease such as malignant lymphoma and cervical lymph-node metastasis.

Besides growth kinetics, other factors to be considered in selecting a diagnostic procedure for cervical lymphadenopathy are the age of the patient, the presence of risk factors for malignancy (e.g., nicotine abuse), and any associated symptoms (e.g., "B symptoms" such as fever, night sweats, and undesired weight loss; see also ☜ 16.5, Malignant Lymphomas).

**History:** In planning the diagnostic algorithm, it is important to ask the patient about risk factors for the causes listed in **Table 16.3**:
- House pets: dogs, cats, rodents, etc.
- Occupational contact with animals or animal products: slaughterhouse worker, butcher, meat seller, cheese production and sales, farm workers, gardeners.
- Eating habits: consumption of raw meat or sheep cheese.
- Trips abroad.
- Institutional settings: medical staff, nursing home workers, kindergarten teachers.

**Palpation** (consistency, mobility relative to skin and underlying tissues) and **B-mode ultrasound** can provide initial clues in making a differential diagnosis.

**Antibiotic trial:** Since it is relatively common for cervical lymph-node enlargement to have a bacterial cause, a broad-spectrum antibiotic (e.g., doxycycline, macrolide) may be tried before proceeding with serologic tests or invasive diagnostic procedures in patients who have no obvious signs of a malignant underlying disease.

☝ Make certain, however, that the patient understands the importance of follow-ups.

**Serology:** The selection of serologic tests should be patient-specific due to the long list of possible causative organisms (detailed history: see also **Table 16.3**).

**Histology:** As a general rule, a surgically removed lymph node will provide the most accurate diagnosis. A histologic work-up should be done in patients with a known immune deficiency (e.g., HIV infection) and in patients on immunosuppressive therapy due to the great many possible (and atypical) causative organisms and the increased incidence of malignant tumors in these subgroups.

Owing to the topographic anatomy of the neck, this type of surgery can usually be done under local anesthesia with relatively low risk. Because the histological architecture of the lymph node provides the best or only indicator of certain diseases such as malignant non-Hodgkin's lymphoma, the most reliable biopsy technique is to excise a complete, representative lymph node rather than perform a partial excision or obtain a core- or fine-needle specimen.

*Special forms and differential diagnoses:*

**Actinomycosis:** This disease is caused by the gram-positive anaerobic bacterium *Actinomyces israelii*. The cervicofacial form of actinomycosis causes a "boardlike" infiltration of the subcutaneous tissue with firm nodules, fistulas, and ulcerations. *Treatment* consists of a prolonged course of antibiotic therapy, which may be supplemented if necessary by surgical measures.

**Table 16.3    Classification of cervical lymphadenitis**

| Classification | | Example or features |
|---|---|---|
| **By time course** | | |
| Acute | Duration of symptoms < 4 weeks | Lymphadenitis in bacterial tonsillitis |
| Chronic | Duration of symptoms > 4 weeks | See listing below |
| **By etiology** | | |
| Infectious | Viral | Numerous pathogens including EBV (infectious mononucleosis), CMV, rubella, HIV |
| | Bacterial, nonspecific | E.g., streptococci, staphylococci |
| | Bacterial, specific | Tuberculosis, atypical mycobacteria, cat-scratch disease, yersiniosis |
| | Fungal | Rare, mainly in immunocompromised patients |
| | Parasitic | E.g., toxoplasmosis |
| Noninfectious lymphadenitis and lymphadenitis of unknown cause | | E.g., sarcoidosis, foreign body reaction, Kawasaki's syndrome, Kikuchi's lymphadenitis, Rosai–Dorfman syndrome |
| **By microbiologic or histologic features** | | |
| Serologic tests | Mononucleosis | Anti-EA, anti-VCA, anti-EBNA |
| | Toxoplasmosis | Sabin–Feldman test, IgG, IgM |
| | Brucellosis | Agglutination test, IgG, IgM |
| | Tularemia | Agglutination test, IgG, IgM |
| | Syphilis | TPHA, FTA-Abs, IgM |
| | Cytomegalovirus | IgG, IgM: relatively unreliable |
| | HIV infection | ELISA, immunofluorescence, western blot, virus load |
| | Cat-scratch disease | IFT, ELISA |
| Culturing or identifying the organism | Tuberculosis | Culture, DNA detection by PCR |
| | Listeriosis | Culture |
| | Cytomegalovirus | Isolation of the virus |
| | Cat-scratch disease | PCR (*Bartonella henselae*) |
| Histologic examination | Nonspecific lymphadenitis | The causative agent cannot be determined from histologic findings |
| | Specific lymphadenitis | The histologic findings provide clues to the causative agent |
| | • Abscess-forming reticular lymphadenitis (pseudotuberculosis-type granulomas) | *Yersinia pseudotuberculosis, Y. enterocolitica, Francisella tularensis, Afipia felis, Bartonella henselae* |
| | • Epithelioid cell lymphadenitis | Toxoplasmosis, sarcoidosis, tuberculosis, atypical mycobacteriosis, sarcoid-like reaction |
| | • Necrotizing histiocytic lymphadenitis | Kikuchi's lymphadenitis |
| | • Sinus histiocytosis with hemophagocytosis | Rosai–Dorfman syndrome |
| | • Angiofollicular lymph-node hyperplasia | Castleman's lymphoma |

Abbreviations: CMV, cytomegalovirus; EA, early antigen; EBNA, Epstein–Barr nuclear antigen; EBV, Epstein–Barr virus; ELISA, enzyme-linked immunosorbent assay; FTA-Abs, fluorescent *treponemal* antibody absorption (test); HIV, human immunodeficiency virus; IgG, immunoglobulin G; IgM, immunoglobulin M; PCR, polymerase chain reaction; TPHA, *Treponema pallidum* hemagglutination; VCA, virus capsid antigen.

**Rosai–Dorfman syndrome** (synonym: sinus histiocytosis with massive lymphadenopathy) is an essentially benign disease occurring in children and young adults and characterized by a (grotesque) enlargement of the cervical lymph nodes. The causative agent of the disease, which is unknown but may be infectious, incites an excessive phagocytosis of hemolymphatic cells, mostly histiocytes. The disease usually runs a self-limiting course of several weeks, but aggressive forms may occur.

**Castleman's lymphoma** (synonym: angiofollicular lymph-node hyperplasia) is a histologically defined entity that occurs in a localized form characterized by a benign course and in a more aggressive multicentric form; the latter is more likely to affect the cervical lymph nodes. The pathogenesis appears to be based on an abnormal regulation of interleukin-6 (IL-6) production, justifying a trial of corticosteroid therapy.

## Deep Neck Infections

Synonym: parapharyngeal abscess.

*Etiology:* Cervical abscesses can develop from various diseases:
- Tonsillogenic infections, peritonsillar abscess (see 5.4, Acute Inflammations).
- Suppurative lymphadenitis.
- Mastoiditis: Bezold's mastoiditis (see **Fig. 11.18**).
- Dentogenic infections: cellulitis of the oral floor (Ludwig's angina).
- Lesions of the pharyngeal mucosa (retropharyngeal abscess, foreign bodies).

*Symptoms:* The characteristic features of cervical abscesses are high fever, tenderness to pressure, and, in some cases, holding the neck and head in a guarded position. The symptoms of the causative underlying disease may also be present.

*Diagnosis:* The diagnosis is established by the typical clinical findings, markedly elevated inflammatory parameters—white blood cell (WBC) count, erythrocyte sedimentation rate (ESR), C-reactive protein (CRP)—and the detection of an abscess by ultrasound or CT.

*Treatment:* Treatment consists of antibiotic therapy specific for the underlying disease and surgical abscess drainage.

**Fig. 16.20 Cervical cellulitis**

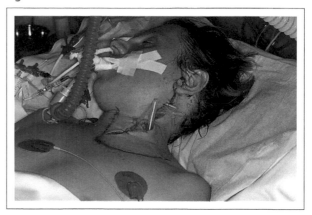

A 17-year-old patient developed cervical cellulitis as a complication of a parotid abscess. The patient is shown following surgical fasciotomy. The drains provide access for irrigation in the septic patient, who is on a ventilator.

## Cervical Cellulitis

Synonym: cervical phlegmon.

Unlike circumscribed cervical abscesses, cervical cellulitis involves a diffuse inflammation of the cervical soft tissues.

⚕ Given the anatomic relationships of the cervical soft tissues and the communication of the parapharyngeal space with the mediastinum, cervical cellulitis is a life-threatening condition (see 16.1).

*Etiology:* Cervical cellulitis may occur as a primary condition in patients with a predisposing underlying disease, or it may complicate an infection of the upper aerodigestive tract.

*Symptoms:* Most patients present with high fever and severe malaise. The cervical soft tissues are diffusely tender to pressure; even imaging studies cannot demonstrate discrete inflammatory foci. The cervical soft tissues appear markedly rarefied, and occasionally there is loss of normal delineation of anatomic structures.

*Treatment:* Treatment with broad-spectrum antibiotics (first- or second-generation cephalosporins, clindamycin, aminopenicillins + b-lactamase inhibitor) should be instituted without delay. All of the compartments in the neck should be broadly opened, and mediastinal drainage may be necessary (see **Fig. 16.20**).

# 16.5 Tumors of the Neck

Benign tumors of the neck are relatively rare. Except for the paragangliomas covered in ✑16.3, the most common benign tumors of the neck are lipomas. A special type of cervical lipoma is Madelung's disease. Very rare disorders are desmoid fibromatosis, fibrosing cervicitis, and rhabdomyoma, which are beyond our present scope. The presence of a malignant disease should always be considered in the differential diagnosis of neck masses. The diagnostic work-up should be planned with this in mind: histologic confirmation should be obtained in patients with a suspicious history or clinical findings and for masses unresponsive to a trial of antibiotic therapy.

## Benign Tumors

### Lipoma

Lipomas present clinically as soft, circumscribed, painless masses. They have a characteristic ultrasound appearance: superficial (subcutaneous) lipomas are usually encapsulated, while deeper lipomas tend to show more aggressive, infiltrative growth. Surgical removal should be considered only for cosmetically objectionable masses.

### Madelung's Disease

Synonyms: benign symmetrical cervical lipomatosis, horse collar, Launois–Bensaude syndrome.
This special form of lipoma occurs predominantly in middle-aged men who often have a history of excessive alcohol consumption (60–90% of patients). Hyperuricemia, diabetes mellitus, disorders of fat metabolism, and obstructive sleep apnea syndrome are common associated features.
**Histologic examination** shows a diffuse, unencapsulated, nonseptate proliferation of univacuolar lipocytes with tonguelike extensions into the surrounding tissue, which may involve a neoplasia of the brown fat. The changes are poorly demarcated from surrounding tissues.
**Course:** The most common "horse collar" form of the disease is characterized by the intermittent, symmetrical proliferation of fatty tissue about the neck (**Fig. 16.21**), nuchal area ("buffalo hump"), and/or the upper arms ("puffed sleeves").
**Treatment** consists of surgical removal of the excess fatty deposits. Recurrences are not uncommon. Any metabolic diseases that are diagnosed should be referred for appropriate therapy.

✂ The risk profile associated with Madelung's disease (increased cancer risk!) requires surveillance by an otolaryngologist.

## Neurinoma

Neurinomas arise from the Schwann cells of the fibrous nerve sheath and are also referred to as schwannomas. Most of these tumors are solitary, circumscribed, and encapsulated.
The most frequent **sites of occurrence** in the neck are the cervical plexus, brachial plexus, and vagus nerve. Neurinoma may also arise from the sympathetic trunk, glossopharyngeal nerve, accessory nerve, or hypoglossal nerve.

*Symptoms:* Occasionally, the tumor causes local pain that is aggravated by palpation. There may also be symptoms relating to dysfunction of the affected nerve.

*Diagnosis:* A neurinoma should be suspected when imaging (ultrasound or CT/MRI) demonstrates a fusiform mass.

*Treatment* consists of surgical resection, which may be followed by a nerve reconstruction.

*Differential diagnosis:* Neurinomas require definitive histologic differentiation from neurofibromas. The latter are particularly common in Recklinghausen's type I disease, which has an autosomal-dominant mode of inheritance. In contrast to neurinomas, it is not unusual for neurofibromas to undergo malignant transformation.

Fig. 16.21 Madelung's disease

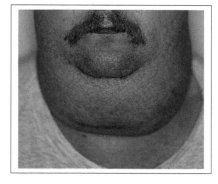

Symmetrical lipomatosis of the neck in a 33-year-old man with a history of alcoholism. The affected areas feel soft on palpation (e.g., like a fatty abdominal wall).

# Malignant Tumors of the Cervical Lymph Nodes

Malignant tumors in the neck are manifested predominantly in the cervical **lymph nodes**. Malignancies such as Hodgkin's disease and non-Hodgkin's lymphoma require differentiation from metastatic tumors with a different histologic origin. **Soft-tissue tumors** (sarcomas) that arise from connective tissue, muscle, or vessels are relatively rare.

## Malignant Lymphomas

Certain subtypes of malignant lymphoma show a predilection for the head and neck region. Solitary or multiple lymph nodes or nodal stations may be involved, depending on the subtype and stage of the disease. Extranodal sites of involvement such as the spleen, liver, lung, skeleton, mucosae—mucosa-associated lymphatic tissue (MALT) lymphoma—Waldeyer's ring (especially with B cell lymphomas), and skin (especially with T cell lymphomas) are not uncommon.

*Diagnosis:* The **history** and **clinical findings** can suggest the presence of a malignant lymphoma. Given the topographic anatomy of the neck, enlarged cervical lymph nodes become conspicuous at a relatively early stage. **B symptoms** (unexplained weight loss of >10% within 6 months and/or unexplained fever >38°C and/or night sweats), while nonspecific, may be suggestive of malignant lymphoma in patients with enlarged cervical lymph nodes and should prompt an immediate **histologic examination**. This is the only way to establish a *diagnosis* and also *identify the tumor subgroup*, which usually has a significant bearing on treatment and prognosis. Immunohistochemical and/or molecular biological techniques are generally applied. The best sites for finding additional, extranodal manifestations of lymphoma are the mucous membranes of the upper aerodigestive tract and particularly the lymphatic structures of Waldeyer's ring.

*Further management:* Once the diagnosis of malignant lymphoma has been confirmed histologically, the patient should be referred at once to a hematologic oncology center so that the disease can undergo Ann Arbor staging (see textbooks of internal medicine) and appropriate management.

## Lymph-Node Metastases

Synonym: malignant lymphadenopathy.

*Etiology:* Lymph-node metastases are predominantly of epithelial origin; the lymphatic metastasis of mesenchymal tumors (sarcomas) is relatively rare. The most common primary tumors are *carcinomas of tributary mucosal areas* of the upper aerodigestive tract, salivary glands, and thyroid gland (**Table 16.4**). But tumors of any other organs may also metastasize to the cervical lymph nodes. It is not uncommon for cancers of the lung, breast, stomach, kidneys, cervix, and prostate to metastasize to cervical nodes. The "sentinel node" (signal node, Virchow's node) in the left supraclavicular fossa is considered a fairly reliable indicator of gastric carcinoma.

Owing to the anatomy of the lymphatic drainage system, the site of a cervical lymph-node metastasis shows some degree of correlation with the site of the primary tumor (see **Fig.16.2**).

*Symptoms:* Cervical lymph-node metastases generally present as a painless, more or less fast-growing swelling on one or both sides of the neck (**Fig. 16.22**). The underlying primary tumor may be asymptomatic, or it may be possible to elicit symptoms of a primary tumor by careful questioning. Information from the patient on the duration of symptoms may be unreliable.

*Diagnosis:* During the *clinical examination*, attention is given to the number and size of enlarged lymph nodes and their mobility relative to their surroundings. *B-mode ultrasound* can provide an accurate size determination and can also help define the relation of the masses to the large vessels and muscles in the neck.

| Table 16.4 | Incidence of cervical lymph-node metastases associated with carcinomas of the upper aerodigestive tract |
|---|---|
| *Tumor location* | *Incidence of cervical lymph-node metastases at diagnosis* |
| Oral cavity | 30–65% |
| Oropharynx | 39–83% |
| Nasopharynx | 60–90% |
| Hypopharynx | 52–72% |
| Supraglottis | 35–54% |
| Glottis | 7–9% |
| Nasal cavity and paranasal sinuses | 10–20% |
| Salivary glands | 25–50% |
| Thyroid gland | 18–84%[a] |

[a]Depends on age and histologic subtype.

**Fig. 16.22 Cervical lymph-node metastasis**

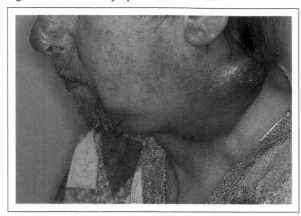

Extensive cervical lymph-node metastasis (N3) of tonsillar carcinoma in a 55-year-old man. The tumor is about to ulcerate.

*Doppler ultrasound* is helpful for investigating vascular compression and infiltration.

**Search for a primary tumor:** Whenever a cervical lymph node is suspicious for metastasis, the upper aerodigestive tract should be screened for a primary tumor by ear, nose, and throat mirror examination, endoscopy, and B-mode ultrasound.

- If a lesion is found that is suspicious for a primary tumor, it should be investigated further as described in 4.2, 4.5, and 5.2.
- If a primary tumor is not detected on clinical examination, it is advisable to remove a suspicious lymph node for histologic examination and use this result to direct further evaluation. If squamous cell carcinoma is found, indirect examination of the upper aerodigestive tract should be supplemented by detailed *endoscopy* of the nasopharynx, pharynx, larynx, trachea, bronchial system, and esophagus. Since the base of the tongue, tonsils, and nasopharynx may harbor a submucous carcinoma that is not accessible to direct visual detection, these sites should be carefully *probed* and also routinely evaluated by *deep biopsies, tonsillectomy,* and also by *curettage* in the nasopharynx. Ultrasound, MRI, and PET (performed before biopsies because biopsy-induced inflammation may result in false-positive PET signs) can also be used to locate a primary tumor. Because even primaries located outside the upper aerodigestive tract may metastasize to the cervical nodes, the search should be extended to other primary sites if a tumor is not detected in that region.
- If a diligent search (see above) fails to disclose a primary tumor (this occurs in ~5–10% of cases and usually involves squamous cell carcinoma), then the metastasis is classified as a "carcinoma of unknown primary" (**CUP syndrome**; see also 16.12). The most common site of involvement in CUP syndrome is a solitary cervical lymph node.

---

**16.12 Carcinoma of unknown primary (CUP) syndrome**

The *etiopathogenesis* of CUP syndrome is uncertain. Four main theories have been advanced:

1. A primary tumor initially present in the mucosa of the upper aerodigestive tract induces regional metastasis and then regresses completely while the regional metastases proliferate (*disappeared primary*).
2. The primary tumor has a weak local growth potential but a strong propensity for metastasis. The primary tumor is not detected by ordinary clinical methods because of its small size, but theoretically it would be detectable if more refined methods were used (*hidden primary*).
3. An ectopic mass of epithelial tissue within a lymph node undergoes malignant degeneration.
4. The lesion is not a lymph-node metastasis but a primary branchiogenic carcinoma.

**Treatment** for CUP syndrome consists of surgery (neck dissection), radiotherapy, and, if necessary, chemotherapy. The *5-year survival rate* is approximately 50% or more. Attention is given to possible metachronous manifestations of the primary tumor during oncologic follow-up.

**Table 16.5 TNM classification of regional lymph-node metastases of head and neck tumors**

| | *All head and neck tumors (except for p16-positive oropharyngeal carcinomas and nasopharyngeal carcinomas, which have a separate classification)* |
|---|---|
| **NX** | Regional lymph nodes cannot be assessed |
| **N0** | No regional lymph-node metastasis |
| **N1** | Metastasis in a single ipsilateral lymph node, ≤ 3 cm without ENE |
| **N2a** | Metastasis in a single ipsilateral lymph node, > 3–6 cm without ENE |
| **N2b** | Metastasis in multiple ipsilateral lymph nodes, none > 6 cm, without ENE |
| **N2c** | Metastasis in bilateral or contralateral lymph nodes, none > 6 cm, without ENE |
| **N3a** | Lymph-node metastasis (metastases) > 6 cm, without ENE |
| **N3b** | Metastasis in a single or multiple lymph nodes with clinical ENE |

Abbreviation: ENE, extranodal extension.
Source: Brierley et al 2017.

**Staging: Table 16.5** reviews the TNM classification system for regional lymph-node involvement by tumors of the upper aerodigestive tract.

***Treatment of the cervical lymphatics in patients with head and neck tumors:*** Most cancers of the upper aerodigestive tract have already metastasized to the cervical lymph nodes at the time of diagnosis (**Table 16.4**). It is necessary, therefore, to include the cervical lymphatics in primary treatment planning.

**Neck dissection:** In most cases, a neck dissection is performed concurrently with surgical treatment of the primary tumor. The *indication* for a neck dissection depends on the location and spread of the primary tumor and on the clinical status of the cervical lymph nodes. A *therapeutic* neck dissection is done in patients with clinically positive cervical nodes (N⁺), while an *elective* neck dissection is done in patients with clinically negative nodes (NO). The need for an elective neck dissection is dictated by the high rate of occult cervical lymph-node metastasis that is associated with many primary tumor sites (even tumors at a low T category).

- A *modified radical ("functional") neck dissection* involves the removal of all cervical lymph nodes on one side (**Fig. 16.23a**). It was developed as a modification of the radical neck dissection described below.
- A *radical neck dissection* additionally removes the sternocleidomastoid muscle, internal jugular vein, and accessory nerve, regardless of whether or not they are involved by tumor (**Fig. 16.23b**). This operation causes limitation of head and shoulder motion due to resection of the accessory nerve and sternocleidomastoid muscle. The resection of one internal jugular vein generally has no adverse sequelae owing to increased compensatory drainage by the vertebral veins, paravertebral plexus, and the internal jugular vein on the opposite side.

🖉 Because these compensatory mechanisms take time to develop, both internal jugular veins should never be resected at the same time, as the resulting acute bilateral decrease in venous outflow would lead to raised intracranial pressure (Monro–Kellie doctrine), with a high mortality.

Within a few weeks after unilateral resection of the jugular vein, the extrajugular venous channels have increased so much in capacity that the contralateral internal jugular vein can also be resected with very little risk.

- The neck dissection may be limited to selected regions (*selective neck dissection*), depending on the location and extent of the primary tumor.

**Radiotherapy:** Postoperative (adjuvant) radiotherapy may be indicated, depending on the extent of the primary tumor and of cervical lymph-node metastasis. With very extensive (inoperable) tumor growth or smaller tumors with no clinical evidence of neck metastasis, the cervical soft tissues can be treated by radiotherapy alone.

**Fig. 16.23  Neck dissection**

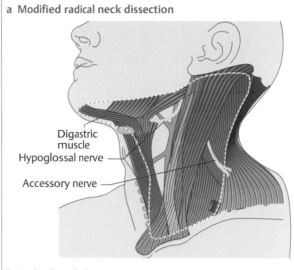

a  Modified radical neck dissection

Digastric muscle
Hypoglossal nerve
Accessory nerve

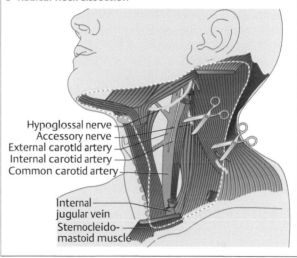

b  Radical neck dissection

Hypoglossal nerve
Accessory nerve
External carotid artery
Internal carotid artery
Common carotid artery
Internal jugular vein
Sternocleido-mastoid muscle

**a** In a modified radical neck dissection, only the cervical lymph nodes on the affected side are removed.
**b** In a radical neck dissection, the sternocleidomastoid muscle, internal jugular vein, and accessory nerve are also removed.

# 17 Larynx and Trachea

## 17.1 Embryology, Anatomy, and Physiology of the Larynx and Trachea

The complex functions of the larynx rely on the precise, coordinated interaction of the intricate anatomic structures that carry out the opposing processes of respiration and phonation. The development of the larynx (⌕ 17.1) is the basis for understanding many diseases of this organ, which in humans is endowed with the unique function of producing speech. Malfor-

mations of the larynx in particular cannot be properly understood without a knowledge of embryology.

The trachea transports the inspiratory air to the lungs and channels the expiratory air from the lungs to the mouth and nose. Although the trachea consists of metameric subdivisions, many tracheal diseases show typical sites of predilection.

### Anatomy of the Larynx

#### Cartilaginous Skeleton, Ligaments, and Muscles

The **skeleton of the larynx** (**Fig. 17.1**) is composed of the hyaline **thyroid cartilage**, **cricoid cartilage**, and **arytenoid cartilages**, as well as the fibroelastic cartilage of the **epiglottis** and the tips of the functionally insignificant accessory cartilages located above the arytenoids (the corniculate and cuneiform cartilages). In males, the thyroid cartilage forms an externally visible prominence also known as the Adam's apple. The laryngeal cartilages begin to ossify at approximately 20 years of age.

Each of the inferior horns of the thyroid cartilage articulates with the cricoid cartilage, forming the hinged **cricothyroid joint**, which permits tilting movements in the sagittal plane (**Fig. 17.2**). Each of the **arytenoid cartilages** has an anterior vocal process, which attaches to the posterior end of the corresponding vocal cord, and a posterolateral muscular process. The base of the arytenoid cartilage articulates with the superior border of the cricoid cartilage, forming a **cricoarytenoid joint** of variable shape, which permits rotation and gliding movements. The muscles that attach to the muscular process are particularly active in rotating the arytenoid cartilage about its longitudinal axis. Changing the position of the vocal cords alters the shape and size of the opening (glottis) between the two vocal folds.

### Fig. 17.1 Laryngeal cartilages

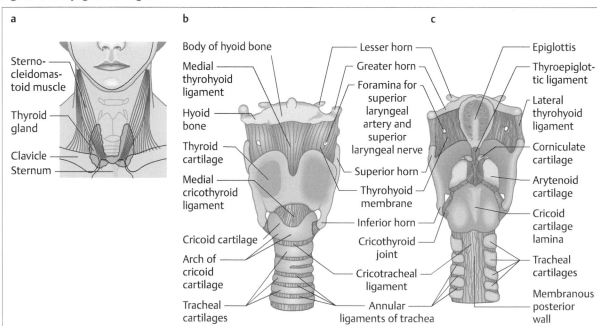

**a** Anterior view of the larynx projected onto the neck. Source: Lumley 1993.
**b,c** Anatomy of the laryngeal skeleton. Source: Tillmann 1997.

Fig. 17.2 Movements of the laryngeal joints

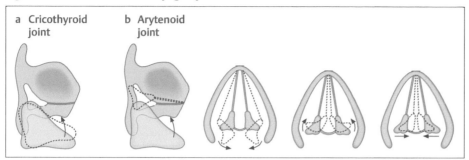

Source: Ferlito 1985.

a Cricothyroid joint  b Arytenoid joint

Fig. 17.3 Laryngeal muscles

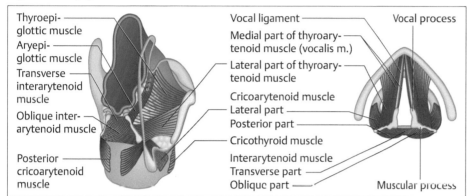

Source: Tucker 1993.

Thyroepi-glottic muscle
Aryepi-glottic muscle
Transverse interarytenoid muscle
Oblique inter-arytenoid muscle
Posterior cricoarytenoid muscle

Vocal ligament
Medial part of thyroary-tenoid muscle (vocalis m.)
Lateral part of thyroary-tenoid muscle
Cricoarytenoid muscle
Lateral part
Posterior part
Cricothyroid muscle
Interarytenoid muscle
Transverse part
Oblique part

Vocal process

Muscular process

The paired **vocal cords** (vocal folds) stretch between the vocal process of the arytenoid cartilage and the inner surface of the thyroid cartilage at the junction of its lower and middle thirds.

The stalk (petiole) of the **epiglottis** is attached to the posterior surface of the thyroid cartilage by the **thyroepiglottic ligament**, which may also contain contractile muscle fibers (thyroepiglottic muscle). The **thyrohyoid membrane** extends from the hyoid bone to the thyroid cartilage. This membrane is traversed by the superior laryngeal artery and vein and by the internal branch of the superior laryngeal nerve, which supplies sensory innervation to the mucosa lining the upper portions of the larynx. The **cricothyroid membrane** (synonym: cricothyroid ligament) connects the cricoid cartilage to the thyroid cartilage and is divided in a *cricothyrotomy* (coniotomy; see **Fig. 17.39**).

Thus, extrinsic ligaments and connective-tissue membranes serve to anchor the larynx to its surroundings, while numerous joints, ligaments, and membranes between the cartilaginous elements interact with the various muscles to ensure the coordinated functional movements of laryngeal structures. Intrinsic laryngeal muscles and one extrinsic muscle (**Table 17.1**, **Fig. 17.3**) open and close the glottis and tense the vocal cords. The muscles that close the glottic plane predominate over the single muscle that opens it (posterior cricoarytenoid muscle) by a force ratio of approximately 3:1.

As noted earlier, the larynx is the narrowest point in the upper respiratory tract, making it particularly susceptible to obstructions. The cricoid cartilage encircles the subglottis like a ring, imparting a mechanical stability that helps to prevent collapse of the laryngeal skeleton (**Table 17.2**). It also ensures that any mucosal swelling at that level will be directed toward the lumen.

This is particularly important in newborns and infants, because a circumferential swelling of the glottic and subglottic mucosa by just 1 mm can cause more than a 60% reduction in total luminal cross section.

It should also be recalled that the airway resistance in a stenotic segment is directly proportional to the length of the stenosis and inversely proportional to the fourth power of the radius (Hagen–Poiseuille law, **Fig. 17.5**).

## Nerve Supply

The larynx and the trachea derive their motor and sensory innervation from the superior laryngeal nerve and recurrent laryngeal nerve, both of which arise from the vagus nerve. The **superior laryngeal nerve** supplies motor innervation to the extrinsic laryngeal muscle (anterior cricothyroid) with its external branch, while its internal sensory branch supplies the

### 17.1 Embryology of the larynx and trachea

The epithelium of the respiratory tract (larynx, tracheobronchial system, lungs) develops as an outpouching of the ventral wall of the foregut (**laryngotracheal groove**, day 26 of gestation) and is therefore of entodermal origin. The **tracheoesophageal septum** forms during the fourth week, completely separating the primordia of the esophagus and the larynx/trachea/lung (laryngotracheal tube) from one another (**Fig. 17.4a–c**). The mesoderm that surrounds the primitive respiratory tract differentiates into cartilaginous, muscular, and connective tissue so that the entodermal respiratory tract is finally encased by mesodermal tissue. The paired **arytenoid eminences** and the unpaired **epiglottic swelling** impart a T-shaped appearance to the laryngeal inlet (**Fig. 17.4d**).

With further chondrogenesis, epithelial proliferation causes a temporary closure of the laryngeal lumen (7th–10th weeks). This is followed by recanalization of the larynx and the development of the mucosal folds (ventricular and vocal folds, starting in the 10th week; **Fig. 17.4e**).

The **hyoid bone** is derived from the second and third branchial arches, and the laryngeal cartilages except for the epiglottis, arytenoid cartilages, and accessory cartilages are derived from the fourth and sixth branchial arches. The epiglottis, arytenoid cartilages, and accessory cartilages develop secondarily from the mesenchyma ("secondary cartilage"). The cells that give rise to the laryngeal muscles migrate to the larynx from the myotomes of the cranial somites.

The associated **branchial arch nerves** are branches of the vagus nerve (fourth branchial arch: superior laryngeal nerve, sixth branchial arch: recurrent laryngeal nerve).

During embryonic and fetal life, the epiglottis is still located behind the soft palate and extends to the nasopharynx. By the time of birth, the epiglottis has already migrated caudally so that its tip is level with the axis dens. The laryngeal skeleton continues to descend with aging, after puberty reaching its definitive position at about the level of the C5 vertebral body. It is no longer believed that the larynx develops from two separate parts that fuse together during development (the buccopharyngeal and tracheobronchial buds), with separation of the supra- and subglottic lymphatic drainage systems (compartmentalization of the larynx). Nevertheless, the **lymphatic drainage of the larynx** is subdivided anatomically into supraglottic, glottic, and subglottic pathways.

**Fig. 17.4  Embryology of the larynx**

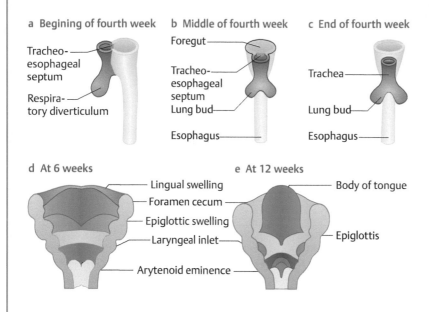

a  Begining of fourth week
Tracheo-esophageal septum
Respiratory diverticulum

b  Middle of fourth week
Foregut
Tracheo-esophageal septum
Lung bud
Esophagus

c  End of fourth week
Trachea
Lung bud
Esophagus

d  At 6 weeks
Lingual swelling
Foramen cecum
Epiglottic swelling
Laryngeal inlet
Arytenoid eminence

e  At 12 weeks
Body of tongue
Epiglottis

Source: Moore and Persaud 1996, Sadler 1998.

mucosa of the upper larynx including the glottic plane. The **recurrent laryngeal nerve** supplies sensory fibers to the laryngeal mucosa below the glottis and to the tracheal mucosa. The recurrent laryngeal nerve also supplies all the intrinsic muscles of the larynx. This means that the muscles that open and close the glottis plane receive their motor innervation from the same nerve.

The course of the recurrent laryngeal nerve differs between the left and right sides. While the larger left recurrent nerve curves around the aortic arch, the right recurrent nerve reaches or winds around the subclavian artery. On each side, the nerve then passes between the trachea and esophagus and enters the larynx behind the inferior horn of the thyroid cartilage (**Fig. 17.6**). The difference in length between the two nerves is a few centimeters. The different calibers of the nerve fibers offset this difference, enabling the impulses to reach the muscles at the same time.

### Vascular Supply

The glottic plane divides the **blood supply** to the larynx into two territories. The blood supply at the

**Table 17.1    Laryngeal muscles**

| Function | Muscle | Origin, insertion, nerve supply, function |
|---|---|---|
| Opening the glottis | Posterior cricoarytenoid muscle (a variable slip from the cricoid cartilage plate to the inferior horn of the thyroid cartilage is termed the ceratocricoid muscle) | **O:** Lamina of cricoid cartilage (posterior surface)<br>**I:** Muscular process of arytenoid cartilage<br>**N:** Recurrent laryngeal nerve<br>**F:** Rotates the arytenoid cartilage outward about a vertical axis, tilts it laterally |
| Closing the glottis | Lateral cricoarytenoid muscle (lateralis muscle) | **O:** Arch of cricoid cartilage<br>**I:** Muscular process of arytenoid cartilage<br>**N:** Recurrent laryngeal nerve<br>**F:** Rotates the arytenoid cartilage inward about a vertical axis |
| | Interarytenoid muscle (transverse and oblique interarytenoid muscles) | **O:** Arytenoid cartilage (posterior surface)<br>**I:** Contralateral arytenoid cartilage<br>**N:** Recurrent laryngeal nerve<br>**F:** Narrows the intercartilaginous part of the vocal fold by adducting the arytenoid cartilages |
| | Thyroarytenoid muscle, lateral part | **O:** Thyroid cartilage (inner surface, laterally adjacent to the vocalis muscle)<br>**I:** Arytenoid cartilage<br>**N:** Recurrent laryngeal nerve<br>**F:** Rotates the arytenoid cartilage inward about a vertical axis |
| Tightening the vocal cords | Cricothyroid muscle | **O:** Arch of cricoid cartilage (outer surface)<br>**I:** Thyroid cartilage<br>**N:** External branch of superior laryngeal nerve<br>**F:** Tilts the cricoid cartilage relative to the thyroid cartilage on a transverse axis |
| | Thyroarytenoid muscle, medial part (vocalis muscle) | **O:** Thyroid cartilage (inner surface)<br>**I:** Vocal process and oblong fovea of arytenoid cartilage<br>**N:** Recurrent laryngeal nerve<br>**F:** Controls the tension on the vocal fold by isometric contraction |

supraglottic and glottic levels is derived from the superior laryngeal artery arising from the external carotid, while the subglottic areas are supplied by the inferior laryngeal artery arising from the subclavian artery and thyrocervical trunk.

**Venous drainage** of the larynx is handled by the superior thyroid vein, which drains into the internal jugular vein, and by the inferior thyroid vein, which drains into the brachiocephalic vein (**Fig. 17.7**).

Except for the glottic region, the **lymphatic vessels** in the larynx are well developed and are more numerous above the glottis than below (see above). The very dense lymphatic capillary network of the supraglottis drains into the vertical cervical lymphatic chains (deep cervical lymph nodes) and especially into the lymph nodes at the junction of the facial and internal jugular veins (junctional nodes). The ipsilateral lymphatic

drainage is complemented by significant contralateral drainage, with the result that even strictly unilateral supraglottic malignancies are very likely to show bilateral lymphogenous metastasis. The prelaryngeal lymph nodes are referred to as "Delphian lymph nodes" ("oracle of the larynx," see also **Fig. 17.7**) owing to their special prognostic significance in patients with laryngeal cancer. Lymphatic capillaries are sparse in the area of the vocal cords, explaining the low potential of glottic malignancies for lymphogenous metastasis. The glottic lymphatic vessels mainly drain cephalad into the supraglottic lymphatic capillary network. The mechanical stresses on the vocal cords normally prevent an exchange of lymph between the supraglottis and subglottis, despite the presence of delicate lymphatic connections between both regions. As soon as the mobility of a vocal cord has been impaired by carcinoma

Table 17.2   Changes in the cricoid cartilage diameter with aging

| Age | Smallest intraluminal diameter (mm) |
| --- | --- |
| 0–3 mo | 3.5 |
| 3–9 mo | 4.0 |
| 9–24 mo | 4.5 |
| 2–4 y | 5.0 |
| 4–6 y | 5.5 |
| 6–8 y | 6.0 |
| 8–9 y | 6.5 |
| 9–12 y | 7.0 |
| Adult women | 7–8 |
| Adult men | 8–9 |

Source: Mostafa 1976.

growth, the risk of lymphogenic metastasis increases due to the absence of a mechanical barrier.

The lymphatic vascular network of the subglottis is less dense than that of the supraglottis (**Fig. 17.8**). The subglottic lymphatic channels also drain into the vertical cervical lymphatic chains in principle, but there are additional, prognostically important connections with the peritracheal and mediastinal nodes. Ipsilateral and contralateral lymphogenous metastasis can occur even with subglottic malignancies.

### Epithelial Lining

Like the trachea, most of the endolarynx is lined by **respiratory epithelium**—a stratified ciliated epithelium with interspersed goblet cells. A stratified, nonkeratinized and sometimes keratinized **squamous**

Fig. 17.5   Swelling of the subglottic mucosa

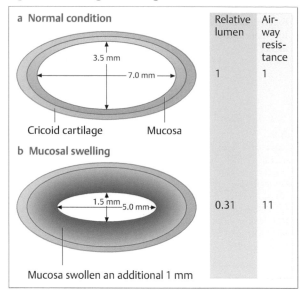

Effect of subglottic mucosal swelling in a newborn on luminal size and airway resistance.

**epithelium** is found with great regularity in the laryngeal epiglottis, ventricular folds, and vocal cords and occasionally in other areas of the larynx. The presence of this squamous epithelium and its expansion with aging are often interpreted as responses to increased mechanical stresses.

### Vocal Cord Histology

The histologic structure of the vocal cord is shown in **Fig. 17.9**. **Reinke's space** is a subepithelial plane in the

Fig. 17.6   Nerve supply to the larynx

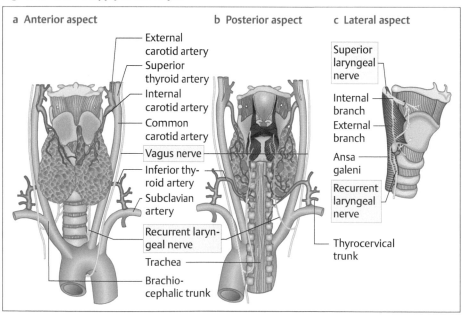

Source: **a, b** Cévese et al 1988; **c** Tucker 1993.

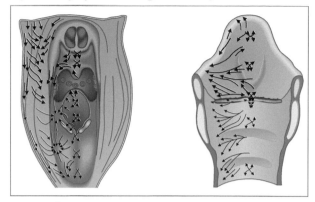

## Fig. 17.7 Blood supply to the larynx

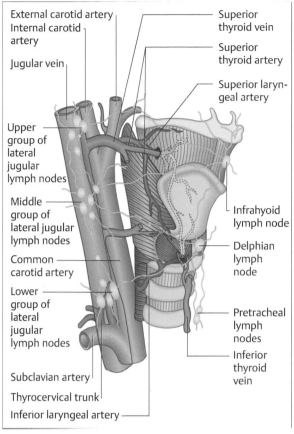

External carotid artery
Internal carotid artery
Jugular vein
Upper group of lateral jugular lymph nodes
Middle group of lateral jugular lymph nodes
Common carotid artery
Lower group of lateral jugular lymph nodes
Subclavian artery
Thyrocervical trunk
Inferior laryngeal artery

Superior thyroid vein
Superior thyroid artery
Superior laryngeal artery
Infrahyoid lymph node
Delphian lymph node
Pretracheal lymph nodes
Inferior thyroid vein

Source: Tucker 1993.

vocal cord that contains no glands or lymphatic capillaries.

## Relations of the Larynx

The larynx is bounded cranially by the free margins of the epiglottis, the aryepiglottic fold, and the interarytenoid eminence. Caudally, the inferior border of the cricoid cartilage marks the junction of the larynx with the trachea. The larynx forms the narrowest point in

## Fig. 17.8 Lymphatic drainage of the larynx

Source: Tillmann 1997.

the respiratory tract between the nasopharynx and trachea.

The laryngeal cavity is divided into three parts in relation to the glottis (**Fig. 17.10**):
- **Supraglottis:** laryngeal inlet to the sinus of Morgagni.
- **Glottis:** plane of the vocal cords plus approximately 1 cm of their subglottic flank.
- **Subglottis:** extending to the lower border of the cricoid cartilage.

📖 The vocal cord consists of the vocal ligament, vocalis muscle, and associated mucosal cover.

The glottis (rima glottidis) is the opening between the vocal cords. It has a membranous part backed by the vocal ligament and a cartilaginous part formed by the vocal process of the arytenoid cartilage. The transglottic space occupies the region from the ventricular folds, or false vocal cords, to the glottis (see **Fig. 17.10**).

## Physiology of the Larynx

The larynx serves as the **organ of phonation** (vocal cords closed = phonation position) and as an **airway**

## Fig. 17.9 Microanatomy of the vocal cord

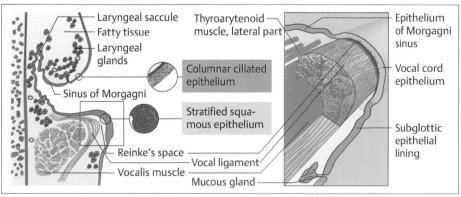

Laryngeal saccule
Fatty tissue
Laryngeal glands
Sinus of Morgagni
Columnar ciliated epithelium
Stratified squamous epithelium
Reinke's space
Vocalis muscle
Vocal ligament
Mucous gland
Thyroarytenoid muscle, lateral part
Epithelium of Morgagni sinus
Vocal cord epithelium
Subglottic epithelial lining

Source: Sternberg 1997, Becker et al 1989.

**Fig. 17.10    Topographic anatomy of the larynx**

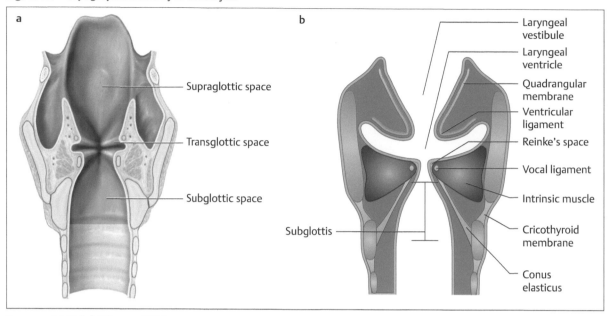

Source: **a** M. Voll; **b** Tillmann 1997.

(vocal cords open = respiratory position). It keeps the foodway and airway separate during food ingestion.

## Protective Mechanisms

The most important protective mechanism is the immediate and complete **reflex closure of the vocal cords** in response to the pharyngeal phase of swallowing (see also **Fig. 5.4**). Simultaneous contraction of the suprahyoid and infrahyoid muscles elevates the entire laryngeal skeleton by 2 to 3 cm, while the base of the tongue bulges over the larynx and presses the epiglottis downward, directing the food bolus past and behind the larynx to the esophageal inlet. The epiglottis itself has no essential importance either in closing off the larynx or in preventing aspiration. If food material does transgress the glottic plane, the **cough reflex** activates another important mechanism that protects the lower airways. After a deep reflex inspiration, the glottis closes tightly, allowing a rise in intrathoracic pressure. The glottis then opens widely and rapidly to allow forceful expulsion of the aspirated material.

🗲 Manipulations within the larynx (e.g., intubation) can stimulate vagovagal reflex pathways that may incite a cardiac arrhythmia, bradycardia, or even cardiac arrest.

## Anatomy of the Trachea

The trachea is suspended from the cricoid cartilage—the narrowest stiff-walled element in the upper respiratory tract—by the **cricotracheal ligament**.

In many cases, however, the upper ring of the trachea is also fused to the cricoid cartilage. The trachea has a length of 10 to 13 cm in adults, extending from the level of the C6–C7 vertebral body to the T4–T5 vertebra, replicating the curvature of the spine and bifurcating at the T4–T5 level into the right and left main bronchi (**Fig. 17.11**). The trachea is very superficial in its upper portion, but as it descends it passes behind the sternum to a depth of 4 to 5 cm. In other important relations, the anterior and posterior walls of the trachea are closely related to the isthmus and lobes of the thyroid gland and to the recurrent laryngeal nerves.

The lumen of the trachea is maintained by 12 to 20 hyaline cartilage "rings" that are horseshoe-shaped (open posteriorly) and are interconnected by strong collagenous and elastic connective-tissue fibers, the **annular ligaments**. The cervical part of the trachea is 6 to 7 cm long and contains six to eight cartilaginous rings. The **membranous posterior wall** of the trachea is related to the anterior wall of the esophagus (**Fig. 17.11b**). Foreign bodies and tumors of the esophagus may impinge upon the posterior surface of the trachea, constricting the airway lumen.

The transverse diameter of the trachea averages 13 to 20 mm (13–16 mm in women, 16–20 mm in men).

The trachea is lined by two rows of **ciliated epithelium** with goblet cells. The mucociliary clearance mechanism in the trachea is directed toward the larynx and contributes to the cleaning, warming, and humidification of the inspired air.

The **blood supply** to the trachea is provided mainly by the inferior thyroid artery (from the thyrocervical trunk) and to a lesser degree by the superior thyroid

**Fig. 17.11** Anatomy of the trachea

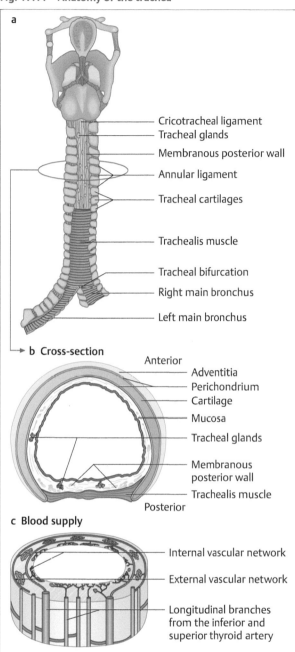

a

Cricotracheal ligament
Tracheal glands
Membranous posterior wall
Annular ligament
Tracheal cartilages

Trachealis muscle

Tracheal bifurcation
Right main bronchus

Left main bronchus

**b Cross-section**

Anterior
Adventitia
Perichondrium
Cartilage
Mucosa
Tracheal glands

Membranous
posterior wall
Trachealis muscle
Posterior

**c Blood supply**

Internal vascular network

External vascular network

Longitudinal branches
from the inferior and
superior thyroid artery

For anterior aspect, see also **Fig. 17.1**.
Source: Tillmann 1997.

artery (see also **Fig. 17.11c**). As in the subglottic region, the **lymphatic drainage** of the trachea is handled by the vertical lymphatic chain in the neck (deep cervical lymph nodes) and by the paratracheal and mediastinal groups of lymph nodes.

The trachea receives its **nerve supply** from the vagus nerve and sympathetic trunk.

# 17.2   Symptomatology and Examination of the Larynx and Trachea

The cardinal symptoms of laryngeal disorders are based on the functions of the larynx as the "mediator" between the airway and foodway and as the organ of phonation. Besides indirect examination with a mirror or endoscope, which yields both morphologic and functional information, diseases of the larynx can be investigated by sectional imaging modalities and function tests (e.g., electromyography).

## Cardinal Symptoms

### Larynx

The main symptoms of laryngeal disorders are inspiratory stridor, dyspnea, phonation problems (e.g., hoarseness), and eating difficulties. These symptoms may occur separately or in combination.

### Trachea

The cardinal symptoms of diseases involving the trachea are **inspiratory stridor**, **cough**, **sputum production**, and **respiratory distress** due to narrowing of the tracheal lumen.

Tracheal stenosis—whether due to inflammation, scarring, or neoplasia—is commonly manifested by an **inspiratory stridor**. When the history is taken, the patient should be questioned about blood in the sputum, exercise-dependence or position-dependence of respiratory problems, exposure to potentially harmful inhalants, and any concomitant diseases of the upper aerodigestive tract.

## Methods of Examination

### Larynx: Inspection and Palpation

**Inspection** of the neck provides initial information on the configuration of the larynx and possible inspiratory jugular retraction due to laryngotracheal obstruction. Also, the mobility of the larynx should be observed during swallowing to exclude inflammatory or neoplastic fixation and any extrinsic mass effects on the laryngeal skeleton (e.g., from tumors in the neck). Bimanual **palpation** of the laryngeal skeleton is done from the front or from behind to check for contour irregularities and sites of tenderness. It may include the thyroid gland, and the cervical soft tissues should be palpated if malignancy is suspected.

## Indirect Laryngoscopy

Indirect examination of the larynx can be performed with a laryngeal mirror or with a rigid or flexible endoscope.

**Classic indirect laryngoscopy** requires a laryngeal mirror of suitable size, a light source, a head mirror, and a gauze sponge (**Fig. 17.12a**). Normally, the examination is done with the patient sitting upright, after any dentures have been removed.

The (right-handed) examiner grasps the protruded tongue with a gauze sponge in the left hand, placing the thumb on top of the tongue and the middle finger under the tongue.

🖉 When the tongue is pulled forward, care is taken not to injure the frenulum on the lower incisors.

The index finger of the left hand is braced on the upper teeth and is used to retract the upper lip. The light from the head mirror is directed toward the uvula.

The reflective surface of the laryngeal mirror should be gently warmed with the hand or wetted with alcohol solution to prevent fogging by the patient's breath and body heat. The examiner holds the laryngeal mirror in the right hand like a pencil and advances it beneath the palate to the uvula. Touching the base of the tongue or the posterior wall of the pharynx may evoke a gag reflex. The uvula is now lifted on the back surface of the mirror, which is angled approximately 45 degrees, and gently pushed backward and upward so that the larynx can be brought into view (**Fig. 17.12a, b**).

The larynx should always be examined in the respiratory position (tell the patient to take a deep breath) and in the phonatory position (have the patient say "Hee") to assess laryngeal function (**Fig. 17.12c, d**). Besides the larynx, the examiner can evaluate the base of the tongue, the oropharynx and hypopharynx, and even the anterior wall of the cervical trachea by viewing through the open glottis in the respiratory position.

The posterior portions of the larynx (the posterior commissure and subglottic space) are best examined with the examiner sitting and the patient standing

**Fig. 17.12  Indirect laryngoscopy**

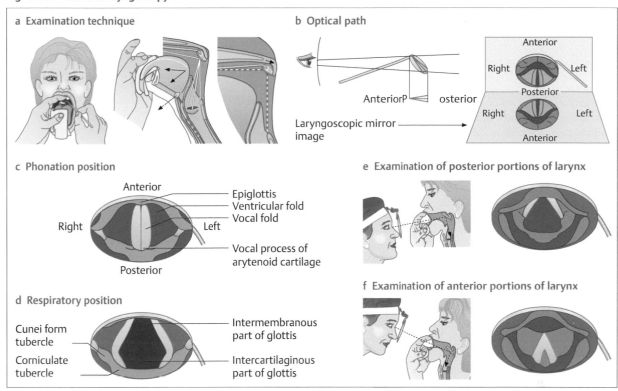

a Examination technique

b Optical path

Anterior
Right   Left
Posterior
Laryngoscopic mirror image
Right   Left
Anterior
AnteriorP osterior

c Phonation position

Anterior
Epiglottis
Ventricular fold
Vocal fold
Right   Left
Vocal process of arytenoid cartilage
Posterior

e Examination of posterior portions of larynx

f Examination of anterior portions of larynx

d Respiratory position

Cunei form tubercle
Corniculate tubercle
Intermembranous part of glottis
Intercartilaginous part of glottis

Source: **a** Birnmeyer 1987, Dedo 1990; **c–f** Tillmann 1997.

with the head tilted forward (**Fig. 17.12e**). The anterior portions of the larynx (the laryngeal epiglottic surface, petiole, and anterior commissure) are best examined with the examiner standing and the patient sitting with the head tilted backward (**Fig. 17.12f**).

 Keep in mind that this examination provides an inverted "mirror image" of the larynx (see **Fig. 17.12b**).

In recent years, routine mirror examination of the larynx has been increasingly superseded by **telescopic laryngoscopy** using a rigid endoscope with a 90-degree wide-angle view that can brightly illuminate and also magnify the area being examined (**Fig. 17.13a**). The telescopic examination is performed in the same way as the mirror examination and yields the same findings, except that the examined areas are not inverted but are displayed in their natural position (**Fig. 17.13b,c**). This true orientation, plus the option for magnification, also makes it easier to perform biopsies and tissue ablation in the conscious patient.
**Flexible endoscopy** (**Fig. 17.14**): In a small number of patients, the larynx cannot be inspected by mirror or telescopic laryngoscopy due to a powerful gag reflex, despite the use of topical anesthesia. The laryngeal structures can be inspected in these patients by using a flexible nasopharyngeal laryngoscope. Another indi-

cation for flexible laryngeal endoscopy, in which the endoscope is passed through the nose into the nasopharynx and then down the oropharynx into the larynx, exists in cases where it is necessary to combine laryngeal inspection with tracheobronchoscopy. The flexible endoscopes used for this purpose have an outer diameter of 2.7 to 6.0 mm but deliver poorer image quality than the rigid telescopes described above. **FEES** (flexible endoscopic evaluation of swallowing) is used for real-time examination of the act of swallowing.

### Direct Laryngoscopy

Direct laryngoscopy, which provides a direct view into the larynx, is most commonly performed under general anesthesia, using either intubation anesthesia or injector ventilation without an endotracheal tube. With the head fully extended, an illuminated rigid tube (laryngoscope) is advanced straight through the mouth to the plane of the larynx (**Fig. 17.15**). The laryngoscope may be held in place by a lever arm supported on the patient's chest or a tray suspended above the patient's chest ("suspension laryngoscopy" or "suspension autoscopy"). Direct laryngoscopy is usually done as a microscope-assisted procedure (microlaryngoscopy or microlaryngoendoscopy, MLE), permitting the detailed scrutiny of laryngeal abnormalities. Other

**Fig. 17.13 Rigid telescopic laryngoscopy**

a Examination technique

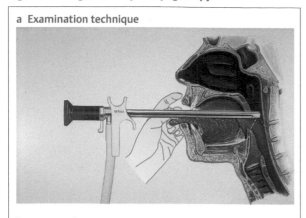

b View in phonation position

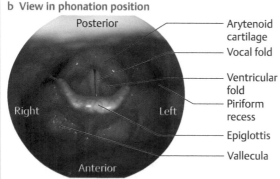

Posterior

Arytenoid cartilage

Vocal fold

Ventricular fold

Piriform recess

Epiglottis

Vallecula

Right

Left

Anterior

c View in respiratory position

Piriform recess

Arytenoid cartilage

Vocal fold

Ventricular fold

Tracheal anterior wall

Epiglottis

Posterior

Right

Left

Anterior

The 90-degree telescope is equipped with an insufflation channel and focusable magnifying lenses. The light source is a halogen or xenon lamp with a fiberoptic cable.
Source: **a** Richard Wolf, Knittlingen, Germany.

instruments such as laser delivery systems (**Fig. 17.15b**) can also be used for many therapeutic applications.

## Imaging of the Larynx and Trachea

Plain radiographs are no longer in use for visualization of laryngeal pathology. **Computed tomography** is the examination of first choice in laryngeal pathology, as magnetic resonance imaging (MRI) needs longer acquisition time with the consequence of motion artifacts.
**Ultrasonography** can be used to evaluate prelaryngeal and paralaryngeal soft tissues and determine whether intralaryngeal masses have eroded through the laryngeal skeleton and spread contiguously to extralaryngeal structures. Given the physical principles of sound propagation ("air is the enemy of ultrasound"), intralaryngeal structures cannot be clearly visualized. The same applies to ultrasound evaluation of the trachea.

### Function Tests

**Electromyography** of the laryngeal muscles is described in ✍17.9. **Phoniatric studies** (stroboscopy, frequency/intensity profile) are covered in ✍18.1.

### Methods of Examining the Trachea

During **inspection**, attention is first given to any cervical masses and their relationship to the trachea and respiratory excursions. The trachea is palpated with the head flexed forward (to relax the airway), and tracheal mobility is assessed in relation to the surrounding structures. Because diseases of the thyroid gland may directly affect the upper respiratory tract (dyspnea caused by a hemorrhagic cyst of the thyroid gland, tracheomalacia due to thyroid enlargement, vocal cord paralysis due to a malignancy), the thyroid gland should also be palpated.

The upper part of the trachea can often be viewed through the glottis during **indirect laryngoscopy**. But in cases where tracheal pathology is strongly suspected, endoscopic inspection of the entire trachea is essential for definitive confirmation. Both flexible and rigid optical systems are available for this purpose.

**Flexible tracheo(broncho)scopy** can, in principle, be performed under topical anesthesia in the conscious patient. The endoscope (2.7–6.0 mm outer diameter) is introduced transnasally or transorally and advanced through the glottis into the trachea (**Fig. 17.14**). This technique not only permits a detailed evaluation of the trachea, but—if necessary—the entire bronchial tree can be inspected out to the level of the subsegmental bronchi. Flexible endoscopes with a working channel and suction-irrigation system can be used for diagnostic procedures (specimen retrieval) and also for therapeutic manipulations (fiberoptic intubation, foreign-body extraction even in the peripheral bronchial tree, stent insertion, laser tumor ablation).

Endoscopic examination of the trachea with rigid, illuminated systems (**rigid tracheobronchoscopy**) is generally performed under general anesthesia, and ventilators can be adapted for this purpose. With the patient's neck fully extended, the endoscope barrel is advanced through the larynx into the trachea. The limited view of peripheral portions of the bronchial system can be somewhat improved by using an oblique scope. Either a flexible or rigid system can be used for foreign-body removal in the tracheobronchial

**Fig. 17.14    Flexible nasopharyngeal laryngoscopy**

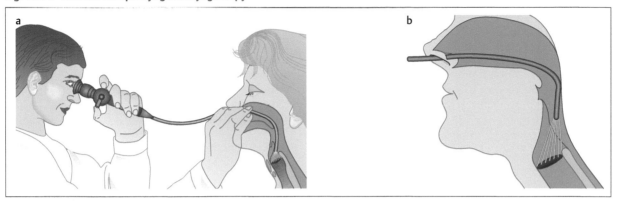

Source: Dedo 1990.

system, depending on the nature, configuration, and location of the foreign body. More extensive manipulations in the tracheobronchial system that require a clear view, due particularly to an increased risk of bleeding, are still within the domain of rigid endoscopy.

**Plain radiographs** of the upper airways in the posteroanterior (PA) and lateral projections can demonstrate the tracheal air column along with any intraluminal lesions or masses that are causing extrinsic tracheal compression. One PA radiograph taken after forced inspiration and another taken during a subsequent **Valsalva maneuver** will show evidence of any abnormal weak spots in the tracheal wall (tracheomalacia). Today, **computed tomography** is the method of first choice in evaluating tracheomalacia. The functional impact of stenotic lesions of the larynx and trachea can be objectively evaluated by **pulmonary function testing** and **body plethysmography** (details can be found in textbooks of internal medicine).

**Fig. 17.15    Microlaryngoendoscopy**

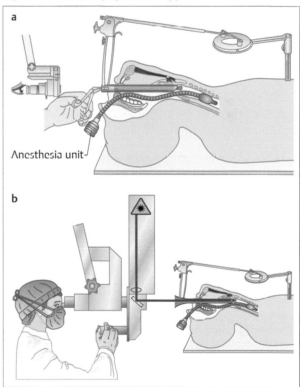

The capabilities of direct laryngoscopy (**a**) can be expanded by using a $CO_2$ laser with a micromanipulator (**b**). This allows for precise tissue resection under microscopic control.

# 17.3 Malformations of the Larynx and Trachea

Laryngeal anomalies have a reported incidence of 1 in 10,000 to 1 in 50,000 newborns. The severity of the malformations ranges from the extremely rare and almost always fatal laryngeal atresia to the very common and usually harmless laryngomalacia. Besides the cardinal symptoms of *inspiratory stridor* and *dyspnea*, other possible features are *dysphonia* and *dysphagia*. The anomalies may be manifested at the supraglottic, glottic, or subglottic level.

As a rule, the clinical suspicion of a laryngeal malformation can be confirmed only by endoscopic examination.

## Malformations of the Larynx

### Laryngomalacia

*Epidemiology:* Laryngomalacia is the most frequent cause of congenital stridor, accounting for 60 to 75% of cases.

*Etiopathogenesis:* The supraglottic structures (epiglottis, arytenoid cartilages) in particular are abnormally soft and pliable, causing them to collapse inward during inspiration. Neurologic abnormalities and infectious processes may also have causal significance.

*Symptoms:* Typically, a low-pitched inspiratory stridor is audible from birth. It may be constant or intermittent and may change with the position of the child, becoming louder in the supine position and quieter in the prone position. Life-threatening airway compromise is extremely rare, but feeding difficulties are occasionally seen.

*Diagnosis:* Laryngoscopy is helpful in making the diagnosis. In typical cases of laryngomalacia, the aryepiglottic folds are shortened and the arytenoid cartilages are bowed anteriorly and toward each other. Another typical finding is a soft, pale, "omega-shaped" epiglottis with its lateral edges curled inward. In extreme cases, the epiglottis completely covers the laryngeal inlet.

*Differential diagnosis:* Rare cleft anomalies of the larynx are distinguished from laryngomalacia by the additional presence of dysphagia with recurrent episodes of aspiration. Other causes of stridor such as congenital cysts and laryngoceles can be excluded by laryngoscopy.

*Treatment:* The stridor should resolve without treatment during the first 2 years of life as the laryngeal skeleton becomes more rigid. Very rare cases may require a temporary tracheotomy, however. It is particularly important to explain the condition to the anxious parents and reassure them that it is usually harmless.

---

### 🔎 17.2 Congenital laryngeal cysts and laryngoceles

**Congenital laryngeal cysts** (saccular cysts) may develop on the laryngeal side of the epiglottis or at the subglottic level. It is particularly common to find cystic dilatations of the ventricular fold and aryepiglottic fold. These intralaryngeal cysts are variously attributed to an appendicular constriction of the laryngeal ventricle or the presence of isolated epithelial rests. They contain mucus and are consistently lined with ciliated, columnar, or squamous epithelium. Sufficiently large cysts can produce the clinical picture of congenital stridor, which may be associated with dyspnea, hoarseness, and occasional dysphagia. Generally, the cysts are removed during microlaryngoscopy without opening the cervical soft tissues.

**Laryngoceles (Fig. 17.16)** are an extremely rare cause of airway obstruction in infants and small children. But if the ventricular fold is displaced medially by a hernialike outpouching of the laryngeal ventricle (*internal laryngocele*), it may cause obstruction of the laryngeal inlet.

In most cases, however, the laryngocele extends past the superior border of the thyroid cartilage and protrudes through the thyrohyoid membrane. Often, this *external laryngocele* is not detected until adolescence or adulthood, presenting as a soft, lateral neck mass that distends with air in response to a Valsalva maneuver and is deflated by external pressure, producing a gurgling sound. This condition is common in players of wind instruments. Surgical treatment is rarely necessary in infants but may be appropriate in adults.

**Fig. 17.16 Internal and external laryngoceles**

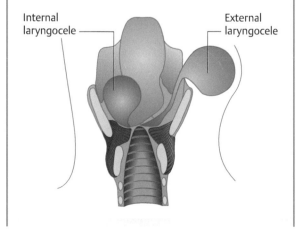

Internal laryngocele — External laryngocele

**Fig. 17.17  Types of tracheoesophageal malformation**

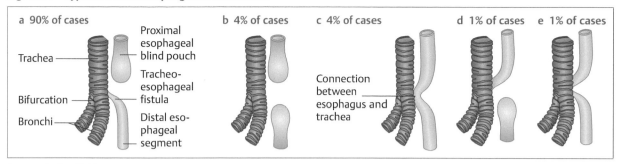

a  90% of cases

Trachea

Bifurcation

Bronchi

Proximal esophageal blind pouch

Tracheo-esophageal fistula

Distal eso-phageal segment

b  4% of cases

c  4% of cases

Connection between esophagus and trachea

d  1% of cases   e  1% of cases

Source: Sadler 1998.

## Congenital Laryngeal Web and Glottic Atresia

Perhaps the best-known laryngeal anomaly, if not the most common, is the **laryngeal web** or glottic web.

*Etiopathogenesis:* This membranelike stenosis of the glottic plane results from incomplete recanalization of the glottic lumen during embryogenesis (see $\wp$ **17.1**). If there is a complete failure of recanalization, the result is glottic atresia.

*Symptoms:* The main symptoms are inspiratory stridor, which is present at rest only with a large web, and a breathy, aphonic voice. In most cases, the web is not diagnosed in infancy but is discovered later when the patient is intubated for general anesthesia or during a routine examination of the larynx (**Fig. 17.18**). A child with glottic atresia is cyanotic at birth and makes scant, ineffectual breathing movements with no respiratory sounds. Only an immediate, emergency tracheotomy can save the life of a newborn with this rare anomaly. In exceptional cases, laryngeal atresia coexists with a tracheoesophageal fistula that permits adequate respiration.

*Diagnosis:* The web is usually visible at laryngoscopy, stretching across the anterior commissure and leaving a residual posterior glottic airway sufficient for respiration.

*Treatment:* In most cases, the web can be endoscopically divided during microlaryngoscopy, although there is a risk of recurrent synechia formation in the anterior commissure. To prevent this, it is occasionally necessary to place a temporary stent (keel) between the vocal folds through an extra-laryngeal approach. In some cases of glottic atresia, performing an EXIT procedure may be indicated.

## Congenital Subglottic Stenosis

*Epidemiology:* Congenital subglottic stenosis is the most common stenosing anomaly of the larynx and,

**Fig. 17.18  Laryngeal web**

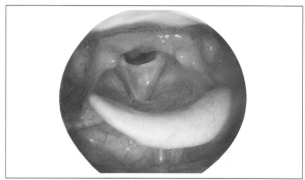

after laryngomalacia, is the second most frequent cause of congenital stridor.

*Etiopathogenesis:* Considered an incomplete form of subglottic atresia, this anomaly usually presents as a ring-shaped narrowing of the larynx approximately 2 to 3 mm below the glottic plane. A **soft stenosis**, composed of thickened fibrous tissue, is distinguished from a **hard stenosis** caused by malformation of the cricoid cartilage.

*Symptoms:* The inspiratory stridor of congenital subglottic stenosis is unaffected by position ("fixed" stridor) and is variable in its degree, depending on the size of the residual lumen. An upper respiratory infection can cause additional mucosal swelling that exacerbates the symptoms.

*Diagnosis:* Laryngoscopy demonstrates narrowing of the laryngeal lumen below the glottic plane.

*Treatment:* The first step after endoscopic confirmation is to establish a secure airway. Although congenital subglottic stenosis tends to resolve as the child grows, the classic wait-and-see approach with a temporary tracheotomy is being superseded more and more by a surgical procedure to enlarge the larynx, which can also be done in infants and small children.

**Table 17.3    Malformations of the trachea**

| Condition | Symptoms and findings | Treatment |
|---|---|---|
| Tracheal agenesis or atresia | Ineffectual breathing efforts by the newborn with no lung ventilation; if a tracheoesophageal fistula is also present, limited ventilation may occur | Generally untreatable; if possible, EXIT procedure |
| Tracheal web | Stridor, depending on the degree of airway obstruction; discrete luminal narrowing by fibrous tissue | Tracheal expansion by perforation and bougie dilation |
| Congenital tracheal stenosis | Stridor, depending on the degree of airway obstruction; luminal narrowing involves a longer segment and deeper layers of the trachea | Bougie dilation is often unsuccessful; patient may require a temporary tracheotomy and resection of the stenotic segment |
| Stenosis with or without a tracheoesophageal fistula (**Fig. 17.17**) | Stridor, depending on the degree of luminal narrowing; airway obstruction during feeding, with cyanosis and signs of aspiration; open connection between the tracheal lumen and esophagus | Surgical correction immediately after birth |
| Tracheomalacia (occurs independently of laryngomalacia) | Biphasic stridor due to luminal narrowing; difficulty in coughing up secretions | Usually self-limiting as the tracheal framework becomes more stable at age 12–18 months; conservative measures may include humidifying the inspired air |
| Tracheal deformities in the setting of vascular malformations | Compression of the trachea by anomalies of the aortic arch or its major branches, causing airway obstruction; concurrent compression of the esophagus leads to dysphagia | Need for surgical intervention depends on the severity of symptoms |
| Malformations of individual tracheal cartilages | Circumscribed narrowing of the trachea, especially on expiration, due to partial absence of supporting structures; expiratory stridor | Conservative, expectant approach; some cases may require a temporary tracheotomy and/or reconstruction |
| Tracheal cysts and tracheoceles | Outpouchings of the tracheal wall; symptoms depend on the degree of luminal narrowing | Surgical excision may be required |

## Neurogenic Disorders: Congenital Vocal Cord Paralysis

*Etiopathogenesis:* Congenital vocal cord paralysis caused by a lesion of the vagus nerve or its laryngeal branches may be unilateral or bilateral. The causes of vocal cord paralysis include diseases of the brain, myelomeningoceles with or without hydrocephalus, Arnold–Chiari syndrome, obstetric head trauma, mediastinal tumors, anomalies of the heart and great vessels (Ortner's syndrome), and anomalies of the lung and esophagus. Hereditary bilateral recurrent laryngeal nerve palsy has also been described. In many cases, however, a specific cause cannot be identified for the neural impairment of laryngeal function (idiopathic recurrent laryngeal nerve palsy).

*Symptoms:* A weak cry in a normally breathing infant is the hallmark of a unilateral recurrent nerve palsy that does not require treatment. The cardinal symptom of bilateral congenital vocal cord paralysis is respiratory distress with inspiratory stridor and cyanosis. Swallowing may also be impaired due to loss of pharyngeal sensation (superior laryngeal nerve).

*Diagnosis and differential diagnosis:* Laryngoscopy reveals unilateral or bilateral vocal cord fixation. If both vocal cords are immobile, the differential diagnosis should include congenital ankylosis of the cricoarytenoid joints. The two conditions can be differentiated by electromyographic testing of the vocalis muscle.

*Treatment:* In cases with bilateral paralysis, the airway can be secured by tracheotomy or by early latero-fixation of one vocal cord, depending on the symptoms and cause.

## Laryngeal Subglottic Hemangioma

*Occurrence:* Cutaneous hemangiomas are a common finding and are often associated with similar lesions in other organs. Hemangiomas are occasionally observed in the subglottic space of newborns. Many cases become symptomatic during the first months of life as the hemangioma enlarges.

***Etiopathogenesis:*** Hemangiomas are growing vascular lesions (ectasias) that belong to the category of hamartomas (= dysontogenetic growth of normally formed tissue).

***Symptoms:*** When luminal narrowing is present, the symptoms may resemble those of congenital subglottic stenosis: respiratory distress and inspiratory stridor. Typically, the stridor increases during crying due to increased engorgement of the lesion with blood. Hoarseness is not a typical feature.

***Treatment:*** The fact that these vascular neoplasms may regress and disappear spontaneously during the first 2 to 4 years of life justifies an initial wait-and-see period, during which local and systemic corticosteroids may be administered. Involution of hemangioma may be induced by the systemic administration of beta blockers such as propranolol. Depending on the size of the lesion, it may be possible to remove the hemangioma with the $CO_2$ laser and avoid tracheotomy. If the lesions do not regress spontaneously during the first years of life, they should be surgically removed.

## Malformations of the Trachea

The *symptoms* of tracheal malformations that develop starting in weeks 4 to 6 of embryonic development are similar to the clinical manifestations of laryngeal anomalies: airway obstruction with **inspiratory stridor**, wheezing, cyanosis, and gasping for breath. The voice is unchanged, however. Most tracheal malformations are accompanied by anomalies of the esophagus, the most common being a tracheoesophageal fistula. Isolated tracheal malformations are rare and usually involve the cervical part of the trachea. These very rare disorders are listed in **Table 17.3** and **Table 17.4**.

***Diagnosis:*** As with laryngeal anomalies, endoscopic examination is of key importance. Certain clinical problems may additionally require radiographic contrast examination of the esophagus and/or bronchial system (e.g., for a suspected tracheoesophageal fistula) or angiography (for suspected vascular malformations).

**Table 17.4  Clinical classification of laryngotracheal malformations**

*Laryngotracheal malformations can be classified as follows based on clinical criteria:*

- Malformations that are (largely) incompatible with life:
  - Aplasia
  - Atresia
- Malformations that cause respiratory impairment (congenital stridor):
  - Laryngomalacia, tracheomalacia
  - Webs, stenosis
  - Congenital recurrent laryngeal nerve palsy
  - Laryngoceles, tracheoceles, cysts
  - Subglottic hemangiomas
  - Cartilaginous anomalies
  - Malformations of the major vessels with tracheolaryngeal compromise
- Malformations that cause dysphagia and respiratory impairment:
  - Cleft anomalies
  - Tracheoesophageal fistulas
- Malformations that have no clinical significance:
  - Epiglottic malformations

Source: Schultz-Coulon 1984.

# 17.4 Infectious Diseases of the Larynx and Trachea in Children

**Airway infections are the most frequent cause of illness and death in infants and children.**
**The airway dimensions in the pediatric upper respiratory tract are small, and even a slight obstruction can lead to critical luminal narrowing (see Fig. 17.5). From 1 to 3 years of age, children come into increasing** contact with a multitude of viruses and bacteria, and various portions of the upper and middle respiratory tracts may be affected. Initial challenges from these organisms often incite much more pronounced disease manifestations than subsequent infections that are acquired in later childhood.

## Diseases Associated with Croup Symptoms

Croup syndrome refers to the inspiratory stridor that is caused by inflammatory laryngeal or subglottic stenosis. It is usually associated with respiratory distress, cough, and hoarseness. A croup syndrome may be caused by various diseases that have different prognostic implications. **True croup** is the term applied to specific laryngitis in the setting of diphtheria. **Pseudocroup** is a collective term for viral, bacterial, and spastic forms of subglottic laryngitis. These entities should be strictly distinguished from acute (usually bacterial) epiglottitis, although the latter is associated with crouplike symptoms.

**Table 17.5** reviews the most common diseases that may be associated with croup symptoms.

### Diphtheria

"True croup" resulting from membrane formation and airway stenosis in diphtheria is very rarely seen today. Diphtheritic laryngitis with typical pseudomembranes occurs as an isolated condition in 25% of cases and is combined with nasopharyngeal diphtheria in 75% of cases. The major symptoms are hoarseness, a barking cough, and inspiratory stridor.

> Mucosal swelling or the separation of pseudomembranes may incite an acute attack of respiratory distress that requires immediate intervention (airway maintenance, tracheotomy if required).

The disease is described more fully in 5.4.

### Acute Subglottic Laryngitis

Synonym: acute laryngotracheobronchitis.

*Epidemiology:* This viral disease, known also as pseudocroup, is by far the most common (90%) form of the croup syndrome. It occurs predominantly in infants and small children from 6 months to 3 years of age.
Acute subglottic laryngitis has a seasonal peak incidence in the spring and fall, is frequently epidemic, and affects up to 5% of the population in this age group.

*Etiopathogenesis:* The disease develops gradually over 1 to 3 days during the course of an upper respiratory viral disease transmitted by droplet infection—

**Table 17.5** Differential diagnosis of the most common infectious diseases associated with croup symptoms in infants and small children

| Criteria | Epiglottitis | Subglottic laryngitis (pseudocroup) | Bacterial (laryngo)tracheitis |
|---|---|---|---|
| Causative organism | *Haemophilus influenzae* b | Viruses | Viruses with bacterial superinfection |
| Age | 2–8 y | 6 mo to 3 y | Infants, small children |
| Onset | Sudden | Gradual | Gradual |
| Stridor | Inspiratory | Inspiratory and expiratory | Inspiratory and expiratory |
| Cough | – | Barking, dry | Productive |
| Voice | Muffled, soft, strained | Harsh, hoarse to aphonic | |
| Swallowing | Difficult, painful | Unaffected | Usually difficult, painful |
| Dysphagia | +, drooling | – | – |
| Fever | High | Usually subfebrile | Moderate |
| Leukocytosis | ++ | – | + |

parainfluenza I–III, influenza, respiratory syncytial (RS) viruses. Measles and varicella zoster and rubella viruses can produce similar symptoms.

*Symptoms:* The voice is hoarse due to vocal cord involvement. Patients typically develop a dry, harsh, barking cough and stridor during the evening hours or at night after a few hours' sleep. The stridor is loudest during inspiration and may progress to severe respiratory distress with cyanosis, depending on the degree of airway compromise. Generally, however, subglottic laryngitis runs a milder course than acute epiglottitis (see below).

*Diagnosis:* The body temperature is only moderately elevated or normal. Leukocytosis is usually absent. Laryngoscopy demonstrates an inflammatory swelling below the vocal cords and in the upper part of the cervical trachea. As the disease progresses, further luminal narrowing occurs due to crusting.

*Treatment:* Emphasis is placed on airway humidification and an adequate fluid intake. Generally, there is no need for antibiotics. The efficacy of rectally or orally administered steroids has not been definitely proven but may be beneficial in patients with increasing stridor. In cases with pronounced stridor and dyspnea, inhalation therapy with epinephrine derivatives will promote the regression of inflammatory swelling. Intubation is necessary only in exceptional cases.

Most cases of acute subglottic laryngitis run a mild course, showing a complete resolution of symptoms and complaints in 3 to 5 days. Acute subglottic laryngitis may recur, however.

### Bacterial (Laryngo)tracheitis

*Epidemiology:* This disease occurs sporadically and without seasonal incidence in infants and small children.

*Etiopathogenesis:* Bacterial (laryngo)tracheitis has a primary viral etiology (parainfluenza, influenza) with subsequent bacterial superinfection by staphylococci, pneumococci, streptococci, or *Haemophilus influenzae.*

*Symptoms and diagnosis:* The gradual onset with rhinitis and pharyngitis initially resembles the features of a mild subglottic laryngitis, but soon additional symptoms appear that do not occur in isolated laryngitis: expiratory and inspiratory stridor, numerous rales over the lungs, and other signs of a pulmonary complication (pneumonia, atelectasis).

Besides inflammatory airway obstruction, there is also a risk of lower airway obstruction by viscous mucus.

Stenotic symptoms develop relatively slowly. The temperature is moderately elevated, and a left shift is often seen in the blood count.

On clinical examination, mucosal redness is noted throughout the upper and lower respiratory tract. The vocal cords appear just as red and swollen as the subglottic and tracheal mucosae.

*Treatment and prognosis:* Antibiotic therapy should be supplemented by treatment with mucolytic agents (e.g., acetylcysteine, ambroxol), airway humidification, and adequate fluid intake. Intubation is indicated in severe cases for tracheobronchial toilet.

The prognosis is good in cases that receive prompt treatment.

### Acute Spasmodic Laryngitis

Synonym: spasmodic croup.

*Epidemiology:* Male infants and small children from 1 to 3 years of age are predominantly affected.

*Etiopathogenesis:* Acute spasmodic laryngitis is a rare disease whose etiology is not yet fully understood. Some authors have proposed an allergic etiology analogous to bronchial hyperreactivity as well as gastroesophageal reflux. The symptoms are based on laryngeal spasms.

*Symptoms:* A child with no previous signs of infection wakes up at night in an extremely anxious state with coughing, stridor, and dyspnea. In contrast to bacterial laryngotracheitis, the symptoms subside completely within a few hours. Similar episodes may recur on subsequent nights.

*Treatment and prognosis:* The symptoms can be quickly relieved by administering ipecac syrup to induce vomiting. Additionally, the room air should be cool and humidified. Severe cases may require hospital observation. Intubation is rarely necessary.

The disease, though recurrent, is self-limiting and has a favorable prognosis.

### Acute Epiglottitis

*Epidemiology:* Epiglottitis occurs sporadically with no seasonal predilection and mainly affects children 2 to 8 years of age. The overall incidence has declined since the introduction of the *H. influenzae* type b vaccine.

*Etiopathogenesis:* Acute epiglottitis is a bacterial inflammation of the pharynx and laryngeal inlet. The most common pathogen is *H. influenzae* (type b). Other causative organisms are pneumococci and β-hemolytic streptococci.

**Fig. 17.19 Acute epiglottitis**

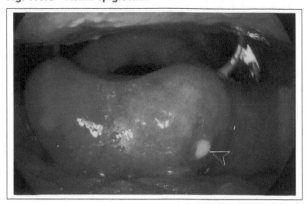

The arrow indicates a site of incipient abscess formation.

*Symptoms:* The disease has a swift onset marked by high fever, a loud inspiratory stridor, and severe respiratory distress. Hoarseness and cough may be absent. Most children complain of very painful swallowing. A muffled "hot potato" voice is a characteristic feature. Progression of the disease is marked by increasing inspiratory retraction in the jugular, sternal, and intercostal areas. The dyspnea may progress rapidly due to increasing inflammatory obstruction of the laryngeal inlet, and death from asphyxia may occur within minutes to a few hours after onset.

∅ The mortality rate is 5 to 10%.

*Diagnosis:* On examination of the oral cavity and pharynx, the posterior pharyngeal wall appears bright red and the epiglottis is swollen and erythematous ("cherry red epiglottis"). Abscess formation may occur (**Fig. 17.19**).

∅ This inspection should be done with extreme care. Never press on the base of the tongue with a tongue blade, as this might reflexly evoke a laryngeal spasm causing total airway obstruction.

More than 50% of affected children develop bacteremia (blood culture). The blood count indicates leukocytosis with a left shift.

*Treatment:* Since intubation is usually unavoidable in children with acute epiglottitis, it should be performed as early as possible, but under controlled conditions (most deaths occur in prehospital settings). Given the short natural history of the disease, a tracheotomy is generally unnecessary. Besides sedation, treatment should include antibiotic therapy with adequate coverage for the spectrum of causative organisms (antibiotics of choice: third-generation cephalosporins). With prompt and adequate treatment, most patients can be extubated after the regression of inflammatory stenosis, usually 1 to 3 days after intubation. The recurrence of acute epiglottitis is very rare.

*Prophylaxis:* The best protection against this potentially life-threatening disease is the universal vaccination of infants and small children against *H. influenzae* after 2 months of age.

## Laryngeal Involvement by Infectious Diseases

Inflammatory involvement of the larynx may occur in the setting of measles, scarlet fever, varicella, or pertussis. It is treated symptomatically.

### Syphilitic Laryngitis

Involvement of the larynx by syphilis has become rare as a result of modern treatment. Although manifestations of syphilis are more common in the mouth and pharynx than in the larynx, laryngeal manifestations may be observed in all three stages of acquired syphilis.

# 17.5 Inflammatory Diseases of the Larynx and Trachea in Adults

Viruses, noxious agents, and extralaryngeal factors are the principal causes of inflammatory laryngotracheal diseases in adults. The cardinal symptom is hoarseness. Less common symptoms are stridor and respiratory distress.

## Acute Laryngitis

*Epidemiology and etiopathogenesis:* Acute laryngitis often occurs in the setting of upper respiratory tract diseases that descend to involve the larynx. It mainly has a viral etiology, and bacterial superinfection may occur.

*Symptoms:* The hallmark of simple laryngitis is hoarseness, occasionally accompanied by a dry, nonproductive cough with no signs of airway obstruction. Dyspnea may occur in rare cases that have unusually severe mucosal swelling.

*Diagnosis:* Inspection of the larynx shows redness and possible thickening or edema of the vocal cords, which are coated with viscous mucus. Besides the glottis, the rest of the intralaryngeal mucosa may also be involved.

▯ A severe form is fibrinous or interstitial laryngitis, marked by homogeneous redness of the vocal cords and possible whitish coatings due to fibrin exudation.

*Treatment:* The treatment of laryngitis consists of voice rest, inhalation therapy, mucolytic agents, and anti-inflammatory agents as required. Antibiotics are prescribed in patients with a concomitant bacterial infection. The systemic infection is an important factor to be considered in treatment planning.
Exogenous irritants (air pollutants, cigarette smoke, climatic influences) should be eliminated and avoided as much as possible.

## Acute Epiglottitis

Synonym: adult supraglottitis.

Acute epiglottitis is a bacterial inflammation, the main causative agents for which are *Haemophilus influenzae*, *Streptococcus pneumoniae*, and β-hemolytic streptococci. The clinical presentation resembles that described in 🔖17.4 (see Acute Epiglottitis and **Fig. 17.19**). Given the risk of airway obstruction, the examination should be performed carefully and with necessary emergency instruments on hand. The patient should be hospitalized for observation and treatment. Early initiation of treatment with intravenous antibiotics (first choice: third-generation cephalosporins) and anti-inflammatory agents (corticosteroids systemically and by inhalation, epinephrine derivatives by inhalation) can frequently avoid the need for intubation.

## Angioneurotic Laryngeal Edema, Acute Laryngeal Edema

*Epidemiology:* This rare, paroxysmal disease predominantly affects adolescents and adults. Occurrence in infants and small children is unusual.

*Etiopathogenesis:* Hereditary angioneurotic edema is caused by a congenital deficiency of C1 esterase inhibitor. An associated rise in esterase levels, often triggered by an infection or other disease process, leads to paroxysmal laryngeal edema.

*Symptoms:* Rapid edematous swelling of the larynx causes a typical inspiratory stridor. Similar edematous changes in the lip, tongue, palate, uvula, throat, or facial skin may accompany the laryngeal edema or may precede it by a variable period of time.

*Diagnosis:* Indirect laryngoscopy reveals edematous changes involving the entire larynx. Serologic testing can confirm the C1 esterase inhibitor deficiency.
The *differential diagnosis* should include allergic reactions (e.g., insect bite, anaphylaxis) and angioedema induced by an angiotensin-converting enzyme (ACE) inhibitor.

*Treatment:* All forms of acute laryngeal swelling benefit from parenteral treatment with corticosteroids and antihistamines and the subcutaneous or local administration of epinephrine (by spray or inhalation). C1 esterase inhibitor products are available for the replacement therapy of C1 esterase inhibitor deficiency. Another option is the administration of bradykinin B2 receptor antagonists such as icatibant.
Intubation is occasionally necessary in patients with increasing airway obstruction unresponsive to these measures.

🔍 **17.3  Rare inflammatory diseases in adults**

### Laryngeal cellulitis and laryngeal abscess

**Etiopathogenesis:** Bacterial infections of the larynx may progress, leading to cellulitis or laryngeal abscess.

**Symptoms:** Laryngeal cellulitis and abscess usually have a sudden onset, often marked by initial chills. Cellulitis in particular is characterized by extremely severe odynophagia, which radiates to the ears. Dyspnea and hoarseness may develop, depending on the location and degree of swelling. Externally, the larynx and hyoid bone may be swollen and tender to pressure. The disease usually reaches its climax in approximately 3 to 5 days. Not infrequently, an abscess will point and rupture spontaneously and resolve quickly after draining. While an inflammation with abscess formation usually runs a harmless course, diffuse cellulitis poses a risk of descending infection with mediastinal involvement, inciting a life-threatening mediastinitis.

**Diagnosis:** Telescopic laryngoscopy shows an *abscess* as a bright red, circumscribed swelling of the laryngeal mucosa with a central, yellowish zone of liquefaction. It is typically located on the epiglottic surface facing the tongue and less commonly within the larynx.

With *cellulitis*, the entire larynx appears markedly reddened. Cellulitic inflammation may not be clearly distinguishable from an abscess.

**Treatment** consists of administering a broad-spectrum antibiotic (third-generation cephalosporin) and securing the airway. Intubation may be unavoidable in some cases and particularly in patients with cellulitic laryngitis.

If an abscess is noted during laryngeal inspection, it should be surgically opened and drained under general anesthesia.

### Laryngeal perichondritis

**Etiopathogenesis:** This inflammatory disease of the larynx has both a primary and a secondary form.

*Primary perichondritis* begins in the perichondrium and spreads from there to the rest of the laryngeal skeleton. In former years, it occurred metastatically in acute infectious diseases such as typhus, spotted fever, and variola. This primary form of laryngeal perichondritis has become rare today.

In *secondary perichondritis*, the cartilage inflammation is preceded by a mucosal disease (e.g., laryngitis, laryngeal abscess, laryngeal cellulitis). It may also be caused by various kinds of trauma (external laryngeal injury, surgery) or by radiotherapy.

**Symptoms:** Besides respiratory distress, voice change, and odynophagia with referred earache, the affected portion of the larynx is usually tender to pressure. Acute perichondritis may be associated with marked systemic symptoms (chills, fever).

**Diagnosis:** Laryngeal perichondritis is easily diagnosed in cases where an external swelling or abscess has already formed. At first, the perichondritis is virtually indistinguishable from a simple edematous process by laryngoscopic examination. Suspicion is raised by more extensive infiltration with limited motion, ulceration, a protracted course, and severe subjective complaints. The formation of sequestered bone fragments confirms the diagnosis. These bony changes are consistently detectable by magnetic resonance imaging (MRI) and are occasionally visible on plain radiographs.

**Treatment:** Antibiotic treatment is of primary importance. Airway obstruction may necessitate a tracheotomy. If signs of liquefaction are seen, the abscess should be surgically drained and any sequestered bone fragments should be removed. Laryngectomy may be necessary in very rare cases. The resolution of perichondritis may leave the patient with significant laryngeal stenosis requiring surgical treatment. The incidence of this complication depends on the location of the inflammatory process in the laryngeal skeleton.

**Fig. 17.20  Causes of chronic laryngitis**

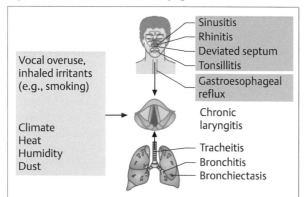

Chronic laryngitis has a multifactorial etiology and is often exacerbated by intercurrent viral and bacterial infections.

## Chronic Nonspecific Laryngitis

**Epidemiology:** Chronic laryngitis is most prevalent in smokers and in persons who abuse their voice. Most patients are men between 50 and 60 years of age.

**Etiopathogenesis:** The principal causes of chronic laryngitis are shown in **Fig. 17.20**. The epithelium responds to the irritants by thickening (hyperplasia and hyperkeratosis) and by developing submucous edema with inflammatory infiltrates and increased mucous glands (*chronic hyperplastic laryngitis*).

This condition is distinguished histologically from the less common chronic atrophic laryngitis ("laryngitis sicca"), which is characterized by a loss of laryngeal mucous glands.

**Symptoms:** Typical symptoms are hoarseness, rapid vocal fatigue, frequent throat clearing, and dry cough. The voice becomes low-pitched.

*Diagnosis:* Telescopic laryngoscopy yields nonspecific findings, often showing a reddened, hyperemic mucosa with a smooth surface. It is not uncommon to find a cobblestone appearance with leukoplakia and exophytic (whitish) keratosis.

📙 Chronic laryngitis often cannot be positively distinguished clinically from an early stage of laryngeal carcinoma.

*Treatment:* The first priority is to identify and eliminate the causal irritants. With chronic laryngitis due to an ascending or descending inflammation (e.g., chronic sinusitis, bronchiectasis), an effort should be made to eradicate the primary focus (e.g., septoplasty, see 📖 3.2, Septal Deviation; paranasal sinus surgery, see 📖 3.8, Acute Sinusitis and 🔍 **3.18**). Inhalation therapy and mucolytics are also beneficial. Acute exacerbations should be treated with antibiotics and, if necessary, with corticosteroid inhalant therapy.

The *prognosis* of chronic laryngitis depends largely on the ability to eliminate exposure to noxious exogenous agents.

📙 Any intractable form of "laryngitis" requires histologic investigation and long-term follow-up.

## Reinke's Edema

Synonym: chronic hyperplastic laryngitis.

*Epidemiology:* Men and women are affected equally, with a peak incidence between 40 and 60 years of age.

*Etiopathogenesis:* A subepithelial fluid collection forms between the glottic epithelium and the vocal ligament (Reinke's space), presumably due to a local disturbance of lymphatic drainage from that space. The main etiologic factors are nicotine abuse and vocal abuse. Reinke's edema is also viewed as a characteristic form of chronic hyperplastic laryngitis, although there is no reported tendency for Reinke's edema to undergo malignant transformation.

*Symptoms:* The typical symptoms are hoarseness, frequent throat clearing, and a decrease in habitual voice pitch with rapid vocal fatigue. Dyspnea is not typically present.

*Diagnosis:* Laryngoscopy shows a glassy, edematous swelling at the level of the vocal cords (**Fig. 17.21**).

*Treatment:* Treatment consists of microsurgical removal of the edema while preserving the vocal ligament, with circumscribed resection of the mucosa. Bilateral Reinke's edema is operated in two stages (6 weeks apart) to prevent the formation of anterior

🔍 **17.4 Fungal infections of the larynx and trachea**

Involvement of the larynx and trachea by fungal diseases is rare. Most cases involve the secondary spread of infection from the oral cavity and pharynx. Primary fungal infections of the larynx and/or trachea are unusual. Predisposing factors are generally present and include wasting diseases, cachexia, vitamin deficiencies, congenital immune defects, acquired immunosuppression by treatment with corticosteroids or cytostatics, steroid inhalants for lung disease, antibiotic therapy, human immunodeficiency virus (HIV) infection, etc.

**Candidiasis**
This disease is caused by yeast fungi of the genus *Candida*. The most important representative, *Candida albicans*, is a normal intestinal saprophyte and becomes virulent only when predisposing host factors are present. In cases with extensive involvement of the oral mucosa, focal or membranelike whitish plagues may also develop at the laryngeal inlet and especially on the epiglottis. A primary infection confined to the larynx is uncommon. Swallowing difficulties and hoarseness may provide subjective evidence of laryngeal involvement.
*Treatment*: Antifungal agents may be applied topically to affected sites (with a brush under local anesthesia) or systemically (e.g., fluconazole).

**Blastomycosis, aspergillosis, sporotrichosis**
Laryngeal or tracheal involvement is rare. All of these fungal infections are marked by the development of superficial, granulomatous, ulcerating mucosal lesions. Differentiation from one another and from tuberculosis, syphilis, and neoplasia is occasionally difficult and requires identification of the causative organism. Treatment relies on antifungal agents specific for the infecting organism. Patients should also be screened for a predisposing underlying disease.

synechiae. Surgical treatment is reinforced by having the patient quit smoking and by referring the patient for voice therapy as needed.

## Posterior Laryngitis

Synonym: gastroesophageal reflux laryngitis (GERL).

**Posterior or reflux laryngitis** is a special form of chronic laryngitis attributed to the (nocturnal) reflux of gastric contents into the esophagus and pharynx. The cardinal symptoms are intractable hoarseness and a laryngopharyngeal foreign-body or globus sensation. As 24-hour esophageal pH measurements have shown, laryngeal acid reflux may occur in patients who have no other typical complaints of reflux disease (see textbooks of internal medicine). The disease, then, results from injury to the laryngeal and pharyngeal mucosa caused by chronic exposure to refluxed gastric acid. Given the anatomic relationship of the esophagus and larynx, the most severe damage occurs to the posterior portions of the larynx (arytenoid area) and to the postcricoid area. Inspection of these areas demonstrates redness, edema, and tissue

**Fig. 17.21 Reinke's edema**

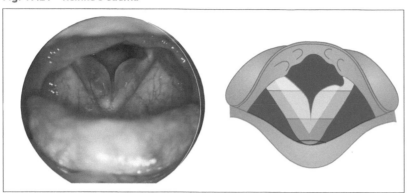

Lobular thickening of both vocal cords is apparent at laryngoscopy.

---

> 🥄 **17.5 Pregnancy-related laryngopathy**
>
> Edematous changes may develop in the laryngeal mucosa beginning in the fifth month of pregnancy as a result of hormonal changes. Laryngoscopy shows mucosal hyperemia and edematous swelling that may assume life-threatening proportions in rare cases. The principal complaint is dysphonia. The changes and their symptoms are reversible following parturition.

proliferation, occasionally causing the interarytenoid area to have a "garden fence" appearance.

Thus, laryngitis in which the morphologic changes are predominantly posterior should always suggest a diagnosis of reflux laryngopathy. A gastroenterologic work-up (esophagogastroduodenoscopy, 24-hour pH-metry) is advised. Treatment follows established medical guidelines for reflux diseases. Proton-pump inhibitors are particularly effective.

## Laryngitis in Chronic Infectious Diseases

### Tuberculous Laryngitis

*Epidemiology:* As the incidence and prevalence of pulmonary tuberculosis have declined, tuberculous laryngitis has also become less common, although a certain rising trend has been documented in recent years.

*Etiology and pathogenesis:* Tuberculous changes in the larynx are almost always secondary to active pulmonary tuberculosis. Bacteria-laden secretions that are coughed up from the bronchi may infect the larynx, showing a special predilection for the posterior larynx, the interarytenoid area, and the laryngeal surface of the epiglottis. Laryngeal involvement usually parallels acute flare-ups of pulmonary tuberculosis. The extent and course of laryngeal tuberculosis, which may also be acquired hematogenously, depend on the efficacy of local host defenses and the

virulence of the infecting organism. Laryngeal perichondritis and foci of liquefaction may develop as the disease progresses, and a secondary infection develops in most cases.

*Symptoms:* Tuberculous laryngitis has a variety of subjective symptoms ranging from mild, frequent throat clearing to severe hoarseness or aphonia. Odynophagia signifies an advanced process with involvement of deeper tissues.

*Diagnosis:* Laryngoscopic inspection shows the characteristic appearance of tuberculous laryngitis: redness and thickening of one vocal cord (**monochorditis**), occasionally with small ulcerations.

> 🖉 Only histologic examination can differentiate tuberculous laryngitis from glottic carcinoma.

Reddish-brown, partially confluent submucous nodules are additionally found in the interarytenoid area and supraglottis.

*Treatment:* The mucosal changes will heal in response to tuberculostatic therapy, with no significant functional sequelae. Sites of cartilage destruction in the larynx will leave residual damage, but the prognosis is still favorable.

### Intubation Granuloma

See 🥄 **17.6**.

### Contact Ulcer

*Epidemiology:* Men are predominantly affected. Contact ulcers are rare in children.

*Etiopathogenesis:* These lesions appear to be caused by chronic vocal abuse. Overuse of the voice leads to the repetitive, forcible adduction of the vocal processes of

Fig. 17.22 Contact ulcer

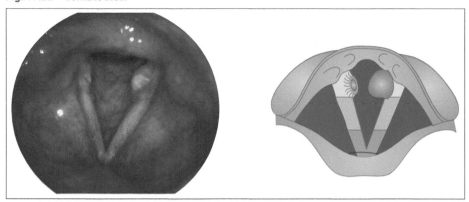

Unilateral epithelial thickening inflicts "hammer blows" to an opposing site on the contralateral vocal cord. This impingement causes ulceration or erosion.

both arytenoid cartilages. The added presence of gastroesophageal reflux further contributes to the pathogenesis of this condition.

*Symptoms:* Typical complaints are hoarseness, a foreign-body sensation, and throat pain.

*Diagnosis:* Laryngoscopy initially shows a superficial mucosal lesion that later gives way to a contact granuloma with unilateral epithelial thickening and a rounded mucosal ulceration on the opposite vocal cord ("hammer-and-anvil" effect; **Fig. 17.22**). A phoniatric examination is indicated.

*Treatment:* Antireflux therapy and voice therapy are the cornerstones of treatment. Surgery (microlaryngoscopic ablation) is necessary only if conservative measures are unsuccessful. Contact granulomas have a strong tendency to recur.

# 17.6    Foreign-Body Aspiration and Injuries to the Larynx and Trachea

Foreign-body aspiration occurs in children as well as adults. It is common for aspirated foreign bodies to enter the lower airways in children, whereas rapid glottic closure in adults is usually sufficient to prevent lower level impaction. For children under 6 years of age, aspirated foreign bodies are the leading cause of death in the home.

External injuries to the larynx or trachea are rare occurrences, as this soft-tissue region is protected by the mandible, sternum, and spinal column. Also, the head is often flexed forward as a reflex response to external trauma.

Internal injuries to the larynx and trachea are more common and can have more serious ramifications. Internal injuries include intubation trauma and also the mucosal lesions and scarring that may be caused by many harmful agents.

Laryngeal and tracheal injuries are almost always internal in children younger than 12 years; external injuries become more common with aging.

## Foreign-Body Aspiration

*Epidemiology:* Foreign-body aspiration is most prevalent in children younger than 3 years, with an approximately 2:1 preponderance of boys over girls.

*Etiology and pathogenesis:* Oropharyngeal swallowing abnormalities predispose to foreign-body aspiration. For anatomic reasons, aspirated foreign bodies are found four times more often in the right main bronchus than in the left main bronchus. They are rarely found in the larynx and trachea.

🖉 Radiolucent foreign bodies are considerably more common than radiopaque objects.

Food items are aspirated with particular frequency, especially peanuts (**Fig. 17.23**; caution: may swell within the airway) and watermelon seeds. Tablets are common (laryngeal) foreign bodies in adults.

*Symptoms:* The initial symptoms of foreign-body aspiration depend on the size, shape, and composition of the foreign body, its location, and the age of the patient. Usually, the object provokes an immediate coughing fit with or without cyanosis, accompanied by dyspnea, stridor, and pain. Larger foreign bodies impacted in the larynx may cause death from asphyxiation, whereas smaller objects lead to hoarseness and cough. The clinical picture of a complete obstruction is that of a cyanotic, aphonic patient with spasmodic breathing movements that do not ventilate the lungs. **Bolus death** refers to acute cardiac arrest caused by a vasovagal reflex evoked by obstruction of the upper airways. Foreign bodies in the trachea cause far greater complaints than objects in a bronchus, ranging from a slight cough to fatal asphyxia. If a foreign body in the trachea moves with respirations, it produces the telltale signs of a small

Fig. 17.23    Aspirated foreign body

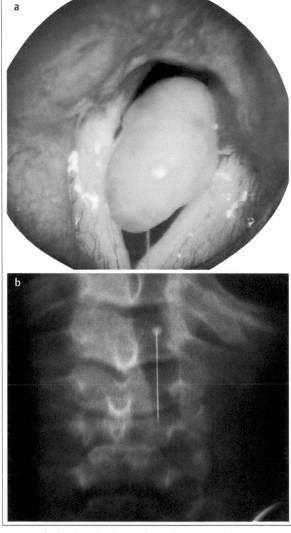

**a** Peanut lodged in the glottic plane of a 4-year-old boy.
**b** Posteroanterior radiograph shows an aspirated needle in the trachea of a 15-year-old girl.

palpable impact, an audible click, and movement of the trachea. A foreign body close to the vocal cords may be manifested by whistling sounds and stridor.

A foreign body lodged in the cervical esophagus may compromise the upper airway by compression, with associated symptoms. Complete obstruction of the esophagus also poses a risk of **overflow aspiration**.

***Diagnosis and treatment:*** Besides the clinical examination with inspection and auscultation, **radiographs** are of key importance in determining the location of an aspirated foreign body. Chest radiographs at end-inspiration and end-expiration and lateral soft-tissue views of the neck are also helpful in locating nonradiopaque foreign bodies.

If there is the least suspicion of an aspirated foreign body, generally there is no substitute for **endoscopy** of the upper aerodigestive tract for diagnostic and therapeutic purposes. Especially with soft, fragile foreign bodies, rigid endoscopy is definitely superior to flexible endoscopy for mobilizing and removing the foreign material. Special instruments are available for snaring and retrieving peanuts and other foreign bodies without breaking them into smaller fragments that could slip down into smaller airways and become lost in peripheral bronchi. Rigid endoscopy also provides the access needed to break sharp-edged or impacted objects into smaller pieces before definitive extraction. The rigid scope eliminates the risks of mucosal injury and perforation that are associated with a flexible endoscope.

With a foreign body completely obstructing the larynx, **Heimlich's maneuver** can be used to expel the object from the airway (see **Fig. 17.24**).

If the larynx is only partially obstructed, allowing some degree of respiration, the recommended treat-ment is endoscopic extraction of the foreign body under controlled conditions.

## External Injuries to the Larynx and Extrathoracic Trachea

***Epidemiology and etiopathogenesis:*** The pediatric larynx is less susceptible to external trauma because it is still very mobile, cartilaginous, and less prominent than in adults. Fractures of the thyroid and/or cricoid cartilages are almost unknown in children. The most frequent causes of laryngotracheal injury are deliberate attacks (strangulation, "karate chops") and other anterior violence that compresses the tissue against the spinal column (e.g., handlebar impact in a bicycle accident, automobile dashboard injury). A life-threatening airway obstruction may occur immediately or with some delay after this kind of trauma.

Ruptures of the extrathoracic trachea are rare. The mechanism is an anterior force acting on the hyperextended neck, causing an outward bending of the posterior ends of the tracheal cartilages with rupture of the membranous posterior wall. The most serious and life-threatening form of blunt neck trauma is a complete avulsion of the larynx from the trachea.

⚠ Attempting intubation in this case could rupture the final connective-tissue attachments between the larynx and trachea, completely disrupting the airway and preventing further ventilation.

***Symptoms:*** Signs indicating a laryngeal or tracheal injury are palpable discontinuities or crepitation in the tracheolaryngeal skeleton, pain, a change in voice, swallowing difficulty, hemoptysis, cutaneous emphysema, and respiratory distress. An airway obstruction may be caused by edema, hemorrhage, injury to the vocal cord or recurrent laryngeal nerve, or mass effect from a tracheal hematoma. Tears in the mucosa and wall of the larynx and/or trachea lead to cutaneous emphysema of the head and nuchal area, with or without a pneumomediastinum and pneumothorax. A tracheal injury can also cause the creation of a tracheoesophageal fistula.

***Diagnosis and treatment:*** Besides the clinical and endoscopic examination, computed tomography also supplies useful information on the location and extent of injuries.

The first priority in the management of external tracheolaryngeal injuries is to establish a secure airway.

⚠ If spontaneous respiration is satisfactory, it is unwise to perform overly aggressive endoscopic intubation in an emergency setting.

**Fig. 17.24 Heimlich's maneuver**

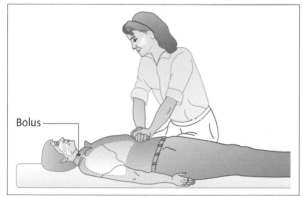

Bolus

Applying a quick upward-and-inward thrust to the epigastric region causes a sudden rise of intrathoracic pressure that expels the obstructing foreign body out of the larynx and mouth. This maneuver is not without hazards, however, and is effective only in patients with a complete luminal obstruction.

Whenever possible, endoscopy of the larynx and trachea should be performed under controlled conditions. Then an endotracheal tube can be introduced, with facilities available for performing a tracheotomy if needed.

**Relatively minor injuries** generally do not require further measures. Severe laryngeal and tracheal injuries should be treated operatively (e.g., cartilage repair) to prevent later stenosis. **Avulsion injuries** should be referred for reconstructive surgery without delay.

## Internal Injuries to the Larynx and Trachea

Internal injuries to the larynx and trachea may be caused by thermal injuries (scalds and burns), chemical agents (caustic ingestion), or mechanical injuries (intubation, endoscopy).

### Thermal Injuries

Thermal injuries to the laryngeal and tracheal mucosa may result from aspiration, burns due to hot foods or liquids, generalized burns, or surgical laser use.

### Chemical Agents

Mucosal injuries by chemical agents most commonly affect the pharynx and supraglottic larynx. The sphincter function of the glottis usually protects the lower airways, although some 50% of pediatric victims will suffer respiratory tract injury due to aspiration, retching, or vomiting. While most lesions involve the supraglottic region, it is also possible for other portions of the endolarynx, the trachea, and the bronchial system to be affected.

*Etiopathogenesis:* Caustic injuries are caused mainly by household cleansers, which are typically ingested by children younger than 4 years. In adults, suicide attempts by acid or alkali ingestion are not altogether uncommon. These agents primarily damage the mucosal surface but may also cause deeper injuries. While acids tend to cause superficial **coagulation necrosis**, alkalis cause deeper **colliquative necrosis**, which has a poorer prognosis.

*Symptoms:* Besides acute airway obstruction due to mucosal swelling, patients are also threatened by the systemic effects of the absorbed chemical compounds.

*Diagnosis and treatment:* The main priority in acute cases is to establish a secure airway and provide systemic therapy for the caustic ingestion, which includes adequate parenteral fluid replacement.

☝ An endoscopic survey should be done only during the first 24 hours due to the risk of perforation.

Primary management should also include immediate high doses of corticosteroids. The benefits of continuing this therapy at a maintenance dosage are uncertain. The causative agent should be identified and secured for therapeutic reasons (possible antidote) and to help in making a prognosis.

Second-look endoscopy should be performed no sooner than 10 to 14 days after the injury. A broad-spectrum antibiotic should be administered due to the risk of bacterial infection.

After the acute lesions have healed, there may be chronic residual changes in the laryngotracheal system marked by stricture formation and laryngeal dysfunction (incomplete glottic closure with recurrent aspiration). Corrective surgical treatments often prove difficult in these cases.

### Mechanical Injuries

Internal mechanical injuries to the larynx and trachea are almost always a result of medical procedures such as intubation, endoscopy, and foreign-body extraction. Even suctioning the trachea with a catheter can lead to mucosal injuries. Acute injuries to the mucosal lining usually heal rapidly without treatment. The more deeply the wound extends toward the submucosa, the greater the tendency for granuloma formation (intubation granulomas, ✐ **17.6**) and the greater the infection risk to cartilage and articular structures. **Table 17.6** shows the Eckerbom scheme for grading the severity of intubation injuries.

It is rare for intubation to cause the fracture or fracture-dislocation of an arytenoid cartilage.

### Effects of (Prolonged) Intubation

The prolonged presence of an endotracheal tube can lead to chronic pathologic changes. There are various primary factors in prolonged intubation that can lead to permanent functional deficits such as stenosis, vocal dysfunction, and dysphagia.

*Etiology and pathogenesis* (**Fig. 17.25**): Besides the duration of intubation, a major pathogenic factor is a

**Fig. 17.25   Causes of intubation injuries**

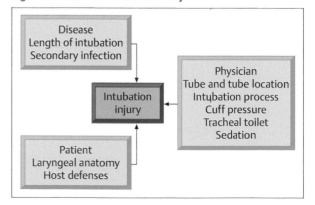

### 🔎 17.6 Intubation granulomas

Orotracheal or nasotracheal intubation may incite circumscribed inflammatory changes that in time can lead to the development of potentially large granulomas. The vocal process of the arytenoid cartilage is a site of predilection for intubation granulomas as a result of tissue damage from the particularly high tube pressure in the posterior glottis. Typically, intubation granulomas do not reach a symptomatic size until several weeks after extubation. Examination of the larynx for increasing hoarseness reveals a smooth, tense, pea-sized to cherry-sized polypoid mass with inflammatory redness (**Fig. 17.26**). Initially, large intubation granulomas may regress spontaneously in 2 to 3 months. Microlaryngoscopic removal is indicated if the changes persist, but recurrences are common.

**Fig. 17.26  Intubation granulomas**

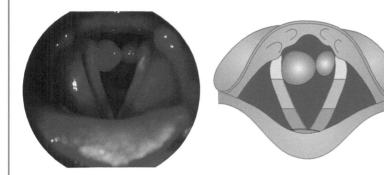

Source: Prof. F. Rosanowski, Nuremberg, Germany; Prof. U. Eysholdt, Oldenburg, Germany.

| Table 17.6 | Classification of acute intubation injuries to the larynx |
|---|---|
| Grade | Symptoms and findings |
| I | Hyperemia, edema, discoloration of the mucosa |
| II | Ulceration and necrosis of the mucosa and lamina propria |
| III | Deep ulceration and necrosis extending to the cartilage |

Source: Eckerbom 1986.

possible disproportion between the caliber of the endotracheal tube and the internal diameter of the cricoid cartilage. The cricoid cartilage encircles the narrowest point in the upper respiratory tract, and it has very little elastic compliance because of its annular geometry. Friction between the tube and larynx—which may occur in restless patients, for example, and especially when ventilator movements are transmitted to the tube—tends to erode through the extremely thin pad of submucosa lining the cricoid cartilage. The exposed cartilage is susceptible to infection, and the resulting perichondritis heals with the formation of granulations and scar tissue. This can result in subglottic stenosis, ankylosis of the arytenoid joints, and scar adhesions between the arytenoid cartilages causing vocal cord fixation in the midline.

Overinflating the tube cuff, or inflating it for too long a period, can also damage the mucosa. Intubation can also have late sequelae that are caused not only by local injury mechanisms but also by a weakening of host defenses that often accompanies the underlying disease and by intervals of hypotension with microcirculatory insufficiency. Patient age is also a significant factor in upper airway lesions following intubation. Because the cricoid cartilage is still soft and compliant in newborns, this is the age group in which intubation is best tolerated. While there have been isolated reports of subglottic stenosis occurring in infants after only one day of intubation, many other infants have been intubated for up to 2 months with no adverse effects. Generally, the risk of intubation-related complications is higher after orotracheal intubation than after nasotracheal intubation, because in the latter technique there is less frictional trauma to mucosal surfaces from the tube.

**Manifestation:** The chronic changes that can result from intubation (stenoses and intubation granulomas) often do not appear until 2 to 6 weeks after removal of the endotracheal tube.

**Treatment:** Generally, these changes, especially subglottic stenoses, can be corrected only by a major surgical procedure (🔎 **17.7**).

**Prophylaxis:** The prevention of these surgically challenging intubation injuries is based on selecting the proper tube size (🔎 **17.8**) and promptly recognizing the need for a tracheotomy where indicated. While tracheotomy should be considered in adult patients when the length of intubation is expected to exceed 3 to 6 days, infants and small children can tolerate 2 to 3 weeks of intubation owing to their compliant laryngeal anatomy. Tracheotomy is recommended in

### 🔎 17.7 Treatment of subglottic and tracheal stenosis

For best results, the surgical treatment of subglottic and tracheal cicatricial stenosis should be deferred until the site is free of inflammation. Generally, there has been sufficient scarring to stabilize the site by 4 to 6 months after the causative event.

A **subglottic stenosis (Fig. 17.27a)** can be expanded simply by splitting the cricoid cartilage and interposing an anterior or posterior autologous (costal) cartilage implant. Increasingly, however, surgeons are favoring a partial resection of the cricoid cartilage with separation of the larynx and trachea and an end-to-end anastomosis of the cervical trachea to the thyroid cartilage (thyrotracheopexy, **Fig. 17.27b**). The inherent tension of the trachea requires that the neck be immobilized in an anteflexed position for 1 to 4 weeks to relieve tension on the anastomosis.

When the operative site is exposed, care is taken to preserve the recurrent laryngeal nerves running between the trachea and esophagus. Ordinarily, a transverse resection cannot be performed if the segment to be resected is more than 5 to 6 cm long, and a different plastic reconstructive technique should be used (e.g., reconstructing the tracheal wall with cartilage grafts). A permanent tracheostomy or permanent intraluminal stent insertion may be unavoidable in some cases. A long-segment cicatricial stenosis should not be treated by repeated bougie dilation or by partial laser resection of the stenosis. These treatments are appropriate only for discrete webs.

**Fig. 17.27 Surgical treatment of subglottic and tracheal stenosis**

a  Subglottic stenosis

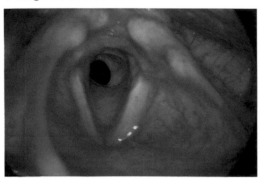

b  Pearson's thyrotracheopexy

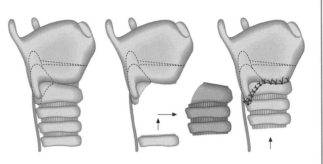

c  Tracheal stenosis

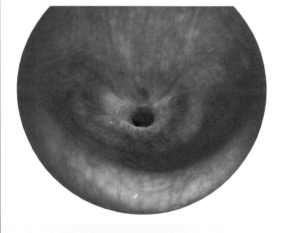

d  Transverse tracheal resection

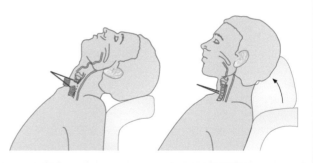

**Table 17.7 Recommended tube sizes**

| Age group | Tube circumference (Ch) | Inside diameter of tube (mm) |
|---|---|---|
| Premature infants | 10–12 | 2.5 |
| Newborns | 12–14 | 3 |
| 1–6 mo | 16 | 3.5 |
| 6–12 mo | 18 | 4.0 |
| 1–2 y | 18–20 | 4.0–4.5 |
| 2–3 y | 20–22 | 4.5–5.0 |
| 3–4 y | 22–24 | 5.0–5.5 |
| 4–5 y | 24–26 | 5.5–6.0 |
| 5–7 y | 26–28 | 6.0–6.5 |
| 7–9 y | 28 | 6.5 |
| 10–11 y | 28–30 | 6.5–7.0 |
| 12–13 y | 32 | 7.5 |
| 14–16 y | 34 | 8.0 |
| Adults (women) | 30–34 | 7–8 |
| Adults (men) | 34–36 | 8–9 |

Source: Larsen 2002.

Based on the relationships that have been described and the
complications that may arise, the size of an endotracheal
tube should be appropriate for the age of the patient.

A good rule of thumb, especially in children, is that the tube
diameter should not exceed the diameter of the patient's
small finger. The figures listed in **Table 17.7** are based on
data from the anesthesiologic literature.

Usually, a somewhat larger ventilation tube can be used in a
tracheostomy, because the trachea has a larger diameter in
that region than at the subglottic level.

Cicatricial stenosis of the trachea requires differentiation
from tracheomalacia, in which the tracheal walls are flaccid
and tend to collapse causing functional stenosis. This condition is attributed to cartilage damage due, for example, to a
pressure-induced deficiency of blood flow (e.g., goiter).

**Treatment** options are tracheopexy (suturing the trachea to
adjacent structures) or intraluminal stent insertion.

**Fig. 17.28   Acquired laryngeal and tracheal stenosis**

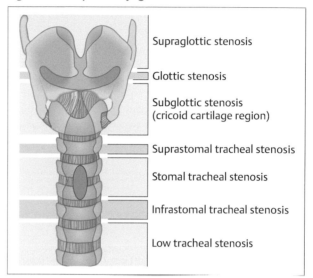

Supraglottic stenosis

Glottic stenosis

Subglottic stenosis
(cricoid cartilage region)

Suprastomal tracheal stenosis

Stomal tracheal stenosis

Infrastomal tracheal stenosis

Low tracheal stenosis

Source: Tillmann 1997, Meyer et al 1982.

older children and adolescents when it is expected
that intubation will exceed 1 to 2 weeks. Tracheotomy
can prevent the aforementioned lesions that can
develop in the larynx as a result of prolonged
endotracheal intubation.

The rare *complications of a correctly performed
tracheotomy* include postinflammatory cicatricial
stenosis of the trachea above the stoma (suprasternal
stenosis, **Fig. 17.28**), below the stoma (infrastomal stenosis), or at the level of the stoma (stomal stenosis).
Tracheal stenosis can also result from mucosal lesions
caused by cuff pressure from the tracheostomy tube
(**Fig. 17.28**). This type of tracheal stenosis is rare, however, compared with the tracheal lesions caused by
orotracheal or nasotracheal intubation.

# 17.7 Tumors of the Larynx and Trachea

The cardinal symptom of all neoplasms of the *larynx*, whether benign or malignant, is persistent hoarseness. Any hoarseness that lasts longer than 2 weeks should be investigated by laryngoscopy. Making risk patients (smokers) more aware of hoarseness as a potential warning sign can aid in the early detection and more effective treatment of glottic carcinoma, which is the most common malignant tumor of the head and neck.

## Benign Neoplasms of the Larynx

Benign tumors constitute the majority of laryngeal neoplasms in both children and adults. They generally present clinically as a mechanical obstruction of the upper airways with coughing, hoarseness, wheezing, and dyspnea.

### Vocal Cord Polyps

*Epidemiology:* Adults in speaking professions are mainly affected, with a preponderance of males.

*Etiopathogenesis:* The most frequent cause is a mechanical alteration of the vocal cords caused by vocal overuse (phonotrauma) and chronic inflammation. Histologic examination reveals a polypoid mucosal hyperplasia with an inflammatory component. Most vocal polyps are unilateral (90%) and are located on the free edge of the anterior two-thirds of the vocal cord.

*Symptoms:* The cardinal symptom is hoarseness. Floating polyps may cause diplophonia.

Similar to laryngeal tumors, neoplasms of the *trachea* may present with cough, inspiratory stridor, and possible dyspnea as a result of airway obstruction. The most common benign neoplasms are papillomas, fibromas, and hemangiomas. Rigid and flexible tracheobronchoscopy has special importance as both a diagnostic and therapeutic tool. Treatment is generally surgical and may include a tracheotomy if required.

*Diagnosis:* Telescopic laryngoscopy demonstrates a grayish-red sessile or pedunculated mass on the vocal cord (**Fig. 17.29**).

*Treatment:* Treatment consists of microsurgical removal, which may be followed by voice therapy.

### Cysts and Mucoceles

*Epidemiology:* These lesions are most common in older patients and are rarely encountered in children.

*Etiopathogenesis: Cystic lesions* originate in the small mucosal glands of the laryngeal mucosa and form in the area of the ventricular fold, sinus of Morgagni, or subepithelial vocal fold. They are usually lined by squamous or columnar epithelium. Mucus-filled *retention mucoceles* and *extravasation mucoceles* may occur anywhere in the larynx and trachea where mucous glands are present. They are lined by respiratory epithelium.

*Symptoms:* Clinical manifestations depend on the size and location of the lesions and may consist of hoarseness, globus sensation, and rarely dyspnea.

Fig. 17.29  Vocal cord polyp

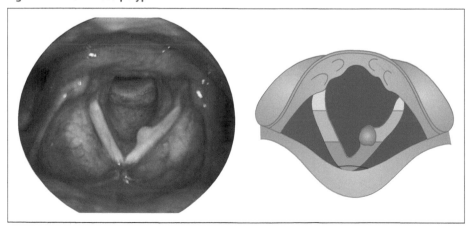

The polyp shows a typical (unilateral) location on the free edge of the anterior two-thirds of the vocal cord.

*Diagnosis:* Telescopic laryngoscopy reveals smooth, epithelium-covered masses of varying size.

*Treatment:* The recommended treatment is removal by endolaryngeal microsurgery.

## Papillomas and Laryngeal Papillomatosis

*Epidemiology:* Papillomas are the most common benign laryngeal tumors in children, juvenile papillomas are most prevalent between the second and fourth years of life. While papillomas in adults (second to fourth decades) are usually solitary, juvenile laryngeal papillomatosis is characterized by multiple lesions that spread to the trachea and bronchial system. Multiple lesions may also be found in adults, however.

*Etiopathogenesis:* Histologically, the papillomas are neoplasms and not a reaction to a chronic inflammatory stimulus. The causal agents are human papillomaviruses (HPVs), most notably HPV 6 and HPV 11. Malignant transformation is rare in juvenile papillomatosis but is more common in the adult form.

*Symptoms:* The initial symptoms are hoarseness and an inspiratory stridor that develops with increasing obstruction. Occasional aggressive growth may cause life-threatening luminal obstruction of the larynx or trachea.

*Diagnosis:* The typical endoscopic appearance is that of multiple soft, reddish-pink, villous, raspberrylike lesions covering a large area of the glottis and supraglottis (**Fig. 17.30**). Generally, the lesions first appear on the vocal cords.

🔖 Regular histologic follow-ups are essential due to the potential for malignant transformation.

*Treatment:* The treatment of choice is $CO_2$ laser surgery, which can remove the frequently recurring lesions with very little bleeding. A potential complication of repeated excisions is glottic webbing. Other treatment modalities (β-interferon, virostatics, photodynamic therapy) have been used with varying success.

**Fig. 17.30 Laryngeal papillomatosis**

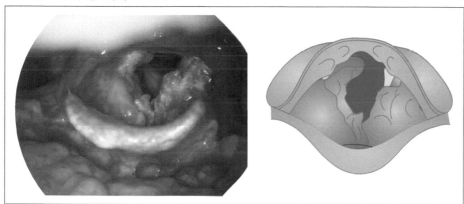

Both vocal cords are covered by multiple, confluent, exophytic papillomas. The gross appearance resembles that of laryngeal carcinoma.

**Fig. 17.31 Vocal nodules**

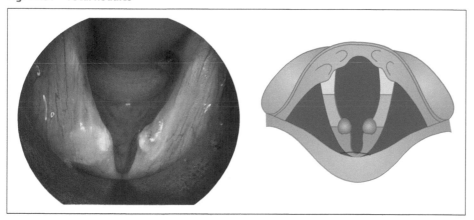

The nodules are bilateral and are typically located at the junction of the anterior and middle thirds of the vocal cords. (See also **Fig.18.9**.)

*Prophylaxis:* HPV vaccination.

*Prognosis:* The papillomas may resolve spontaneously in rare cases, or may recur after an asymptomatic interval.

## Vocal Nodules

*Epidemiology:* Vocal nodules can occur in children (screamer's nodules), singers (singer's nodules), and in patients who speak professionally, especially younger women.

*Etiopathogenesis:* The underlying cause is harmful vocal habits (vocal abuse) causing bilateral nodules to form at opposing sites at the junction of the anterior and middle thirds of the vocal cords (maximum vibrational amplitude; **Fig. 17.31** and **Fig. 18.9**). Histologic examination reveals fibrosis with epithelial thickening and submucosal connective-tissue proliferation.

*Symptoms:* Typical symptoms are hoarseness, diplophonia, habitual throat clearing, and a foreign-body sensation.

*Treatment:* The treatment of choice is voice therapy. Surgical removal is indicated only in patients with exceptionally large nodules and for whom voice therapy has failed. Vocal nodules in puberty generally regress spontaneously due to longitudinal growth of the vocal cords.

## Malignant Laryngeal Tumors

### Laryngeal Carcinoma

*Epidemiology:* Malignant tumors of the larynx are the most common head and neck malignancies, accounting for approximately 40% of these cancers and for 1 to 2% of all malignant tumors. The reported incidence in the United States is 4 to 6 per 100,000 population per year. Internationally, incidence rates range from 2.5 to 17.1 per 100,000 population per year in men and from 0.1 to 1.3 per 100,000 population per year in women.

*Etiopathogenesis:* Besides the epithelial changes described in 🔍 **17.10**, chronic laryngitis must be considered a predisposing factor for laryngeal carcinoma based on the presence of the same risk factors.

*Histology, sites of occurrence, and classification:* The great majority of laryngeal malignancies are keratinized or nonkeratinized squamous cell carcinomas (90–95%). The rest consist of undifferentiated carcinomas, well-differentiated verrucous carcinomas, and other rare entities.

Sixty percent of laryngeal carcinomas are located in the glottic plane, 40% in the supraglottic region, and only approximately 1% in the subglottis. A carcinoma of the glottis, Morgagni's pouch, and ventricular fold that has an indeterminate site of origin is called a **transglottic carcinoma**.

The growth of supraglottic malignancies into the preepiglottic fat pad, extension to the glottic plane, the spread of glottic malignancies to the anterior commissure with possible thyroid cartilage invasion, and paraglottic extension down along the thyroid cartilage not only worsen the prognosis but also limit the possibilities for larynx-conserving surgery. Vocal cord fixation by invasion of the muscles inserting on the arytenoid cartilage or by infiltration of the cricoarytenoid joint signifies the very advanced growth of a glottic or subglottic cancer and critically affects

---

🔍 **17.10  Carcinogenesis**

Malignant tumors of the upper aerodigestive tract are mostly squamous cell carcinomas (95%) and are caused mainly by exposure to exogenous carcinogens. The prime offender is tobacco, which contains polycyclic aromatic hydrocarbons, N-nitroso compounds, and aromatic amines as its principal mutagens. Alcohol abuse, especially the consumption of high-alcohol beverages, also has causal significance. Several industrial agents (soot, tar, nickel, heat) have been identified as potential laryngeal carcinogens. Particular importance is assigned to asbestos, and asbestos exposure has been recognized as an occupational disease.

Carcinogenesis in the upper aerodigestive tract is described as a **multistep process**. The exogenous agents cited above cause epithelial injury that evokes an epithelial response consisting of (hyper)regeneration (**hyperplasia**) and/or **hyperkeratosis (Fig. 17.32a–f)**.

With continued exposure to the noxious agents, there is a growing likelihood that foci of epithelial dysplasia will develop, spread, and eventually progress to intraepithelial neoplasia. Once this has taken place, regression of the lesions can no longer occur. In the next step, the in-situ lesion penetrates the basement membrane, becoming an invasive cancer with metastatic potential (**Fig. 17.32 g**).

Multiple epithelial changes or even malignancies occur concurrently or consecutively at different sites in the upper aerodigestive tract (synchronous or metachronous tumors) in up to 20% of patients. We can explain this by noting that all of the mucosa in the upper aerodigestive tract is exposed to exogenous carcinogens (**field cancerization**). For this reason, patients with upper aerodigestive tract malignancies should undergo comprehensive endoscopic scrutiny of this region at the time of diagnosis and at regular intervals after the conclusion of treatment.

The different line thickness of the black arrows represents the likelihood of regression of the dysplastic epithelial changes or the development of invasive carcinoma. The red arrows represent inevitable, irreversible processes.

**17.10 Carcinogenesis** (*continuation*)

**Fig. 17.32  Stepwise development of squamous cell carcinoma from dysplasia**

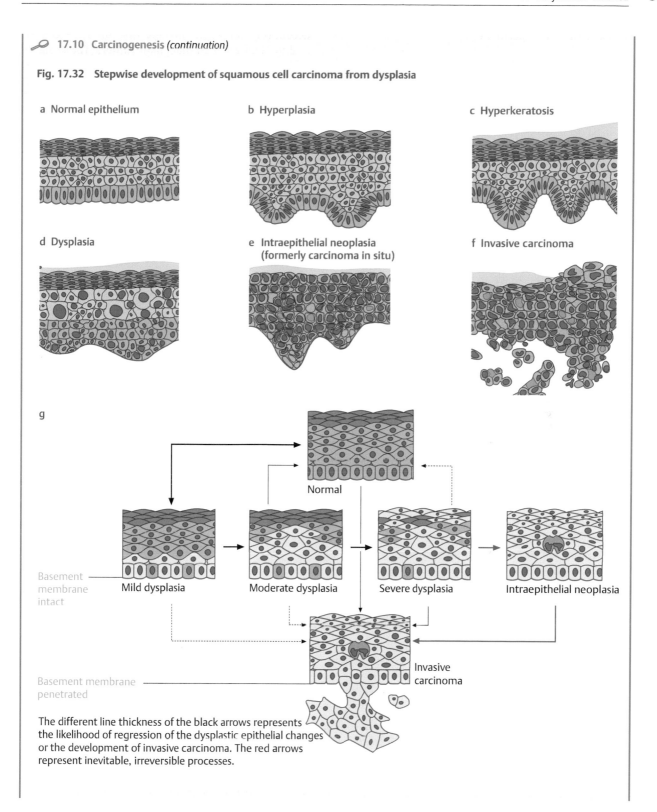

a  Normal epithelium

b  Hyperplasia

c  Hyperkeratosis

d  Dysplasia

e  Intraepithelial neoplasia
(formerly carcinoma in situ)

f  Invasive carcinoma

g

Normal

Basement membrane intact

Mild dysplasia

Moderate dysplasia

Severe dysplasia

Intraepithelial neoplasia

Invasive carcinoma

Basement membrane penetrated

The different line thickness of the black arrows represents the likelihood of regression of the dysplastic epithelial changes or the development of invasive carcinoma. The red arrows represent inevitable, irreversible processes.

### 17.11 Premalignant lesions

Premalignant (precancerous) lesions are epithelial changes that may give rise to carcinoma. The gross clinical appearance of potentially premalignant lesions in the larynx is highly variable. The degree of dysplasia is a histologically defined criterion that cannot be assessed clinically.

- **Leukoplakia** (**Fig. 17.33**): whitish patch of mucosa that cannot be rubbed away; may be circumscribed or more diffuse. Gross appearance does not permit reliable benign–malignant differentiation.
- **Erythroplakia**: reddish, nonkeratinized epithelial lesion with a strong likelihood of malignant transformation. In many cases, carcinoma in situ is already present.
- **Pachydermia**: area of epithelial thickening, more or less completely covered by keratin scales.

In all of these lesions, the degree of dysplasia should be evaluated histologically based on the World Health Organization staging system for epithelial dysplasia (see also **Fig. 17.32** in **17.10**):

- Hyperplasia.
- (Hyper)keratosis.
- Dysplasia (three grades: mild, moderate, severe).
- Intraepithelial neoplasia.

In principle, squamous cell carcinoma of the larynx can develop from all histologic grades of epithelial dysplasia (see **Fig. 17.32** in **17.10**). In a smaller percentage of laryngeal cancers, especially at the supraglottic level, normal epithelium may also undergo a direct malignant transformation.

These epithelial changes may be asymptomatic but often cause complaints in the form of hoarseness, dry cough, or a foreign-body sensation. The lesions are nine times more common in men than in women.

The changes visible by indirect laryngoscopy most commonly affect the vocal cords but may involve any portion of the larynx. Microlaryngoscopy is indicated for tissue sampling and histologic evaluation and may involve complete removal of the affected mucosa. In cases with vocal cord involvement, the histologic degree of dysplasia will determine whether it is possible to remove the epithelium of the vocal folds while leaving the vocal ligament intact.

All cases require regular follow-ups and particularly the elimination of causal agents (cessation of smoking).

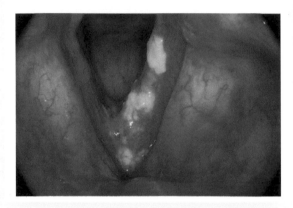

**Fig. 17.33   Laryngeal leukoplakia: this may be an (invasive) glottic carcinoma**

management. Like all head and neck tumors, laryngeal carcinoma is staged according to international UICC guidelines (**Table 17.8**).

Glottic malignancies have a considerably better *prognosis* than supraglottic or subglottic cancers, not only because of earlier diagnosis but also because of their limited lymphatic drainage (see 17.1, Vascular Supply). Up to 60% of supraglottic and subglottic malignancies already have ipsilateral lymph-node metastases at the time of diagnosis, and up to 30% have bilateral or contralateral regional nodal metastases, which imply a very poor prognosis. By contrast, less than 10% of tumors confined to the glottic plane are accompanied by regional metastases when diagnosed. Distant metastases, which most often spread hematogenously to the lung and then require differentiation from a second primary (bronchial carcinoma), are unusual with laryngeal malignancies, and asymptomatic patients require no screening tests for distant metastases other than a computed tomography of the chest. As with all other tumors of the upper aerodigestive tract, the simultaneous or metachronous occurrence of second tumors in the upper foodway and airway is of major significance in patients with laryngeal cancer. The UICC staging system displayed in **Table 17.9** is based on local tumor extent (T category),

regional lymph-node involvement (N category, see **Table 16.5**), and distant metastasis (M category).

*Symptoms:* The symptoms of laryngeal malignancies—foreign-body sensation, habitual throat clearing, dysphagia, respiratory distress, hemoptysis—depend on the location and extent of the tumor. Glottic malignancies, even when small, are likely to cause voice change (hoarseness) as their initial symptom, enabling them to be diagnosed at an earlier stage than supraglottic malignancies, which often remain silent for some time. The cardinal symptoms of subglottic cancers are dyspnea and inspiratory stridor.

Hoarseness that persists longer than 2 to 3 weeks should be investigated by laryngoscopy.

Earache in the absence of otoscopic abnormalities, known as referred otalgia, may signify tumor-related irritation of the vagus nerve in the larynx and hypopharynx.

*Diagnosis:* Suspicious cases are initially evaluated by indirect laryngoscopy, giving particular attention to vocal cord mobility. The examiner should also palpate the laryngeal skeleton (for extralaryngeal tumor

**Table 17.8** Classification of laryngeal carcinoma according to the Union for International Cancer Control (UICC) system

| T | Primary tumor |
|---|---|
| TX | Primary tumor cannot be assessed |
| T0 | No evidence of primary tumor |
| Tis | Carcinoma in situ |
| **Supraglottis** | |
| T1 | Tumor limited to one subsite of supraglottis with normal vocal cord mobility |
| T2 | Tumor invades more than one adjacent subsite of supraglottis or glottis or region outside the supraglottis (e.g., mucosa of the base of the tongue, vallecula, medial wall of the piriform sinus), without fixation of the larynx |
| T3 | Tumor limited to larynx with vocal cord fixation and/or invasion of postcricoid area, preepiglottic space, paraglottic space, and/or inner cortex of thyroid cartilage |
| T4a | Tumor invades through the thyroid cartilage and/or invades soft tissues beyond the larynx, e.g., trachea, soft tissues of the neck including deep/extrinsic muscle of tongue (genioglossus, hyoglossus, palatoglossus, and styloglossus), strap muscles, thyroid, or esophagus |
| T4b | Tumor invades prevertebral space, mediastinal structures, or encases carotid artery |
| **Glottis** | |
| T1 | Tumor limited to vocal cord(s) (may involve anterior or posterior commissure) with normal mobility |
| T1a | Tumor limited to one vocal cord |
| T1b | Tumor involves both vocal cords |
| T2 | Tumor extends to supraglottis and/or subglottis, and/or with impaired vocal cord mobility |
| T3 | Tumor limited to the larynx with vocal cord fixation and/or invades paraglottic space, and/or inner cortex of thyroid cartilage |
| T4a | Tumor invades through the outer cortex of the thyroid cartilage and/or invades tissues beyond the larynx, e.g., trachea, soft tissues of the neck including deep/extrinsic muscle of tongue (genioglossus, hyoglossus, palatoglossus, and styloglossus), strap muscles, thyroid, esophagus |
| T4b | Tumor invades prevertebral space, mediastinal structures, or encases carotid artery |
| **Subglottis** | |
| T1 | Tumor limited to the subglottis |
| T2 | Tumor extends to vocal cord(s) with normal or impaired mobility |
| T3 | Tumor limited to the larynx with vocal cord fixation |
| T4a | Tumor invades cricoid or thyroid cartilage and/or invades tissues beyond the larynx, e.g., trachea, soft tissues of the neck including deep/extrinsic muscle of tongue (genioglossus, hyoglossus, palatoglossus, and styloglossus), strap muscles, thyroid, esophagus |
| T4b | Tumor invades prevertebral space, mediastinal structures, or encases carotid artery |
| N | Regional lymph nodes |
| N1 | Metastasis in a single ipsilateral lymph node, < 3 cm without ENE |
| N2a | Metastasis in a single ipsilateral lymph node, 3–6 cm without ENE |
| N2b | Metastasis in multiple ipsilateral lymph nodes, none > 6 cm, without ENE |
| N2c | Metastasis in bilateral or contralateral lymph nodes, none > 6 cm, without ENE |
| N3a | Metastasis in a lymph node > 6 cm without ENE |
| N3b | Metastasis in single or multiple lymph nodes with clinical ENE |
| M | Distant metastasis |
| M0 | No distant metastasis |
| M1 | Distant metastasis |

Abbreviation: ENE, extranodal extension.
Source: Brierley et al 2017.

extension) and the soft tissues of the neck (for lymph-node metastases). Ultrasonography of the cervical soft tissues is an essential part of the basic work-up to detect possible regional metastasis. Computed tomography and MRI can be helpful in verifying tumor extent.

Microlaryngoscopy (**Fig. 17.34**) is used to define the precise tumor extent and to obtain histologic tissue samples that can differentiate cancer from other laryngeal pathology such as chronic laryngitis or benign endolaryngeal neoplasms. This procedure should include panendoscopy (inspection of the nasopharynx, oropharynx, hypopharynx, tracheobronchial passages, and esophagus) to exclude second tumors.

*Treatment:* The main therapeutic options are surgery and radiotherapy, **in some cases with simultaneous chemotherapy**. Surgery remains the primary treatment of choice, however.

**Table 17.9  TNM categories of laryngeal carcinoma**

| Stage | T | N | M |
|---|---|---|---|
| 0 | Tis | N0 | M0 |
| I | T1 | N0 | M0 |
| II | T2 | N0 | M0 |
| III | T3 | N0 | M0 |
|  | T1–3 | N1 | M0 |
| IV A | T4a | N0–1 | M0 |
|  | T1–T4a | N2 | M0 |
| IV B | T4b | Any N | M0 |
|  | Any T | N3 | M0 |
| IV C | Any T | Any N | M1 |

Source: Brierley et al 2017.

A larynx-sparing and voice-sparing partial resection can be done in a large percentage of patients, depending on the tumor location and extent. This is a particularly good option with circumscribed tumors.

With more extensive tumors (T3, T4), which may broadly infiltrate adjacent structures, complete removal of the larynx (laryngectomy) is occasionally unavoidable for oncologic reasons.

Generally, a neck dissection is unnecessary with small glottic carcinomas (Tis, T1), but it is indicated for higher tumor categories and especially for supraglottic and subglottic cancers. The need for postoperative radiotherapy will depend on the location and extent of the tumor and on lymphogenous metastasis. ⏧ **17.12** illustrates several partial laryngectomy techniques in current use.

**Fig. 17.34  Laryngeal carcinomas**

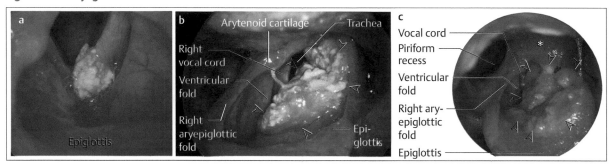

**a** Glottic carcinoma involving the anterior third of the left vocal cord (T1a).
**b** Glottic–supraglottic carcinoma involving the left side of the larynx (T3; arrows).

**c** Supraglottic carcinoma (arrows) arising from the epiglottis. Note the edematous swelling of the arytenoid region on the affected side (*).

---

⏧ **17.12  Surgical treatment options for laryngeal carcinoma**

**Glottic carcinoma**

*Voice-sparing procedures*

Vocal cord stripping (**Fig. 17.35a**):
*Principle:* removal of the vocal cord epithelium.
*Approach:* endolaryngeal by microlaryngoscopy.
*Indication:* epithelial dysplasia, intraepithelial neoplasia.

Partial or complete cordectomy (**Fig. 17.35b**):
*Principle:* removal of the tumor-involved portion of the vocal cord.
*Approach:* endolaryngeal by microlaryngoscopy with $CO_2$ laser resection or external access via thyrotomy (incision of thyroid cartilage).
*Indication:* T1a laryngeal carcinoma.

More extensive partial laryngectomies (**Fig. 17.35c**):
*Principle:* supraglottic, glottic, or subglottic tissue resection for bilateral and advanced glottic malignancies, may include resection of cartilaginous structures from the thyroid and/or cricoid cartilage; can be extended to a hemilaryngectomy.
*Approach:* external via thyrotomy (incision or resection or thyroid cartilage) or endolaryngeal by microlaryngoscopy with $CO_2$ laser resection.
*Indication:* T1b or T2 glottic carcinoma; can be extended under certain conditions to remove more extensive tumors.

*Non–voice-sparing procedure*

Total laryngectomy (**Fig. 17.35d**):
*Principle:* complete removal of the larynx with separation of the airway and foodway and construction of a permanent tracheostomy.
*Approach:* external.
*Indication:* advanced laryngeal tumors that cannot be adequately removed by other procedures in accordance with oncologic principles.

**Supraglottic laryngeal carcinoma**

*Voice-sparing procedure*

Horizontal partial laryngectomy (**Fig. 17.35e**):
*Principle:* removal of the supraglottic larynx with preservation the glottic plane and arytenoid cartilages.
*Approach:* external via horizontal partial laryngectomy or endolaryngeal by microlaryngoscopy with $CO_2$ laser resection.
*Indication:* T1 and T2 supraglottic malignancies; may be suitable for more extensive tumors.

*Non–voice-sparing procedure*

Laryngectomy (**Fig. 17.35d**):
*Principle and approach:* see above.
*Indication:* advanced laryngeal tumors that cannot be adequately removed by other procedures in accordance with oncologic principles.

⚬ **17.12  Surgical treatment options for laryngeal carcinoma** *(continuation)*

**Fig. 17.35  Surgical treatment of laryngeal carcinoma**

a  Vocal cord stripping

b  Excision of vocal cord

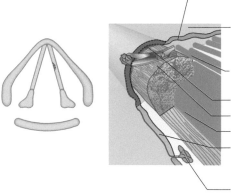
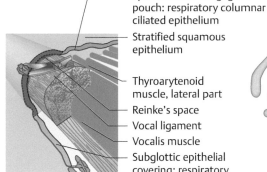
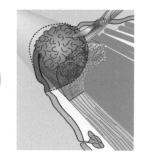

- Epithelium of Morgagni's pouch: respiratory columnar ciliated epithelium
- Stratified squamous epithelium
- Thyroarytenoid muscle, lateral part
- Reinke's space
- Vocal ligament
- Vocalis muscle
- Subglottic epithelial covering: respiratory columnar ciliated epithelium
- Mucous gland

c  More extensive partial laryngectomy

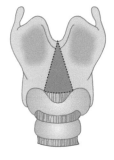
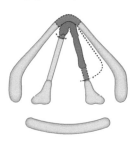
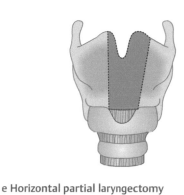
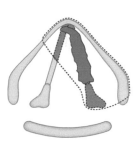

d  Laryngectomy

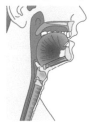
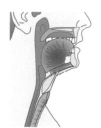

Before laryngectomy    After laryngectomy

e Horizontal partial laryngectomy

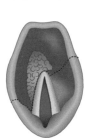
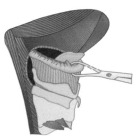

Source: **a, b** Becker et al 1989; **e** Naumann 1998, Naumann et al 1995.

Early glottic cancers are sometimes treated with radiotherapy alone, the major advantage being superior voice quality after treatment. Disadvantages are the necessary length of treatment (~6 weeks), a higher complication rate in surgery for recurrent or residual disease, and the risk of radiation-induced malignancy. In patients with advanced tumors, radiotherapy alone has so far been used only as a palliative treatment. Modern fractionation schemes for radiotherapy, combined with the use of cytostatics, may open up new possibilities in the future.

Today, the highest cure rates for laryngeal malignancies are achieved with surgery, which may be followed by radiotherapy in patients with advanced tumors and especially metastases.

*Prognosis*: The prognosis depends on the location and stage of the disease. While T1 glottic carcinomas have a 5-year survival rate of up to 100%, the rates associated with advanced glottic cancer (T4) decline to about 50%. Supraglottic carcinoma has a considerably poorer prognosis even in T1 cases, which have a 5-year survival rate of 70 to 80%. The 5-year survival with advanced tumors is 30 to 40%.

### Functional Sequelae of Surgery for Laryngeal Malignancies

Permanent voice change is a very common sequel to partial laryngectomy, depending on the resection technique. But a much more serious problem for patients is the swallowing difficulty that can result from impairment of the laryngeal sphincter function following a very extensive partial laryngectomy. This can lead to chronic aspiration with recurrent bouts of pneumonia and may ultimately require separating the respiratory and digestive tracts by performing a total laryngectomy.

Swallowing function is generally not impaired after a total laryngectomy, but laryngeal voice production is lost.

### Laryngectomy Effects and Voice Rehabilitation

Since a total laryngectomy completely separates the respiratory tract from the digestive tract, laryngectomized patients have respiratory anosmia due to the absence of nasal airflow but still have intact gustatory olfaction. They can no longer sneeze, blow their nose, or perform a Valsalva maneuver. The nose and pharynx can no longer condition the inspired air, and so the air inhaled through the tracheostomy is neither warmed nor humidified, especially at certain times of the year. This can lead to irritation of the trachea mucosa (tracheitis) with crusting. Shields can be worn to protect the tracheostomy while bathing or showering. Various options are available for voice rehabilitation after laryngectomy, all of which require intensive speech training by a therapist. It is always helpful to teach the patient esophageal speech, which is produced by swallowing air into the esophagus and forcing it back up against folds of mucosa in the upper esophagus and hypopharynx.

Another method of voice restoration is to create a tracheoesophageal fistula through which air can be forced into the upper part of the esophagus, with mucosal folds in the pharyngoesophageal segment functioning as a speech generator. The tracheoesophageal fistula may be surgically constructed ("neoglottis," with risk of aspiration during swallowing), or a valve prosthesis may be placed between the trachea and esophagus (**Fig. 17.36**). Another option is to use electronic devices for speech production. In this method, an external sound generator transmits vibrations to the pharyngeal wall and oral floor, setting the air in the resonant chambers (pharynx, mouth, nose) into vibration and producing speech. The role of these devices is limited, however, by the relatively poor quality and mechanical nature of the sound.

It is extremely helpful to refer laryngectomized patients to self-help groups (e.g., the International Association of Laryngectomees) once they have been made aware of the options for voice rehabilitation after laryngectomy.

### Oncologic Follow-Up

Regular oncologic follow-up visits are scheduled chiefly for the purpose of detecting a local or regional tumor recurrence while it is still asymptomatic. The high incidence of metachronous second tumors in the upper aerodigestive tract is also a major concern, requiring that all risk-exposed mucosal areas be examined during each follow-up. The standard follow-up examination includes a specific history, a complete

Fig. 17.36 **Speech valve prosthesis**

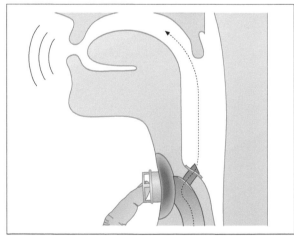

Principle of a speech valve prosthesis for voice rehabilitation after laryngectomy, illustrated here for a Provox valve.

otolaryngologic examination, and palpation and ultrasound scanning of the cervical soft tissues. If the findings raise the suspicion of a tumor, or if all mucosal areas cannot be reliably evaluated, it may be necessary to proceed with panendoscopy under general anesthesia.

In scheduling the follow-up intervals, it should be kept in mind that the great majority of locoregional recurrences are diagnosed within 2 years after the primary treatment.

## Tracheal Tumors

### Chondroma, Osteochondroma, Osteoma

These cartilaginous and bony neoplasms may be manifested in the trachea and the main bronchi. They appear endoscopically as a thickening of tracheal or bronchial cartilages and are surrounded by a capsule. Endoscopic biopsy is often unsuccessful due to the hardness of the tumors. They grow very slowly but have the potential to cause extensive bronchopulmonary destruction. Sarcomatous transformation has been described. Treatment consists of partial or—if possible—complete surgical removal.

### Tracheopathia osteochondroplastica

This condition is based on a malformation of the tracheal and bronchial cartilages. Abnormal deposits of cartilaginous tissue in the endotracheal mucosa during embryonic development present postnatally as numerous small bony or cartilaginous tumors that project into the tracheal lumen and may cause progressive airway obstruction. There is no causal treatment for this disease, which is manifested by wheezing, coughing, hemoptysis, and increasing respiratory distress.

Progressive airway obstruction is relieved by debulking or removing the lesions that cause the greatest degree of luminal narrowing.

### Malignant Tumors of the Trachea

Primary malignancies of the trachea are very rare. The most common type is adenoid cystic carcinoma (**Fig. 17.37**). It is much more common, however, for

**Fig. 17.37   Adenoid cystic carcinoma of the trachea**

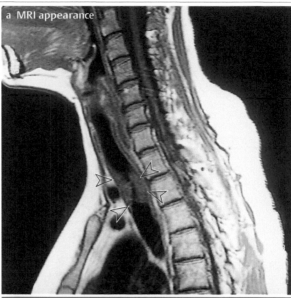
a MRI appearance

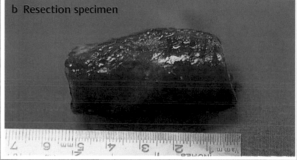
b Resection specimen

**a** Arrows indicate the carcinoma.
**b** Surgical specimen following resection and end-to-end anastomosis.
Source: Prof. B. Kramann, Homburg, Saar, Germany.

malignant tumors to invade the trachea from adjacent structures (larynx, hypopharynx, esophagus, thyroid gland). Surgical treatment is the best option whenever it can be done with curative intent. Otherwise, radiotherapy and/or chemotherapy should be considered, depending on the tumor histology. An essential palliative measure is airway maintenance. This can be done by repeated (laser) tumor debulking, stent insertion, or tracheotomy.

# 17.8 Airway Management

The principal methods of airway management—establishing an airway, stenting, preventing blood aspiration, ventilation—are intubation (see textbooks of anesthesiology and emergency medicine), cricothyrotomy, and tracheotomy. Special care measures are needed in tracheotomized patients.

## Tracheotomy and Cricothyrotomy

Tracheotomy refers to an incision of the trachea below the larynx. In the technique that is now most favored, the isthmus of the thyroid gland is transected and an opening is made between the second and third tracheal rings.

### Elective Tracheotomy

An elective tracheotomy (indications: **Table 17.10**) is performed under controlled surgical conditions. The opening in the cartilage should not exceed a critical size; otherwise, subsequent closure of the tracheotomy could lead to tracheal stenosis due to the loss of cartilaginous substance. It is particularly important in children to avoid resecting any cartilaginous structures, as this could lead to refractory postoperative complications.

The anterior wall of the trachea is sutured to the skin of the neck to create an epithelialized tract (**Fig. 17.38**). Unlike a nonepithelialized tracheostomy, this type of tracheostomy eliminates the danger of false passage during cannula changes and avoids the risk of a descending pretracheal inflammation.

### Emergency Tracheotomy

Orotracheal or nasotracheal intubation is the usual primary method of airway intervention in patients with acute respiratory distress caused by an upper airway obstruction between the dental arch and larynx. Today, this method is rapidly available, largely standardized, and has a low complication rate (see textbooks of anesthesiology). Occasionally, however, intubation is unsuccessful even when done under operative conditions and endoscopic control (fiberoptic intubation), and it may be necessary to open the trachea to establish a secure airway. When the head is fully extended and neck anatomy is undistorted, the cervical trachea is palpable and visible in the midline beneath the skin. In a highly acute emergency situation, incision of the trachea may be hampered by subcutaneous tissue layers and especially by bleeding from the thyroid isthmus.

**Table 17.10   Indications for elective tracheotomy**

- Laryngeal stenosis caused by:
  - Tumors
  - Swelling (e.g., postirradiation)
  - Bilateral vocal cord paralysis
  - Subglottic stenosis
- Tracheal stenosis above the proposed stoma site
- Prolonged mechanical ventilation (see 17.6, Effects of [Prolonged] Intubation)
- Pulmonary diseases (to facilitate bronchial toilet and reduce dead space)
- Postoperative airway management following upper respiratory tract surgery

In children, very strict criteria should be applied in assessing the need for tracheotomy.

**Fig. 17.38   Principle of elective tracheotomy**

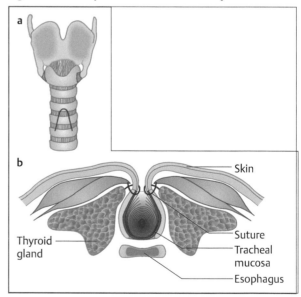

**a** Incision of the anterior tracheal wall.
**b** Schematic cross section of an epithelialized tracheostomy.

## Cricothyrotomy

Synonym: coniotomy.

Cricothyrotomy, in which the airway is opened through the cricothyroid ligament between the thyroid cartilage and cricoid cartilage, is still an important procedure in emergency situations (**Fig. 17.39**). This area of the larynx is subcutaneous, is easily palpated, and can be opened with a transverse incision. The instrument used to make the luminal incision (e.g., pocketknife) should be held perpendicular to the skin and should not be withdrawn until the tube has been introduced between the thyroid and cricoid cartilages; otherwise, the tissue planes would shift and block access to the lumen. It is very helpful to include a ready-to-use cricothyrotomy set in every emergency kit (**Fig. 17.39**). A cricothyrotomy should be converted to a standard tracheotomy as soon as possible due to the danger of cricoid cartilage injury with intralaryngeal stenosis.

## Percutaneous Tracheotomy

In this technique, a needle is inserted between the tracheal rings, a guidewire is introduced, the tract is dilated, and finally the tracheotomy tube is introduced over the guidewire into a palpable area of the trachea. Percutaneous tracheotomy is most commonly used in emergency medicine and to establish a temporary tracheostomy in intensive-care settings.
Commercial sets are available for percutaneous tracheotomy, which requires a familiarity with cervical anatomy.

## The Tracheotomized Patient

Tracheotomized patients with an intact larynx can speak by plugging the tracheotomy tube with a finger or cap. Voice quality will depend on the extent of pathology in the laryngeal region. A *speaking tube* with a valve suspended in the inspiratory/expiratory air stream will also allow for phonation. **Fig. 17.40** shows an assortment of commonly used tracheostomy tubes. Tracheotomized patients and their families should be taught the specifics of tracheostomy care before leaving the hospital. This includes accessories for tracheotomized patients such as a suction device, an inhalation and/or room-humidifier unit, dressings, and tube care materials. The selection of the tube material (plastic, silver, cuffed or noncuffed) depends on the underlying disease, the necessary duration of the tracheostomy, and local findings.
Respiratory distress in tracheotomized patients usually signifies obstruction of the trachea due to crusting. Initial emergency measures are decannulation, tracheoscopy, and removal of the crusts as needed.
In a temporary tracheotomy, the tube is withdrawn at the end of the tracheotomy period and the stoma is

Fig. 17.39  Cricothyrotomy

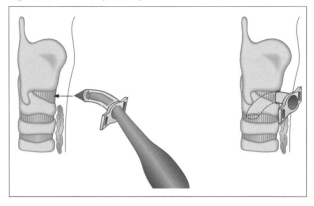

Fig. 17.40  Tracheostomy tubes

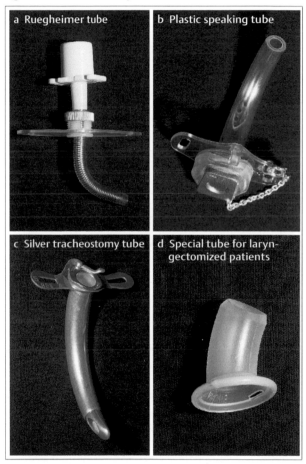

Essential criteria that distinguish different tubes are diameter, material, length, curvature, and the presence of an inflatable cuff.

closed with an airtight adhesive seal to make certain that the patient can breathe adequately on his own. This tentative closure, combined with removal of the tube, will cause the stoma to shrink and facilitate surgical closure. Especially with an epithelialized tracheostoma, plastic surgical technique should be used in making the definitive closure.

# 17.9    Neurogenic Disorders of the Larynx

Paralysis of the vocal cord muscles supplied by the recurrent laryngeal nerves often has an iatrogenic cause (e.g., thyroid gland surgery) as well as unknown idiopathic causes. The cardinal symptom of unilateral vocal cord paralysis is hoarseness, whereas bilateral paralysis is manifested by dyspnea, which often necessitates emergency intervention. Isolated paralysis of the superior laryngeal nerve and vagus nerve is relatively rare.

## Recurrent Laryngeal Nerve Paralysis

It is necessary to distinguish between unilateral and bilateral recurrent laryngeal nerve paralysis due to their different cardinal symptoms and treatment strategies.

### Unilateral Recurrent Laryngeal Nerve Paralysis

*Epidemiology and etiopathogenesis:* The typical causes of recurrent laryngeal nerve paralysis are listed in **Table 17.11**. The most frequent cause is a lesion sustained during **thyroid surgery**, with reported lesion rates of 0.14 to 5.0% in initial operations and up to 20% in revision procedures. These figures pertain to unilateral recurrent laryngeal nerve lesions detected immediately after surgery. With lesions that do not disrupt the continuity of the nerve, it is reasonable to expect that functional recovery will occur within weeks or months in a certain percentage of cases. Intraoperative exposure of the recurrent laryngeal nerves during thyroid surgery lowers the lesion rate.
"Idiopathic" vocal cord paralysis is diagnosed by exclusion upon the completion of comprehensive diagnostic tests (see below). This condition is more common in men than women, has a peak incidence at 20 to 30 years of age, and affects the left side more often than the right side. It is assumed to have a viral etiology, as it is often preceded by an upper respiratory infection.

*Symptoms:* The chief complaint of unilateral recurrent laryngeal nerve paralysis is hoarseness. Respiratory distress is generally not observed.

*Diagnosis:* At telescopic laryngoscopy, unilateral vocal cord immobility is noted *during respiration*. Usually, the vocal cord is fixed in a **paramedian position** (**Fig. 17.41** and **Fig. 17.42**), but the vocal cord position alone is not a reliable indicator of lesion location. If a cause cannot be identified, a diagnosis of "idiopathic" paralysis should not be made until further tests have been performed. These include examination of the thyroid gland and neck (ultrasonography), the mediastinum (computed tomography or MRI), serologic tests, and a possible history of exposure to harmful agents.

| Table 17.11    Causes of recurrent laryngeal nerve paralysis |
|---|
| **Unilateral** |
| • Iatrogenic nerve injury, especially in thyroid operations (most frequent cause, usually affecting the left side) and surgery of the esophagus, trachea, mediastinum, lung, or heart. Variations in the course of the nerve (e.g., a "nonrecurrent" recurrent nerve) are a predisposing factor |
| • Infiltration or compression of the nerve by tumors of the thyroid gland, larynx, trachea, or mediastinum |
| • Laryngeal trauma |
| • Nerve compression by mediastinal masses (known as Ortner's syndrome, e.g., cardiac hypertrophy, aortic aneurysm, malignant lymphoma, sarcoidosis) |
| • Infectious or toxic neuritis (e.g., influenza viruses, herpes viruses, alcohol, lead, arsenic, vinca alkaloids) |
| • (Poly)neuritis in the setting of a rheumatoid or (auto)immune disease |
| • Infectious diseases: Lyme disease, syphilis, mononucleosis |
| • Diabetic (poly)neuropathy |
| • Idiopathic (~20% of cases; viral and other etiologies have been proposed) |
| **Bilateral** |
| • Preexisting unilateral recurrent laryngeal nerve paralysis, with one of the above causes supervening |
| • Both recurrent laryngeal nerves affected by one of the above causes |
| • Iatrogenic bilateral nerve injury (usually in thyroid operations, especially malignant tumor resections and resections of large or recurrent goiters; also surgery of the trachea and esophagus) |
| • Simultaneous bilateral recurrent nerve paralysis caused by infectious or toxic agents is relatively rare but may occur |

**Electromyography (EMG)**, which may employ needle electrodes inserted transorally or transcervically into the vocal cords under local or general anesthesia without muscle relaxation, supplies information useful in assessing the cause, extent, and prognosis of the lesion. EMG is also helpful in differentiating a recurrent laryngeal nerve lesion from the rare conditions of *arytenoid dislocation*, which is usually caused by intubation trauma, and *arytenoid fixation* by scar tissue (detectable muscle activity).

An examination of the larynx to assess vocal cord mobility is essential before and after thyroid surgery (strumectomy, thyroidectomy).

*Treatment:* The treatment of unilateral recurrent laryngeal nerve paralysis depends chiefly on its cause. If the paralysis occurs immediately after a surgical procedure in the territory of the nerve, it should first be determined whether the nerve is transected or whether it still has continuity and may have been functionally compromised due to pressure (hematoma, nerve caught in a stitch). Because the recurrent laryngeal nerve supplies nerve fibers to both agonistic and antagonistic muscles (abductors and adductors), there is little hope of success in reapproximating a completely severed nerve, even if the ends can be found, due to the erratic nature of regeneration by axonal sprouting. But if continuity of the nerve is preserved, an immediate revision procedure can be done to decompress the nerve and promote regeneration. Whenever possible, causal therapy should be attempted first for nontraumatic nerve lesions, depending on the established or presumed cause. An unsevered nerve can regenerate, and it is very likely that recovery will occur within 6 to 12 months. It is rare for spontaneous recovery to occur after 1 year.

Long-term unilateral recurrent laryngeal nerve paralysis leads to muscular atrophy with excavation of the vocal cord and persistent vocal dysfunction.

Voice therapy may help to reduce hoarseness in patients with persistent unilateral vocal cord paralysis. Other options are augmentation of the paralyzed vocal cord by the injection of Teflon or autologous collagen and a medialization procedure to improve vocal cord position (see 18.2).

### Bilateral Recurrent Laryngeal Nerve Paralysis

*Etiology:* See **Table 17.11**.

*Symptoms:* The chief complaint is dyspnea—ranging in severity from resting dyspnea to dyspnea on exertion—because the paralyzed vocal cords assume an almost closed position due to the relative predominance of the adductor muscles over the abductors (see **Table 17.1**). The severity of the dyspnea depends on the residual glottic gap. Additional mucosal swelling due to intubation or infection can exacerbate the respiratory distress.

*Diagnosis:* Telescopic laryngoscopy *during respiration* usually shows the vocal cords fixed in a paramedian position and displaying only passive motion in response to transglottic airflow. The diagnostic methods described under unilateral recurrent laryngeal nerve paralysis should be applied as needed.

**Fig. 17.41 Vocal cord position in laryngeal paralysis**

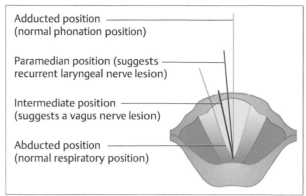

The vocal cord position can be a useful suggestive sign, but it does not indicate the precise location of the nerve lesion.

**Fig. 17.42 Vocal cord position in recurrent laryngeal nerve paralysis**

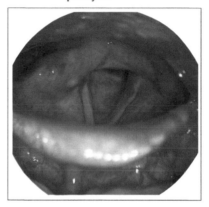

Laryngoscopic appearance of the vocal cords during respiration in a patient with right-sided recurrent laryngeal nerve paralysis. While the left vocal cord is well abducted, the right vocal cord is fixed in a paramedian position.

*Treatment:* When bilateral vocal cord paralysis is noted immediately after a surgical procedure (e.g., strumectomy), it should first be determined whether it is advisable to perform an immediate revision procedure with neurolysis of one or both nerves. If the nerves have not definitely been severed, this type of surgery is generally indicated.

An immediate tracheotomy is unavoidable in the great majority of cases.

The next step is to wait and see if one or both nerves regenerate. A prognosis can be offered based on the EMG findings.

Surgical procedures to widen the glottis should be considered no earlier than 6 months after the onset of paralysis.

With persistent bilateral recurrent laryngeal nerve paralysis, the goal of further treatment is to widen the glottic gap and eliminate the need for tracheotomy. This can be done either by suturing portions of one vocal cord in a lateralized position (laterofixation,

**Fig. 17.43    Laterofixation of a vocal cord**

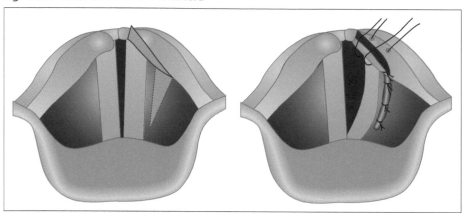

In cases of persistent bilateral recurrent laryngeal nerve paralysis, the glottic aperture can be sufficiently widened for respiration by lateralizing one of the vocal cords. The drawings illustrate a technique in which two narrow mucosal triangles are resected in the false vocal cord and over the arytenoid cartilage, which is also removed.
Source: Naumann 1972.

**Fig. 17.43**) or by partially resecting one vocal cord and/or an arytenoid cartilage. This may be done internally through an endolaryngeal approach or externally through an extralaryngeal approach, using any of several available techniques (over 100 have been described). When postoperative swelling has subsided and the patient is doing well, the tracheostomy can be closed in a separate sitting.

The goal is to achieve a glottic width of 3 to 5 mm, which represents a compromise between good respiration and acceptable voice quality. As the glottic width increases, respiration improves, while phonation becomes poorer.

▯ Laterofixation always aims for the best tradeoff between voice quality and respiratory function for the individual patient. The surgical procedure should also be tailored to the specific patient (age, desired voice quality).

## Superior Laryngeal Nerve Paralysis

Paralysis of the superior laryngeal nerve may be iatrogenic following thyroid surgery (usually affects only the motor component) or laryngeal surgery (also affects the sensory component). It is less common than recurrent laryngeal nerve paralysis and usually does not produce motor symptoms. Only singers and professional speakers will notice the (unilateral) loss of innervation to the cricothyroid muscle (**Table 17.12**). The vocal cord on the affected side appears flaccid at laryngoscopy because the posterior commissure is deviated toward the side of the paralysis, causing a slight length discrepancy between the vocal cords. Voice therapy may be appropriate in some cases. A more serious concern is the impairment of laryngeal sensation that occurs in cases with internal branch involvement. Bilateral lesions are particularly likely to cause dysphagia with aspiration, and care should be taken to avoid these lesions during laryngeal surgery. If these symptoms fail to improve with swallowing exercises,

**Table 17.12    Symptoms of unilateral paralysis of the superior laryngeal nerve**

- Low-frequency vocal range
- Deeper, monopitched speaking voice
- Inability to sing higher notes
- Breathy voice that fatigues easily
- Decrease in maximum phonation time

Source: Berendes 1982.

laryngectomy may be considered as a final recourse on functional grounds.

## Vagus Nerve Paralysis

*Etiology and pathogenesis:* Vagus nerve lesions are much less common than recurrent laryngeal nerve paralysis. Possible causes are listed in **Table 17.13**.

*Symptoms:* The symptoms basically represent a combination of the symptoms associated with recurrent laryngeal nerve paralysis and superior laryngeal nerve paralysis. In the rare cases with bilateral vagus nerve lesions, the dominant feature is dyspnea. The chief complaint in unilateral paralysis is hoarseness.

*Diagnosis:* Telescopic laryngoscopy again shows an immobile vocal cord, which is usually described as being fixed in an **intermediate position**. This may be true in the early phase, but as other factors supervene (e.g., atrophy of the denervated muscles) the vocal cord position is not a reliable site-of-lesion indicator. Depending on the presumed location of the lesion, the patient should be referred for a neurologic work-up that includes cranial imaging and/or an examination of the neck (ultrasound, computed tomography, MRI).

*Treatment:* Treatment is tailored to the established or presumed etiology. The treatment options described for recurrent laryngeal nerve paralysis are also appropriate for vagus nerve paralysis.

| Table 17.13 Causes of vagus nerve paralysis |
| --- |

**Intramedullary** (see also textbooks of neurology)
- Congenital: Arnold–Chiari syndrome, Dandy–Walker syndrome, syringobulbia, myelomeningocele, Klippel–Feil syndrome, aplasia of vagal nuclei (Gerhardt's syndrome)
- Inflammatory: poliomyelitis, herpes zoster, Guillain–Barré syndrome, diphtheria, tabes dorsalis
- Vascular: thrombosis, hemorrhage, angioma, Wallenberg's syndrome
- Tumors of the brainstem and floor of the fourth ventricle
- Disseminated encephalomyelitis

**Extramedullary**
- Tumors in the area of the jugular foramen (e.g., paragangliomas)
- Basal skull fractures
- Vagus neurinomas (cardinal symptom: coughing fit triggered by palpation of the mass)
- Trauma: stab wounds and gunshot injuries, iatrogenic lesion caused by local anesthesia, neck dissection, revascularizing procedures on the carotid artery

### 17.13 Superior laryngeal neuralgia

Shooting, throbbing pain lasting seconds to hours or a constant ache lasting several hours or days in the side of the neck may be caused by superior laryngeal neuralgia (Avellis' syndrome). The point of maximum pain intensity is usually at the site where the internal branch enters the thyrohyoid membrane. The pain may radiate to the ear, tongue, and throat. Differentiation is mainly required from dentogenic causes, sialolithiasis, and glossopharyngeal neuralgia (which may coexist with superior laryngeal neuralgia).

The treatment of first choice is local infiltration of the nerve with a long-acting local anesthetic. Pregabalin, gabapentin, and carbamazepine have also proved beneficial. Another option is surgical division of the nerve (for functional sequelae, see Superior Laryngeal Nerve Paralysis above).

# 18    Voice Disorders

## 18.1    Clinical Voice Physiology and Diagnostic Procedures

Verbal communication is the essential foundation for interpersonal contacts and for human culture in general. It is inextricably linked to the integrity of receptive language function (hearing and understanding) and of expressive language abilities. In this textbook of otolaryngology, we are concerned mainly with the laryngologic aspects of communication disorders.

### Basic Principles of Speech Production

#### Physiology

The most important anatomic structures for speech production are the vocal cords (vocal folds), which form the lateral boundaries of the glottis (see also ✏17.1).

The **primary voice signal** is produced in the larynx by the vibrations of the vocal cords and is sustained by a dynamic equilibrium between the expiratory air pressure and the muscular tone of the vocal cords.

Vocal cord vibration consists of a complex three-dimensional motion:

- The basic motion is produced by the predominantly mediolateral vibration of the vocalis muscle and vocal ligament (**Fig. 18.1a**).
- The mobility of the superficial mucosa relative to the vocalis muscle during phonation generates a surface wave in the epithelium. This "traveling wave motion" is superimposed over the transverse vibrations of the vocalis muscle (**Fig. 18.1b**). Normal traveling wave motion is a prerequisite for what is subjectively perceived as "good" voice quality. As the voice becomes louder, the glottis remains closed for a relatively longer time during the vibratory cycle, which maintains a constant period (**Fig. 18.2**).

Based on a simple concept called the *source-filter model*, the primary voice signal is modulated by the resonant cavities of the pharynx, mouth, and nose (the "vocal tract") and is emitted from the mouth as a **complex voice sound** (**Fig. 18.3**). In an ordinary speaker, no interaction takes place between the vocal cord vibrations and the vocal tract. Trained singers or professional speakers learn how to manipulate these interactions to enhance the quality and timbre of their voices.

#### Pathophysiology

Changes in the elasticity of the connective tissue, the tone of the vocalis muscles, and the properties of the epithelium can significantly limit and alter the normal traveling wave motion of the vocal folds. This change is clearly audible, even to laypersons, as a voice disorder.

If the vocal cords snap together too forcefully due to pathology, the vibratory cycle becomes jerky and the voice sounds harsh and grating. If the cords adduct too weakly or are unable to meet, the voice sounds weak and breathy and its loudness cannot be increased. In this case, the vocal cord vibrations can become temporarily desynchronized, causing the right and left sides to vibrate at different fundamental frequencies.

### Changes in the Voice with Aging

When an infant cries for the first time, the larynx begins to function as an organ of phonation. The voice of infants and small children has a very high fundamental frequency (400 Hz), which decreases to approximately 300 Hz as the larynx continues to grow. Laryngeal growth undergoes a sex-specific response to hormonal changes during puberty. As a result, the fundamental frequency of the voice in girls decreases by a third to a fifth to 220 to 250 Hz, while in boys it falls by more than an octave to 110 to 140 Hz (**Fig. 18.4**). This physiologic change or "breaking" of the voice is termed **mutation**.

In adults as well, the phonatory function of the larynx is influenced by hormonal changes (e.g., during pregnancy and menopause). By approximately 70 years of age, the voice acquires a similar pitch in males and females ("senile voice") and loses much of its variety of expression.

### Diagnostic Procedures

All diagnostic evaluation of the voice is based on an endoscopic examination of the larynx. Other basic tests involve the recording, measurement, and evaluation of voice quality and performance. Optional tests such as electromyography (EMG) and respiratory function may also be added.

## Fig. 18.1 Vibratory pattern of the vocal cords

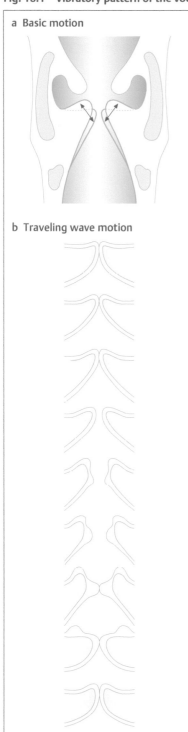

a Basic motion

b Traveling wave motion

**a** The basic vibratory pattern of the vocal cords is antero-lateral motion.
**b** A traveling wave motion of the mucosa is essential for a "normal" sounding voice.

## Fig. 18.2 Phase relationships at different loudness levels

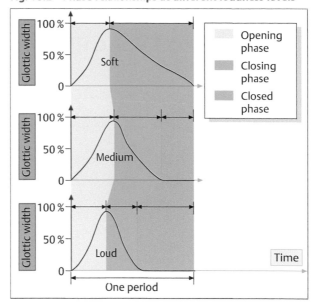

Soft

Medium

Loud

Opening phase

Closing phase

Closed phase

Time

One period

As the voice becomes louder, the relationship between glottic opening and closure is changed. As the sound becomes louder, the vocal cords are adducted more rapidly, and the glottis remains closed for a longer portion of the vibratory cycle.

### Endoscopic Examination

Today, the larynx is always examined with the aid of endoscopic illumination and magnification (rigid telescopic laryngoscope with a 90- or 70-degree viewing angle; see also 17.2). Vocal cord vibrations at a fundamental frequency of 100 to 400 Hz cannot be observed with an ordinary light source, but they can be viewed by **stroboscopy** (**Fig. 18.5**). In this technique, the vibrating vocal cords are illuminated with a strobe light flashed at a rate that is matched to the fundamental frequency of the voice.

An experienced examiner can evaluate the muscular tone and organic symmetry of the vocal cords based on the stroboscopic examination. The findings can be recorded on videotape for analytical playback and can help patients understand the nature of their condition.

### Perceptual Evaluation of the Voice

Despite the availability of quantitative test procedures, the quality of a voice is still evaluated mainly by subjective auditory perception. The following dimensions of voice quality are evaluated in the **RBH system**:

- **R**oughness.
- **B**reathiness.
- **H**oarseness.

Fig. 18.3 Voice production

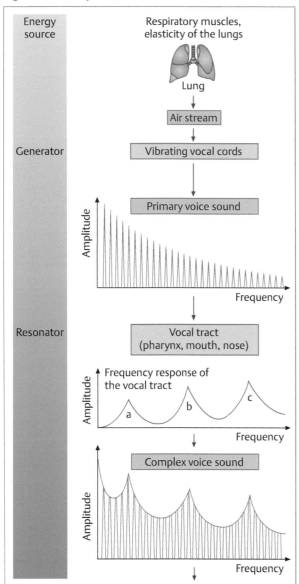

The lung emits an air stream that sets the vocal cords into vibration. The primary voice sound from the vocal cords is transformed by the pharynx, mouth, and nose into a complex voice sound. Peaks a, b, and c represent the formants produced in the supraglottic vocal tract (formant = characteristic component of a sound).

These properties are described more fully in **Table 18.1** and, with a little practice, are easy to distinguish from one another. They are graded on a four-point scale:
**0** = no disorder.
**1** = mild disorder.
**2** = moderate disorder.
**3** = severe disorder.

It should be noted that in the RBH system, roughness and breathiness are rated separately from each other, while hoarseness is considered an "overall measure" of voice quality. Thus, the value of H is always equal to the greater of the R and B values.

**Hoarseness** is the end result of a voice disorder. Because of this, the quality and degree of hoarseness depend little on the specific cause—i.e., various disorders can produce the same hoarseness. Conversely, a particular disease in a patient can cause different types of hoarseness that may vary at different times of day, for example.

🗹 Rating voice quality and identifying the cause of a voice disorder are inherently ambiguous, therefore.

The standard clinical work-up can be supplemented by the **voice range profile**, in which the subject's pitch and loudness ranges are plotted against each other in a two-dimensional graph called a phonetogram. Connecting the upper and lower points in the graph outlines the area within which normal phonation can occur (**Fig. 18.6**). The larger the enclosed area, the greater the "capacity" of the voice.

🗹 This test requires a cooperative patient who can sing musical notes, and so it is subject to uncontrolled influences.

| Table 18.1 Dimensions of voice quality in the RBH system: definition and source | | |
|---|---|---|
| *Sound impression* | *Acoustic definition* | *Source* |
| **R**oughness | Noise components caused by aperiodicities in the fundamental vibration of the voice sound, with superimposed components | Irregularities of vocal cord vibrations, additional sound sources |
| **B**reathiness | Noise components caused by turbulence of unmodulated expiratory airflow | Incomplete glottic closure |
| **H**oarseness | Noise components in speech | All deviations from the normal vibratory pattern of the vocal cords, additional sound sources |

Source: Wendler et al 1996.

**Fig. 18.4 Habitual pitch of the speaking voice before and after puberty**

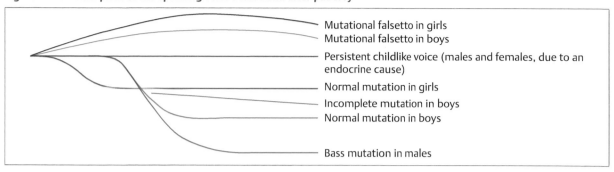

The voice mutates differently in girls and boys during puberty. Mutation disorders (described in 📖18.2) can result in an abnormally high-pitched or low-pitched voice.

**Fig. 18.5 Principle of stroboscopy**

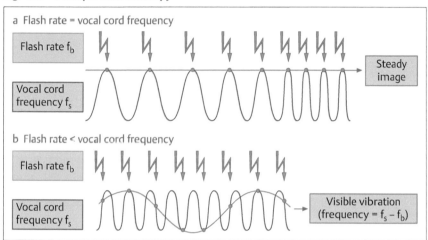

**a** If the flash rate of the stroboscope exactly matches the vocal cord frequency, a steady image is produced.
**b** If the flash rate is slightly different from the vocal cord frequency, the position of the vocal cords in one image is slightly shifted relative to the previous image. The vocal cords appear to move in slow motion.

**Fig. 18.6 Phonetogram**

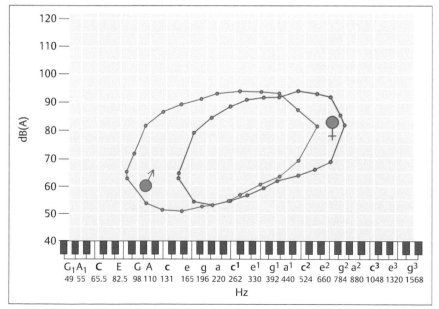

# 18.2 Clinical Aspects of Voice Disorders

A basic distinction is drawn between organic and functional voice disorders (dysphonias). The organic correlates of voice disorders involving the larynx are covered in 🕭17.3–17.7 and 🕭17.9. The present 🕭 deals with the functional aspects of these disorders.

## Organic Dysphonia

*Classification:* Organic voice disorders are distinguished from functional voice disorders and are classified under the following etiologic headings (**Table 18.2**):
- Malformations ("dysplastic dysphonia").
- Trauma.
- Inflammation.
- Tumors.
- Functional disorders.

**Laryngeal malformations** are very rare and may be manifested by the *cardinal symptoms* of dyspnea, dysphonia, and dysphagia. The main functional problem in newborns with laryngeal anomalies is dyspnea (see 🕭17.3, Laryngomalacia), while dysphonia and dysphagia become more important with aging. The main functional priority in children is airway maintenance. The main goal in teenagers and adults is to compensate for the disorder or adapt to the functional deficit. Generally, this is accomplished by functional training and in rare cases by surgical intervention.

The functional sequelae of **laryngeal trauma** depend on the extent of the trauma. They can range from hoarseness to aphonia, from respiratory distress to apnea, from odynophagia to dysphagia, and from coughing to hemoptysis. The degree of residual dysfunction depends on the extent of the primary injury. Treatment in the acute stage focuses on airway maintenance and if necessary may include the surgical reconstruction of structures that have been destroyed. In patients who have residual dysfunction, the only option is symptomatic therapy aimed at promoting compensatory mechanisms. Surgical procedures such as adhesiolysis are of very limited value.

Voice disorders in **acute laryngitis** generally resolve with regression of the organic lesion. From a functional standpoint, it is important to maintain voice rest during the inflammatory stage to prevent maladaptive compensation. Patients in certain occupations may require a 7- to 10-day leave of absence. If hoarseness persists after acute laryngitis has subsided, the patient should be referred for voice therapy to keep the hoarseness from becoming chronic. Twenty sessions are generally sufficient, preferably in an outpatient setting (inpatient therapy is rarely necessary). In **chronic laryngitis**, only a few selected patients will require voice therapy to optimize compensatory mechanisms.

The hoarseness associated with a **benign laryngeal neoplasm** will generally improve after treatment of the neoplasm. In exceptional cases, the voice disorder may persist in an attenuated form due to maladaptive compensation, necessitating voice therapy. Postoperative voice therapy may also be tried in patients with residual dysfunction, which is relatively common after the surgical removal of extensive Reinke's edema. This therapy has only a modest success rate, however, in terms of compensating for the dysfunction.

The surgical resection of **malignant laryngeal neoplasms** is almost invariably followed by dysphonia. From a phoniatric standpoint, voice therapy should be initiated as soon after the surgery as possible since a more extensive resection does not necessarily imply a poorer prognosis in terms of vocal function. Surgical techniques of glottic reconstruction after a unilateral vocal cord removal, for example, have only a very limited prospect of success.

## Functional Dysphonia

*Definition:* Functional dysphonia is a category of voice disorders in which there is no obvious organic change affecting the phonatory structures.

*Etiopathogenesis:* Functional voice disorders usually have a multifactorial etiology (**Fig. 18.7**). Constitutional, habitual, stress-related, and psychogenic causal factors have been identified. It is difficult in any given case to determine the relative contribution of specific factors to the overall picture. Usually, multiple factors can be identified that may reinforce one another under certain conditions. A vicious cycle may perpetuate a chronic voice disorder, which may later give rise to morphologic changes (vocal nodules, known also as screamer's or singer's nodules; see below and **Fig. 18.9**). It is customary to subdivide functional dysphonias into hyperfunctional and hypofunctional disorders.

*Symptoms:* These disorders may be associated with a general impairment of all aspects of voice function.

*Diagnosis:* Every examination for dysphonia should begin with a detailed *history*. Besides the objective information contained in the history, a perceptual evaluation of the patient's voice during speech and the observation of overall posture, muscular tone,

**Table 18.2  Differential diagnosis of voice disorders**

| Cause | Special features | For description see: |
|---|---|---|
| **Malformations** | | |
| Internal and external laryngoceles | Can have a very broad range of symptoms, depending on size | 🔍 **17.2** |
| Hemangiomas | | 📖 17.3, Laryngeal Subglottic Hemangioma |
| Laryngomalacia | | 📖 17.3, Laryngomalacia |
| Congenital webs | | 📖 17.3, Congenital Laryngeal Web and Glottic Atresia |
| Laryngeal stenosis | | 📖 17.3, Congenital Subglottic Stenosis |
| Vocal cord sulcus | Rarely presents with other laryngeal symptoms | 🔍 **18.1** |
| **Posttraumatic** | | |
| Arytenoid dislocation | Post intubation | 📖 17.6, Effects of (Prolonged) Intubation |
| Intubation granuloma | | 🔍 **17.6** |
| Laryngeal stenosis | | 🔍 17.7 |
| **Inflammatory** | | |
| Acute laryngitis | | 📖 17.5 |
| Chronic nonspecific laryngitis | | 📖 17.5 |
| Epiglottitis | Typical: muffled speech ⚠ Emergency with no prior history | 📖 17.5 |
| Laryngeal edema | | 📖 17.5 |
| Pseudocroup | | 📖 17.4, Diseases Associated with Croup Symptoms |
| **Neoplasms** | | |
| Vocal nodules | Organic lesion secondary to a functional disorder | 📖 17.7, Benign Neoplasms of the Larynx |
| Reinke's edema | Hoarseness, habitual throat clearing, low-pitched voice | 📖 17.7, Benign Neoplasms of the Larynx |
| Cysts | Postinflammatory | 📖 17.7, Benign Neoplasms of the Larynx |
| Laryngeal papillomas | Besides vocal nodules, this is the most important differential diagnosis in pediatric dysphonia | 📖 17.7, Benign Neoplasms of the Larynx |
| Contact granuloma | Most common in hypofunctional dysphonia, often associated with laryngeal reflux | 📖 17.7, Benign Neoplasms of the Larynx |
| Vocal cord polyps | | 📖 17.7, Benign Neoplasms of the Larynx |
| **Functional** | Vocal abuse | |
| **Neurogenic** Recurrent laryngeal nerve paralysis | | 📖 17.9, Recurrent Laryngeal Nerve Paralysis |

mimetics, and gestures can provide further clues to possible causal factors. Information on occupational voice use is essential for evaluating a voice disorder.

*Laryngoscopy* and *stroboscopy* (see 📖 18.1, Diagnostic Procedures) supply important information on the nature of the voice impairment and on secondary morphologic changes.

*Psychogenic dysphonia and aphonia:* Much experience is needed to assign a psychogenic cause to a voice disorder. These cases present with uncharacteristic laryngoscopic and stroboscopic findings. It is helpful to note, however, that most patients with psychogenic voice disorders can cough and laugh normally.

**Fig. 18.7    Causes of functional voice disorders**

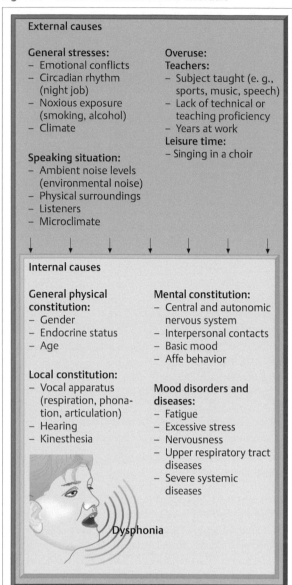

External causes

**General stresses:**
- Emotional conflicts
- Circadian rhythm (night job)
- Noxious exposure (smoking, alcohol)
- Climate

**Overuse:**
Teachers:
- Subject taught (e. g., sports, music, speech)
- Lack of technical or teaching proficiency
- Years at work

Leisure time:
- Singing in a choir

**Speaking situation:**
- Ambient noise levels (environmental noise)
- Physical surroundings
- Listeners
- Microclimate

Internal causes

**General physical constitution:**
- Gender
- Endocrine status
- Age

**Mental constitution:**
- Central and autonomic nervous system
- Interpersonal contacts
- Basic mood
- Affe behavior

**Local constitution:**
- Vocal apparatus (respiration, phonation, articulation)
- Hearing
- Kinesthesia

**Mood disorders and diseases:**
- Fatigue
- Excessive stress
- Nervousness
- Upper respiratory tract diseases
- Severe systemic diseases

Dysphonia

🗝 **18.1    Vocal cord sulcus**

With a vocal cord sulcus (**Fig. 18.8**), the mucosa at the free edge of the vocal cord(s) is indrawn and fixed (arrow heads), making the epithelium less mobile or immobile in relation to the vocalis muscle and vocal ligament. Apparently, this disorder is caused by muscle fibers inserting on the vocal cord mucosa or by residual dysfunction following a previous inflammation. The *result* is a hoarse voice. *Treatment* consists mainly of symptomatic voice therapy. Surgical release of the muscle fibers from the mucosa or resection of the affected mucosa is not widely practiced due to the risk of postoperative scarring.

**Fig. 18.8    Laryngoscopic picture of a vocal cord sulcus (arrows)**

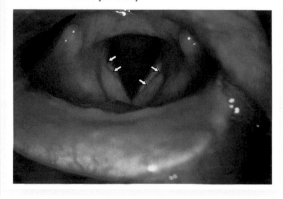

skills. For workers in most occupations, the voice is an indispensable tool for communication.

🔖 Many patients with pronounced dysphonia can keep their jobs only by undergoing an intensive, rigorous course of voice therapy, which may even require an inpatient program.

*Children*, as a rule, are not good candidates for formal voice therapy because they are not cooperative enough to follow the protocol. A better focus of treatment in these patients is to optimize motor functions while improving concentration and play behavior (e.g., ergotherapy).

**Treatment of secondary organic changes:** Vocal nodules may be an indication for surgical treatment, depending on whether they are hard or soft. This assessment requires much experience and very careful consideration.

🔖 Once vocal nodules have been surgically removed, it is essential to identify and treat the underlying cause of the lesions—e.g., with conservative voice therapy.

🔖 Psychogenic dysphonia or aphonia should never be dismissed as a trivial condition.

Psychogenic dysphonia is a *psychosomatic disorder* whose true significance is often appreciated only during a prolonged course of therapy.

*Treatment:* Causal factors and underlying diseases should be corrected or eliminated as completely as possible before treatment is initiated. The actual **voice therapy** consists of an individualized program of vocal exercises. Today, numerous competing methods known collectively as "functional voice training" take into account not just the laryngeal aspects of voice production but also breathing, posture, and personality issues. The basic goal is the rapid restoration of physiological and economical phonation and general communication

Surgical ablation is not indicated for vocal nodules *in children*. These lesions have a strong tendency to regress spontaneously by puberty, especially in boys.

**Treatment of psychogenic voice disorders:** Psychotherapy alone is unlikely to relieve hoarseness in

**Fig. 18.9 Vocal cord nodules**

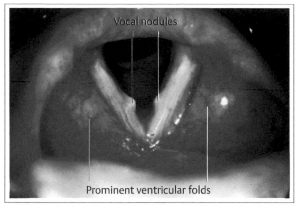

Vocal nodules

Prominent ventricular folds

These lesions are secondary to an underlying functional disorder (long-term vocal overuse or misuse). Voice therapy is the mainstay of treatment (see also 🔍 **18.1**).

these patients, and the plan of treatment should always include somatically oriented voice therapy. An essential task of the physician confronted with psychogenic dysphonia is first to motivate the patient to recognize the psychogenic nature of the complaint and accept the need for help.

Formerly, it was common for speech-language pathologists to use "surprise tactics" with the object of provoking a normal voice.

🛇 Surprise tactics are not fair to the patient and are purely of historical interest today.

## Hyperfunctional Dysphonia

*Epidemiology:* Hyperfunctional dysphonia appears to be most prevalent in talkative, extroverted individuals, especially women.

*Pathogenesis:* A dynamic balance normally exists between subglottic pressure and muscular tone in the larynx. In hyperfunctional dysphonia, this balance is shifted toward higher pressures and tone values, causing the system to function at an uneconomical and inefficient level.

When the patient uses this uneconomical phonation mechanism for an extended period of time, sites of connective-tissue hyperplasia develop at the junction of the anterior and middle thirds of the vocal cords.

These **vocal nodules** (synonyms: screamer's nodules, singer's nodules; **Fig. 18.9**) represent secondary morphologic changes based on the primary functional disorder.

*Symptoms:* The speaking voice is often raised to a higher pitch. Usually, the voice sounds harsh, scratchy, and strained and is reduced in its ability to be raised or modulated. It is also common to find symptoms such as a general increase in muscular tension

with neck and throat problems. In many patients, pronounced movements of the shoulder girdle can be observed during breathing (unphysiologic "upper chest breathing").

*Diagnosis:* **Laryngoscopy** often shows incomplete glottic closure with an hourglass-shaped glottis and adduction of the false vocal folds during phonation, which may even prevent the true vocal folds from being seen. The epiglottis may be displaced posteriorly and may assume an almost vertical position. The vocal cords may be hyperemic, mimicking their appearance in laryngitis. **Stroboscopy** often shows a suppression of vibrational amplitudes and traveling wave motion.

## Hypofunctional Dysphonia

Hypofunctional dysphonia may result from prolonged voice use or from a habitual tendency to speak with too little effort. The dynamic balance of vocal cord vibrations is shifted downward toward low pressures and tone values.

The body posture is marked by decreased muscular tension, the breathing is shallow, and the voice sounds weak and breathy.

The glottic insufficiency in this condition is often not appreciated with conventional laryngoscopy and is seen only during stroboscopy. This study also shows increased amplitudes and an amplified traveling wave motion due to a decrease in vocal cord tension.

## Mixed Dysphonia

Mixed forms of dysphonia may exhibit both hyperfunctional and hypofunctional features. The mixed pattern can be explained by various mechanisms of decompensation or maladaptive compensation. For example, compensatory participation of the ventricular folds in phonation may occur in a patient with hypofunctional glottic insufficiency. It is very difficult to establish the nature of the primary disorder in any given case.

## Mutational Voice Disorders

The most common of these disorders involve a **prolonged voice mutation** or **incomplete mutation. A premature voice change** may reflect a serious hormonal disorder and should be investigated by a pediatric endocrinologist.

A **mutational falsetto** results from increased cricothyroid muscle tension and always has a psychological cause. External downward pressure on the thyroid cartilage (the Gutzmann maneuver) will often evoke a normal-sounding voice. Generally, however, this condition requires a prolonged course of treatment to give the adolescent time to adapt to a normal chest voice. Even if the disorder is presumed to have a psychogenic cause, there is no need for specific psychotherapy in most cases. It is extremely important to educate the parents about the nature of the condition.

## Endocrine Dysphonia

Endocrine dysphonia very often presents clinically as a harsh, cracking, low-pitched voice, frequently combined with loss of the singing voice and rapid fatigability. It is much more common in women than in men.

Endocrine voice disorders may be caused by a disease-related hormonal imbalance or, more commonly, by exogenous hormone administration (therapeutic or for athletic doping). The voice may fluctuate during the course of the ovarian cycle. A common disorder in pregnancy is laryngopathia gravidarum. Menopausal women may also develop voice changes.

The examiner should give particular attention to any signs of virilization that may reflect an abnormal androgen excess (e.g., due to a hormonally active tumor). **Treatment** aims at reestablishing a normal hormonal balance. Often, however, these voice disorders respond poorly to treatment, and therapeutic exercises are prescribed to achieve optimum compensation.

**Fig. 18.10   The glottis in unilateral vocal cord paralysis**

| Vocal cord position | Respiration | Phonation |
|---|---|---|
| a Paramedian | | |
| b Intermediate | | |
| c Lateral | | |

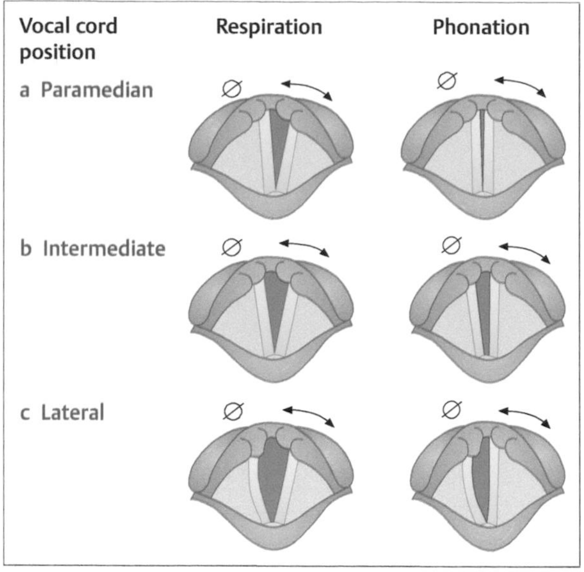

The position of the paralyzed vocal cord is described in relation to an imaginary midline: paramedian, intermediate, or lateral.

---

### 🔎 18.2  Phonosurgical procedures

**Isshiki's type I thyroplasty**
*Indication:* unilateral vocal cord paralysis.
*Principle:* This procedure is based on the concept that the dynamic equilibrium of vocal cord vibrations can be modified indirectly by altering the cartilaginous framework without causing direct trauma to the vocal cords. The surgery is done under local anesthesia. A piece of thyroid cartilage is excised at the level of the paralyzed vocal cord (**Fig. 18.11a**). While the patient phonates, the cartilage is pressed inward until the voice improves (**Fig. 18.11b**). The cartilage is then fixed in that position with tissue adhesive or a silicone shim (**Fig. 18.11c**).

**Nawka's arytenoidectomy**
*Indication:* bilateral vocal cord paralysis.
*Principle:* The glottis is widened by excising the arytenoid cartilage (**Fig. 18.11d**) and the posterior part of the vocalis muscle (**Fig. 18.11e**), usually on one side. The vocal cord mucosa is sutured to the mucosa of the ventricular fold (**Fig. 18.11f**).
*Result:* Usually, an acceptable compromise can be achieved between ventilation and phonation.

**Fig. 18.11   Surgical procedures in unilateral (a–c) and bilateral (d–f) recurrent nerve palsy.**

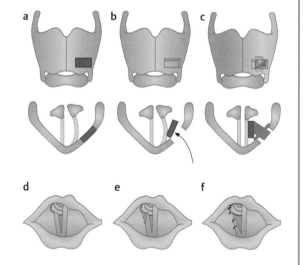

**a–c** Isshiki's type 1 thyroplasty: medialization of the paralyzed vocal cord.
**d–f** Nawka's arytenoidectomy: endoscopic resection of the posterior part of one paralyzed vocal cord.

## 18.3 Phonosurgery

*Definition*: Phonosurgery involves the use of surgical procedures to improve the voice.
The following *phonosurgical guidelines* should be observed:

**A normal traveling wave motion requires integrity of various structures: Reinke's space, the free edge of the vocal cords, and the vocal cord mucosa.**

**An effort should be made to obtain adequate contact between the vocal cords during the closed phase of the vibratory cycle.**

**A favorable working point should be found between generating a certain minimum subglottic pressure and speaking without undue force. This is not just a surgical task, however, because effective vocalization can be trained over a broad range with voice therapy.**

**Every phonosurgical procedure should be preceded by the detailed documentation of findings and adequate informed consent.**

*Options*:
**Indirect laryngoscopy**:
*Indication*: Removal of vocal cord polyps, some cysts, and especially discrete marginal edema of the vocal cords.
*Principle*: The patient is conscious and holds the tongue forward with a gauze swab. Topical anesthesia is applied, and the lesions are removed with fine instruments. The vocal cords are observed with a microscope via a laryngoscopic mirror or with an endoscope linked to a video monitor.

*Advantage*: Preserving the muscular tone of the vocal cords makes it easier to see subtle changes and evaluate the immediate functional result by checking the voice intraoperatively.
**Direct laryngoscopy**:
The *indications* for this technique are relatively extensive organic lesions that need to be palpated, removed, or biopsied. It can also be used to remove (pre)malignant lesions that are unrelated to phonosurgical criteria.
*Principle*: General anesthesia is induced by either intubating the patient (see 🔎 **17.14**) or using a jet ventilation laryngoscope.
*Advantage*: General anesthesia permits a longer, unhurried operation that allows very precise work.
*Disadvantage*: The quality of the voice cannot be assessed intraoperatively.
**Transcutaneous laryngeal framework surgery**: The principal options are the Isshiki type I thyroplasty described in 🔎 **18.2** and arytenoid rotation.
**Injection techniques**: Collagen and other materials can be injected for the augmentation of vocal cords that are atrophic due to recurrent laryngeal nerve paralysis, and botulinum toxin can be injected for spasmodic dysphonia. These techniques are reserved for highly selected indications.
**Laryngeal reinnervation techniques** are currently in development and are still classified as experimental procedures.

## Vocal Cord Paralysis

Synonym: laryngeal palsy.

*Symptoms:* **Unilateral vocal cord paralysis** is characterized by a breathy, hoarse, weak voice that is markedly restricted in its pitch and volume range. The voice may deteriorate further over time due to the use of improper compensatory mechanisms.
With **bilateral vocal cord paralysis,** severe respiratory distress may be the dominant feature. Often the voice sounds almost normal.

*Diagnosis:* The paralyzed vocal cord is fixed in a paramedian position (**Fig. 18.10**). It may be "excavated" as a result of muscular atrophy. The stroboscopic findings depend on the degree of vocal cord tension. With incomplete paralysis, the traveling wave motion may be detectable even in the absence of respiratory motion.

*Treatment:* Unilateral vocal cord paralysis is treated initially with *conservative voice exercises*, which should be supported by synchronous *electrical stimulation* to prevent muscular atrophy.

⚡ Electrical stimulation alone is of no value without synchronous voice therapy.

If conservative voice therapy fails to give satisfactory improvement, *phonosurgical procedures* should be considered: thyroplasty (see 🔎 **18.2**) and arytenoid rotation. As a rule, surgery is not undertaken until at least 1 year after the onset of vocal cord paralysis to allow time for possible spontaneous recovery. Earlier phonosurgery may be considered for older patients in whom conservative voice therapy is ineffectual due to general physical weakness.
**Bilateral vocal cord paralysis** with serious respiratory distress should be managed in the acute stage by intubation or tracheotomy. Tracheotomized patients should be fitted with a *speaking tube*. This type of tube keeps the tracheostomy open and allows free respiration. On expiration, a small flap valve occludes the tube and the exhaled air can be used for phonation in the usual way. In chronic cases with satisfactory respiration that does not require a tracheotomy, an attempt can be made to widen the glottis with a minor surgical procedure on the vocal cords (arytenoidectomy, see 🔎 **18.2**). However, this almost always causes some degree of voice deterioration due to incomplete glottic closure.

# 19 Speech and Language Disorders

## 19.1 Principles of Normal and Abnormal Language Development

According to conservative estimates, around 10 to 15% of all children younger than 6 years have a developmental language disorder. Ultimately, this type of disorder can profoundly impair the child's psychosocial integration. To prevent this, it is essential to know the normal patterns of language development, the possible causes of developmental disorders, necessary test procedures, and the indications and options for treatment.

### Normal Language Development

The milestones of normal language development are outlined in **Fig. 19.1**.

### Abnormal Language Development

#### Causes

The causes of abnormal language development are numerous and diverse. When multiple components are present, it is no longer possible in many cases to determine the contribution of individual factors to the overall disorder. The classification of Nickisch and Gross (**Table 19.1**) summarizes the main causes and is helpful in understanding the etiopathogenesis of developmental language disorders.

#### Symptoms

Abnormal language development can have various clinical presentations. The possible deficits may involve:
- Sound recognition, articulation, and distinguishing sounds (dyslalia, stuttering).
- Expressive and receptive vocabulary.
- Speech comprehension.
- The observance of syntactical and grammatical rules (dysgrammatism).
- The comprehension and formulation of spoken or written sentences, reading.
- The contextually appropriate use of language.
- Other disturbances of nonverbal communication, perception, motor skills, and overall cognitive-intellectual and social development.

#### Diagnosis

If a developmental language problem is suspected, it is generally necessary to conduct a comprehensive diagnostic evaluation covering all developmental aspects of the affected child. This includes the testing of speech and language in addition to nonlinguistic areas (general and manual motor skills, cognitive-intellectual development) and social interactions. Play behavior, communicative behavior, and social conduct are assessed based on personal observation or reports from others. Nonlinguistic areas of development are generally investigated by a pediatrician.

> ✐ Every child with a speech or language problem should be tested for a hearing disorder.

The **diagnostic target areas** for speech and language disorders are as follows:
- Spontaneous speech.
- General communicative behavior.
- Speech comprehension.
- Active vocabulary.
- Grammar.
- Ability to distinguish and use sounds that differentiate word meanings.
- Articulation.
- Language learning ability.

#### Treatment

Impaired language development in children can be treated only by a structured exercise program that is tailored specifically to individual deficits and is administered by a speech-language pathologist. The program is based on a combination of play-therapy principles and pedagogic elements, depending on the age of the child.

> ✐ Treatment should be instituted as soon as possible after the causes have been identified and should incorporate the child's caregivers.

For children **up to 2 years of age**, initial intervention is generally indirect and consists of parental counseling. Children **older than 2 years** can receive direct therapeutic intervention, but parenteral counseling is still important.

Psychosocial conditions appropriate for language acquisition should be present or created therapeutically. The scheme for improving language abilities follows the normal sequence of language development: language comprehension–vocabulary–grammar–articulation.

Table 19.1  Causes of developmental language disorders

| Classification | Causes |
|---|---|
| **Isolated developmental language disorder** | • Familial language impairment<br>• Psychosocial causes: overprotection, deprivation, bilingualism, lack of language stimulation<br>• Disturbance of peripheral speech organs<br>• Abnormal central coordination of peripheral speech organs (e.g., oral dyspraxia) |
| **Developmental language disorder (DLD) combined with other disorders** | |
| DLD combined with at least two of the listed disorders and not associated with intellectual impairment | • Peripheral hearing disorders<br>• Auditory perception disorder<br>• Peripheral visual disorder<br>• Visual perceptual disorder<br>• Peripheral or central motor disease with normal speech organs<br>• Mental disorder (e.g., autism) |
| DLD in the setting of global developmental disorders | • Congenital (prenatally acquired or hereditary) intellectual disability<br>  – With associated physical anomalies (syndrome)<br>  – Without physical anomalies<br>• Perinatally or postnatally acquired intellectual disability (traumatic, inflammatory, hypoxic, metabolic, neurodegenerative) |

Source: Nickisch and Gross 1987.

The **goal of treatment** is to correct the developmental language deficit before the child enters school to permit mainstream schooling or prevent a delay in school enrollment.

## Prognosis

The prognosis depends on the individual causes, the severity of the disorder, and the prompt initiation of services and treatment. *Primary deficits* can be compensated as the child grows older. *Secondary disorders* such as social withdrawal or aggressive modes of behavior may affect the overall picture. Children who have no severe, progressive, or refractory underlying diseases will generally have a good prognosis.

**Fig. 19.1 Milestones of language development**

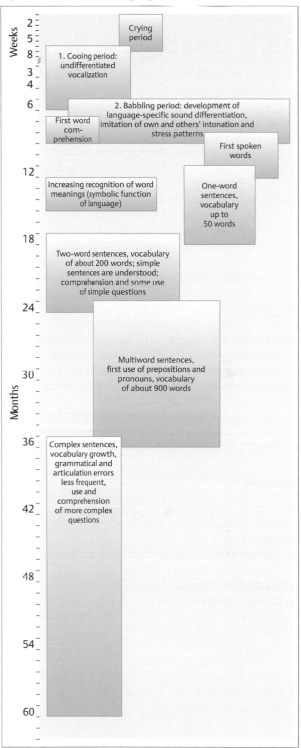

# 19.2    Important Types of Speech and Language Disorders

Given the fundamental importance of speech in all forms of human interaction, many branches of science and several medical specialties are concerned with the phenomena of normal and abnormal speech and language development, viewing speech and language disorders from varying perspectives and with various goals.

Several main types of language disorders can be characterized to facilitate a systematic approach to these disorders and create a basis for routine clinical work.

## Dyslalia

*Definition:* Dyslalia refers to any of several articulation disorders characterized by errors of pronunciation. Individual vocal sounds may be omitted, distorted, or replaced by other sounds. Dyslalia includes the inability to use sounds or sound combinations in a way that clearly differentiates word meanings.

*Classification:* Dyslalia can be classified on the basis of various criteria:

**Quantity**:
- Isolated dyslalia: defective pronunciation of a sound.
- Partial dyslalia: defective pronunciation of certain sounds.
- Multiple dyslalia: defective pronunciation of many sounds.
- Universal dyslalia: defective pronunciation of virtually all sounds.

**Constancy**:
- Constant dyslalia: the error is always present.
- Inconstant dyslalia: the error is sometimes present.

**Variability**:
- Consistent dyslalia: the nature of the error is always the same.
- Inconsistent dyslalia: the errors or substitute sounds may vary.

**Quality:** Specific articulation errors are named for the Greek letter equivalents of the affected consonants, with the ending "ism" or "tism" added: sigmatism, rhotacism, etc. Dyslalia most commonly affects the *sibilants*, particularly the "s" sound—a condition known as sigmatism or lisping.

The prefix "para" indicates the use of a substitute sound, while the prefix "a" denotes the absence of a sound ("asigmatism"). When clinical findings are interpreted, moreover, it should be noted whether the articulation error occurs in sound groupings—i.e., in syllables, words, or sentences. Thus, while one sound may be correctly pronounced in isolation, it may be mispronounced within the context of syllables or words. In some cases, this can result in universal dyslalia.

**Extent:** A key distinction in the diagnostic classification of dyslalia is whether the patient has an isolated ("pure") articulation disorder or a general impairment of language development. Isolated dyslalia in a child younger than 3 to 4 years with a normal vocabulary and normal grammar is classified as *developmental dyslalia* or *physiologic dyslalia*. **Fig. 19.1** reviews the normal timetable for the acquisition of vocal sounds.

**Etiology:** *Organic dyslalia* is the term applied to articulation disorders caused by congenital or acquired defects at the peripheral receptive level (hearing impairment), central level, or peripheral expressive level (teeth). Central defects generally cause more complex deficits than just dyslalia, however. This is also true of intellectual disability, general physical developmental disorders, and serious systemic diseases. Insufficient language stimulation (deprivation) also tends to cause a more comprehensive disturbance of language development.

## Dysgrammatism

*Definition:* Dysgrammatism is an inability to speak grammatically due to errors of word morphology (tense, number, gender) and syntax (sentence structure).

*Occurrence:* Within the context of normal language acquisition, dysgrammatic elements occur physiologically during the second and third years of life. However, after 3 years of age a marked deviation from the age-specific norm usually indicates a significant developmental language disorder. As a rule, dysgrammatism is associated with other abnormalities of language acquisition. Dysgrammatism rarely occurs as a dominant complaint; when it does, it is often the cardinal symptom of an auditory disorder.

*Diagnosis:* The evaluation of general language development includes testing for dysgrammatism. The extent of the disorder is assessed on the basis of various tasks (spontaneous speech, repeating sentences, telling a story based on a series of pictures, retelling a story shown in pictures).

**Treatment:** The treatment of dysgrammatism is integrated into a complex, overall treatment plan that is patterned after physiologic language development. The *prognosis* depends on the extent of the overall disorder. Dysgrammatism may persist for some time as a refractory residual symptom. The prognosis is usually favorable, however.

## Rhinolalia

Synonyms: rhinophonia, rhinism.

**Definition and pathogenesis:** Rhinolalia is altered speech caused by abnormal airflow through the nose during phonation. It may have an organic or functional cause. While it is technically correct to distinguish between **altered voice sounds (rhinophonia)** and **altered sound production (rhinolalia)**, both terms are often used interchangeably. Several types of rhinolalia are distinguished based on the voice sound:

**Hypernasal speech** (rhinophonia aperta): Nasal resonance is increased during speech as a result of velopharyngeal dysfunction, creating an ineffectual seal between the oral cavity and nasopharynx. The underlying cause may be a cleft palate or paralysis of the soft palate in a setting of myasthenia. Functional hypernasality may reflect nonuse of the soft palate following a tonsillectomy.

**Hyponasal speech** (rhinophonia clausa): Nasal resonance is decreased during speech. Usually, this has an organic cause based on obstructive lesions such as adenoid vegetations in the nose or nasopharynx.

**Mixed nasality** (rhinophonia mixta): Both hyponasal and hypernasal features are present.

**Diagnosis:** The initial goal in diagnosis is to identify the specific type of rhinolalia that is present. In the *mirror test,* a cold mirror or a device called a Czermak plate is held beneath the nose while vowels are pronounced. Fogging of the mirror indicates the nasal air escape that characterizes hypernasal speech. A Czermak plate has rings that show the extent of fogging, permitting a semiquantitative assessment of nasal air escape.

In the "ah-ee test," the vowel sounds "ah" and "ee" are spoken in succession. With hypernasal speech, the tester will hear a nasal-sounding change in the vowel sound. This does not occur in hyponasal speech.

The *cheek inflation test* (with the tongue protruded) can detect an **organic** cause of hypernasal speech. If the soft palate is shortened due to an incomplete cleft, the patient will be unable to inflate the cheeks with air while the tongue is protruded.

The "backdrop sign" is an important finding in patients with paralysis of the soft palate. Hypernasal speech can be *accentuated by head turning* toward the unaffected side.

🖉 An underlying neurologic disease may also have to be excluded in some cases.

**Treatment:** The initial treatment for **functional disorders** is an intensive voice therapy program, which may be long and arduous in some patients.

The treatment for **organic hypernasal speech** due to a cleft palate is integrated into a comprehensive plan for treating the underlying disorder.

**Organic hyponasal speech** due to an obstructive lesion in the nose or nasopharynx is easily corrected with surgery.

## Speech Fluency Disorders

### Stuttering

**Definition:** Stuttering is an impairment of speech fluency that is independent of the will of the speaker. The strict classification of stuttering into tonic and clonic forms is no longer considered essential due to a lack of therapeutic implications.

Disfluency occurs physiologically during language acquisition between 2.5 and 4 years of age.

**Epidemiology:** The incidence of stuttering is about 1% in the overall population and about 4% in children, regardless of language and culture. Males are predominantly affected.

**Etiology:** The etiology of stuttering is uncertain. *Organ theories* stress the causal significance of genetic components as well as hyperexcitability of the central nervous system. There are also *learning theory models* of causation, and there is evidence to support a *psychogenic* cause in specific cases. For clinical purposes, it is useful to postulate a multifactorial etiology with hereditary influences along with organic, psychological, and environmental factors.

**Symptoms: Tonic stuttering** is characterized by a *blocking* of speech at the beginning of words or sentences, usually associated with a generalized rise in body tension. **Clonic stuttering** is characterized by *repetitions* of sounds, syllables, or words.

**Secondary characteristics** include changes in breathing, mimetics, gestures, and autonomic responses that accompany stuttering.

**Diagnosis:** The diagnostic evaluation of stuttering should cover the following specific points:

- Basic symptoms and accompanying features by number and severity, fear of speaking and avoidance behavior, body image, variability of symptoms,

situations that elicit or exacerbate stuttering, or situations that elicit fluent speech.
- Causal factors and progression over time, social milieu (family, friends, acquaintances, work environment).
- Awareness of the stuttering by self and others, attitude toward the stuttering (self-consciousness).
- Speaking demands, quality of information, emotionality, and motivation.

In **children**, diagnosis should begin by assessing the relative importance of the stuttering symptom within the framework of a general developmental language disorder, which is usually present.

*Treatment:* Based on the assumption of a multifactorial etiology, the treatment of stuttering combines symptom-oriented elements with psychotherapeutic–psychosocial treatment strategies to create an integrative, multidimensional program. The focus of the program is on improving self-perception, desensitizing the stutterer to his or her own disorder, modifying the symptom by the use of specific speaking techniques, generalizing the new speaking techniques into spontaneous communication, and establishing support by referring the patient to a self-help group, for example. Tranquilizers and other medications may be helpful as adjuncts.
In **children**, an effort is made to direct the patient's attention to fluent episodes and reduce any fears that are associated with speaking. In exceptional cases, elements of adult therapy may be applied in this age group for the purpose of direct symptom modification. Parental counseling is also emphasized.

*Prognosis*: Regardless of the age group, approximately one-third of patients will recover completely, one-third will improve, and one-third will experience no change.

## Cluttering

Cluttering is a fluency disorder characterized by an abnormally rapid and irregular rate of speech delivery. The speech may be difficult to understand due to the omission of sounds, syllables, or even entire words. The symptoms are improved (even with strangers) by concentrating on the verbal output and deliberately slowing the rate of speaking. The clutterers themselves rarely perceive their speech as being abnormal. The *etiopathogenesis* of cluttering is as poorly understood as that of stuttering.
After potential causes have been investigated, the main task in *diagnosis* is to differentiate cases that require treatment from cases that have no pathologic significance.

As a rule, no specific *treatment* is necessary in adults because usually they are not self-conscious about their disorder. Cluttering in children is usually part of a general developmental language disorder and is treated within that context.

## Aphasia

*Definition:* Aphasia refers to the partial or complete loss of speech (formulation, memory, comprehension) after the completion of language acquisition.

*Epidemiology:* The *incidence* of aphasic syndromes is estimated at 60 new cases per 100,000 persons per year, with a rising trend.

*Etiology and pathogenesis:* Predisposing underlying diseases are arterial hypertension, disorders of fat metabolism, diabetes mellitus, and generalized atherosclerosis. More than 80% of cases have a cerebrovascular cause. More than 90% of these cases are caused by a thrombotic or embolic vascular occlusion and less than 10% by an intracranial hemorrhage.

*Symptoms:* Aphasia may present clinically as a disturbance of both written and spoken language, meaning that all the coding functions for the same information may be impaired. All linguistic components—phonology, lexicon, syntax, and semantics—may be affected. Based on the cerebrovascular etiology, various patterns of injury may be encountered in aphasic patients, and other cognitive deficits such as altered consciousness or a decline in intelligence may accompany the language disorder.

The peripheral speech organs and especially the peripheral auditory apparatus are not directly affected by aphasia.

*Classification:* There is still no universally accepted scheme for the classification of aphasia. The classification of Poeck et al, based on the dominant features of different aphasias, is perhaps the most widely used system in German-speaking countries. It is the classification upon which the *Aachen Aphasia Test (AAT)* is based, of which an English-language version (EAAT) is also in use.
**Global aphasia** is the most common cerebrovascular type of aphasia and is considered the most severe form. It results from damage to the brain in the territory of the middle cerebral artery. Regardless of the affected hemisphere, global aphasia is characterized by a severe impairment of all receptive and expressive language functions.

The term *Wernicke's aphasia* is currently preferred over older terms such as "sensory," "receptive," "acoustic," and "posterior" aphasia, because the latter terms do not reflect the potential complexity of the disorder and are not helpful in directing treatment. Wernicke's aphasia results from lesions in the territory of the posterior temporal artery. The cardinal symptoms are poor speech comprehension and a fluent but often unintelligible output ("fluent nonsense"). Thus, Wernicke's aphasia bears a close resemblance to global aphasia from the standpoint of language comprehension.

**Amnestic aphasia** is caused by damage to the temporoparietal area of the brain. The principal causative lesions are brain tumors, temporal lobe abscesses, and degenerative processes. Its cardinal symptom is word-finding difficulty, and the patient tries to compensate for this by paraphrasing. As a rule, amnestic aphasia has the best prognosis of all the aphasias, barring progression of the underlying disease.

The term *Broca's aphasia* is preferred over the older terms *motor* and *expressive aphasia*, which do not accurately describe the nature of the disorder. The main features of Broca's aphasia are a marked increase in speaking effort combined with poor articulation and altered prosody (the "melody" of speech). The disturbance is never confined to language expression and always includes comprehension difficulties. Dysgrammatism or agrammatism is also present.

The classification also includes **special forms** of aphasia, which are beyond our present scope.

*Diagnosis:* Regardless of the type of aphasia present, it is currently believed that every aphasic patient is fundamentally impaired at all language levels, and that different forms differ mainly in the predominance of certain features. The **Aachen Aphasia Test (AAT)** is among the instruments that can be used to differentiate and quantify these features.

**Audiologic-phoniatric testing** is performed in aphasic patients for the classification and quantification of language disorders in both receptive and expressive functions.

*Differential diagnosis:* Aphasia requires differentiation from **dysarthria,** which results from the paralysis or incoordination of respiratory, voice, and speech muscles due to an organic brain lesion. Differentiation is also required from **developmental language disorders, language disorders in psychiatric conditions,** and **apraxia,** which is an inability to perform voluntary and intentional movements with one part of the body in the absence of muscular weakness or paralysis.

*Treatment:* The goal of treatment in aphasia is to restore the communication skills needed to cope with everyday situations, achieve social reintegration, and ideally return the patient to work. The overriding goal is to restore overall communication more than rehabilitate its separate components. The treatment of aphasia can be divided into three phases:

During the **activation phase** in the first 6 months after the onset of aphasia, treatment focuses on the general acti-vation of seeing, listening, reading, and writing. Automatic terms such as number sequences, days of the week, and months can be used to stimulate more voluntary words and phrases. Intact abilities are used to "unblock" impaired functions, proceeding, for example, from speaking with the therapist to repeat-ing words after the therapist and finally naming objects.

In the **exercise phase**, which begins after the aphasic syndrome has stabilized, the therapy consists of exercises tailored to the specific disorder. Largely intact modalities are used as an access point, linguistic principles are conveyed, and drills are performed to condition and improve certain language skills. Compensatory strategies are developed to cope with irreversible deficits.

In the **consolidation phase**, further disorder-specific work will no longer improve the patient's language skills. The emphasis in this phase is on reintegrating the patient into everyday life and reestablishing contact with the environment.

## Dysarthria

Synonym: dysarthrophonia.

*Definition:* Dysarthria is a speech disorder based on an impairment of the neural mechanisms that control speech movements.

*Etiopathogenesis and symptoms:* Given its neurologic cause, dysarthria may affect one or more of the systems involved in the production of speech: respiration, phonation, and articulation. Prosody, or the melody of speech, is also affected in most cases. The speech of dysarthric patients is characterized by altered muscular tone, weakness, slowing, incoordination, or hyperkinetic symptoms.

Several forms of dysarthria can be distinguished based on clinical criteria:

**Spastic dysarthria**:

*Etiopathogenesis:* Spastic dysarthria is the most common form occurring after severe craniocerebral trauma. It appears to involve a spastic paralysis caused by damage to the first motor neuron, leading to acceleration-dependent muscular hypertonicity with a decrease in strength and fine motor skills. Reflex functions (swallowing, coughing, gagging) are preserved.

*Symptoms:* The voice sounds strained, consonants are pronounced imprecisely, and the speech has a slow, monotonic quality. Unilateral lesions may be associated with subtle clinical findings.

**Rigid hyperkinetic dysarthria**:

*Etiopathogenesis:* The most frequent cause is Parkinson's disease, in which rigid hyperkinetic dysarthria is an early symptom.

*Symptoms:* The voice sounds soft and breathy and has a limited range.

**Ataxic dysarthria**:

*Etiopathogenesis:* This form is presumably based on deficits in cerebellar motor functions.

*Symptoms:* Patients typically have variable articulation errors and uncontrolled variations in vocal pitch and loudness. The voice may sound harsh and strained, and voice breaks are frequent.

**Hyperkinetic and dystonic forms**:

*Etiopathogenesis:* The causes are diverse and include brainstem lesions as well as rare neurologic disorders such as Huntington's disease or athetosis.

*Symptoms:* Tremor and myoclonias can cause variable impairment of the voice and speech, depending on the affected muscle group.

**Hypotonic dysarthria**:

*Etiopathogenesis:* Hypotonic dysarthria is a characteristic feature of bulbar palsy like that occurring in association with brainstem lesions (e.g., amyotrophic lateral sclerosis). A lesion of the second motor neuron leads to a flaccid paralysis of the affected muscles.

*Symptoms:* Characteristic features are muscular hypotonicity, loss of strength, and the limitation or abolition of voluntary and reflex movements. The voice sounds soft, breathy, and hypernasal. Consonant articulation is slowed and imprecise.

*Diagnosis:* The diagnosis of dysarthria is always based on a **neurologic** examination to investigate possible causes, determine the location of the lesion, and assess the extent of the underlying neurologic disease.

**Phoniatric** tests evaluate phonation and articulation, oral communication, reading, and writing. A quantitative assessment can be made by rating the degree of various criteria on a point scale, such as:

- Ability for voiced phonation.
- Voice quality (harsh, breathy, strained?).
- Habitual pitch and volume.
- Voice stability (pitch and loudness fluctuations, trembling?).
- Jaw movements (visual assessment).
- Vowel and consonant articulation.
- Resonance (nasality?).
- Slow or rapid rate of speech during repetition or reading.
- Fluency of speech (pauses, iterations, voice arrests?).
- Intonation, accent (monopitched speech?).

*Treatment:* Initial treatment is directed toward improving the underlying disease. Treatment planning should take into account the individual circumstances of the patient (**Table 19.2**). The cornerstones of treatment are reviewed in **Table 19.3**.

Various techniques are used to promote the motor functions essential for speech: special exercises, therapeutic aids (e.g., bite block or pointing board), prosthetic measures (e.g., palatal lift prosthesis), adaptive measures (changing the mode of communication, technical aids such as a PalmPilot), or surgical procedures (velopharyngoplasty, posterior pharyngeal wall augmentation to improve nasopharyngeal closure).

The *prognosis* in all forms of dysarthria depends on the underlying neurologic disease. Generally, the disorder cannot be corrected but often it can be improved.

| Table 19.2 Factors that influence treatment planning | |
|---|---|
| *Classification* | *Description* |
| Neurologic status and prior history | Location, nature, and extent of brain damage, time since lesion onset, progression or stability of the disease |
| Age | Younger patients usually have more rehabilitation potential owing to a better health status and psychosocial conditions |
| Personality | Optimistic, goal-oriented patients benefit more from treatment than uncompromising, less confident, or perfectionistic patients |
| Psychosocial status | A stimulating social environment and the availability of helpers will reinforce the transfer of relearned skills |
| Associated neuropsychiatric deficits | Deficits of attention, memory, learning, planning, language, affect, disease insight, perception, drive, and motivation can adversely affect therapeutic response |
| Degree of impairment | This assessment is based on individual requirements and on social and occupational demands |

Source: Ziegler et al 1998.

| Table 19.3 Guidelines for the treatment of dysarthria | |
|---|---|
| *Guidelines* | *Description* |
| Begin treatment early | To prevent maladaptive responses. Muscular functions that are more intact tend to become overactive and thus inhibit the recovery of other motor skills. Optimize residual skills in progressive diseases |
| Focus on the key disorders | First work on the function that is uppermost in the hierarchy of the causal chain |
| Modify the underlying disorder | Start with measures to restore physiologic function: regulation of muscle tone, postural correction, etc. |
| Promote compensatory behavior | Compensation is necessary for the maximum utilization of residual motor capacities |
| Promote speech awareness | The patient can no longer rely on speaking "automatically" or without special effort |
| Differentiate self-perception Create motivation for treatment | The ability for self-perception needs to be developed Motivation should not be confused with hope for recovery |

Source: Ziegler et al 1998.

# Appendix:
# Emergencies and Primary Measures

# Overview and Referrals for Detailed Information

Emergency situations are common in the head and neck region due to the complex anatomical relationships and the broad spectrum of possible diseases. They may present as life-threatening conditions associated with one or more of the following symptoms: hemorrhage, respiratory distress (dyspnea, stridor), acute dysphagia, and signs of local or systemic inflammation. Acute hearing loss, acute tinnitus, acute vertigo, and facial nerve paralysis are not life-threatening but still represent an acute situation. Skull fractures are also classified as emergencies. The diseases that are relevant in emergency medicine are covered in separate chapters and are reviewed in Table 1, which lists not only life-threatening events but also diseases and injuries in which immediate intervention is necessary to prevent complications or permanent disability.

## Otologic Emergencies

Life-threatening **hemorrhages** are extremely rare, but any bleeding from the ear canal should be investigated in order to determine its cause and confirm the integrity of the tympanic membrane, ossicular chain, and inner ear. Injuries to the tympanic membrane and ossicular chain require immediate evaluation by a specialist, one reason being to exclude a lesion of the inner ear (damage to the auditory and/or vestibular apparatus).

**Inflammations** of the ear are mainly considered emergencies when the process transcends the boundaries of the ear (mastoiditis, brain abscess, meningitis, sepsis), there is evidence of facial nerve paralysis, and/or there are definite signs of inner ear involvement (labyrinthitis, hearing loss, vertigo). This not only applies to acute inflammations but also to **cholesteatoma**, which is likely to produce complications. Auricular inflammations and trauma carry a risk of cartilage damage.

Acute **vestibulocochlear** dysfunction that presents with hearing loss, tinnitus, and/or vertigo generally requires immediate diagnostic and therapeutic intervention. The same applies to **paralysis** of the facial muscles, which requires immediate investigation and treatment regardless of whether the facial nerve damage has an idiopathic, inflammatory (otitis media, cholesteatoma), neoplastic (parotid malignancy, vestibular schwannoma), or traumatic cause (temporal bone fracture).

## Sinonasal Emergencies

**Nosebleed** (epistaxis) is the most common emergency, although life-threatening bleeding is relatively rare. Acute **sinusitis** becomes an emergency when the inflammation spreads to involve the orbit or eye and/or the meninges or frontal lobes of the brain, and immediate action is required.

**Inflammations of the external nose** can lead to cartilage liquefaction and requires appropriate treatment due to the risk of angular vein thrombosis and cerebral venous thrombosis.

**Septal hematomas and abscesses** can occur after nasal trauma and generally require immediate intervention. Emergencies in the broad sense include **fractures** of the nasal bone, zygoma, or orbital floor and intranasal **foreign bodies.**

## Oropharyngeal Emergencies

Besides the **inflammatory complications** of tonsillitis (peritonsillar and parapharyngeal abscess), **postoperative bleeding** after tonsillectomy is a typical emergency situation. The erosion of blood vessels by **malignant tumors** can also provoke massive bleeding. **Impalement injuries** may create a nidus for abscess formation.

**Bilateral choanal atresia** in newborns generally requires immediate intubation because newborns are obligate nose breathers, especially while feeding.

## Laryngotracheal Emergencies

**Obstruction of the airways** by swelling, a tumor, a foreign body, and/or blood and secretions necessitates emergency airway intervention (intubation, cricothyrotomy, tracheotomy).

## Neck Emergencies

The most common emergencies in the neck are **injuries** (stabbing, gunshot, strangulation, blunt trauma), which are marked by bleeding and airway obstruction, and **inflammations** (parapharyngeal abscess, cervical cellulitis), which may progress to mediastinitis.

Table    Otorhinolaryngologic emergencies that require immediate diagnostic and/or therapeutic intervention

| Emergencies | See page | Caution |
|---|---|---|
| **Ear** | | |
| Acute tinnitus | 256, 263 | |
| Acute vertigo, including Ménière's attack | 282–284, 286 | |
| Acute labyrinthitis | 264 | Deafness |
| Acute mastoiditis and its complications | 244 | |
| Acute sensorineural hearing loss: sudden hearing loss (p. 269), acoustic trauma, shock-wave trauma, explosion trauma (pp. 262–264), barotrauma (p. 251) | | Rupture of the round window |
| Auricular injuries: laceration, avulsion, auricular hematoma | 211 | Cartilage necrosis |
| Tympanic membrane and middle ear injuries (p. 250), temporal bone fractures (p. 304) | | Inner ear lesion, facial nerve lesion |
| **Nose** | | |
| Inflammations of the external nose (e.g., nasal furuncle) | 46 | Angular vein thrombosis |
| Complications of acute sinusitis, especially orbital complications | 58 | Vision loss, brain abscess |
| Nasal bone fracture, nasal injuries with cartilage involvement | 38 | Cartilage liquefaction |
| Frontobasal injuries, especially with CSF leak | 42 | Ascending meningitis |
| Septal hematoma, septal abscess, septal fracture | 38 | Cartilage liquefaction |
| Epistaxis | 30 | Aspiration of blood |
| Intranasal foreign body | | Aspiration |
| **Face** | | |
| Furuncle of the upper lip | 46, 70 | Angular vein thrombosis |
| Facial nerve paralysis: idiopathic, traumatic, inflammatory, neoplastic | 297 | Keratitis due to lagophthalmos |
| Fractures: orbital floor fractures, zygomatic arch fractures, midfacial fractures | 39 | Vision, ocular motility, sensation, masticatory muscles |
| **Oral cavity and pharynx** | | |
| Complications of acute tonsillitis, especially peritonsillar abscess, parapharyngeal abscess | 115, 117 | Airways, mediastinitis |
| Inflammation of the tongue base ("lingual tonsillitis") | 112 | Airways |
| Bleeding after tonsillectomy or tumor resection; erosive vascular hemorrhage | | Aspiration |
| Impalement injuries | 110, 122 | Abscess formation |
| Bilateral choanal atresia | 26 | Asphyxiation |
| **Larynx and trachea** | | |
| Nontraumatic laryngeal edema | 357 | Airways |
| Subglottic laryngitis (in children) | 354 | |
| Acute epiglottitis | 355, 357 | Laryngospasm |
| Laryngeal trauma: laryngeal fracture, tracheal laceration or avulsion, caustic ingestion, airway obstruction (foreign body, bleeding, tumor, laryngotracheal fistula with obstruction), obstructed tracheostomy, tracheitis with crusting, bilateral lesions of the recurrent laryngeal nerve or vagus nerve | 362 | Airway obstruction, asphyxiation |
| Acute aphonia, especially psychogenic aphonia | 389 | |
| **Esophagus** | | |
| Foreign bodies, caustic ingestion | 122 | |
| Bleeding (e.g., bleeding esophageal varices) | | Aspiration |
| **Neck** | | |
| Cervical cellulitis, necrotizing fasciitis, mediastinitis | 333 | |
| Lymphadenitis with abscess formation | 333 | |
| Blunt and sharp neck injuries | 363 | |

Abbreviation: CSF, cerebrospinal fluid.

# Sources

## Chapter 2

**Fig. 2.6**    Adapted from Rasp G. Allgemeine rhinologische Untersuchungsmethoden. In: Grevers G, ed. Praktische Rhinologie. Munich: Urban & Schwarzenberg; 1997

**Fig. 2.11**    Reproduced from Grevers G, Leunig A, Klemens A, Hagedorn H. CAS of the paranasal sinuses—technology and clinical experience with the Vector-Vision-Compact-System in 102 patients [in German]. Laryngorhinootologie 2002;81(7):476–483

**Fig. 2.12**    Courtesy of Dr. A. Grevers-Kürten, HNO-Zentrum Neuss, Neuss, Germany

**Table 2.3**    Hummel T, Landis BN, Hüttenbrink KB. Dysfunction of the chemical senses smell and taste [in German]. Laryngorhinootologie 2011;90(Suppl 1):S44–S55

## Chapter 3

**3.14**    Fokkens WJ, Lund VJ, Mullol J, et al. European Position Paper on Rhinosinusitis and Nasal Polyps 2012. Rhinol Suppl 2012;(23):1–298

**Fig. 3.38**    Adapted from Schaub B. Perinatal influences on the development of allergic rhinitis. In: Global Atlas of Allergic Rhinitis and Chronic Rhinosinusitis. Zurich: European Academy of Allergy and Clinical Immunology; 2015:80–82

**Fig. 3.40**    Reproduced from Roecken M, Grevers G, Burgdorf W. Color Atlas of Allergic Diseases. Stuttgart: Thieme; 2003

**Fig. 3.46**    Reproduced from Grevers G, Leunig A. Interaktiver Atlas der HNO-Heilkunde 1.0, CD-ROM. Stuttgart: Thieme; 1999

**Fig. 3.50c**    Grevers G, Königsberger R. Ausgedehnte Mukozele der linken Kieferhöhle. HNO-Nachrichten 2015;45(4):16

**Table 3.4**    Adapted from Brierley JD, Gospodarowicz MK, Wittekind C. TNM Classification of Malignant Tumours. 8th ed. Chichester: John Wiley & Sons; 2017

## Chapter 4

**Fig. 4.5b,c**    Courtesy of Prof. U. Welsch, Institute for Anatomy, Ludwig Maximilian University Munich, Munich, Germany

**Fig. 4.6**    Reproduced from Rauber A, Kopsch F. Anatomie des Menschen. In: Leonhardt H, Töndury G, Ziles K, eds. Nervensystem, Sinnesorgane. Vol. III. Stuttgart: Thieme; 1987

**Table 4.2**    Adapted from Brierley JD, Gospodarowicz MK, Wittekind C. TNM Classification of Malignant Tumours. 8th ed. Chichester: John Wiley & Sons; 2017

## Chapter 5

**Fig. 5.4**    Adapted from Netter FH. The CIBA Collection of Medical Illustrations (Vol. 3, Part I), Upper Digestive Tract. New York, NY: CIBA Pharmaceutical Company; 1975

**Table 5.2**    Adapted from Günther E. Schnarchen und Schlafapnoe - die Rolle des HNO-Arztes. In: Grevers G, ed. Praktische Rhinologie. Munich: Urban & Schwarzenberg; 1997

**Table 5.4**    Adapted from Günther E. Schnarchen und Schlafapnoe - die Rolle des HNO-Arztes. In: Grevers G, ed. Praktische Rhinologie. Munich: Urban & Schwarzenberg; 1997

**Table 5.5**    Adapted from Brierley JD, Gospodarowicz MK, Wittekind C. TNM Classification of Malignant Tumours. 8th ed. Chichester: John Wiley & Sons; 2017

## Chapter 6

**Fig. 6.16**    Adapted from Becker W, Naumann HH, Pfaltz CR. Hals-Nasen-Ohren-Heilkunde. 4th ed. Stuttgart: Thieme; 1989

## Chapter 16

**Fig. 16.4**    Adapted from Whitaker H, Borley NR. Anatomiekompaß. Stuttgart: Thieme; 1997

**Fig. 16.5**    Adapted from Whitaker H, Borley NR. Anatomiekompaß. Stuttgart: Thieme; 1997

**Fig. 16.6**    Adapted from Whitaker H, Borley NR. Anatomiekompaß. Stuttgart: Thieme 1997

**Fig. 16.12c-f**    Adapted from Otto HD. Teratogenetische und klinische Aspekte bei Mißbildungen des Kopf- und Halsbereiches. Eur Arch Oto-Rhino-Laryngol 1994;(Suppl 1):15–100

**Table 16.5**    Adapted from Brierley JD, Gospodarowicz MK, Wittekind C. TNM Classification of Malignant Tumours. 8th ed. Chichester: John Wiley & Sons; 2017

## Chapter 17

**Fig. 17.1a**    Adapted from Lumley JSP. Oberflächenanatomie. Stuttgart: Gustav Fischer; 1993

**Fig. 17.1b,c**    Adapted from Tillmann B. Farbatlas der Anatomie; Zahnmedizin - Humanmedizin. Stuttgart: Thieme; 1997

**Fig. 17.2**   Adapted from Ferlito A. Neoplasms of the Larynx. Churchill-Livingstone; 1985

**Fig. 17.3**   Adapted from Tucker HM. The Larynx. 2nd ed. Stuttgart: Thieme; 1993

**Fig. 17.4**   Adapted from Moore KL, Persaud TVN. Embryologie. Lehrbuch und Atlas der Entwicklungsgeschichte des Menschen. 4th ed. Stuttgart: Schattauer; 1996; and Sadler W. Medizinische Embryologie. 9th ed. Stuttgart: Thieme; 1998

**Fig. 17.6a,b**   Adapted from Cévese PG, D'Amico D, Favia G. Piccin Surgical Technique Series. Vol. XII Surgery of the Neck. Piccin; 1988

**Fig. 17.6c**   Adapted from Tucker HM. The Larynx. 2nd ed. Stuttgart: Thieme; 1993

**Fig. 17.7**   Adapted from Tucker HM. The Larynx. 2nd ed. Stuttgart: Thieme; 1993

**Fig. 17.8**   Adapted from Tillmann B. Farbatlas der Anatomie; Zahnmedizin - Humanmedizin. Stuttgart: Thieme; 1997

**Fig. 17.9**   Adapted from Sternberg SS. Histology for Pathologists. 2nd ed. Philadelphia, PA: Lippincott-Raven; 1997; and Becker W, Naumann HH, Pfaltz CR. Hals-Nasen-Ohren-Heilkunde. 4th ed. Stuttgart: Thieme; 1989

**Fig. 17.10a**   M. Voll

**Fig. 17.10b**   Adapted from Tillmann B. Farbatlas der Anatomic; Zahnmedizin - Humanmedizin. Stuttgart: Thieme; 1997

**Fig. 17.11**   Adapted from Tillmann B. Farbatlas der Anatomie; Zahnmedizin - Humanmedizin. Stuttgart: Thieme; 1997

**Fig. 17.12a**   Adapted from Birnmeyer G. HNO-ärztlicher Spiegelkurs. 4th ed. Stuttgart: Thieme; 1987; and Dedo HH. Surgery of the Larynx and Trachea. Philadelphia, PA: B. C. Decker; 1990

**Fig. 17.12c-f**   Adapted from Tillmann B. Farbatlas der Anatomie; Zahnmedizin - Humanmedizin. Stuttgart: Thieme; 1997

**Fig. 17.13a**   Courtesy of Richard Wolf, Knittlingen, Germany

**Fig. 17.14**   Adapted from Dedo HH. Surgery of the Larynx and Trachea. Philadelphia, PA: B.C. Decker; 1990

**Fig. 17.17**   Adapted from Sadler W. Medizinische Embryologie. 9th ed. Stuttgart: Thieme; 1998

**Fig. 17.26**   Courtesy of Prof. F. Rosanowski, Nuremberg, Germany; and Prof. U. Eysholdt, Oldenburg, Germany

**Fig. 17.28**   Adapted from Tillmann B. Farbatlas der Anatomie; Zahnmedizin - Humanmedizin. Stuttgart: Thieme; 1997; and Meyer R, Flemming I, Stell PM. Reconstructive surgery of the trachea. Stuttgart: Thieme; 1982

**Fig. 17.35a,b**   Adapted from Becker W, Naumann HH, Pfaltz CR. Hals-Nasen-Ohren-Heilkunde. 4th ed. Stuttgart: Thieme; 1989

**Fig. 17.35e**   Adapted from Naumann HH. Head and neck surgery. In: Panje WR, Herberhold C. eds. Neck. Vol. 3. 2nd ed. Stuttgart: Thieme; 1998; and Naumann HH, Helms J, Herberhold C. Oto-Rhino-Laryngologie in Klinik und Praxis. Vol. 3 Hals. Stuttgart: Thieme; 1995

**Fig. 17.37**   Courtesy of Prof. B. Kramann, Radiologische Universitätsklinik Homburg, Saar, Germany

**Fig. 17.43**   Adapted from Naumann HH. Kopf- und Hals-Chirurgie. Vol. 1. Stuttgart: Thieme; 1972

**Table 17.2**   Adapted from Mostafa SM. Variation in subglottic size in children. Proc R Soc Med 1976;69(11):793–795

**Table 17.4**   Adapted from Schultz-Coulon HJ. Clinical course and therapy of congenital malformations of the larynx [in German]. HNO 1984;32(1):135–148

**Table 17.6**   Adapted from Eckerbom B, Lindholm CE, Alexopoulos C. Airway lesions caused by prolonged intubation with standard and with anatomically shaped tracheal tubes. A post-mortem study. Acta Anaesthesiol Scand 1986;30(5):366–373

**Table 17.7**   Larsen R, Anästhesie. 7th ed. Munich: Urban & Fischer; 2002

**Table 17.8**   Adapted from Brierley JD, Gospodarowicz MK, Wittekind C. TNM Classification of Malignant Tumours. 8th ed. Chichester: John Wiley & Sons; 2017

**Table 17.9**   Adapted from Brierley JD, Gospodarowicz MK, Wittekind C. TNM Classification of Malignant Tumours. 8th ed. Chichester: John Wiley & Sons; 2017

**Table 17.12**   Adapted from Berendes J. Organisch bedingte Funktionsstörungen des Kehlkopfes. In: Berendes J, Link R, Zöllner F. Hals-Nasen-Ohrenheilkunde in Praxis und Klinik, part IV, Vol. I, Kehlkopf I. 2nd ed. Stuttgart: Thieme; 1982

## Chapter 18

**Table 18.1**   Adapted from Wendler J, Seidner W, Kittel G, Eysholdt U. Lehrbuch der Phoniatrie und Pädaudiologie. Stuttgart: Thieme; 1996

## Chapter 19

**Table 19.1**   Adapted from Nickisch A, Gross M. Diagnosis in disorders of speech development [in German]. HNO 1987;35(11):445–450

**Table 19.2**   Adapted from Ziegler W, Vogel M, Gröne B, Schröter-Morasch H. Dysarthrie. Stuttgart: Thieme; 1998

**Table 19.3**   Adapted from Ziegler W, Vogel M, Gröne B, Schröter-Morasch H. Dysarthrie. Stuttgart: Thieme; 1998

# Index